EUS Pathology
with
Digital Anatomy Correlation

EUS Pathology with Digital Anatomy Correlation
Textbook and Atlas

Manoop S. Bhutani, MD, FASGE, FACG, FACP, AGAF
Professor of Medicine and Experimental Diagnostic Imaging
Eminent Scientist of the Year 2008, International Research Promotion Council
Director of Endoscopic Research and Development
Department of Gastroenterology, Hepatology and Nutrition
UT MD Anderson Cancer Center
Houston, Texas, USA

John C Deutsch, M.D.
Department of Gastroenterology and Cancer Center
St Mary's Duluth Clinic
Duluth, MN, USA

2010
PEOPLE'S MEDICAL PUBLISHING HOUSE
SHELTON, CONNECTICUT

People's Medical Publishing House–USA
2 Enterprise Drive, Suite 509
Shelton, CT 06484
Tel: 203-402-0646
Fax: 203-402-0854
E-mail: info@pmph-usa.com

© 2010 PMPH–USA, Ltd.

PMPH-USA

All rights reserved. Without limiting the rights under copyright reserved above, no part of this publication may be reproduced, stored in or introduced into a retrieval system, or transmitted, in any form or by any means (electronic, mechanical, photocopying, recording, or otherwise), without the prior written permission of the publisher.

09 10 11 12 13/PMPH/9 8 7 6 5 4 3 2 1

13-digit ISBN: 978-1-60795-028-8
10-digit ISBN: 1-60795-028-6
Printed in China by People's Medical Publishing House of China
Copyeditor/Typesetter: Spearhead; Cover Designer: Mary McKeon

Sales and Distribution

Canada
McGraw-Hill Ryerson Education
Customer Care
300 Water St
Whitby, Ontario L1N 9B6
Canada
Tel: 1-800-565-5758
Fax: 1-800-463-5885
www.mcgrawhill.ca

Foreign Rights
John Scott & Company
International Publisher's Agency
P.O. Box 878
Kimberton, PA 19442
USA
Tel: 610-827-1640
Fax: 610-827-1671

Japan
United Publishers Services Limited
1-32-5 Higashi-Shinagawa
Shinagawa-ku, Tokyo 140-0002
Japan
Tel: 03-5479-7251
Fax: 03-5479-7307
Email: kakimoto@ups.co.jp

United Kingdom, Europe, Middle East, Africa
McGraw Hill Education
Shoppenhangers Road
Maidenhead
Berkshire, SL6 2QL
England
Tel: 44-0-1628-502500
Fax: 44-0-1628-635895
www.mcgraw-hill.co.uk

Singapore, Thailand, Philippines, Indonesia, Vietnam, Pacific Rim, Korea
McGraw-Hill Education
60 Tuas Basin Link
Singapore 638775

Tel: 65-6863-1580
Fax: 65-6862-3354
www.mcgraw-hill.com.sg

Australia, New Zealand
Elsevier Australia
Locked Bag 7500
Chatswood DC NSW 2067
Australia
Tel: +61 (2) 9422-8500
Fax: +61 (2) 9422-8562
www.elsevier.com.au

Brazil
Tecmedd Importadora e Distribuidora
de Livros Ltda.
Avenida Maurilio Biagi 2850
City Ribeirao, Rebeirao, Preto SP
Brazil
CEP: 14021-000
Tel: 0800-992236
Fax: 16-3993-9000
Email: tecmedd@tecmedd.com.br

India, Bangladesh, Pakistan, Sri Lanka, Malaysia
CBS Publishers
4819/X1 Prahlad Street 24
Ansari Road, Daryaganj, New Delhi-110002
India
Tel: 91-11-23266861/67
Fax: 91-11-23266818
Email: cbspubs@vsnl.com

People's Republic of China
PMPH
Bldg 3, 3rd District
Fangqunyuan, Fangzhuang
Beijing 100078
P.R. China
Tel: 8610-67653342
Fax: 8610-67691034
www.pmph.com

Notice: The authors and publisher have made every effort to ensure that the patient care recommended herein, including choice of drugs and drug dosages, is in accord with the accepted standard and practice at the time of publication. However, since research and regulation constantly change clinical standards, the reader is urged to check the product information sheet included in the package of each drug, which includes recommended doses, warnings, and contraindications. This is particularly important with new or infrequently used drugs. Any treatment regimen, particularly one involving medication, involves inherent risk that must be weighed on a case-by-case basis against the benefits anticipated. The reader is cautioned that the purpose of this book is to inform and enlighten; the information contained herein is not intended as, and should not be employed as, a substitute for individual diagnosis and treatment.

■ ■ ■ ■ ■

This book is dedicated to our wives Anjali Bhutani and Joan Deutsch for their patience and support during the countless hours spent by us on this project.

Manoop S. Bhutani and John Deutsch

■ ■ ■ ■ ■

Contributors

Sharmila Anandasabapathy, M.D.
Mount Sinai Medical Center
New York, New York, USA

Jouke T. Annema, M.D., Ph.D.
Department of Pulmonary Diseases
Leiden University Medical Center
Leiden, Netherlands

Paolo Giorgio Arcidiacono, M.D.
Gastorenterology and Gastrointestinal Endoscopy Unit
Vita Salute San Raffaele University
San Raffaele Scientific Insitute
Milan, Italy

Everson L.A. Artifon, M.D.
Department of Gastroenterology
University of Sao Paulo
Sao Paulo, Brazil

Subhas Banerjee, M.D.
Division of Gastroenterology and Hepatology
Stanford University School of Medicine
Stanford, California, USA

Olga Barkay, M.D.
Division of Gastroenterology and Pediatric Gastroenterology Unit
Tel Aviv Sourasky Medical Center
Tel Aviv, Israel

Kirk P Bernadino, MD
Center for Digestive Diseases
SMDC Health Systems
Duluth, Minnesota, USA

Manoop S. Bhutani, M.D.
Department of Gastroenterology, Hepatology and Nutrition
The University of Texas M. D. Anderson Cancer Center,
Houston, TX, USA

William Brugge, M.D.
Division of Gastroenterology
Massachusetts General Hospital
Boston, Massachusetts, USA

Giancarlo Caletti, M.D.
Division of Gastroenterology and Digestive Endoscopy
Hospital of Castel S. Pietro Terme/AUSL of Imola
Castel S. Pietro Terme, Bologna, Italy

Silvia Carrara, M.D.
Division of Gastroenterology & Gastrointestinal Endoscopy
Vita-Salute San Raffaele University
Scientific Institute San Raffaele
Milan, Italy

Marc F. Catalano, M.D.
Department of Gastroenterology
St. Luke's Medical Center
Milwaukee, Wisconsin, USA

Suresh T. Chari, M.D.
Division of Gastroenterology and Hepatology
Mayo Clinic
Rochester, Minnesota, USA

Jennifer Chennat, M.D.
Center for Endoscopic Research and Therapeutics (CERT)
University of Chicago Medical Center
Chicago, Illinois, USA

Jacques Van Dam, M.D., Ph.D.
Division of Gastroenterology and Hepatology
Stanford University Medical Center
Stanford, California, USA

John C. Deutsch, M.D.
Gastroenterology and Cancer Center
SMDC Health Systems
Duluth, Minnesota, USA

John M. DeWitt, M.D.
Gastroenterology Division
Indiana University Medical Center
Indianapolis, Indiana, USA

Mohamad A. Eloubeidi, M.D.
Division of Gastroenterology
University of Alabama at Birmingham Medical Center
Birmingham, Alabama, USA

Douglas O. Faigel, M.D.
Division of Gastroenterology
Oregon Health and Science University
Portland, Oregon, USA

Annette Fritscher-Ravens, M.D.
Department of Interdisciplinary Endoscopy
University Hospital Schleswig-Holstein/Campus Kiel
Kiel, Germany

Norio Fukami, M.D.
Division of Gastroenterology and Hepatology
University of Colorado
Denver, Colorado, USA

Pietro Fusaroli, M.D.
University of Bologna
Division of Gastroenterology and Digestive Endoscopy
Hospital of Castel S. Pietro Terme/AUSL of Imola
Castel S. Pietro Terme, Bologna, Italy

Eugenio Giovannini, M.D.
University of Bologna
Division of Gastroenterology and Digestive Endoscopy
Hospital of Castel S. Pietro Terme/AUSL of Imola
Castel S. Pietro Terme, Bologna, Italy

Marc Giovannini, M.D.
Department of Medical Oncology
Paoli-Calmettes Institute
Marseille, France

Antonino Grillo, M.D.
University of Bologna
Division of Gastroenterology and Digestive Endoscopy
Hospital of Castel S. Pietro Terme/AUSL of Imola
Castel S. Pietro Terme, Bologna, Italy

Nadim G. Haddad, M.D.
Division of Gastroenterology
Georgetown University Hospital
Washington, D.C., USA

Lyndon V. Hernandez, M.D.
Department of Gastroenterology
St Luke's Medical Center
Milwaukee, Wisconsin, USA

Franc H. Hetzer, M.D.
Department of Surgery
Division of Coloproctology
Cantonal Hospital
St. Gallen, Switzerland

Brenda Hoffman, M.D.
Division of Gastroenterology and Hepatology
Medical University of South Carolina
Charleston, South Carolina, USA

Joo Ha Hwang, M.D., Ph.D.
Division of Gastroenterology
University of Washington Medical Center
Seattle, Washington, USA

Atsushi Irisawa, M.D., Ph.D.
Department of Internal Medicine 2
Fukushima Medical University School of Medicine
Fukushima City, Japan

Takao Itoi, M.D., Ph.D.
Department of Gastroenterology and Hepatology
Tokyo Medical University
Tokyo, Japan

Kunal Jajoo, M.D.
Division of Gastroenterology and Hepatology
Weill Cornell Medical College
New York, New York, USA

Akio Katanuma, M.D.
Department of Gastroenterology
Teine-Keijinkai Hospital
Hokkaido, Japan

Murli Krishna MD
Dept. of Laboratory Medicine and Pathology
Mayo Clinic College of Medicine
Jacksonville, Florida, USA

Jeffrey H. Lee, M.D.
Department of Gastroenterology, Hepatology, and Nutrition
UT M.D. Anderson Cancer Center
Houston, Texas, USA

Michael J. Levy, M.D.
Department of Gastroenterology and Hepatology
Mayo Clinic
Rochester, Minnesota, USA

Christa Meyenberger, M.D.
Division of Gastroenterology and Hepatology
Cantonal Hospital
St. Gallen, Switzerland

Katsutoshi Obara, M.D., Ph.D.
Department of Internal Medicine 2
Fukushima Medical University Hospital
Fukushima City, Japan

Hiromasa Ohira, M.D., Ph.D
Department of Internal Medicine 2
Fukushima Medical University School of Medicine
Fukushima City, Japan

Maria Chiara Petrone, M.D
Gastorenterology and Gastrointestinal Endoscopy Unit
Vita Salute San Raffaele University
San Raffaele Scientific Insitute
Milan, Italy

Klaus F. Rabe, M.D.
Department of Pulmonary Diseases
Leiden University Medical Center
Leiden, Netherlands

Nischita K. Reddy, M.D., M.P.H.
Department of Gastroenterology and Hepatology
University of Texas Medical Branch
Galveston, Texas, USA

William Ross, M.D., MBA
Department of Gastroenterology, Hepatalogy, & Nutrition
The University of Texas M. D. Anderson Cancer Center
Houston, TX, USA

Stephen J. Rulyak, M.D.
Division of Gastroenterology
The Everett Clinic
Everett, Washington, USA

Adrian Săftoiu, M.D., Ph.D.
Department of Gastroenterology
Research Center of Gastroenterology and Hepatology
University of Medicine and Pharmacy
Craiova, Dolj, Romania

Paulo Sakai, M.D., Ph.D.
Department of Gastroenterology
University of Sao Paulo
Sao Paulo, Brazil

Erwin Santo, M.D.
Department of Gastroenterology
Tel Aviv Sourasky Medical Center
Tel Aviv, Israel

Thomas J. Savides, M.D.
Division of Gastroenterology
University of California San Diego
San Diego, California, USA

Max A. Shapiro, M.D.
Department of Medicine
Division of Gastroenterology
Georgetown University Hospital
Washington, D.C., USA

Goro Shibukawa, M.D.
Department of Internal Medicine 2
Fukushima Medical University School of Medicine
Fukushima City, Japan

Chan Sup Shim, M.D., Ph.D.
Digestive Disease Center
KonKuk University Medical Center
Seoul, Korea

Gerard A. Silvestri, M.D., M.S.
Department of Medicine
Medical University of South Carolina
Charleston, South Carolina

Assaad M. Skoury, M.D.
Division of Gastroenterology
American University of Beirut, Medical Center
Beirut, Lebanon

Thomas C. Smyrk, M.D.
Department of Clinical Pathology & Anatomic Pathology
Mayo Clinic
Rochester, Minnesota

Assaad M. Soweid, M.D.
Division of Gastroenterology
American University of Beirut
Beirut, Lebanon

Tadayuki Takagi, M.D.
Department of Internal Medicine 2
Fukushima Medical University School of Medicine
Fukushima City, Japan

Naoki Takahashi, M.D.
Department of Radiology
Mayo Clinic
Rochester, Minnesota, USA

Eric P. Tamm, M.D.
Department of Radiology
UT M.D. Anderson Cancer Center
Houston, Texas, USA

Alberto Herreros de Tejada, M.D., PhD
Center for Endoscopic Research and Therapeutics (CERT)
University of Chicago Medical Center
Chicago, Illinois, USA

Nundhini Thukkani, M.D.
Division of Gastroenterology and Hepatology
Oregon Health and Sciences University
Portland, Oregon

Theodoros Topalidis, M.D.
Cytological Institute of Hannover
Hannover, Germany

Shyam Varadarajulu, M.D.
Division of Gastroenterology-Hepatology
University of Alabama at Birmingham Medical Center
Birmingham, Alabama

M. Veseliç, M.D.
Department of Pathology
Leiden University Medical Center
Leiden, Netherlands

Shivakumar Vignesh, M.D.
Division of Gastroenterology
H. Lee Moffitt Cancer Center & Research Institute
Tampa, Florida

Peter Vilmann, M.D.
Department of Surgical Gastroenterology
Gentofte University Hospital
Hellerup, Denmark

Brad Vincent, M.D.
Department of Pulmonary, Critical Care and Sleep Medicine
Medical University of South Carolina
Charleston, South Carolina, USA

Michael B. Wallace, M.D., M.P.H.
Division of Gastroenterology
Mayo Clinic
Jacksonville, Florida, USA

Irving Waxman, M.D.
Center for Endoscopic Research and Therapeutics (CERT)
University of Chicago Medical Center
Chicago, Illinois, USA

Lutz Welker, M.D.
Centre for Pneumology and Thoracic Surgery
Hospital Groflhansdorf
Groflansdorf, Germany

Brian R. Weston, M.D.
Division of Gastroenterology
University of Washington Medical Center
Seattle, Washington, USA

C. Mel Wilcox, M.D.
Division of Gastroenterology-Hepatology
University of Alabama at Birmingham Medical Center
Birmingham, Alabama, USA

Brian Yan, M.D.
Division of Gastroenterology and Hepatology
Stanford University Medical Center
Stanford, California, USA

Tony E. Yusuf, M.D.
Division of Gastroenterology
Director of GI Endoscopy
Kings County Hospital Center
Brooklyn, New York, USA

Foreword

It is with a certain irony that I have been asked to write the foreword to the *EUS Pathology with Digital Anatomy Correlation*, edited by Manoop Bhutani and John Deutsch. Stated in its most simple terms, I myself do not perform endoscopic ultrasound (EUS). Which is not to say that EUS has not done more to change my practice patterns than any other technology, including magnetic resonance cholangiopancreatography (MRCP). For, from the gastroesophageal standpoint, how does one treat a superficial malignancy with mucosectomy, endoscopic submucosal dissection (ESD), or Radio frequency (RF) current without assurance that the lesion being resected or ablated is truly superficial? In acute relapsing pancreatitis without a definable etiology after conventional laboratory testing and imaging, would anyone rush into an endoscopic retrograde cholangiopancreatography (ERCP), with or without manometry, unless that patient had first undergone an EUS?

Indeed, in unresectable patients with distal malignant obstructive jaundice, there is at least a twofold increase in sensitivity with EUS-guided fine needle aspiration (EUS-FNA) compared with ERCP and brush cytology. Moreover, our group has demonstrated cost-efficacy and comparable sensitivity and specificity using EUS as opposed to computed tomography (CT)-guided tissue acquisition. In addition, EUS, multiplane CT scan, and magnetic resonance imaging (MRI)/MRCP have revolutionized our approach to cystic lesions of the pancreas. Finally, EUS plays a role, in conjunction with CT scan, in defining the staging of rectal cancer and depth of tumor in patients with extensive tubulovillous adenoma of the rectum.

From a therapeutic standpoint, EUS has expanded our access to peripancreatic fluid collections (pseudocyst, necrosis, abscess), has been used investigationally in an attempt to ablate cystic lesions of the pancreas, has allowed access into the pancreaticobiliary tree to facilitate transgastric/duodenal stenting or rendezvous procedure after unsuccessful ERCP, and has been variably used for gastric variceal sclerosis and gallbladder stenting and to allow peritoneal access for a variety of natural orifice (NOTES) procedures. I have previously stated and stand by my remark that EUS may ultimately assume therapeutic ascendancy at a time that other endoluminal procedures have peaked or may be replaced by other techniques and technologies.

So this brings me back to *EUS Pathology with Digital Anatomy Correlation*, a composite of high-resolution digital images, taken at necropsy, presented in conjunction with EUS images of these anatomic structures. This correlation is not a technical parlor trick but a sophisticated attempt by the editors to adequately define anatomic landmarks with EUS scope position or direct therapy in an attempt to improve diagnostic accuracy of intra- or extraluminal pathology. The editors have assembled a superb cast of authors and logically divided the text into the upper gastrointestinal (GI) tract and mediastinum, including intrinsic and extrinsic mass lesions, varices, and other vascular anomalies; hepatobiliary disorders and disorders of the abdomen including stone disease, pancreaticobiliary (PB) neoplasms, cysts, acute and chronic pancreatitis, and liver, adrenal, and splenic lesions; colorectal lesions including tumors, ovarian and prostatic lesions, and inflammatory bowel disorders; and a miscellaneous section looking at recent studies of EUS contrast agents and EUS elastography.

What a wonderful smorgasbord of images, disorders, and evolving EUS treatment modalities. This atlas is nothing less than a compendium of endoscopically accessible GI and non-GI pathology and is a "must-have" for the therapeutic endoscopist, whether or not they perform EUS. At my institution, I am fortunate to have five excellent EUS physicians who can perform the vast majority of procedures described in this atlas. Were I not so fortunate, I might be enticed to spend a year or two with Drs. Bhutani and Deutsch, or one of the other talented ultrasonographers who have contributed to this text.

Richard A. Kozarek, MD
Executive Director, Digestive Disease Institute
Virginia Mason Medical Center
Clinical Professor of Medicine
University of Washington
Seattle, Washington

Preface

Endoscopic Ultrasonography (EUS) has become a mainstream gastrointestinal procedure. Whereas EUS was previously restricted to some selected academic centers, it is now available in many communities throughout the world. The role of EUS has expanded beyond gastroenterology as an interventional technique in many other branches of medicine. This work is intended to serve as a teaching tool about various abnormalities and pathologic lesions that one may encounter during EUS from "mouth to anus". The list of authors demonstrates the utilization of EUS by the global community. This text and atlas also demonstrates the value of EUS by illustrating the various EUS findings that can be encountered in practice. We want to thank all of our authors for their efforts and excellent work. We want to thank the scientists at the Center for Human Simulation at the University of Colorado for allowing us access to their high quality digital anatomy resources. We finally want to thank the efforts made by our publisher to ensure the quality of the final product. This is truly a work that was accomplished by efforts by individuals including authors from around the world. It is the editors' hope that this work will serve as a useful resource, not only for novice students of endoscopic ultrasonography, but experienced endosonographers as well. "*An image is worth a thousand words*" but this is true only when one can make sense of the image and it is interpreted accurately since "*what the mind does not know the eyes do not see*".

Manoop S. Bhutani
Houston, Texas

John C. Deutsch
Duluth, Minnesota

Acknowledgments

We are indebted to Vic Spitzer, Karl Reinig and David Rubinstein at the University of Colorado, Denver - Center for Human Simulation for providing us methods to access the Visible Human DataSets™. We thank and appreciate all the authors and contributors to this book from around the world without whom this work would not have been possible.

Contents

Chapter 1
Introduction and Overview — 1

SECTION I / UPPER GI TRACT/MEDIASTINUM — 5

Chapter 2
Early Esophageal Cancer — 7

- Introduction — 8
- Factors Affecting Tumor Staging — 9
  - *Operator expertise* — 9
  - *Technique* — 9
  - *Equipment* — 10
  - *Tumor-Related Factors* — 11
- Eus Staging in Early Esophageal Cancer — 12
  - *EUS Depiction of Early Esophageal Cancer* — 12
  - *Accuracy of EUS in Staging Early Esophageal Cancer* — 13
  - *Over-and Understaging* — 15
  - *Barrett's Esophagus: (HGD Tis, T1m and T1sm)* — 15
- Conclusion — 17

Chapter 3
EUS in Barrett's Esophagus and High Grade Dysplasia/Early Carcinoma — 19

- Introduction — 20
- EUS in Barrett's Metaplasia and Low-Grade Dysplasia — 20
- EUS in High-Grade Dysplasia and Early Carcinoma — 21

Chapter 4
Advanced Esophageal Cancer — 25

- Radial Versus Linear Scanners — 26
- T-Staging — 27
- N-Staging — 28
- M-Staging — 29
- Dilation of Strictures — 29
- EUS After Neoadjuvant Radiochemotherapy — 29

Chapter 5
Early Gastric Cancer — 33

- Introduction — 34
- Instruments and Techniques — 34
  - *Instruments* — 34
  - *EUS Techniques* — 35
- EUS Findings of Early Gastric Cancer — 35
  - *Mural Structure of the Normal Gastric Wall Using Endosonography* — 35
- Future Perspectives of EUS — 45
- Conclusion — 47

Chapter 6
Advanced Gastric Cancer — 49

- Introduction — 50
- EUS and Gastric Cancer — 50
- Summary — 54

Chapter 7
Large Gastric Folds — 57

- Introduction — 58
- EUS for Differential Diagnosis — 59
- EUS for Staging of Malignancies — 60
- EUS Features According to Various Etiologies of LGF — 62
  - *Lymphoma* — 62
  - *Linitis Plastica* — 66
  - *Menetrier's Disease* — 69
  - *Zollinger-Ellison Syndrome* — 70
  - *Gastric Varices* — 71
  - *Other Causes of LGF* — 72

Chapter 8
Subepithelial Lesions of the Upper GI Tract — 79

- Introduction — 80
- Diagnostic Techniques — 80
  - *Endoscopy* — 80
  - *Endosonography* — 80
  - *Tissue Diagnosis* — 81
  - *EUS-Guided Fine Needle Aspiration* — 81
  - *EUS-Guided Core Needle Biopsy* — 81
  - *Stacked Forceps Biopsy* — 82
  - *Endoscopic Submucosal Resection (ESMR) and Dissection (ESD)* — 82
- Differential Diagnosis — 82
  - *Extramural Lesions* — 83
  - *Intramural Lesions* — 83
- Conclusions — 91

Chapter 9
Esophageal and Gastric Varices — 95

- Introduction — 96
- Observational Method 4 — 96
- Vascular Anatomy — 96
- EUS Imaging — 98
  - *Esophagus 4, 5, 6* — *98*
  - *Stomach* — *103*
- Conclusion — 105

Chapter 10
Vascular Anomolies — 107

- Aortic Arch Anomolies — 108
- Acquired Vascular Lesions — 111
- Dieulafoy Lesions — 115
- Conclusion — 116

Chapter 11
EUS for Mediastinal Lymph Nodes and Masses — 117

- EUS Technique — 118
- Benign Posterior Mediastinal Lymph Nodes and Masses — 119
  - *EUS Appearance of Normal Benign Reactive Posterior Mediastinal Lymph Nodes* — *119*
  - *Granulomatous Lymph Nodes* — *119*
  - *Mediastinal Cysts* — *121*
- Malignant Posterior Mediastinal Lesions — 122
  - *EUS Appearance of Malignant Posterior Mediastinal Lymph Nodes* — *122*
- Risks of Mediastinal EUS FNA — 126
- Overall Impact of EUS FNA for Mediastinal Lesions — 126
- Conclusion — 127

Chapter 12
EUS Imaging and FNA of Primary Lung Tumors — 129

- Introduction — 130
- Diagnosis of Primary Lung Tumors by EUS-FNA — 130
- Cytopathology of Lung Tumors — 133
  - *Tissue Handling* — *133*
  - *Cytological Analysis* — *133*
  - *Tumor Types* — *134*
- Detection of Tumor Invasion by EUS — 134
- Conclusion — 135

Chapter 13
Transbronchial Ultrasound — 137

- Background — 138
- Noninvasive Staging Modalities — 138

Invasive Staging Modalities ... 138
Endobronchial Ultrasound Guided Fine Needle Aspiration (EBUS-TBNA) ... 140
EBUS-TBNA: Diagnostic Yield and Impact on Management ... 142
Combined Yield of EUS FNA with EBUS TBNA ... 143
Other Therapeutic Applications of EBUS ... 143
Conclusion ... 143

SECTION II / HEPATOPANCREATOBILIARY/ABDOMEN ... 147

Chapter 14
Pancreatic Carcinoma: Detection and Staging ... 149

Background ... 150
Description of Equipment and Techniques of CT, MRI, and EUS ... 150
   CT ... *150*
   MRI ... *150*
   EUS ... *150*
Diagnosis and Staging by CT, MRI, and EUS ... 151
   CT ... *151*
   MRI ... *156*
   EUS ... *158*
Conclusion ... 161

Chapter 15
Pancreatic Neuroendocrine Tumors ... 165

Localized Functional Pancreatic Neuroendocrine Tumors ... 167
Localized Nonfunctional Pancreatic Neuroendocrine Tumors ... 168
Metastatic Pancreaticneuroendocrine Tumors ... 169
Luminal Neuroendocrine Tumors ... 170

Chapter 16
Pancreatic Metastases ... 173

Introduction ... 174

Chapter 17
Cystic Pancreatic Lesions ... 183

Pseudocysts ... 185
Serous Lesions ... 185
Mucinous Lesions ... 185
Other Cystic Neoplasms ... 186
Summary ... 188

Chapter 18
Endoscopic Ultrasonography in Intraductal Papillary Mucinous Tumors of the Pancreas ... 191

Introduction ... 192
Classification ... 192
Clinical Manifestations ... 192

Pathology	193
Differential Diagnosis	193
Diagnosis	194
Role of Endoscopic Ultrasonography	*194*
Role of EUS with Fine Needle Aspiration	*199*
Role of Intraductal Ultrasound and 3-Dimentional EUS	*200*
Outcome and Therapy	202
Conclusion	202

Chapter 19
Chronic Pancreatitis — 205

EUS Features of Chronic Pancreatitis	206
Ductal Features of Chronic Pancreatitis	211
Parenchymal Features of Chronic Pancreatitis	211
Conclusion	211

Chapter 20
Autoimmune Pancreatitis — 213

Introduction	214
Diagnostic Criteria	214
Histological Findings	214
Pancreatic Imaging	215
Computed Tomography (CT) and Magnetic Resonance Imaging (MRI)	*215*
Endoscopic Retrograde Cholangiopancreatography (ERCP)	*216*
Endoscopic Ultrasound (EUS) and Tissue Sampling	*216*
Serology	219
Other Organ Involvement	220
Response to Steroids	220
Discussion	220
Summary	221

Chapter 21
Pancreas Divisum and Other Pancreaticobiliary Anomalies — 225

Pancreas Divisum	226
Annular Pancreas	227
Santorinicele	231
Anomalous Pancreaticbiliary Junction	231
Partial or Complete Pancreatic Agenesis	233
Biliary Cysts	233
Duodenal Duplication Cysts	236
Miscellaneous Extrahepatic Biliary Anomalies	238

Chapter 22
Choledocholithiasis and Other Benign Bile Duct Lesions — 243

Introduction	244
Instruments and Techniques	244
Uses of EUS	244

The Problem of Choledocholithiasis	245
EUS for CBD Stones	246
EUS Compared to Other Imaging	246
Intraductal US and ERCP	248
Conclusion	248

Chapter 23
Malignant Bile Duct Lesions: Cholangiocarcinoma — 249

Introduction	250
EUS Equipment and Techniques	250
EUS and EUS-FNA Technique	250
Intraductal Ultrasound	*251*
EUS-FNA Technique	252
Role of EUS and IDUS	253
Role of EUS-FNA in Cholangiocarcinoma	*254*
Conclusion	256

Chapter 24
Benign and Malignant Lesions of the Gallbladder — 257

Gallbladder	258
Pathologic Findings	259
Cholesterolosis/Cholesterol Polyp	*259*
Adenomyomatosis	*259*
Cholecystitis	*260*
Inflammatory Polyp	*264*
Adenoma	*264*
Adenocarcinoma	*264*

Chapter 25
Ampullary Lesions — 273

Introduction	274
EUS Exploration	274
Benign Lesions	275
Malignant Lesions	277
Therapeutic Endoscopy	282
Interventional EUS	283
Conclusion	285

Chapter 26
Liver Lesions — 287

Benign Tumors and Tumor-Like Lesions	288
Cavernous Hemangioma	*288*
Focal Nodular Hyperplasia	*288*
Liver Cell Adenoma	*288*
Bile Duct Adenomas and Hamartomas	*288*

  Cystic Lesions   291
  Malignant Tumors   291
   Hepatocellular Carcinoma   *291*
   Fibrolamellar Hepatocellular Carcinoma   *292*
   Intrahepatic Cholangiocarcinoma   *292*
   Combined Hepatocellular and Cholangiocarcinoma   *293*
   Lymphoma   *293*
   Epithelioid Hemangioendothelioma   *294*
   Angiosarcoma   *294*
  Metastatic (Secondary) Liver Tumors   294

Chapter 27
Splenic Lesions   299

  Methods   301
  Pathology   302
   Benign Splenic Lesions   *303*
   Malignant Diseases   *306*
   Accessory Spleen   *310*
  Conclusion   310

Chapter 28
Adrenal Lesions   313

  Identification of the Left Adrenal Gland   314
  Glandular Morphology   315
  EUS-Guided FNA   316
  Summary   317

Chapter 29
Portal Vein Thrombosis   319

  Portal Vein Thrombosis   320
  Splenic Vein Thrombosis   322

Chapter 30
Peritoneal and Pleural Fluid   325

  Introduction   326
  EUS Findings   326
  Pleural Effusions   326
  Pericardial Effusions   326
  Ascites   326
  EUS-Guided Fine-Needle Aspiration   327
  Technique   329
  Fluid Analysis   329
  Complications and Their Avoidance   330
  Outcome   330
  Conclusions   330

SECTION III / COLORECTAL — 333

Chapter 31
Rectal Cancer — 335

- Introduction — 336
- Rectal Anatomy — 336
- Rectal Cancer — 336
  - *Equipment and Technique* — 337
  - *ERUS Staging of Rectal Cancer* — 338
  - *EUS Tumor Stage* — 338
  - *EUS Lymph Node Staging* — 339
- Accuracy of EUS in Staging Rectal Cancer — 339
- Restaging After Neoadjuvant Therapy — 340
- EUS for Local Recurrence of Colorectal Carcinoma — 340
- Three-Dimentional EUS — 341
  - *Tracked Free-Hand Systems* — 341
  - *3-D Reconstruction* — 341
  - *Visualization of 3-D Ultrasound Images* — 341
- Conclusion — 342

Chapter 32
Perirectal Abscesses — 345

- Introduction — 346
- Endoanal Ultrasound in Perirectal Abscess — 351

Chapter 33
Anorectal Fistulae — 355

- Introduction — 356
- Endoanal Ultrasound in Nonspecific Anorectal Fistula — 356
- Endoanal Ultrasound in Specific Anorectal Fistula — 359

Chapter 34
Anal Sphincter Defects — 361

- Introduction — 362
- Endoanal Ultrasound in Fecal Incontinence — 363

Chapter 35
Ovarian and Gynecological Lesions — 369

- Pelvic Inflammatory Disorders — 372
- Conclusion — 374

Chapter 36
Subepithelial Colorectal Lesions/Colon Polyps/Adenomas — 375

- Introduction — 376

Colonic Polyps and Adenomas	376
Endoscopic Ultrasound in Colonic and Rectal Adenomas	378
Anatomy and Technique Tips	*378*
Applications of EUS	*379*
Villous Adenomas	*379*
Other Clinical Applications of EUS of Colonic/Rectal Polyps	*379*
Subepithelial Colorectal Lesions	380
Gastrointestinal Stromal Tumors	*380*
Leiomyomas/Leiomyosarcomas	*380*
Schwannomas, Paragangliomas, and Fibrosarcomas	*381*
Lipomas	*381*
Carcinoids	*381*
Lymphangiomas	*383*
Endometriosis	*383*
Summary	383

Chapter 37
Prostate Lesions — 387

Urologic Echoendoscopy	388
Echoendoscopy in Benign Prostate Pathologies	388
Benign Prostate Hyperplasia (BPH)	*388*
Cysts	*389*
Other Lesions	*389*
Echoendoscopy in Loco-Regional Prostate Cancer Staging	389
Histopathologic Aspects of Prostate Cancer	*390*
Echoendoscopic Examination Technique of the Prostate and Adnexa	*390*
Discussion and Critical Analysis	*394*

Chapter 38
Endoscopic Ultrasound (EUS) in Inflammatory Bowel Disease (IBD) — 397

Fistulae and Abscesses	398
Luminal Inflammatory Bowel Disease	398

SECTION IV / MISCELLANEOUS — 401

Chapter 39
EUS Elastography — 403

Introduction	404
Real-Time Elastography	404
Method	404
EUS Applications	406
Lymph Nodes	*406*
Pancreatic Diseases	*407*
Focal Liver Lesions	*408*
Other Tumors	*408*

Perspectives	409
3-D Applications	*409*
Virtual Palpation	*409*

Chapter 40
EUS Contrast Agents — 413

Contrast Agents	414
Mechanisms of Action	414
Clinical Uses of Contrast Enhanced Endoscopic Ultrasonography (CE-EUS)	414
Differentiating Benign from Malignant Mediastinal Lymphadenopathy	*414*
Esophageal and Gastric Cancer	*415*
Gallbladder Diseases	*415*
Pancreatic Diseases: First Generation	*415*
Pancreatic Diseases: Second Generation	*415*
Esophageal Varices and Portal Hypertension	*417*
Future Perspectives	417

CHAPTER 1

Introduction and Overview

Dr. Manoop S. Bhutani
Dr. John C. Deutsch

EUS Pathology with Digital Anatomy Correlation is a text dedicated to learning about pathologic images seen during endoscopic ultrasonography (EUS). The digital anatomy correlation used in this work is the natural continuation of efforts to apply the University of Colorado's Visible Human Data Set to gastroenterology.

The Visible Human Data Set was created by Dr. Vic Spitzer and colleagues at the University of Colorado and is currently housed at the university's Center for Human Simulation. The data set consists of high-resolution, transaxial digital images captured as cadavers were abraded away at depths of 1 mm or less. These images are compiled into blocks of data, and each structure is identified. This information can be used to pull out and manipulate 3-D structures; it can also allow for the review of planar anatomy in any orientation. An example is shown in Figure 1–1, in which a model of the pancreas, spleen, aorta, hepatic artery, and splenic artery have been taken out from the data set. Another example can be seen in Figure 1–2, where

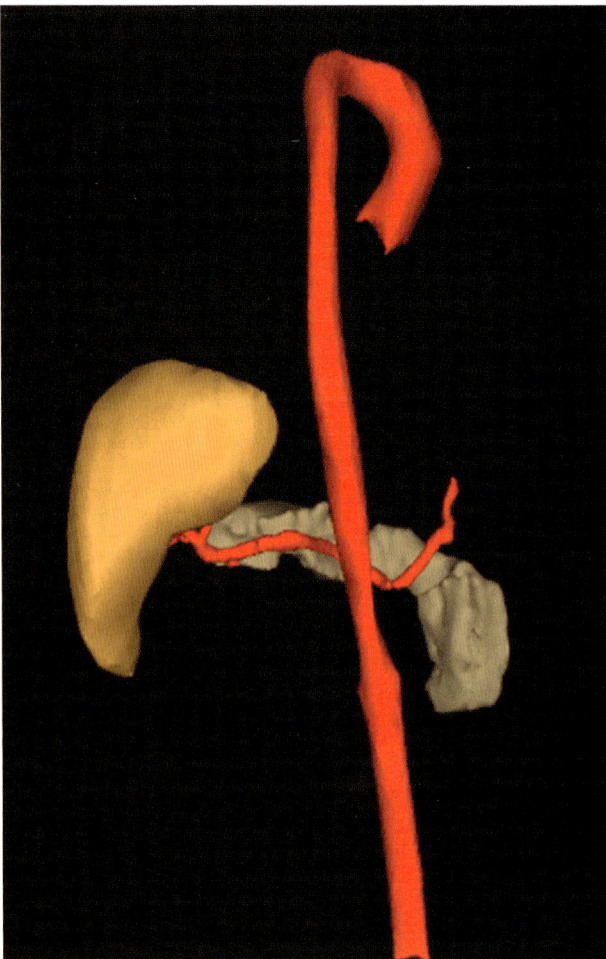

FIGURE 1–2. Visible Human Model of pancreas, spleen, aorta, and splenic artery rotated to a posterior view.

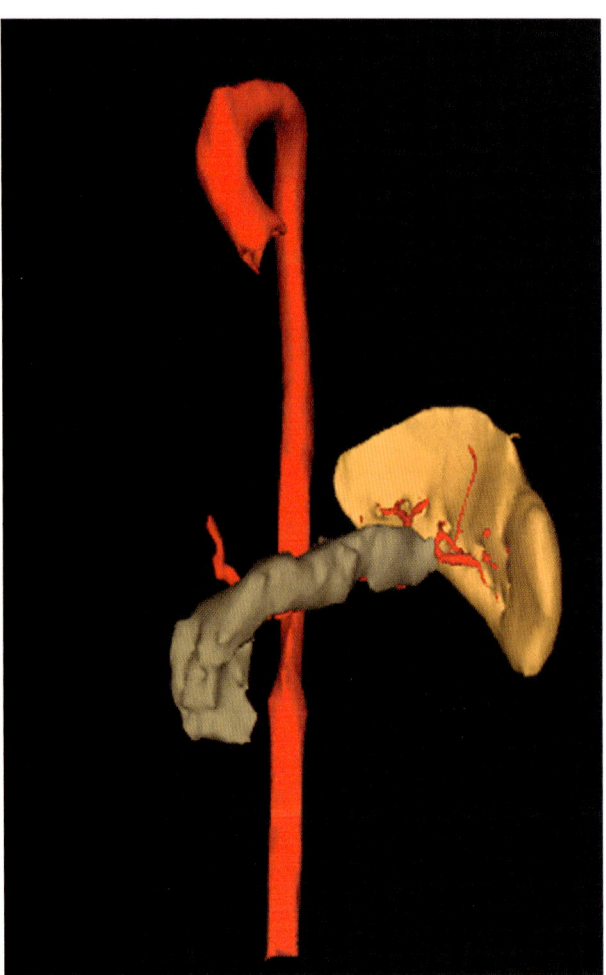

FIGURE 1–1. Visible Human Model of pancreas, spleen, aorta and splenic artery from an anterior view.

that model has been rotated. In Figure 1–3 a plane is shown going through the model. In Figure 1–4, the planar anatomy contained within the plane is visible.

For more details regarding the Visible Human Data Set and applications in gastroenterology, please see the introductory chapters by Dr. Vic Spitzer and Dr. Karl Reinig in Bhutani, M. S., Deutsch, J (Editors): Digital Human Anatomy and Endoscopic Ultrasonography. Hamilton, London: B. C. Decker,Inc., 2005.

Access to anatomy in this manner should have an intuitive appeal to endosonographers, who generate planar images in a variety of nearly random orientations. Using the Visible Human Data Set, one should be able to find a normal anatomy correlation to any image found during an EUS examination.

However, as important as normal anatomy is, the abnormal features are the crux of any EUS examination. Endosonographers are asked to define lumps, bumps, and cysts, and to find correlations

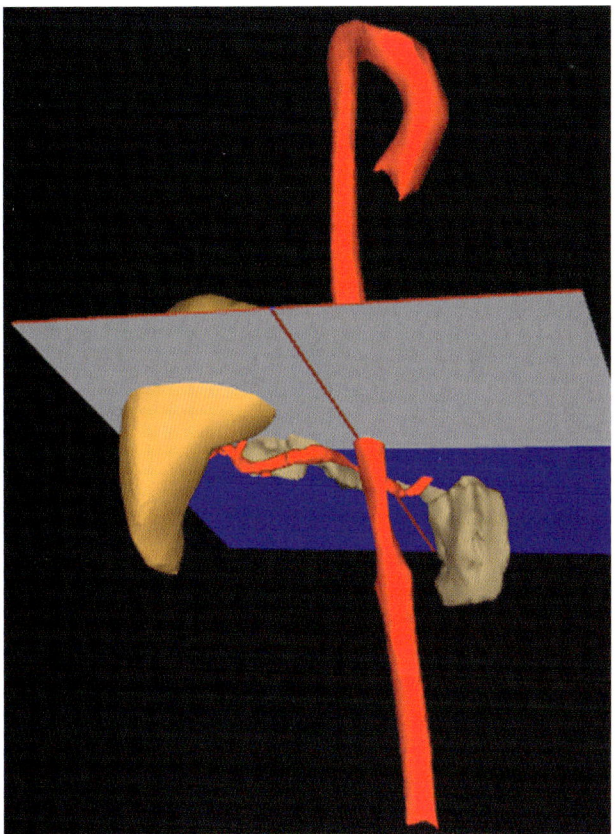

FIGURE 1–3. Visible Human Model of pancreas, spleen, aorta, and splenic artery rotated to a posterior view containing a plane.

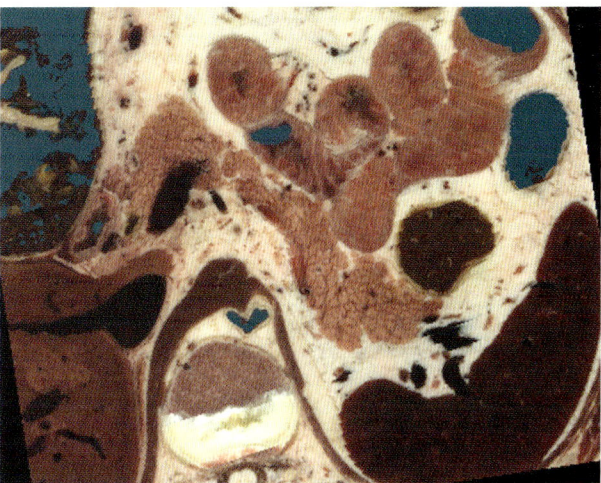

FIGURE 1–4. Anatomy from Visible Human Data Set that is contained in the plane shown in Figure 1-3.

between symptoms and abnormal laboratory findings. Accuracy requires a tremendous amount of skill and experience. To help in this task, we have assembled chapters from a worldwide group of expert endosonographers. These authors have shared their insight and images to help readers better see and understand some of the complexities uncovered during an EUS evaluation. After reviewing each of these excellent chapters, we have selectively added images derived from the Visible Human Data Set in places where we thought we could highlight information provided by our authors. To that end, we would like to thank all of our participating authors and the scientists at the University of Colorado Center for Human Simulation for allowing us to assemble this atlas and textbook of abnormal EUS findings.

SECTION I

Upper GI tract/ Mediastinum

CHAPTER 2

Early Esophageal Cancer

Dr. Brian Yan
Dr. Jacques Van Dam
Dr. Subhas Banerjee

Introduction

Esophageal cancer is the sixth-leading cause of cancer mortality worldwide, with an estimated 14,000 deaths occurring from this cancer in the United States alone in 2006.[1] Approximately 75% of patients have advanced stage cancer at diagnosis, with lymph node involvement noted in 80% and distant metastases in 50%. Staging of esophageal cancer is based on the TNM classification of the American Joint Committee on Cancer (Tables 2-1 and 2-2A).[2] Survival is strongly stage dependent (Table 2-2B), with a five-year survival rate of greater than 90% seen with Stage 1 disease, but a range of only 10% five-year survival rate with Stage 3 disease.[3] Staging strongly guides the therapeutic approach to this cancer.

Staging is typically initiated with a computerized tomography (CT) scan to rule out the presence of distant metastases. However, CT scans are unsatisfactory for loco-regional staging. When distant metastases are not evident on CT, endoscopic ultrasound (EUS) improves loco-regional staging and should therefore be obtained. EUS has established itself as the most accurate imaging modality for staging of tumor depth (T-staging) and regional lymph nodes (N-staging), with a T-staging accuracy of 85–90%, and N-staging accuracy of 75-89%.[4,5] In contrast to CT, which can only provide information regarding lymph node size, EUS is able to evaluate lymph node shape, border characteristics, and central echogenicity, all of which may additionally assist in distinguishing malignant from reactive lymph nodes. Moreover, EUS offers the advantage of allowing fine needle aspiration of lymph nodes, which increases N-staging accuracy rates to more than 98%.[6]

Early esophageal cancers are defined as Stage 0 or 1 (Tis or T1 tumors). T1 tumors may be limited to the mucosa (T1m) or extend into the submucosa (T1sm). Detection of early esophageal cancers with increasing

Table 2-1. AJCC TNM Definitions for Esophageal Cancer[2]

Primary Tumor (T)

Tx	Primary tumor cannot be assessed.
T0	No evidence of primary tumor.
Tis	Carcinoma in situ.
T1	Tumor invades lamina propria or submucosa.
T2	Tumor invades muscularis propria.
T3	Tumor invades adventitia.
T4	Tumor invades adjacent structures.

Regional Lymph Nodes (N)

Nx	Regional lymph nodes cannot be assessed.
N0	No regional lymph node metastasis.
N1	Regional lymph node metastasis

Distant Metastases (M)

Mx	Distant metastasis cannot be assessed.
M0	No distant metastasis.
M1	Tumors of the lower thoracic esophagus
M1a:	Metastasis in celiac lymph nodes
M1b:	Other distant metastasis
	Tumors of the midthoracic esophagus
M1a:	Not applicable
M1b:	Nonregional lymph nodes and/or other distant metastasis
	Tumors of the upper thoracic esophagus
M1a:	Metastasis in cervical lymph nodes
M1b:	Other distant metastasis

Table 2-2A. AJCC Stage Groupings for Esophageal Cancer

Stage	T	N	M
0	Tis	0	0
1	1	0	0
2a	2	0	0
	3	0	0
2b	1	1	0
	2	1	0
3	3	1	0
	4	Any	0
4	Any	Any	1
4a	Any	Any	1a
4b	Any	Any	1b

Table 2-2B. Staging and Prognosis

Stage	Percent of Patients*	Five-Year Survival (%)[3]
0	1	>95
1	10	50-80
2	21	
2a		30-40
2b		10-30
3	18	10-15
4	26	
4a		<5
4b		<1
Unstaged	23	

* Data based on U.S. National Cancer Society SEER Database of 11,154 patients diagnosed in 1998.

frequency may be anticipated over future years. Factors contributing to this trend include the widespread increase in surveillance of patients with Barrett's esophagus, and the increasing availability of endoscopic technology aiding detection of early lesions, such as narrow band imaging, chromoendoscopy (iodine dye, methylene blue, acetic acid staining), high magnification, and confocal endoscopy.

In addition, nonsurgical therapies, such as endoscopic mucosal resection (EMR), endoscopic submucosal dissection (ESD), or photodynamic therapy (PDT), may increasingly be considered for patients with esophageal cancer as they are frequently elderly and often have significant co-morbid diseases, which increase operative risk. Encouraging results have been reported with EMR, making it a viable alternative to surgery in these patients.[7] Accurate EUS staging will therefore play an increasingly important role in the triaging of patients with esophageal cancer to the most appropriate management regimen. In particular, high frequency EUS will be crucial in determining which patients with early esophageal cancer are suitable for nonsurgical therapeutic options, such as EMR.

Factors Affecting Tumor Staging

Operator Expertise

Accurate EUS staging of esophageal cancer requires experienced operators, due to a significant learning curve, as demonstrated initially by Rice et al. Their accuracy in T-staging of their first 28 patients was only 59%, improving subsequently to 81% over the next 52 patients.[8] Similar improvements in accuracy with increasing experience have since been reported by others.[9,10] An experience of 75–100 examinations appears necessary to achieve an acceptable staging accuracy rate of 80-90%.[9,10] Performing a high volume of EUS staging examinations for esophageal cancer also positively impacts accuracy rates. A recent study confirmed that a low volume center had a lower sensitivity (58% vs 75%-90%) and specificity (87% vs 94%-97%) for T1 or T2 stages than several high-volume centers.[11] Similarly, the low-volume center had a lower sensitivity for regional (45% vs 63%-89%) and celiac (19% vs 72%–83%) lymph nodes.[11]

Technique

Operator technique can significantly affect the accuracy of T-staging. The endoscope water balloon should ideally be inflated until optimal acoustic coupling is achieved, while avoiding significant compression of the esophageal wall. Overdistension of the water balloon compresses the layers of the esophageal wall, which may result in inaccurate T-staging. The depth of penetration of tumors may vary over their length and the potential for understaging therefore exists. Time should be taken to carefully locate the maximum depth of tumor invasion, in a scanning plane perpendicular to the surface of the tumor. Scanning in an oblique plane ("Salami Effect") can result in localized thickening or blurring of wall layers and may lead to erroneous overstaging of the tumor.

Achieving satisfactory and safe acoustic coupling for HFPs has been problematic. The esophageal

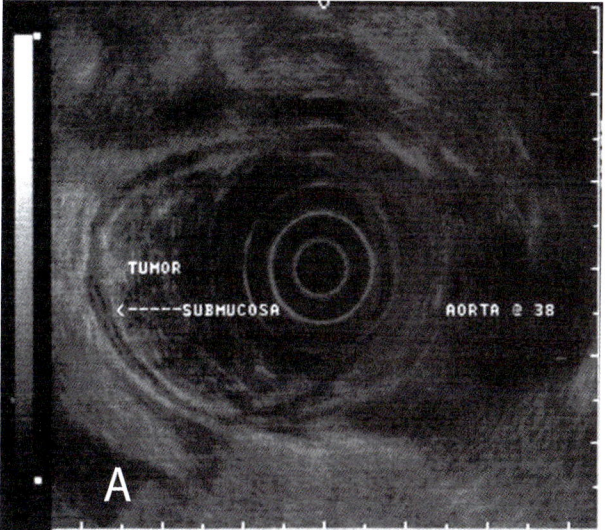

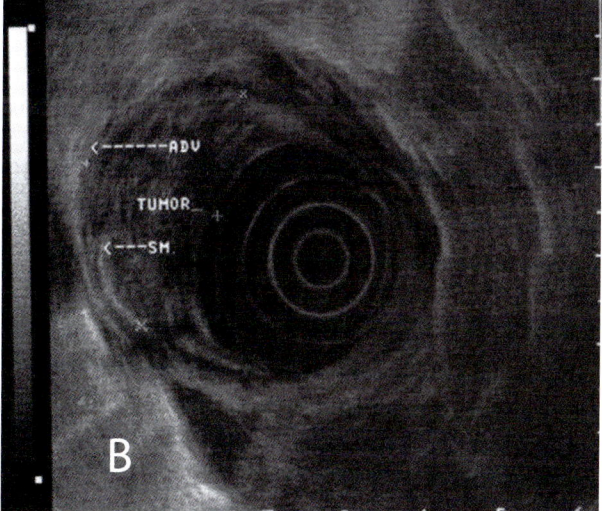

FIGURE 2–1. *A and B* (A) This was a T2 lesion appearing in this image to be T1 submucosal with intact muscularis propria (mechanical radial echoendoscope, 7.5MHz, 6cm range). (B) At a different level of the esophagus, the tumor clearly invades through the muscularis propria but not the adventitia, indicating a T2 lesion.

lumen has been filled with deaerated water to facilitate examination by HFPs.[12] Due to concerns regarding the possibility of aspiration, alternative techniques have evolved, each with their own advantages and disadvantages. Soft, translucent latex condoms have been attached to the distal end of the endoscope and inflated with water after esophageal intubation and prior to advancement of the HFP.[13] This allows for superior acoustic coupling. However, air pockets within the condom are sometimes problematic. This issue has been overcome using a double channel scope, with the second channel used to aspirate air and instill water.[14] The translucent condoms limit visualization, necessitating a separate prior intubation for initial endoscopic evaluation of the lesion, leading to prolongation of procedure time. A balloon sheath has been incorporated into some HFPs to improve imaging.[15] This allows for endoscopic and EUS evaluation with a single intubation. However, problems with acoustic coupling may remain, due to the disparities in size between the balloon sheath and the esophageal lumen. Furthermore, once the HFP has been advanced through the endoscope, suctioning and luminal water instillation are no longer possible. HFPs with balloon sheaths have therefore been used with a double-channel endoscope, with the second channel used to aspirate air and to instill small volumes of water into the esophagus to optimize acoustic coupling.[16] A balloon device that attaches proximal to the tip of the endoscope has been described; it is inflated to occlude the esophageal lumen.[17] The stomach and esophagus distal to the balloon may then be filled with a large volume of water (around 400 ml), with aspiration prevented by the lumen-occluding balloon. More recently, Esaki et al have described a technique of instilling 30–40 ml of echo jelly into the esophageal lumen at the lesion, to enhance acoustic coupling. This removes the need for a balloon. Superior accuracy for T staging of early squamous esophageal cancer was noted, compared with the water-filled condom method.[18]

Equipment

Technology has improved steadily since EUS was first performed more than 30 years ago. Comparison of performance rates between earlier and later studies is therefore confounded by the increasingly sophisticated technology available with advancing time. EUS with older echoendoscopes at frequencies of 7.5 or 12 MHz depicted the esophageal wall in five layers (Table 2–3). EUS at higher frequencies (20 or 30 MHz) depicts the esophageal wall in nine echo layers (Table 2–4), allowing for more precise T-staging. Higher frequency scanning previously required the use of high frequency probes (HFPs), which offer superior resolutions and are positioned under direct endoscopic visualization.[19] Hasegawa et al demonstrated an insignificant trend toward superior accuracy in T1-m and T1-sm staging with HFPs (92%) compared with standard echoendoscopes (76%).[17] Newer echoendoscopes offer a range of frequencies from 5 to 20 MHz allowing higher frequency scanning for accurate T-staging and lower frequency scanning for N-staging. These new echoendoscopes offering high-frequency EUS have not been prospectively compared with HFPs in the staging of early esophageal cancer.

With HFPs, the mucosa is visualized as four layers comprising the epithelium (m1 and m2), the lamina propria (m3), and the muscularis mucosa (m4). Imaging with radial, linear and switchable linear-

Table 2–3 The Esophageal Wall Using 7.5MHz EUS

Echolayer	Histological layer
first hyperechoic layer	superficial mucosa
second hypoechoic layer	deep mucosa
third hyperechoic layer	submucosa
fourth hypoechoic layer	muscularis propria
fifth hyperechoic layer	adventitia

Table 2–4 The Esophageal Wall Using 20 MHz EUS

Echolayer	Histological layer
first hyperechoic layer (m1)	superficial mucosa
second hypoechoic layer (m2)	deep mucosa
third hyperechoic layer (m3)	lamina propria
fourth hypoechoic layer (m4)	muscularis mucosa
fifth hyperechoic layer	submucosa
sixth hypoechoic layers (p1)	inner circular muscle
seventh hyperechoic layer (p2)	intermuscular connective tissue
eighth hypoechoic layer (p3)	outer longitudinal muscle
ninth hyperechoic layer	adventitia

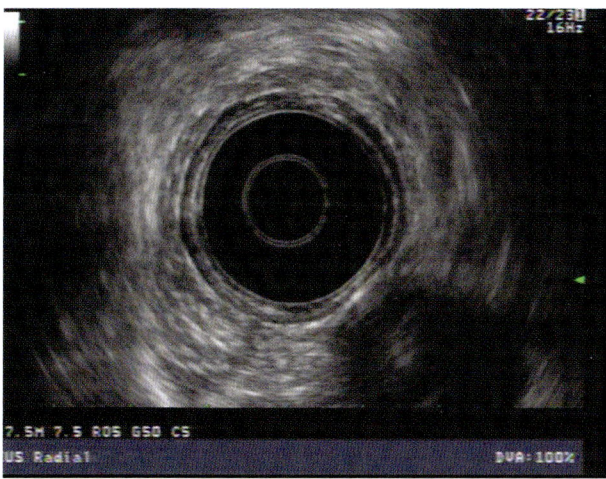

FIGURE 2–2. Normal esophaegal wall at 7.5 MHz (5 layers) (Courtsey of Dr. Manoop Bhutani)

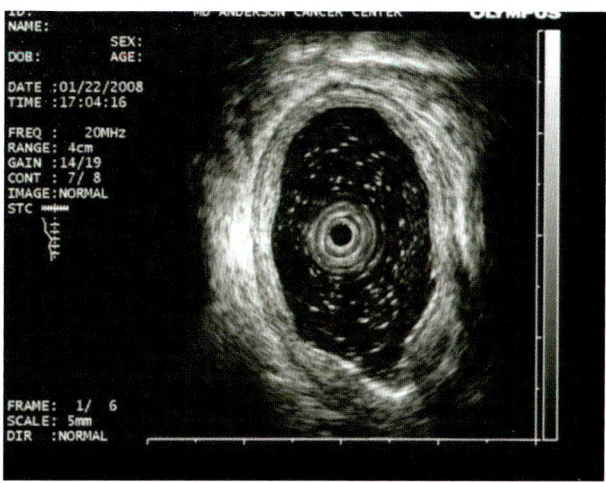

FIGURE 2–3. Normal esophageal wall at 20MHz (9 layers) (Courtsey of Dr. Manoop Bhutani)

radial HFPs has been described.[20] The linear HFP has been reported to be better at depicting the m4 layer (90% frequency) compared with the radial HFP (70% frequency).[12] HFPs allow for finer T-stage discrimination of early tumors into Tm and Tsm, because they provide better resolution over the shallow depths of involvement of these early lesions.[12,17] However, HFPs have a limited depth of penetration and are therefore unsatisfactory for lymph node staging. Thus N-staging should be performed at lower frequency, using a standard echoendoscope. HFPs should be viewed as complementary to echoendoscopes.

Similarly, evaluation of large lengths of involved esophagus may be better performed using standard echoendoscopes. HFPs are best suited for evaluation of focal discrete abnormalities, such as those arising in Barrett's esophagus. Here they have the advantage of allowing accurate interrogation of the abnormality under direct endoscopic control, using a forward-viewing scope. In contrast, accurate localization of a small abnormality may be difficult with the oblique viewing standard echoendoscope. Prototypes on forward-viewing echoendoscopes are now in development, which may resolve this problem. HFPs also do not cause the compression artifact seen with the standard echoendoscope, which can be problematic when determining if a T1 tumor is Tm or Tsm. Disadvantages of HFPs include their lack of durability and their cost (Table 2–5).

Tumor-Related Factors

Normal histological structures, relatively deep early tumors, the presence of nodules or ulcers at the site of cancer, and scarring at prior biopsy sites have all led to errors in staging. These are discussed in more detail in the next section of this chapter.

Table 2–5 Comparison of Dedicated Echoendoscope and High Frequency Probe

	Dedicated Echoendoscope	High Frequency Probe
Advantages	• Wide range scanning frequencies allowing T- and N-staging • Balloon for acoustic coupling • Easier to examine longer tumors • FNA capability	• High frequency allowing high-resolution T-staging • Direct endoscopic positioning of probe to assess small lesions
Disadvantages	• Oblique endoscopic view resulting in difficult localization of small lesions • Compression of tumor from balloon overdistension can lead to inaccurate staging	• Difficult acoustic coupling • Limited depth of signal penetration (inaccurate N-staging) • Cost • Durability

EUS Staging in Early Esophageal Cancer

The bar for T-staging accuracy has been set higher over recent years. Older echoendoscopes scanning at lower frequencies satisfactorily differentiated T1 from T2 tumors. However, the expectation today is for differential T1 staging, at least into T1-m (or T1-a) and T1-sm (or T1-b) tumors. Some centers have further subdivided and staged early cancers based on tumor involvement of the epithelium, lamina propria, muscularis mucosa, or submucosa.[12,20]

EUS Depiction of Early Esophageal Cancer

In the nine-layer echo-image provided by HFPs, tumors involving the first four echolayers are deemed mucosal cancers; with involvement of the fifth hyperechoic layer, they are deemed submucosal cancers. More detailed staging has been described by Murata et al.[12] A Tis lesion is typically depicted as a hypoechoic mass within the m1 and m2 layers, with preservation of the m3 layer (Figure 2–4). With invasion of the lamina propria (T1-lpm), the hypoechoic mass will be seen extending into and involving the m3 layer, while the muscularis layer (m4) remains uninvolved. With involvement of the muscularis mucosa (T1-mm), the hypoechoic mass will be noted extending through the m1, m2, and m3 layers, and involving the m4 layer. The fifth hyperechoic layer depicting the submucosa remains uninvolved. With invasion of the submucosa (T1-sm), the hypoechoic mass will be seen involving m1 through m4 layers and the fifth hyperechoic layer, while the sixth layer (p1 layer of muscularis propria) will remain uninvolved.

An important factor driving the need for increasing accuracy in T-staging of early esophageal cancers is the option of nonsurgical therapies for patients with Tm disease. Endoscopic approaches include EMR and

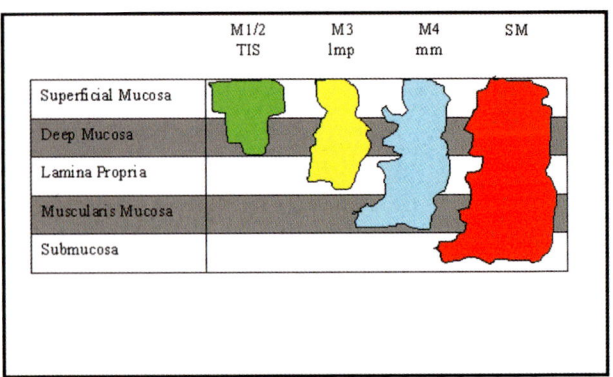

FIGURE 2–4. Subclassification of T1 tumors.

ESD. Disease confined to the mucosa (Stage T1m) has a low risk of lymph node involvement of less than 2%.[21,22] In contrast, with submucosal involvement (T1-sm), the risk of lymph node metastases increases to 30–40%, reflecting the rich lymphatic drainage of the submucosa.[23] Lymph node metastases are increasingly likely with increasing depth of submucosal involvement. Buskens, et al demonstrated a 23% and 69% lymph node involvement rate when the middle and deepest third of the submucosa respectively were involved, compared to tumors limited to the mucosa or to the superficial third of submucosa, where no lymph node involvement was seen.[24] Endoscopic therapy with curative intent should therefore only be considered for T1-m lesions. Accurate differentiation between mucosal (T1m) and submucosal (T1sm) involvement is crucial in selecting patients for nonsurgical therapies.

Encouraging results have been described with the use of EMR in selected patients with early esophageal cancer. A recent study describes EMR successfully performed in 100 consecutive patients with T1m adenocarcinoma arising in Barrett's metaplasia, with no major complications and achievement of complete local remission in 99 of the 100 patients. Over a subsequent follow-up period of 37 months, recurrent or metachronous carcinomas developed in 11% of the patients, but again, successful EMR was possible in all cases.[7]

Table 2–6 Staging of Early Esophageal (T1) cancer: Different Nomenclatures in Use

	I	II	III	IV	IV	Histological Layer	Echo-Layer
Mucosal:	T1m	T1a m2	m1	m1	Tis	Epithelium	1st Hyperechoic 2nd Hypoechoic
			m3	m2	T1-lmp	Lamina propria	3rd Hyperechoic
			m4	m3	T1-mm	Muscularis mucosa	4th Hypoechoic
Submucosal:	T1sm	T1b	sm	sm	T1-sm	Submucosa	5th Hyperechoic

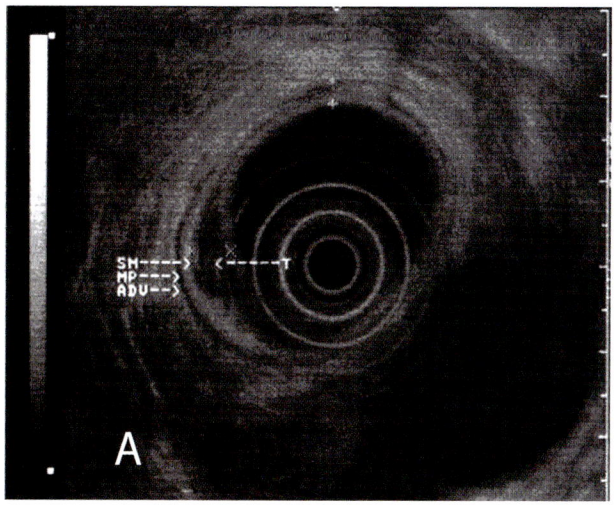

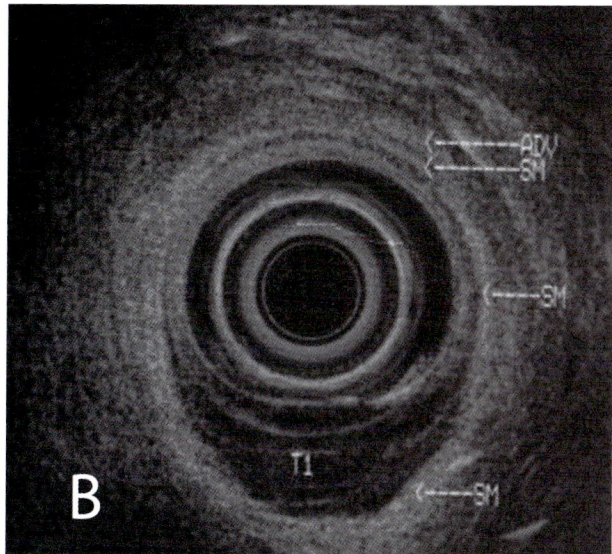

FIGURE 2–5. *A and B* T1 mucosal lesions with intact submucosa layer (mechanical radial echoendoscope, 7.5MHz, 6cm range).

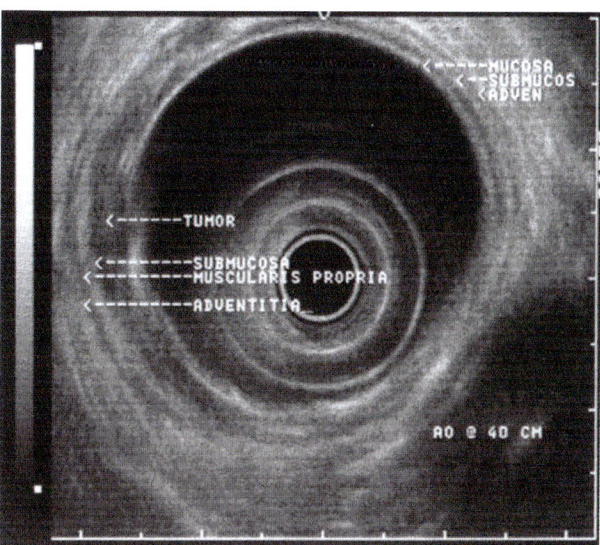

FIGURE 2–6. T1 lesion (12MHz, 4cm range). Often it is difficult to determine T1 mucosal from submucosal invasion with the mechanical radial echoendoscope at lower frequencies. In this image, it is not clear if the tumor involves the submucosa. Imaging with a high frequency probe may better delineate mucosal layers.

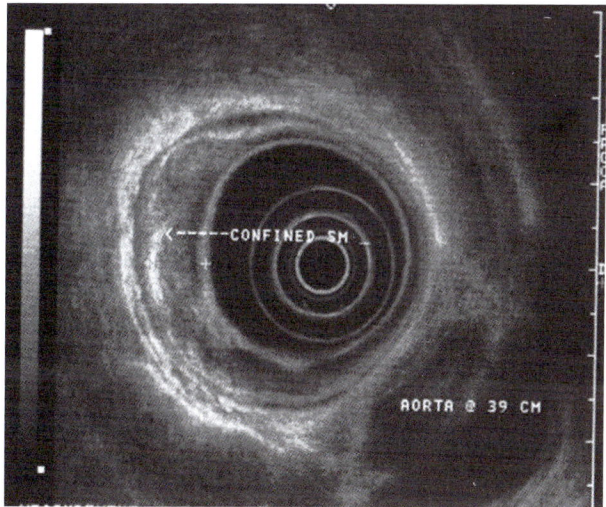

FIGURE 2–7. T1 submucosal lesion (mechanical radial echoendoscope, 12MHz, 6cm range). The submucosa is clearly involved without penetration through the muscularis propria.

Accuracy of EUS in Staging Early Esophageal Cancer

Early reports of mechanical radial echoendoscopes in the evaluation of superficial cancer demonstrated an accuracy rate of 67% and 79% for mucosal and submucosal involvement respectively, with an overall accuracy of 75%.[25]

A number of studies have been published evaluating the accuracy of HFP in staging early esophageal cancer (Table 2–7).[12,16,17,20,26,27,28] Murata et al have described EUS findings in early esophageal cancer using 15–20 MHz HFPs.[12] They found an overall accuracy of 75% for T-staging of early esophageal cancer. However, superior accuracy was noted for predicting cancer limited by the lamina propria (84%) and distinguishing cancers limited to the mucosa from those extending into the submucosa (94%). Using a 15MHz HFP, Hasegawa et al achieved 86% and 94% accuracy rates respectively for T1m and T1sm cancers, with an overall accuracy rate of 92% for all T lesions. In contrast, standard EUS (7.5 and 12 MHz) achieved accuracy rates of 71% and 78% for mucosal and submucosal tumors respectively, with an overall accuracy rate of 76%.[17] Yanai et al achieved lower accuracy rates of 64.7% for Tm and Tsm lesions using a 20MHz HFP.[20]

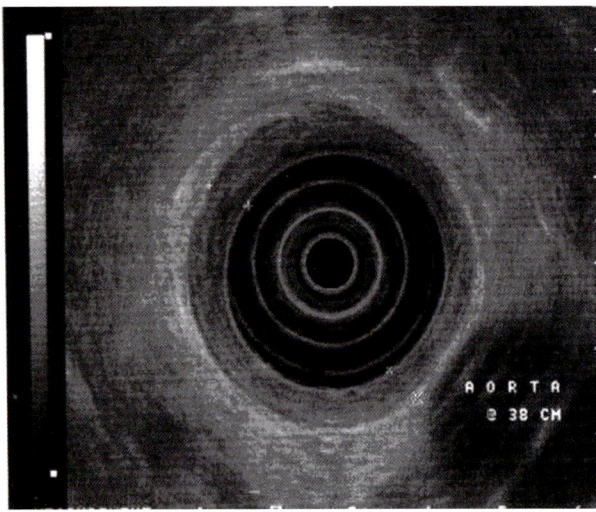

FIGURE 2–8. T1 submucosal lesion (mechanical radial echoendoscope, 7.5MHz, 6cm range) showing circumferential submucosal involvement and intact muscularis propria.

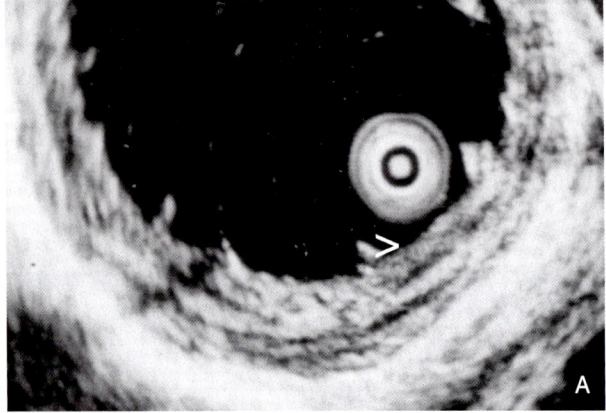 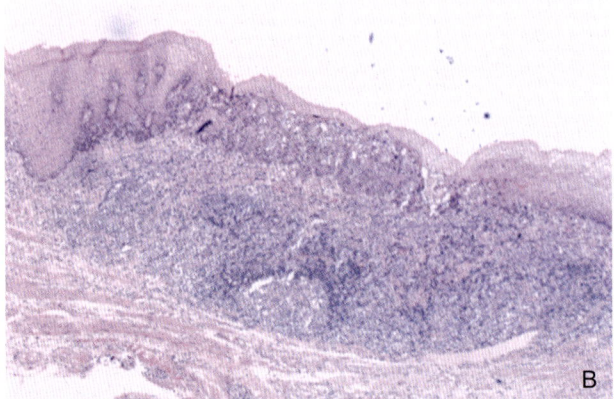

FIGURE 2–9. *A and B* (A) T1 mucosal esophageal cancer with HFP with corresponding histopathology. Esophageal wall was identified with seven layers on EUS, third layer on EUS corresponds to submucosal layer. Hypoechoic lesion is the tumor (arrowhead). (Courtsey of Dr. Atsushi Irisawa) (B) Corresponding histopathology to the lesion in Figure 2–9A. .(Courtsey of Dr. Atsushi Irisawa)

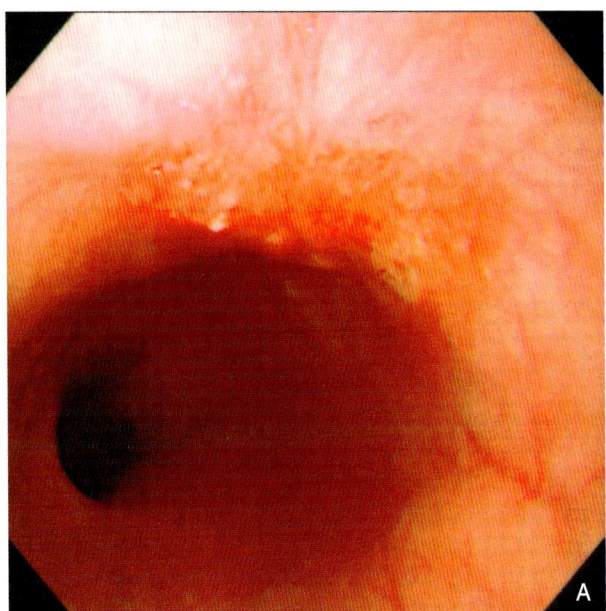 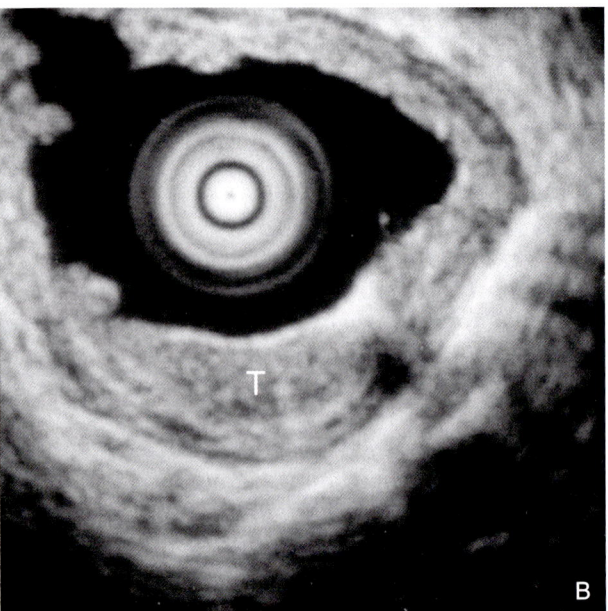

FIGURE 2–10. *A and B* (A) Endoscopic view of an early, superficial cancer. (Courtsey of Dr. Atsushi Irisawa) (B) HFP EUS shows the lesion in Figure 2–10A to be a T1 submucosal esophageal cancer. Esophageal wall was identified with seven layers on EUS, third layer on EUS corresponds to submucosal layer. The tumor infiltrates (T) into the submucosa. (Courtsey of Dr. Atsushi Irisawa)

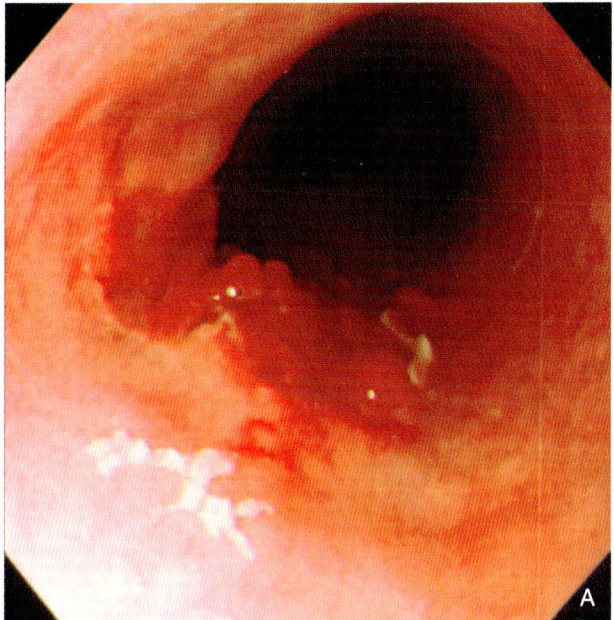
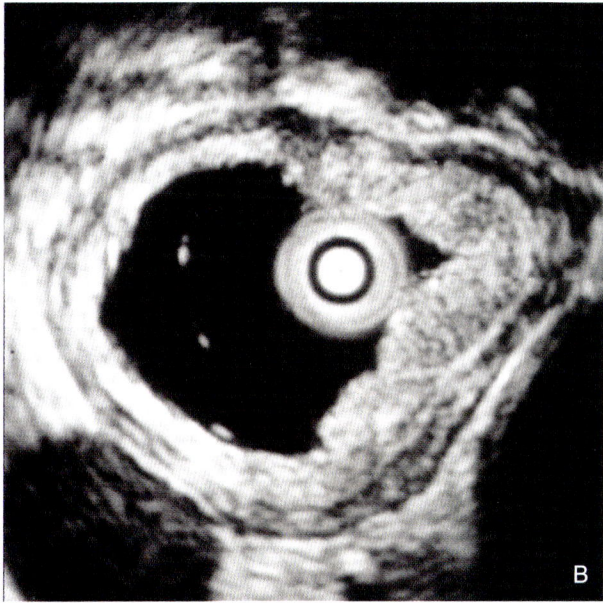

FIGURE 2–11. *A and B* (A) Endoscopic view of an a flat, nodular, esophageal cancer. (Courtsey of Dr Atsushi Irisawa) (B) HFP EUS shows T1 submucosal esophagus cancer. Esophageal wall was identified with seven layers on EUS, third layer on EUS corresponds to submucosal layer. The tumor infiltrates into the deep submucosa. (Courtsey of Dr Atsushi Irisawa)

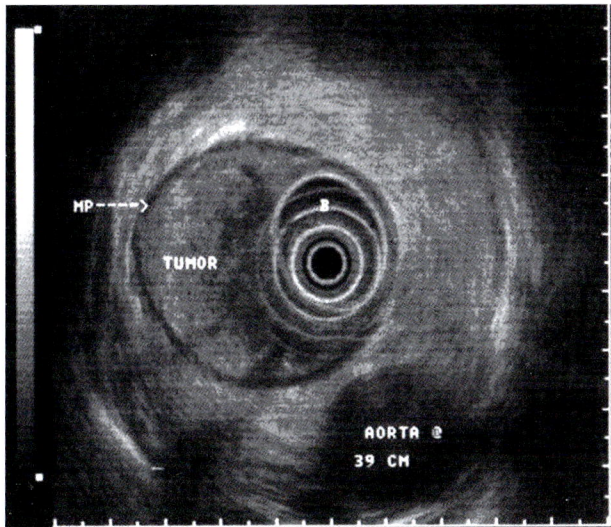

FIGURE 2–12. T2 lesion marginally invading into the muscularis propria (mechanical radial echoendoscope, 7.5MHz, 4cm range).

Over-and Understaging

Overstaging of early esophageal cancers appears more likely than understaging.[12,20] Overstaging of T-is cancer as T1-lpm has been reported due to adjacent hypoechoic lymph follicles or inflammatory infiltration being mistaken for tumor extension. Similarly, overstaging of T1-lpm cancers as T1-sm has been reported due to adjacent hypoechoic collections of mucosal esophageal glands being mistaken for tumor extension. Tm tumors have been overstaged as Tsm lesions due to ambiguous images caused by attenuation of the ultrasound or vibration of the HFP.[20] Scarring caused by previous endoscopic biopsy may lead to obliteration of superficial layers focally, leading to overstaging. T1-sm tumors may be overstaged to T2 where the tumors are relatively large with resultant thinning of the muscularis propria, or with attenuation of ultrasound signal with tumor depth. In the setting of Barrett's esophagus, the presence of a nodule or exophytic growth has been associated with overstating of T1m lesions to T1sm.[24] Similarly, the presence of esophageal ulcers may affect the reliability of staging. Understaging is rare but may occasionally occur where early microscopic invasion of deeper layers has not yet lead to changes in echogenicity detectable by HFPs.[17]

Barrett's Esophagus: (HGD Tis, T1m and T1sm)

Esophagectomy is typically recommended for patients with Barrett's esophagus (BE) and high grade dysplasia (HGD), because coexistent, undiagnosed esophageal cancer is found in a high proportion (30–47%) of these patients. However, a proportion of patients will not be suitable candidates for surgery, due to advanced age and/or co-morbid diseases. In patients with BE and HGD, EUS may complement aggressive biopsy techniques and allow selection of patients appropriate for endoscopic management with EMR.

Table 2-7 — Accuracy of High Frequency EUS for Differentiation of T1m and T1sm for Superficial Esophageal Carcinoma Staging

Study	N	Equipment	Frequency (MHz)	Accuracy T1m	Accuracy T1sm	Total Accuracy (%)
Simizu[26] 1995	40	HFP	20	77.8	NA	82.5
Hasegawa[17] 1996	22	Aloka MP-PN15-08M probe	15	86	94	92
Yanai[20] 1996	16	Fujinon Sp501 Sonoprobe	20	50	100	64.7
Murata[12] 1996	54	Fujinon Sp101, Sp501 Sonoprobes	15 or 20	M1: 38% M2: 64% M3: 100%	83%	75
Vazquez-Sequeiros[16] 2002	4	Olympus UM-3R-2 CUS Probe	20	100	100	100
Kawano[27] 2003	85	Fujinon Sp101, Sp501 Sonoprobes	20	95	89	93
May[28] 2004	93	Fujinon Sp501 Sonoprobe	20	91.2	48	79.6

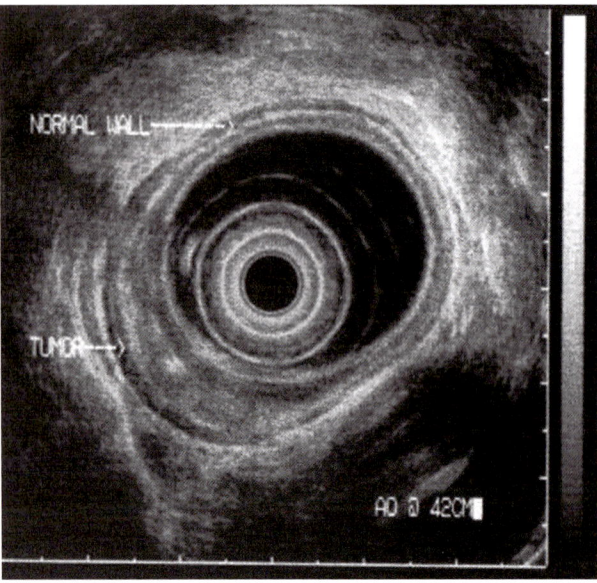

FIGURE 2–13. T1 versus T2. In this image (mechanical radial echoendoscope, 12MHz, 6cm range), the majority of the tumor appears to involve submucosa, however the muscularis propria appears to be invaded at the 6 o'clock position.

An older study by Falk et al found that EUS (standard echoendoscope imaging at 7.5 and 12MHz) was not helpful in determining the need for surgery in patients with BE and HGD. It did not reliably differentiate between benign and malignant wall thickening, leading to frequent overstaging.[29] Recent studies have been more encouraging. Scotionotis et al prospectively assessed 22 preoperative BE patients with HGD or intramucosal carcinoma.[30] EUS at 7.5 and 12MHz using a standard echoendoscope correctly identified all 16 patients with mucosal disease (100%) and 5 of 6 patients with submucosal invasion. Unlike the study of Falk et al, the presence of mucosal nodules did not affect the accuracy of staging in the Scotionotis study. However, the presence of mucosal nodules or strictures in patients with early cancer was associated with a high prevalence (42%) of submucosal involvement.[30] Thus, in the setting of BE and HGD, EUS may allow identification of patients suitable for nonoperative therapies. Buskens et al reached similar conclusions in a small retrospective study using a combination of echoendoscopes and HFPs, where the negative predictive value of EUS for submucosal invasion was 95%.[24]

Pech et al prospectively assessed 66 patients with Barrett's esophagus who had elevated and/or depressed lesions.[31] Histological confirmation of T-staging was possible in 62 of these patients. 7.5MHz frequency probes were used in all patients, and 12.5 or 20MHz probes in those with elevated or depressed lesions. When compared to histology, EUS differentiated T1 from less than T1 cancers in all cases. The sensitivity of EUS probes for detecting mucosal cancer was 89%, but with a low specificity of 27%. The sensitivity for submucosal cancer was only 27% with a specificity of 89%. EUS was clearly superior to CT, which could not adequately differentiate T1 from less than T1 cancers. However, EUS—even with HFPs—could not reliably differentiate between Tm and Tsm cancers. EMR with prior EUS to rule out infiltration of the muscularis propria may provide the most exact T staging. The mixed data on the reliability of EUS in staging of early esophageal cancer in this setting mandates careful histological assessment of the resection specimen, to confirm staging histologically.

Larghi et al performed EUS using a standard echoendoscope (5-20MHz) on 48 patients with Barrett's esophagus and HGD—and possible early cancer.[32] Focal lesions were further assessed with a 20MHz HFP. EUS diagnosed submucosal involvement in 8 of these patients, correctly in 7. When compared to pathologic staging on surgical or EMR specimens, the overall T staging accuracy for EUS was 85%, with one patient overstaged, and 6 patients understaged (diagnosed as T1m on EUS, but found to be T1sm on pathology). Whereas the distinction between mucosal and submucosal invasion was performed with a relatively satisfactory accuracy, difficulty was noted in making distinctions between the various levels of mucosal invasion even at 20 MHz.[32]

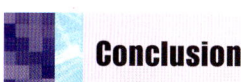

Conclusion

EUS is a highly accurate modality for T-staging of esophageal tumors. Although differentiation between T1 and T2 cancers is accurately achieved with EUS, the goal for the future is achieving consistently reliable distinction between mucosal (T1-m) and submucosal (T1-sm) tumors, because this impacts both prognostically, and allows selection of patients for endoscopic therapies such as EMR. With the increasing availability of HFPs and standard echoendoscopes imaging at 20 MHz, this goal should be achievable. At present, EUS to rule out infiltration of the muscularis propria, followed by EMR with histological examination of the resection specimen, offers the most exact T-staging.

References:

1. http//seer.cancer.gov/statfacts/html/esoph.html
2. Greene, F. L.P. D., Fleming, I. D., Fritz, A., Balch, C. M., Haller, D. G., Morrow, M .(eds.): AJCC Cancer Staging Manual. New York: Springer, 2002.
3. Enzinger, P. C., Mayer, R. J.: Esophageal cancer. N Engl J Med 2003;349:2241–2252.
4. Van Dam, J.: Endosonographic evaluation of the patient with esophageal cancer. Chest 1997;112:184S–190S.
5. Rosch, T.: Endosonographic staging of esophageal cancer: a review of literature results. Gastrointest Endosc Clin N Am 1995;5:537–547.
6. Catalano, M. F., Sivak, M. V. Jr., Rice, T., Gragg, L. A., Van Dam, J.: Endosonographic features predictive of lymph node metastasis. Gastrointest Endosc 1994;40:442–446.
7. Ell, C., May, A., Pech, O., Gossner, L., Guenter, E., Behrens, A., Nachbar, L., Huijsmans, J., Vieth, M., Stolte, M.: Curative endoscopic resection of early esophageal adenocarcinomas (Barrett's cancer). Gastrointestinal Endoscopy 2007;65:3–10.
8. Rice, T. W., Boyce, G. A., Sivak, M. V.: Esophageal ultrasound and the preoperative staging of carcinoma of the esophagus. Journal of Thoracic & Cardiovascular Surgery 1991;101:536-43; discussion 543–544.
9. Schlick, T., Heintz, A., Junginger, T.: The examiner's learning effect and its influence on the quality of endoscopic ultrasonography in carcinoma of the esophagus and gastric cardia. Surg Endosc 1999;13:894–898.
10. Fockens, P., Van den Brande, J. H., van Dullemen, H. M., van Lanschot, J. J., Tytgat, G. N.: Endosonographic T-staging of esophageal carcinoma: a learning curve. Gastrointest Endosc 1996;44:58–62.
11. van Vliet, E. P., Eijkemans, M. J., Poley, J. W., Steyerberg, E. W., Kuipers, E. J., Siersema, P. D.: Staging of esophageal carcinoma in a low-volume EUS center compared with reported results from high-volume centers. Gastrointest Endosc 2006;63:938–947.
12. Murata, Y., Suzuki, S., Ohta, M., Mitsunaga, A., Hayashi, K., Yoshida, K., Ide, H.: Small ultrasonic probes for determination of the depth of superficial esophageal cancer. Gastrointestinal Endoscopy 1996;44:23–28.
13. Inoue, H., Kawano, T., Takeshita, K., Iwai, T.: Modified soft-balloon methods during ultrasonic probe examination for superficial esophageal cancer. Endoscopy 1998;30 Suppl 1:A41–43.
14. Wallace, M. B., Hoffman, B. J., Sahai, A. S., Inoue, H., Van Velse, A., Hawes, R. H.: Imaging of esophageal tumors with a water-filled condom and a catheter US probe. Gastrointest Endosc 2000;51:597–600.
15. Fockens, P., van Dullemen, H. M., Tytgat, G. N.: Endosonography of stenotic esophageal carcinomas: preliminary experience with an ultra-thin, balloon-fitted ultrasound probe in four patients. Gastrointest Endosc 1994;40:226–228.
16. Vazquez-Sequeiros, E., Wiersema, M. J.: High-frequency US catheter-based staging of early esophageal tumors. Gastrointestinal Endoscopy 2002;55:95–99.
17. Hasegawa, N., Niwa, Y., Arisawa, T., Hase, S., Goto, H., Hayakawa, T.: Preoperative staging of superficial esophageal carcinoma: comparison of an ultrasound probe and standard endoscopic ultrasonography. Gastrointestinal Endoscopy 1996;44:388–393.
18. Esaki, M., Matsumoto, T., Moriyama, T., Hizawa, K., Ohji, Y., Nakamura, S., Hirakawa, K., Hirahashi, M., Yao, T., Iida, M.: Probe EUS for the diagnosis of invasion depth in superficial esophageal cancer: a comparison between a jelly-filled method and a water-filled balloon method. Gastrointestinal Endoscopy 2006;63:389–95.
19. Bhutani, M. S.: "Probing" the endoscopic ultrasound (EUS) catheter probe: a small step for EUS or a giant leap? Gastrointest Endosc 1998;48:542–545.
20. Yanai, H., Yoshida, T., Harada, T., Matsumoto, Y., Nishiaki, M., Shigemitsu, T., Tada, M., Okita, K.,

Kawano, T., Nagasaki, S.: Endoscopic ultrasonography of superficial esophageal cancers using a thin ultrasound probe system equipped with switchable radial and linear scanning modes. Gastrointestinal Endoscopy 1996;44:578–582.
21. Rice, T. W., Zuccaro, G., Jr., Adelstein, D. J., Rybicki, L. A., Blackstone, E. H., Goldblum, J. R.: Esophageal carcinoma: depth of tumor invasion is predictive of regional lymph node status. Ann Thorac Surg 1998;65:787–792.
22. Holscher, A. H., Bollschweiler, E., Schneider, P. M., Siewert, J. R.: Early adenocarcinoma in Barrett's oesophagus. Br J Surg 1997;84:1470–1473.
23. Westerterp, M., Koppert, L. B., Buskens, C. J., Tilanus, H. W., ten Kate, F. J., Bergman, J. J., Siersema, P. D., van Dekken, H., van Lanschot, J. J.: Outcome of surgical treatment for early adenocarcinoma of the esophagus or gastro-esophageal junction. Virchows Archiv 2005;446:497–504.
24. Buskens, C. J., Westerterp, M., Lagarde, S. M., Bergman, J. J., ten Kate, F. J., van Lanschot, J. J.: Prediction of appropriateness of local endoscopic treatment for high-grade dysplasia and early adenocarcinoma by EUS and histopathologic features. Gastrointestinal Endoscopy 2004;60:703–710.
25. Yoshikane, H., Tsukamoto, Y., Niwa, Y., Goto, H., Hase, S., Shimodaira, M., Maruta, S., Miyata, A., Yoshida, M.: Superficial esophageal carcinoma: evaluation by endoscopic ultrasonography. American Journal of Gastroenterology 1994;89:702–707.
26. Simizu, Y., Tsukagoshi, H., Nakazato, T., Kawarazaki, M., Sai, K., Oikawa, Y., Mera, K., Hosokawa, M., Oohara, M., Fujita, M.: Clinical evaluation of endoscopic ultrasonography (EUS) in the diagnosis of superficial esophageal carcinoma (Japanese). Rinsho Byori. 1995;43:221–226.
27. Kawano, T., Ohshima, M., Iwai, T.: Early esophageal carcinoma: endoscopic ultrasonography using the sonoprobe. Abdominal Imaging 2003;28:477–485.
28. May, A., Günter, E., Roth, F., Gossner, L., Stolte, M., Vieth, M, Ell, C.: Accuracy of staging in early oesophageal cancer using high resolution endoscopy and high resolution endosonography: a comparative, prospective and blinded trial. Gut 2004;53:634–640.
29. Falk, G. W., Catalano, M. F., Sivak, M. V., Jr., Rice, T. W., Van Dam, J.: Endosonography in the evaluation of patients with Barrett's esophagus and high-grade dysplasia. Gastrointestinal Endoscopy 1994;40:207–212.
30. Scotiniotis, I. A., Kochman, M. L., Lewis, J. D., Furth, E. E., Rosato, E. F., Ginsberg, G. G.: Accuracy of EUS in the evaluation of Barrett's esophagus and high-grade dysplasia or intramucosal carcinoma. Gastrointestinal Endoscopy 2001;54:689–696.
31. Pech, O., May, A., Gunter, E., Gossner, L., Ell, C.: The impact of endoscopic ultrasound and computed tomography on the TNM staging of early cancer in Barrett's esophagus. American Journal of Gastroenterology 2006;101:2223–2229.
32. Larghi, A., Lightdale, C. J., Memeo, L., Bhagat, G., Okpara, N., Rotterdam, H.: EUS followed by EMR for staging of high-grade dysplasia and early cancer in Barrett's esophagus. Gastrointestinal Endoscopy 2005;62:16–23.

CHAPTER

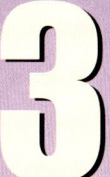

EUS in Barrett's Esophagus and High Grade Dysplasia/Early Carcinoma

Dr. Sharmila Anandasabapathy

Introduction

Barrett's esophagus (BE) is a metaplastic change in which intestinalization occurs in the squamous esophagus above the gastroesophageal (GE) junction. The anatomy of the region is shown in Figure 3-1. BE is the most important risk factor in the development of esophageal adenocarcinoma (EAC), a cancer whose incidence has increased dramatically in the last few decades.[1] The mean annual incidence of the development of esophageal adenocarcinoma in BE is approximately 0.5–1%[2] and usually arises through the progression of dysplastic, or precancerous, changes in the esophagus. From intestinal metaplasia, progression typically occurs through the development of low-grade dysplasia (LGD), high-grade dysplasia (HGD), and ultimately esophageal adenocarcinoma. Because carcinoma has been shown to occur in 30% of resection specimens in individuals with an endoscopic diagnosis of HGD,[3] esophagectomy has traditionally been recommended for individuals with either HGD or intramucosal adenocarcinoma. Esophagectomy, however, carries a mortality rate of between 3 and 20%, depending upon institutional volume.[4] Because of this, endoscopic alternatives to surgery (endoscopic mucosal resection (EMR), radio-frequency ablation, etc. have become increasingly more appealing for individuals with HGD or intramucosal adenocarcinoma. In these individuals, where cancer may be suspected, EUS is invaluable in ruling out submucosal invasion and malignant adenopathy. Indeed, studies have shown that EUS is superior to computed tomography and MRI in the preoperative staging of subjects with Barrett's adenocarcinoma.[5,6,7]

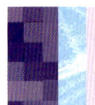
EUS in Barrett's Metaplasia and Low-Grade Dysplasia

The normal esophageal wall consists of four distinct histologic layers: the mucosa, submucosa, muscularis propria, and adventitia. On EUS, this is represented as five alternating bands (Figure 3-1). On both standard and high-resolution EUS, Barrett's esophagus, both with and without dysplasia, is associated with thickening of the mucosal (second) and submucosal (third) layers.[8] When compared to normal controls, patients with Barrett's esophagus have been shown to have a greater mean wall thickness (3.3 mm vs. 2.6 mm).[9] However, among Barrett's patients, there is no statistically significant difference between individuals with dysplasia (4 mm) and those without (Figure 3-2). While a thickened esophageal wall is consistent with Barrett's esophagus, EUS plays no diagnostic role in the identification of dysplasia (Figures 3-3A and B). In an attempt to overcome the sampling limitations of four-quadrant biopsies and enhance mucosal changes that may be suggestive of high-grade dysplasia or intramucosal cancer, other endoscopic imaging modalities are under evaluation, such as magnification chromoendoscopy and narrow band imaging (Figure 3-4 A and B). While these techniques show great promise, they still require validation in large clinical trials.

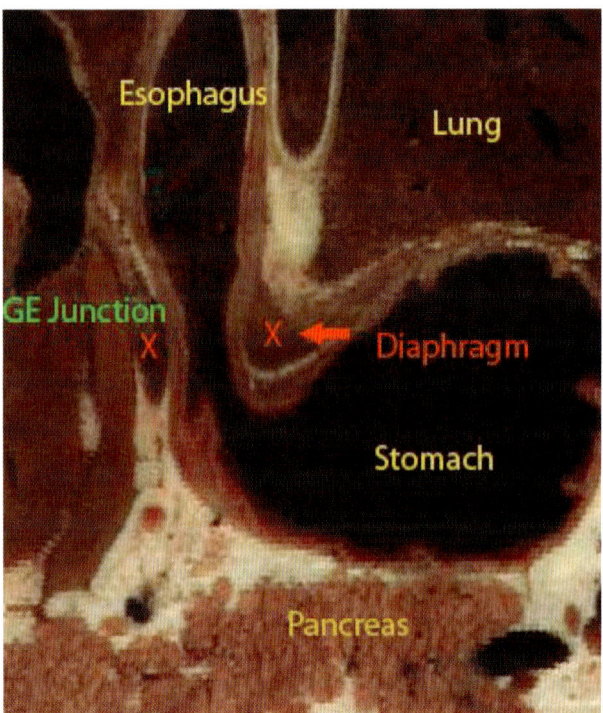
FIGURE 3-1. Visible Human Anatomy showing the gastroesophageal (GE) junction. The diaphragm is marked with orange "x"

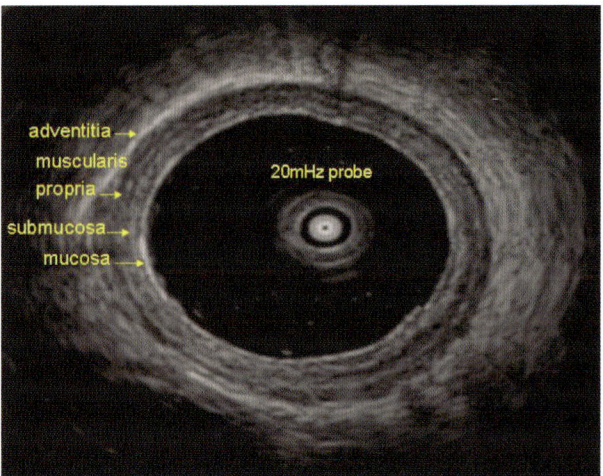
FIGURE 3-2. Normal esophageal wall as seen with a high-frequency (20 MHz) miniprobe

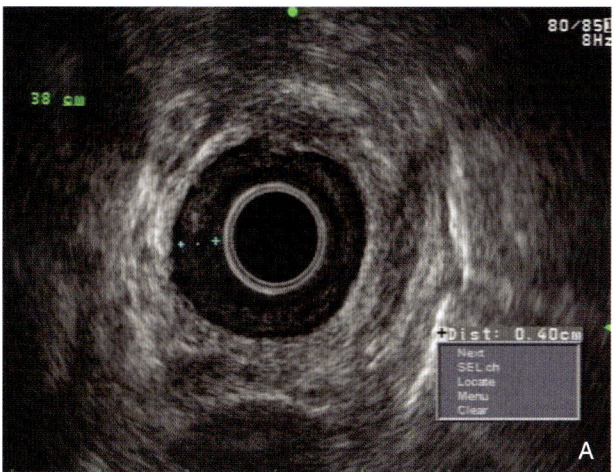 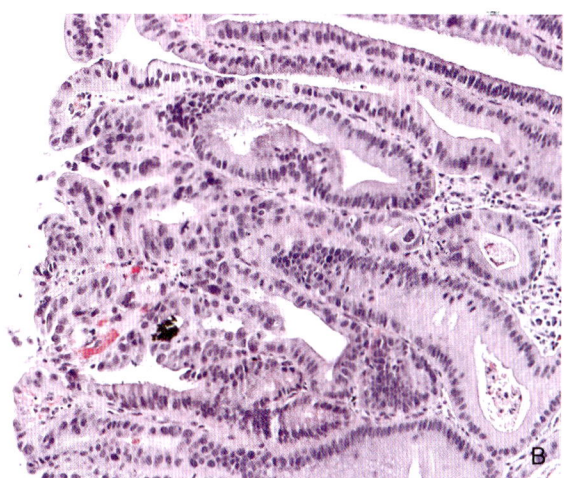

FIGURE 3–3. *A and B* (A) Nonspecific thickening of the mucosal and submucosal layers in Barrett's esophagus as seen with a 7.5 MHz radial echoendoscope. (B) Biopsy of the area showed evidence of high-grade dysplasia. However, such thickening can be seen in Barrett's without dysplasia.
Photo courtesy of John Liang, M.D., Department of Gastrointestinal Pathology, Anderson Cancer Center.

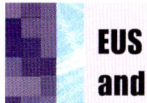 EUS in High-Grade Dysplasia and Early Carcinoma

The primary role of EUS in patients with Barrett's high-grade dysplasia and early carcinoma is to identify individuals who are candidates for endoscopic therapies, such as EMR, radio-frequency ablation, or PDT. Given the dramatically increased risk of lymph node metastases with submucosal invasion,[10] accurate staging is critical in differentiating patients with mucosal disease (T1a) from those with submucosal involvement (T1b). In patients with HGD or IMC imaged with endoscopic ultrasound, the sensitivity, specificity, and negative predictive values of preoperative EUS for submucosal invasion has been shown to be 100%, 94%, and 100% respectively; the values for lymph node involvement were 100%, 81%, and 100%, respectively.[11] Other series, however, have shown lower accuracy rates with sensitivities as low as 61%.[12,13] Despite this, EUS has been shown to be beneficial in selecting patients for endoscopic therapy.[14,15] Use of high-frequency miniprobes (Figure 3–5), has been shown to improve this accuracy somewhat.[16]

The accuracy of EUS may be improved with the addition of EMR (Figure 3–5A–C). In one series, cap-assisted EMR identified submucosal invasion in 40% of patients with intramucosal adenocarcinoma staged by EUS.[17] (Figure 3–6A and B) EMR provides accurate pathologic staging, and is both diagnostic and therapeutic in individuals with disease confined to the mucosa.

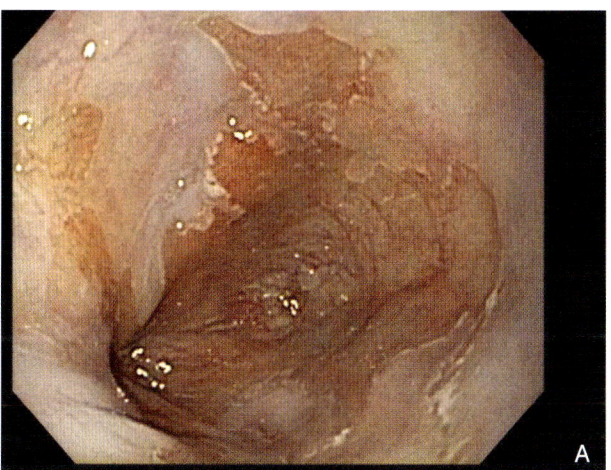 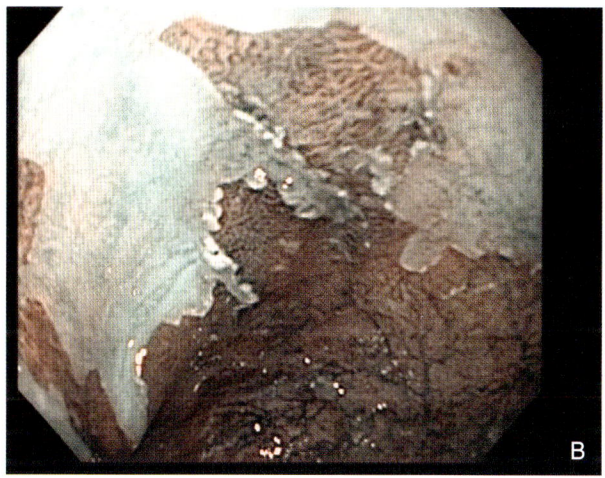

FIGURE 3–4. *A and B* The same segment of Barrett's esophagus seen on both standard white light endoscopy and with narrow band imaging (NBI).

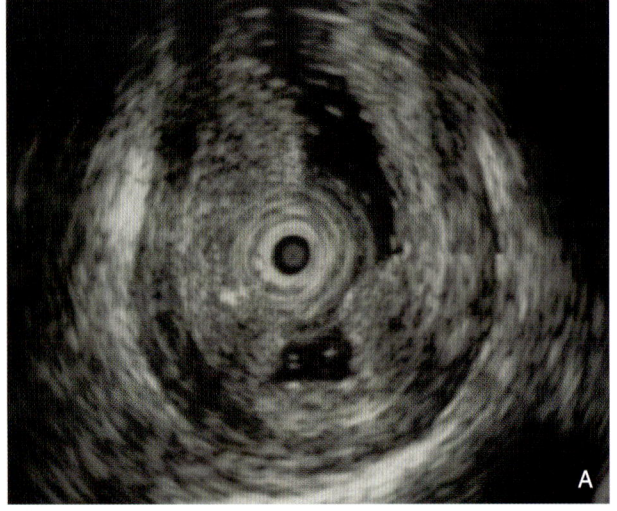
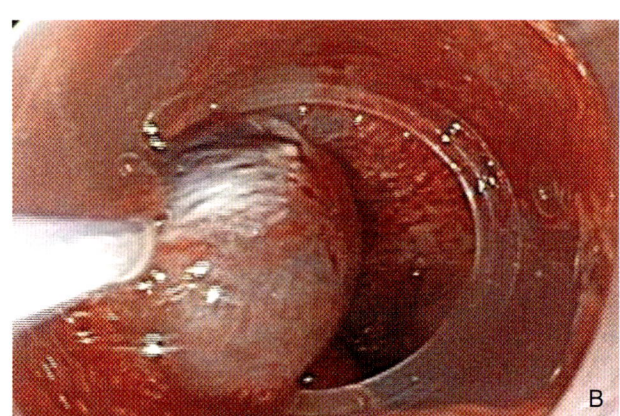
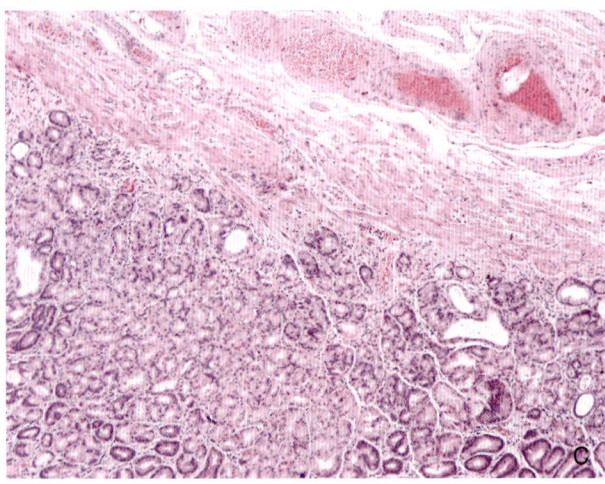

FIGURE 3–5. *A to C* (A) Nodularity in Barrett's esophagus, EUS with a 20 MHz miniprobe suggested the presence of intramucosal cancer. (B) Suction-cap EMR was then performed. (C) Pathology confirmed disease localized to the mucosal layer (T1a).
Barrett's with intramucosal carcinoma. Photo courtesy of John Liang, M.D., Department of Gastrointestinal Pathology, M.D. Anderson Cancer Center

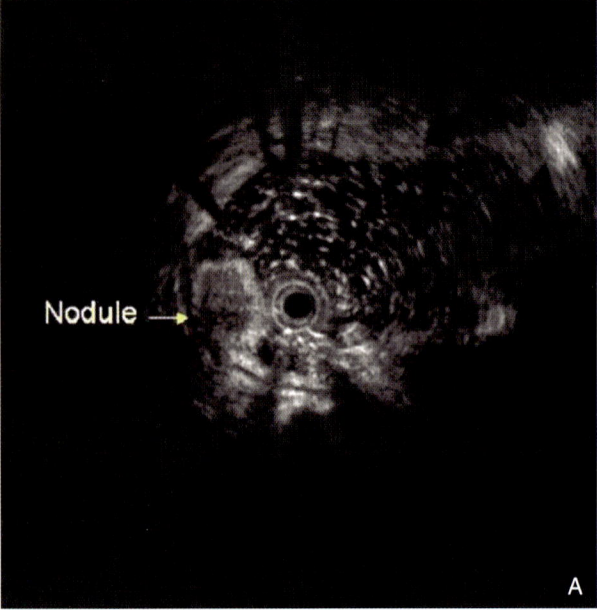
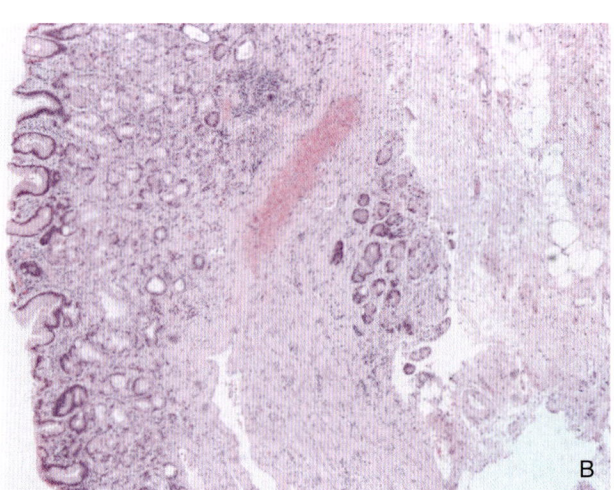

FIGURE 3–6. *A and B* (A) Nodule in the setting of high-grade dysplasia. EUS with a 20-MHz miniprobe confirmed the presence of submucosal involvement (T1 b). (B) Pathology confirmed the presence of submucosal involvement (T1b). T1b adenocarcinoma in Barrett's esophagus. Photo courtesy of John Liang, M.D., Department of Gastrointestinal Pathology, Anderson Cancer Center.

References

1. Crew, K. D., Neugat, A. I.: Epidemiology of Upper Gastrointestinal Malignancies. Semin Oncol 2004; 31(4):450–464.
2. Heath, E. I., Canto, M. I., Wu, T. T., et al.: Chemoprevention for Barrett's Esophagus Trial. Design and Outcome Measures 2003; 16:177–186.
3. Clark, G. W. B., Smyrk, T. C., Burdiles, P., et al.: Is Barrett's metaplasia the source of adenocarcinomas of the cardia? Arch Surg 1994;129: 609–614.
4. Spechler, S. J.: Dysplasia in Barrett's esophagus: Limitations of current management strategies. Am J Gastroenterol 2005; 100:927–935.
5. Botet, J. F., Lightdale, C. J., Zauber, A. G., et al.: Preoperative staging of esophageal cancer: comparison of endoscopic US and dynamic CT. Radiology 1991; 181: 419–425.
6. Romagnuolo, J., Scott, J., Hawes, R. H., et al.: Helical CT versus EUS with fine needle aspiration for celiac nodal assessment in patients with esophageal cancer. Gastrointest Endosc 2002;55:648–654.
7. Caletti, G., Ferrari, A.: Endoscopic ultrasonography. Endoscopy 1996; 28: 156–173.
8. Srivastava, A. K., Vanagunas, A., Kamel, P., et al.: Endoscopic Ultrasound in the evaluation of Barrett's esophagus: a preliminary report. Am J Gastroenterol 1994; 89: 2192–2195.
9. Gangarosa, L. M., Halter, S., Mertz, H.: Methylene blue staining and endoscopic ultrasound evaluation of Barrett's esophagus with low-grade dysplasia. Dig Dis Sci. 2000; 45:225–229.
10. Rice, T. W., Zuccaro, G. Jr., Adelstein, D. J., et al.: Esophageal carcinoma: depth of tumor invasion is predictive of regional lymph node status. Ann Thorac Surg 1998; 65: 787–792.
11. Scotiniotis, I. A., Kochman, M. L., Lewis, J. D., et al.: Accuracy of EUS in the evaluation of Barrett's esophagus and high-grade dysplasia or intramucosal carcinoma. Gastrointest Endosc 2001;54:689–696.
12. Canto, M.: Barrett's Esophagus. Gastrointest Endoscopy Clin N Am 2005; 15: 83–92.
13. Buttar, N., Wang, K., Lutzke, L., et al.: The use of endoscopic ultrasonography in Barrett's esophagus (abstract). Gastrointest Endosc 2001; 53: AB 172.
14. Sharma, P.: Endoscopic mucosal resection of early cancer and high-grade dysplasia in Barrett's esophagus. Gastrointest Endosc 2002; 55:137–139.
15. Wolfsen, H. C., Woodward, T. A., Raimondo, M.: Photodynamic therapy for dysplastic Barrett's esophagus and early esophageal adenocarcinoma. Mayo Clin Proc 2002; 77: 1176–1181.
16. Chak, A., Canto, M., Stevens, P. D., et al.: Clinical applications of a new through-the-scope ultrasound probe: prospective comparison with an ultrasound endoscope. Gastrointest Endosc 1997; 45: 291–295.
17. Larghi, A., Lightdale, C. J., Memeo, L., et al.: EUS followed by EMR for staging of high-grade dysplasia and early cancer in Barrett's esophagus. Gastrointest Endosc 2005; 62: 16–23.

CHAPTER 4

Advanced Esophageal Cancer

Dr. Erwin Santo
Dr. Olga Barkay
Dr. William Ross
Dr. Manoop S. Bhutani

Esophageal cancer is the eighth-leading cause of cancer with worldwide estimates of more than 400,000 new cases and over 300,000 cancer-related deaths annually.[1] Treatment and outcome for patients with esophageal cancer is stage dependent. The TNM system is based on the determination of depth of tumor invasion (T), the presence or absence of regional lymph node metastases (N), and presence or absence of distant metastases (M).[2] Most patients have advanced disease at the time of symptom presentation because the esophagus has a rich lymphovascular supply and lacks a serosal lining. This chapter deals with the role of EUS in the assessment and management of these patients. Please refer to Table 2–1 in Chapter 2 regarding esophageal cancer staging by AJCC classification. Since its introduction in the early 1980s, EUS has played a central role in the staging of esophageal cancer. Although EUS is better then PET and CT for locoregional staging (T and N),[3] the latter modalities are better for detecting distant metastases (e.g. lung, liver). Therefore, it is logical to perform EUS when PET and CT scan have not revealed distant metastases.

Radial Versus Linear Scanners

Radial echoendoscopes use either a rotating or solid-state ultrasound probe and provide high-quality images in a transverse plane. However, they cannot guide biopsy of malignant-appearing lymph nodes. Linear echoendoscopes are solid state and provide longitudinal images and enable FNA. Historically, the vast majority of staging EUS procedures have been performed using radial echoendoscopes. A few studies suggest that linear EUS may be as accurate as radial EUS for staging of esophageal cancer.[4,5] In a more recent prospective randomized trial of 43 patients with upper gastrointestinal malignancies, radial and linear EUS provided similar results of T staging.[6] However, the number of lymph nodes detected by radial EUS was more than that detected by linear EUS.

The authors retrospectively evaluated diagnostic accuracy of linear EUS in 58 consecutive patients with esophageal cancer: accuracy of T-staging was 85.3 %, and that of N-staging was 68%. (Santo EM, Kariv R, Kashtan H, Yakubowicz M, unpublished data). These results were similar to diagnostic accuracy of T- and N-staging with radial echoendoscopes previously reported in the literature. A choice between a linear and a radial echoendoscope should be a matter of personal experience. However, when, based on other diagnostic modalities, EUS-FNA is likely to be needed (e.g. enlarged lymph nodes on CT and/or PET), a linear echoendoscope may be chosen to enable biopsy and shorten the procedure duration.

Some of the relevant anatomy of the region is shown by the Visible Human model and Visible Human transaxial cross-section shown in Figure 4–1.

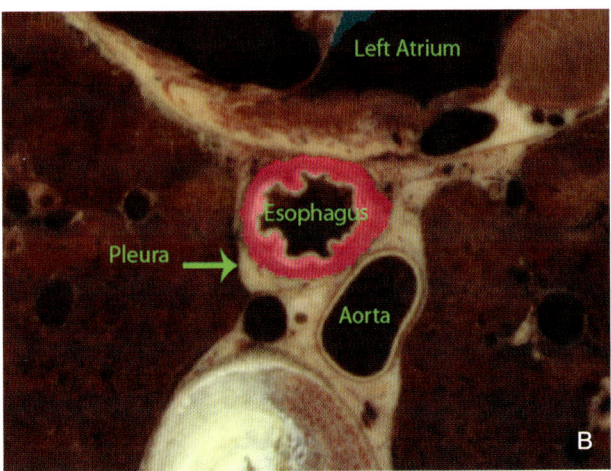

FIGURE 4–1. *A and B* (A) Visible Human model showing the relation of the esophagus to local nodes and the celiac artery. (B) Visible Human transaxial cross-section showing the relation of the esophagus to aorta, pleura, and left atrium

The model shows the relation to local nodes compared to those that would be found near the celiac artery. The cross-section shows the proximity of the esophagus to the pleura, aorta, and heart.

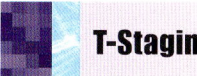

T-Staging

EUS is most accurate in identifying T3 or T4 stage (Figures 4–2- 4–5, Video 4–1). The designation of T2 stage is less accurate (Figure 4–6): equal number of lesions are understaged and overstaged. The most frequent contributors to inaccurate T-staging are microscopic tumor invasion, peritumorous inflammatory changes, luminal stenosis, and oblique scanning artifacts.

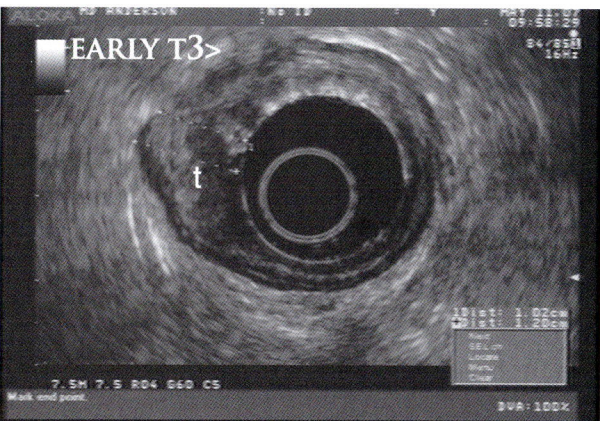

FIGURE 4–2. Radial EUS view of an esophageal cancer (T) that appears to be an early T3 lesion in the upper half of the image (arrowhead) with minimal penetration into the adventitia.

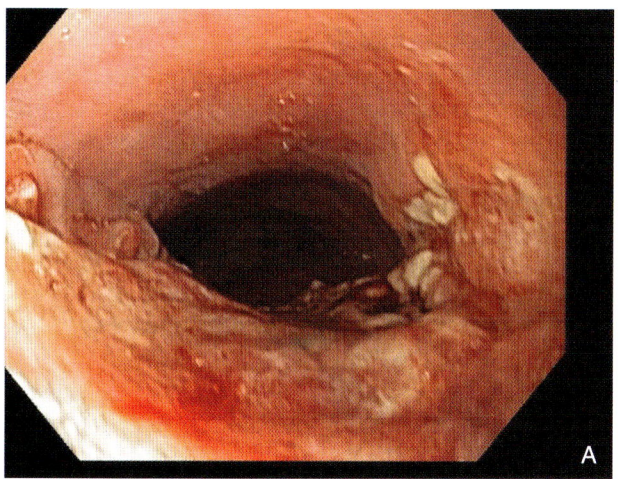

FIGURE 4–3. A and B (A) Endoscopic view of a squamous cell cancer of the esophagus (B) Radial EUS of the cancer in Figure 4–3A showing it to be a T3 lesion with clear penetration into the adventitia and disruption of the muscularis propria.

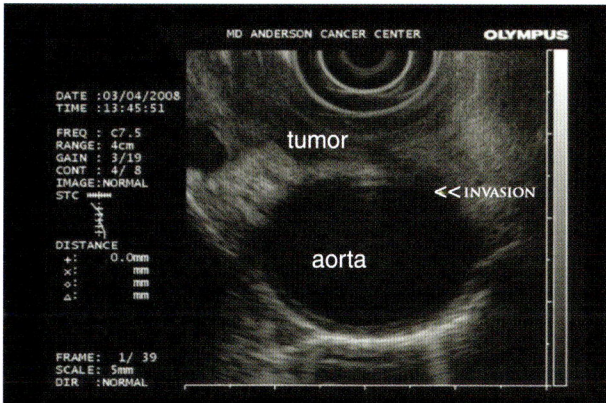

FIGURE 4–4. Radial EUS of esophageal cancer that is invading the wall of the aorta (T4 stage) with obliteration of the echogenic interface between the tumor and the aorta on the left half of the image.

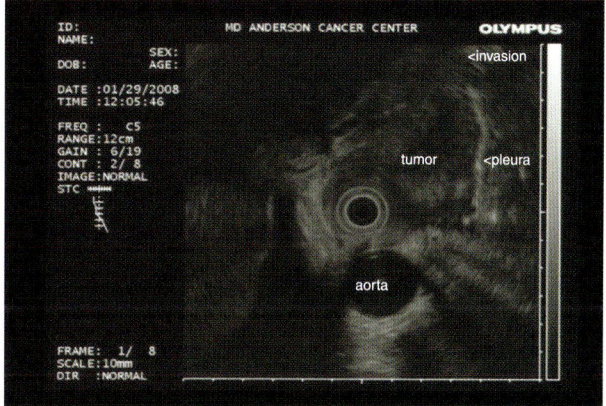

FIGURE 4–5. Radial EUS of a large esophageal carcinoma that is abutting the pleura (thin, white, echogenic line) with invasion of the pleura resulting in its interruption.

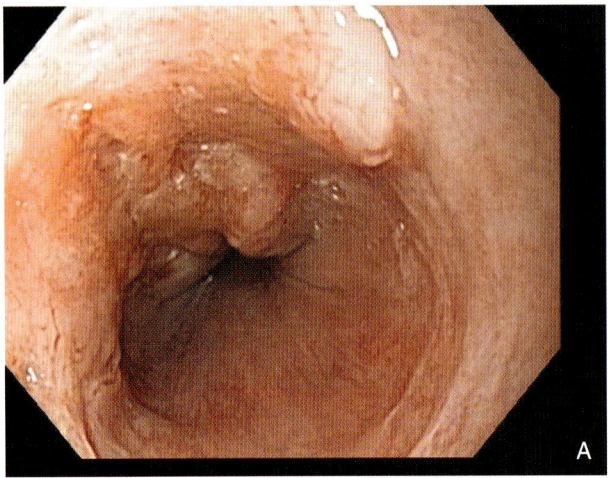
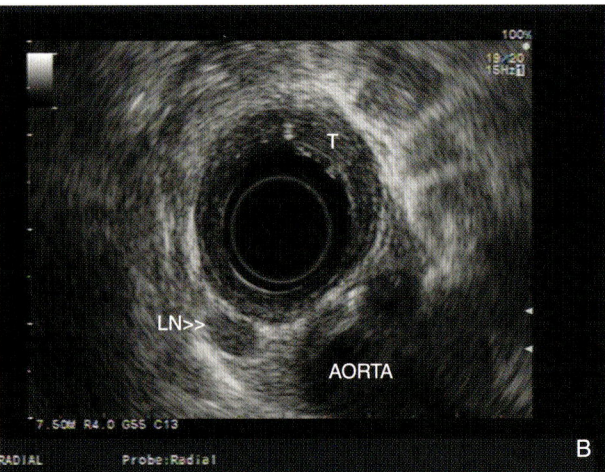

FIGURE 4–6. *A and B* (A) Endoscopic view of an esophageal squamous cell carcinoma (B) Radial EUS of the carcinoma in Figure 6A showing it to be a T2 lesion. The tumor (T) has penetrated into the muscularis propria. It cannot be discerned anymore in the region of the tumor but the outer margin of the tumor is smooth without evidence of penetration into the adventitia. A small peritumrous lymph node (LN) is also seen.

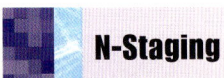

N-Staging

Because of rich esophageal lymphatics, esophageal cancer has the propensity to spread early to local lymph nodes. Patients with local nodal involvement (N1) (Figure 4–7) disease have poorer survival rates compared to those with no involved nodes (N0)[7] and would typically receive preoperative therapy. EUS is superior in detecting peritumoral and celiac lymph nodes compared to CT and PET.[8-10]

Four EUS features have classically been proposed as suggestive of malignancy: size greater than 10 mm, round shape, hypoechoic pattern, and smooth border.[11,12]

When all four features are present, there is 80-100% probability that the lymph node is malignant, but only 25% of malignant lymph nodes will present all four criteria.[11,12]

Recently, modified EUS malignant node criteria were proposed.[13] These modified criteria consist of the four classical ones plus three additional criteria that include lymph node location (celiac region), number of lymph nodes identified by EUS (more than 5), and presence of an advanced T-stage (T3/T4). Sensitivity and specificity reached 100% when a cut off value of less than 1 and more than 6 modified criteria were used: all patients with more than 6 criteria had N1 stage disease, and none of the patients with less than 1 positive modified EUS criteria had N1 disease.

Identification of celiac lymph nodes is especially important. Eloubeidi et al have shown that, regardless of all other features, 90% of all detected celiac lymph were malignant, and 100% of those greater than 1 cm in diameter were malignant.[14] Others have also confirmed that enlarged lymph nodes in this location are almost always malignant.[15,16]

However, biopsy of enlarged celiac nodes (Figure 4–8) may still be needed, because malignant

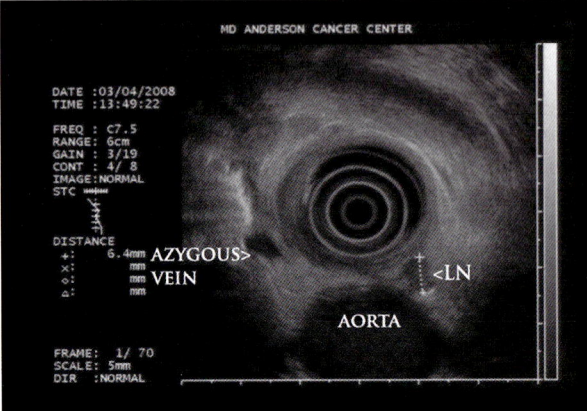

FIGURE 4–7. Radial EUS of the mediastinum in a patient with esophageal cancer, showing a lymph node just proximal to the tumor.

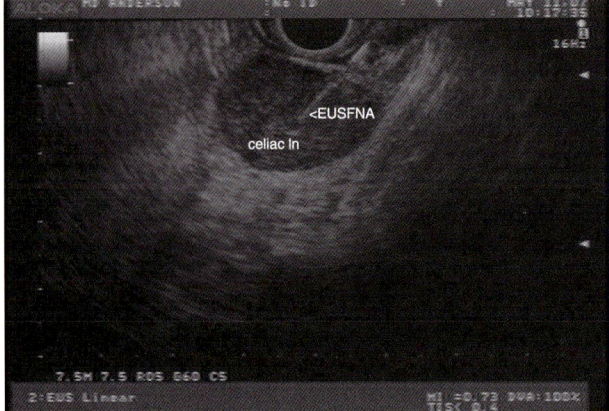

FIGURE 4–8. A large celiac axis lymph node in a patient with esophageal cancer being subjected to EUS FNA with a linear echoendoscope.

involvement of lymph nodes in this location has a dramatic influence on the patient's management and prognosis and, therefore, should be proved histologically.

Large reactive lymph nodes may be present adjacent to the primary tumor or at the subcarina, particularly in smokers,[17] leading to overstaging of the disease. On the other hand, a number of technical factors, such as balloon over-inflation, oblique scanning, and inadequate use of high-frequency scanning may lead to understaging of lymph node involvement in inexperienced hands.[18-21]

A number of studies have shown that EUS-FNA is highly accurate in documenting peritumoral and celiac lymph node involvement in patients with esophageal cancer.[14,22-24]

EUS-FNA has been shown to be superior to lymph node echofeatures.[25] In a retrospective study of Vazquez-Sequerios,[24] the addition of FNA increased the accuracy of nodal staging from 70% to 93%, largely by increasing the sensitivity. (Video 4–2).

Unfortunately, EUS FNA of lymph nodes has limitations. It's not always technically feasible (e.g .peritumoral nodules or high-grade stenosis), prolongs the length of the procedure, may cause complications, and raises the cost of the examination. In addition, a luminal tumor can theoretically contaminate an FNA specimen, leading to a false-positive aspiration. Therefore, some authors have proposed avoiding routine FNA in patient with a high probability of nodal involvement, as defined by "modified" criteria and/or presence of large (greater than 1 cm) celiac lymph nodes,[13,26] while others perform EUS FNA in all esophageal carcinoma patients with identified lymph nodes.[27]

The decision to perform EUS-FNA should depend on a careful assessment of whether or nor the information gained is likely to result in a clinically meaningful change in management. (For example, patients with T4 stage have uniformly poor prognosis irrespective of whether or not they undergo surgery. Therefore, T4 disease is an indication for palliative treatment). When there is more than one suspicious lymph node, it is usually advisable to biopsy a node that has had the greatest uptake on FDG-PET (which, again, should be performed before EUS).

M-Staging

A few studies have demonstrated the ability of EUS to detect small hepatic metastases in the left lobe, which have been missed in CT with consequent upstaging and a major impact on management.[28,29] However, EUS cannot exclude metastatic disease in all areas of the liver because it does not provide imaging of right liver lobe. If liver metastases are identified during EUS examination, FNA can usually be done easily, providing prove of malignant involvement prior to chemotherapy.

Dilation of Strictures

Roughly one-third of esophageal carcinoma patients in Western countries have stenosis at presentation significant enough to prevent passage of a standard echoendoscope.[30] Pre-EUS dilatation has been associated with significant risk of perforations in the past.[31,32] More recent studies reported much lower rates of perforation in this setting.[33-35]

However, one should remember that tumor perforation dramatically worsens survival.[36]

On the other hand, complete staging after dilatation might only be achieved in 62% of cases,[37] and, when achieved, may be less accurate than in "a regular" patient.[38]

Therefore, a decision to perform dilatation should only be made after a careful consideration of the information achieved by an incomplete examination.

Stricturing tumors are rarely less than T3, and positive nodes might be expected in 77–81% of such cases. Sixty percent of involved nodes will be found proximal to the obstruction.[30] In light of these data, the staging problem presented by strictures is limited to relatively few cases, particularly taking into account those unfit for surgery (20%).[39]

If a complete examination is likely to significantly change a patient's management, then sequential dilation up to 14–16 mm may be performed with subsequent passage of a standard echoendoscope.[33,34]

An alternative option is miniprobe, or endobronchial, EUS, which is advanced through the tumor over a previously placed guidewire. This option enables adequate staging without dilatation.[40] However, FNA is not possible with miniprobe.

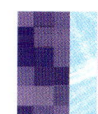
EUS After Neoadjuvant Radiochemotherapy

Given the uniformly poor results achieved with surgery alone, treatment in many centers has shifted to a multimodality approach that incorporates pre-operative chemoradiotherapy in patients with advanced disease, who are potential candidates for subsequent surgical resection.[41] However, results from available studies evaluating the role of neoadjuvant therapy in this setting are still equivocal.[42-44] Therefore, identification of the subset of patients who respond to neoadjuvant therapy and would benefit from subsequent surgical resection is especially important.

EUS has a potential to predict response to chemoradiation. However, T-staging accuracy of EUS postchemotherapy is lower than initial staging accuracy, due to the inability to differentiate residual tumor from inflammatory or fibrotic changes.[45-47] In several small studies, more than 50% reduction of tumor thickness postchemotherapy was associated with better survival.[45,48,49]

Because patients with persistent nodal involvement after neoadjuvant chemoradiotherapy have poor survival,[50] it is important to assess for nodal response after neoadjuvant therapy. Accuracy of EUS N-staging without FNA is suboptimal.[46,47] EUS-guided FNA of suspicious lymph nodes improves accuracy of N-staging.[29] In general, with restaging by EUS, accuracy of N-staging is thought to be higher than T-staging.[51]

PET-CT has been recently shown to be effective in assessing response of esophageal cancer to neoadjuvant therapy.[52] Taken together, this data suggests that performance of EUS in this setting should be restricted to only few selective cases, and PET-CT should be preferred in evaluating a response to chemoradiotherapy.

Videos: Available at www.pmph-usa.com/bhutani
Video 4–1: Radial EUS of an esophageal cancer. Initially the cancer appears to be T2 because the outer margin is smooth, and muscularis propria cannot be clearly defined under the tumor. However, as the transducer is moved back and forth (in the later half of the video), clear evidence of a T3 lesion is seen with penetration into the adventitia.
Video 4–2: Linear EUS FNA of a subcarinal lymph node in a patient with esophageal cancer to determine malignant invasion.

References

1. Parkin, D. M.: International variation. Oncogene 2004;23:6329–6340.
2. Enzinger, P. Z., Page, D. L., Fleming, I. D., et al.: AJCC Cancer Staging Manual (ed 6). New York: Springer, 2000
3. Pfau, P. R., Perlman, S. B., Stanko, P., Frick, T. J., Gopal, D. V., Said, A., Zhang, Z., Weigel, T.: The role and clinical value of EUS in a multimodality esophageal carcinoma staging program with CT and positron emission tomography. Gastrointest Endosc 2007;65(3):377–384.
4. Brugge, W. R., Lee, M. J., Carey, R. W., et al.: Endoscopic ultrasound staging criteria for esophageal cancer. Gastrointest Endosc 1997;45:147–152.
5. Siemsen, M., Svendsen, L. B., Knigge, U., Vilmann, P., Jensen, F., Rasch, L., Stentoft, P.: A prospective randomized comparison of curved array and radial echoendoscopy in patients with esophageal cancer. Gastrointest Endosc 2003;58:671–676.
6. Mattes, K., Bounds, B. C., Collier, K., Gutierrez, A., Brugge, W. R.: EUS staging of upper GI malignancies: results of a prospective randomized trial. Gastrointest Endosc 2006;64:496–502.
7. Eloubeidi, M. A., Wallace, M. B., Hoffmann, B. J., et al.: Predictors of survival for esophageal cancer patients with and without celiac lymph node lymphadenopathy: impact of staging endosonography. Ann Thorac Surg 2001;72:212–219.
8. Rosch, T.: Endosonographic staging of esophageal cancer: a review of literature results. Gastrointest Endosc Clin N Am 1995;5:537–547
9. Romagnuolo, J., Scott, J., Hawes, R. H., et al.: Helical CT versus EUS with fine needle aspiration for celiac nodal assessment in patients with esophageal cancer. Gastrointest Endosc 2002;55:648–654.
10. Akdamar, M., Cerfolio, R., Ojha, B., Tamhane, A., Eloubeidi, M. A.: A prospective comparison of computerized tomography (CT), 18 fluoro-deoxyglucose positron emission tomography (FDG-PET) and endoscopic ultrasonography (EUS) in the preoperative evaluation of potentially operable esophageal cancer (ECA) patients [abstract]. Am J Gastroenterol 2005;98:S5
11. Catalano, M. F., Sivak, M. V., Jr., Rice, T., Gragg, L. A., van Dam, J.: Endosonographic features predictive of lymph node metastasis. Gastrointest Endosc 1994;40:442–446.
12. Bhutani, M. S., Hawes, R. H., Hoffman, B. J.: A comparison of the accuracy of echo features during endoscopic ultrasound (EUS) and EUS-guided fine needle aspiration for diagnosis of malignant lymph node invasion. Gastrointest Endosc 1997;45:474–479.
13. Vazquez-Sequeiros, E., Levy, M. J., Clain, J. E., Schwartz, D. A., Harewood, G. C., Salomao, D., Wiersema, M. J.: Routine vs. selective EUS-guided FNA approach for preoperative nodal staging of esophageal carcinoma. Gastrointet Endosc 2006;63:204–211.
14. Eloubeidi, M. A., Wallace, M. B., Reed, C. E., et al.: The utility of EUS and EUS guided fine needle aspiration in detecting celiac lymph node metastasis in patients with esophageal cancer: a single-center experience. Gastrointest Endosc 2001;54;714–719.
15. Williams, D. B., Sahai, A. V., Aabakken, L., Penman, I. D., van Velse, A., Webb, J., et al.: Endoscopic ultrasound guided fine needle aspiration biopsy: a large single centre experience. Gut 1999;44:720–726.
16. Reed, C. E., Mishra, G., Sahai, A. V., Hoffmann, B. J., Hawes, R. H.: Esophageal cancer staging: improved accuracy by endoscopic ultrasound of celiac lymph nodes. Ann Thorac Surg 1999;67:319–321.
17. Penman, I. D., Shen, E. F.: EUS in advanced esophageal cancer. Gastrointest Endosc 2002;56:S2-6.
18. Catalano, M. F., Sivak, M. V., Jr., Bedford, R. A., Falk, G. W., van Stolk, R., Presa, F., Van Dam, J.: Observer variation and reproducibility of endocopic ultrasonography. Gastrointest Endosc 1995;41:115–120.
19. Palazzo, L., Burtin, P.: Interobserver variation in tumor staging. Gastrointest Endosc Clin North Am 1995;5:559–567.

20. Fockens, P., Van den Brande, J. H., van Dullemen, H. M., van Lanschot, J. J., Tytgat, G. N.: Endosonographic T-staging of esophageal carcinoma: a learning curve. Gastrointest Endosc 1996;44:58–62.
21. Massari, M., Cioffi, U., De Simone, M., Lattuada, E., Montorsi, M., Segalin, A., Bonavina, L.: Endoscopic ultrasonography for preoperative staging of esophageal carcinoma. Surg Laparosc Endosc 1997;7:162–165.
22. Eloubeidi, M. A., Vilmann, P., Wiersema, M. J.: Endoscopic ultrasound guided fine-needle aspiration of celiac lymph nodes. Endoscopy 2004;36:901–908.
23. Vazquez-Sequeiros, E., Wiersema, M. J., Clain, J. E., et al.: Impact of lymph node staging on therapy of esophageal carcinoma. Gastroenterology 2003;125:1626–1635.
24. Vazquez-Sequeiros, E., Norton, I. D., Clain, J. E., et al.: Impact of EUS-guided fine-needle aspiration on lymph node staging in patients with esophageal carcinoma. Gastrointest Endosc 2001;53:751–757.
25. Chen, V. K., Eloubeidi, M. A.: Endoscopic ultrasound-guided fine needle aspiration is superior to lymph node echofeatures: a prospective evaluation of mediastinal and peri-intestinal lymphadenopathy. Am J Gastroenterol 2004;99:628–633.
26. Vazquez-Sequeiros, E.: Nodal staging: Number or site of nodes? How to improve accuracy? Is FNA always necessary? Junctional tumors- what's N and what's M? Endoscopy 2006;38(S1):S4–S8.
27. Eloubeidi, M. A.: Routine EUS-guided FNA for preoperative nodal staging in patients with esophageal carcinoma: is the juice worth the squeeze? Gastrointest Endosc 2006;63:212–214.
28. Prasad, P., Schmulewitz, N., Patel, A., Varadarajulu, S., Wildi, S. M., Roberts, S., Tutuian, R., King, P., Hawes, R. H., Hoffmann, B. J., Wallace, M. B.: Detection of occult liver metastases during EUS for staging of malignancies. Gastrointest Endosc 2004;59:49–53.
29. Cerfolio, R. J., Bryant, A. S., Ohja, B., Bartolucci, A. A., Eloubeidi, M. A.: The accuracy of endoscopic ultrasonography with fine-needle aspiration, integrated positron emission tomography with computed tomography, and computed tomography in restaging patients with esophageal cancer after neoadjunant chemoradiation therapy. J Thorac Cardiovasc Surg 2005;129:1232–1241.
30. Meenan, J.: Staging stenotic oesophageal tumors: Are CT and/or PET enough? Dilate or not? Endoscopy 2006;38:S8–12.
31. Van Dam, J., Rice, T. W., Catalano, M. F., Kirby, T., Sivak, M. Jr.: High grade malignant stricture is predictive of esophageal tumor stage. Risks of endosonographic evaluation. Cancer 1993;71:2910–2917
32. Catalano, M. F., Van Dam, J., Sivak, M. V. Jr.: Malignant esophageal strictures: staging accuracy of endoscopic ultrasonography. Gastrointest Endosc 1995;41:535–539.
33. Wallace, M. B., Hawes, R. H., Sahai, A. V., Van Velse, A., Hoffmann, B. J.: Dilatation of malignant esophageal stenosis to allow EUS guided fine-needle aspiration: safety and effect on patient management. Gastrointest Endosc 2000;51:309–313.
34. Pfau, P. R., Ginsberg, G. G., Lew, R. J., Faigel, D. O., Smith, D. B., Kochman, M. L.: Esophageal dilatation for endosonographic evaluation of malignant esophageal strictures is safe and effective. Am J Gastroenterol 2000;95:2813–2815.
35. Kallimanis, G. E., Gupta, P. K., Al-Kawas, F. H., Tio, L. T., Bejamin, S. B., Bertagnolli, M. E., et al.: Endoscopic ultrasound for staging esophageal cancer, with or without dilatation, is clinically important and safe. Gastrointest Endosc 1995;41:540–546.
36. Jethwa, P., Lala, A., Powell, J., McConkey, C. C., Gillison, E. W., Spychal, R. T.: A regional audit of iatrogenic perforation of tumors of the oesophagus and cardia. Aliment Pharmacol Ther 2005;21:479–484.
37. Vazquez-Sequeiros, E., Wiersema, M. J., Clain, J. E., Norton, I. D., Levy, M. J., Romero, Y., Salomao, D., Dierkhising, R.: Impact of lymph node staging on therapy of esophageal carcinoma. Gastroenterol 2003;125:1626–1635.
38. Catalano, M. F., Van Dam, J., Sivak, M. V., Jr.: Malignant esophageal strictures: staging accuracy of endoscopic ultrasonography. Gastrointest Endosc 1995;41:535–539.
39. Gockel, I., Kneist, W., Junginger, T.: Incurable esophageal cancer: patterns of tumor spread and therapeutic consequences. World J Surg 2006;30:183–190.
40. Mallery, S., Van Dam, J.: Increased rate of complete EUS staging of patients with esophageal cancer using the nonoptical, wire-guided echoendoscope. Gastrointest Endosc 2005; 50:53–57.
41. Kelsen, D. P.: Multimodality therapy of local regional esophageal cancer. Semin Oncol 2005;32:S6–10.
42. Cunningham, D., Allum, W. H., Stenning, S. P., et al.: Perioperative chemotherapy in operable gastric and lower esophageal cancer: Final results of a randomized controlled trial (the MAGIC trial, ISRCTN 93793971) [abstract]. J Clin Oncol 2005;23:308s.
43. Medical Research Council Esophageal Cancer Working Group. Surgical resection with or without preoperative chemotherapy in esophageal cancer: a randomized controlled trial. Lancet 2002;359:1727.
44. Kelsen, D. P., Ginsberg, R., Pajak, T. F., et al.: Chemotherapy followed by surgery compared with surgery alone for localized esophageal cancer. N Engl J Med 1998;339:1979.
45. Ribeiro, A., Franceschi, D., Parra, J., Livingstone, A., Lima, M., Hamilton-Nelson, K., Ardalan, B.: Endoscopic ultrasound restaging after neoadjuvant chemotherapy in esophageal cancer. Am J Gastroenterol 2006;101(6):1216–1221.
46. Zuccaro, G., Jr, Rice, T. W., Goldblum, J., Medendorp, S. V., Becker, M., Pimentel, R., et al.: Ensdoscopic ultrasound cannot determine suitability for esophagectomy after aggressive chemoradiotherapy for esophageal cancer. Am J Gastroenterol 1999;94:906–412.
47. Kalha, I., Kaw, M., Fukami, N., Patel, M., Singh, S., Gagneja, H., Cohen, D., Morris, J.: The accuracy of endoscopic ultrasound for restaging esophageal carcinoma after chemoradiation therapy. Cancer 2004;101(5):940–947.
48. Hirata, N., Kawamoto, K., Ueyama, T., Masuda, K., Utsunomiya, T., Kuwano, H.: Using endosonography to assess the effects of neoadjuvant therapy in patients with advanced esophageal cancer. Am J Roentgenol 1997;169:485–491.
49. Chak, A., Canto, M. I., Cooper, G. S., Isenberg, G., Willis, J., Levitan, S., et al.: Endosonographic assessment of multimodality therapy predicts survival of esophageal carcinoma patients. Cancer 2000;88:1788–1795.
50. Rice, T. W., Blackstone, E. H., Adelstein, D. J., Zuccaro, G., Jr., Vargo, J. J., Goldblum, J. R., Rybicki, L. A.,

Murthy, S. C., Decamp, M. M.: N1 esophageal carcinoma: the importance of staging and downstaging. J Thorac Cardiovasc Surg 2001;121:454–464.

51. Das, A., Chak, A.: Reassessment of patients with esophageal cancer after neoadjuvant therapy. Endoscopy 2006;38:S13–17.

52. Mamede, M., Abreu-E-Lima, P., Oliva, M. R., Nos, V., Mamon, H., Gerbaudo, V. H.: FDG-PET/CT tumor segmentation-derived indices of metabolic activity to assess response to neoadjuvant therapy and progression-free survival in esophageal cancer: correlation with histopathology results. Am J Clin Oncol 2007;30: 377–388.

CHAPTER 5

Early Gastric Cancer

Dr. Chan Sup Shim

Introduction

Gastric cancer, a common cancer of the digestive tract, occurs worldwide. Whereas it is relatively uncommon in Western countries, the incidence of this form of cancer is extremely high in Japan, China, Chile, Iceland, and Korea.[1] The overall five-year survival rates for gastric cancer are still discouraging, although considerable advances in diagnostic modalities and chemotherapy regimens have been made in recent decades. Improvement in survival rates depends primarily on early detection and treatment. Many large-scale clinical trials show that the majority of patients are at an advanced stage at the time of diagnosis, indicating a poor outcome.

Accurate preoperative staging is not only important for predicting the prognosis, but also essential for establishing individualized cancer therapy. Early gastric cancer is defined as a gastric carcinoma that does not infiltrate beyond the submucosa. This definition is not influenced by the absence or presence of lymph node metastases or by the diameter of the tumor.

The role of endoscopic ultrasonography (EUS) is to evaluate the changes in the gastrointestinal wall due to carcinoma, based on the ultrasonic layered structure of the wall. This assessment is an important factor in choosing the optimal treatment, such as endoscopic mucosal resection (EMR), endoscopic submucosal dissection (ESD), laparoscopic surgery, or conventional treatment. The diagnostic accuracy of the depth of carcinoma invasion is approximately 80% when lesions are divided into mucosal (m) carcinoma, submucosal (sm) carcinoma, carcinoma invading the muscularis propria (pm), and carcinoma deeper than the subserosal layer (ss).[2]

In recent years, endoscopic surgery has been widely used as a radical therapy for early gastric cancers. However, endoscopic treatment is not indicated for lesions with metastasis to lymph nodes or other organs because it is only a local therapy. EUS can help to distinguish whether lesions are treatable using endoscopic resection. The distinction between mucosal and submucosal carcinomas has important clinical implications with respect to endoscopic surgery. Both are early gastric cancers, but the frequency of node involvement and the prognosis differ. If a small tumor is diagnosed as mucosal carcinoma using some reliable method, it is sufficient to remove it endoscopically using laser ablation, photocoagulation, microwave coagulation, polypectomy, or endoscopic resection. The possibility of lymph node metastasis is almost zero in these tumors. In contrast, if a tumor is diagnosed as submucosal carcinoma, the risk of lymph node metastasis is much higher. Sano et al.[3] reported that 3.3% of cancers limited to the mucosa and 19.6% of cancers invading the submucosa showed lymph node involvement. Because of its ability to distinguish distinct wall layers and lymph node enlargement, EUS can provide extremely useful information on the choice of treatment and the prognosis of early gastric cancer.

Instruments and Techniques

Instruments

Two types of EUS instruments are currently available for endosonography of gastric cancer: conventional echoendoscopes with a radial scan transducer at the tip and miniprobes with a small radial scan transducer that can be used through the working channel of a standard endoscope.

There are two types of conventional EUS: a radial array echo scanner and a linear array echo scanner. Radial array echo scanning is used more commonly used than linear array instruments. Radial array echo scanning provides an image perpendicular to the longitudinal axis that is analogous to computed tomography (CT), thereby making radial images easier to interpret. The linear array echoendoscope has side-viewing optics that provide imaging in a parallel plane. It is especially useful for imaging gastric cardia cancers and the esophagus. However, the linear echoendoscope is generally thought to be more difficult to use. The greatest experience in staging gastric cancer using a radial array EUS has been with echoendoscopes, which have switchable frequencies from 5 to 20 MHz. Recently developed solid-state radial array instruments enable advanced imaging techniques, such as color Doppler, power Doppler, and tissue harmonic echo.

Although conventional echoendoscopes are being used increasingly for staging upper gastrointestinal malignancies and for ultrasound-guided fine-needle aspiration of lesions, visualization of large lesions in curved areas is difficult. In addition, optical control of such a large instrument for small lesions is difficult, and the resolution is insufficient for the precise observation of superficial lesions.

The miniprobe is an ultrathin probe with a diameter of 2.5 mm, which is compatible with scope channels of 2.8 mm and above. Miniprobes provide 12-, 20-, and 30-MHz images. Miniprobes enable us to perform high-resolution target scanning of very small gastric cancer lesions under endoscopic control. The miniprobe image provides 360° images of the gastric wall through the instrument channel and allows real-time assessment while the catheter is moved over the tumor region. The examination can be performed as a single-step procedure during diagnostic endoscopy. High-resolution miniprobes passed through the working channel of an endoscope are better than conventional echoendoscopes for staging early cancer. The use of higher frequencies should allow higher-resolution images, but the concomitant reduction in signal penetration has limited its use by gastroenterologists.

EUS Techniques

Obtaining a detailed transmural anatomy depends on the frequency of the probe used and on good contact between the EUS scanner and mucosa, without the presence of luminal air. To avoid intraluminal air, either a water-filled balloon can be used with its outer rim lying against the mucosal surface, or the stomach can be filled with water.

For the examination, the tip of the endoscope is placed at the proximal end of the tumor. To achieve acoustic coupling between the transducer and gastric wall, either the lumen can be filled with 200–300 ml of water or a balloon over the transducer on the tip of the endoscope is filled with water. Subsequently, the transducer is advanced across the tumor. The infiltration depth and lymph node status of the tumor are assessed in real time as the transducer is moved over the tumor.

In principle, filling the lumen with water allows excellent definition of the gastric wall structure, but it is frequently difficult to cover the wall of the cardia and prepyloric areas with water. In this case, the water-filled balloon method is particularly helpful. It may be necessary to move the patient to the prone or right oblique position to submerge the desired area.

The major challenge in performing miniprobe ultrasonography of the stomach is obtaining adequate acoustic coupling between the transducer and gastric wall. The most commonly used scanning method for gastric lesions is the water-immersion technique (Table 5–1). Before instilling water into the stomach, any gastric juice and mucus should be removed because they interfere with clear endosonographic imaging. Usually, suctioning all of the air out of the stomach is all that is needed. After reducing the gastric volume with suction, water is instilled until the lesion is flooded completely. The use of a two-channel endoscope facilitates the ultrasonographic examination. When scanning, the miniprobe should be placed 3–5 mm from the lesion vertically. The antrum, pylorus, and angle may be more difficult to fill. When the region of interest is not filled with water, despite adequate instillation of water into the stomach, aspirating the air may help to fill the antrum with water. Raising the head of the bed to put the antrum in a more dependent position may also be helpful.

Table 5–1 Water Immersion Technique Using the Miniprobe

Elimination of Gastric Juice and Mucus

Water is instilled after reducing the gastric volume by air suction.
Water is instilled until the lesion is completely covered (usually 200-300 mL).
A two-channel endoscope is convenient.

Scanning

The lesion is scanned vertically.
An adequate distance from the lesion should be maintained when scanning (3-5 mm).

Because the antrum lies anterior to the gastric body, or body of the stomach and fundus, rolling the patient into a prone position similar to that used for endoscopic retrograde cholangiopancreatography (ERCP) will fill the antrum with water when other maneuvers fail. With the patient in the left lateral decubitus position, water will fill the body easily due to its location. For lesions located in these areas, this provides excellent acoustic coupling and high-quality imaging. Similar to the stomach body, water fills the fundus and cardia easily when the patient is in the left lateral decubitus position. It is particularly important to try to obtain a perpendicular view of the lesion (Figure 5–1). Imaging a lesion obliquely will produce a tangential image and cause errors in staging or assessing lesion size. To obtain a perpendicular view of the lesion, the endoscopist must control the angle of the scope, regulate the water volume, and use the patient's respiration and peristalsis of the stomach. The tip of the endoscope should be angulated acutely when scanning a lesion on the angle or lesser curvature of the antrum (Figure 5–2). When scanning lesions of the cardia, sometimes it is necessary to make a U-turn at the end of the scope to obtain a perpendicular view of the lesion. However, the posterior wall of the cardia can be scanned using a straight scope (Figure 5–3).

EUS Findings of Early Gastric Cancer

Mural Structure of the Normal Gastric Wall Using Endosonography

Generally, the mural structure of the gastric wall is examined using an echoendoscope or a 12–20 MHz miniprobe. The normal gastric wall is visualized as five

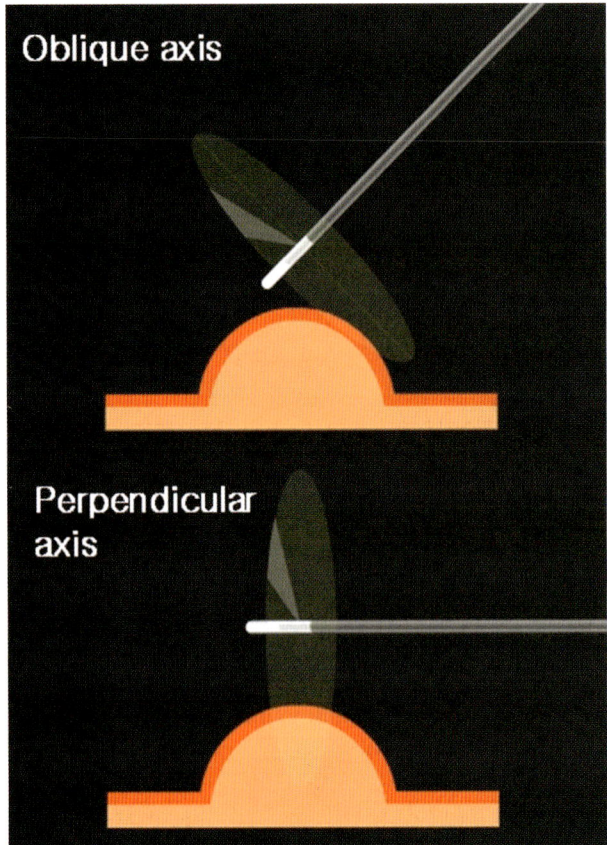

FIGURE 5–1. Obtaining a perpendicular view with the endoscopic ultrasonography probe. The lesion should be scanned in a plane perpendicular to the axis of the scope. Imaging a lesion obliquely will produce a tangential image and cause errors in staging or assessing the size of the lesion.

distinct echo layers (Figure 5–4). The mucosa corresponds to the hyperechoic first layer and hypoechoic second layer, whereas the submucosa corresponds to the hyperechoic third layer. The muscularis propria is visualized as the hypoechoic fourth layer; it is usually one layer, but can be visualized as two layers at high frequency. The hyperechoic fifth layer is the subserosa and serosa. The fine hypoechoic layer between the second and third layers is thought to correspond to the muscularis mucosa. When the muscularis mucosa and intermuscular interface of the muscularis propria are visualized using a frequency of 20 MHz, the normal gastric wall is observed as a seven- or nine-layered structure (Figure 5–5).[4] The muscularis mucosa may be visualized in approximately 30% of cases in the stomach and esophagus.[5]

Endoscopic ultrasonography images should be interpreted in terms of tumor invasion based on the five-layer architecture of the gastric wall. Lesions are classified as mucosal, submucosal, or advanced. In the latter, the tumor has invaded the muscularis propria or deeper. On EUS imaging, early gastric cancer is

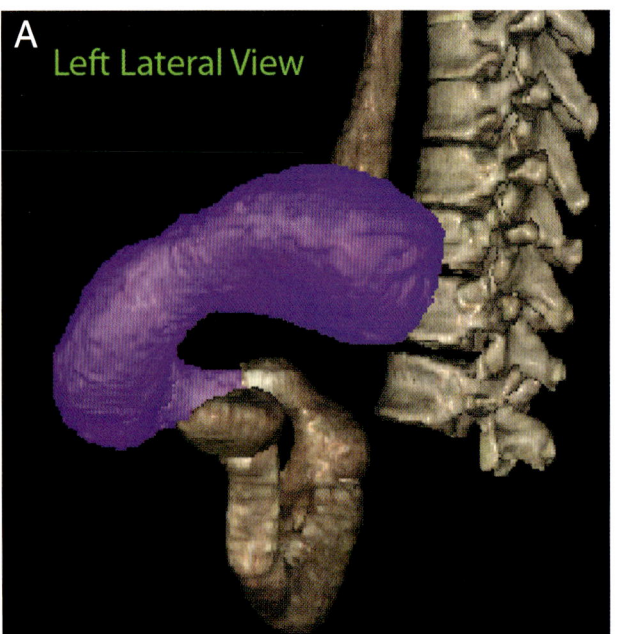

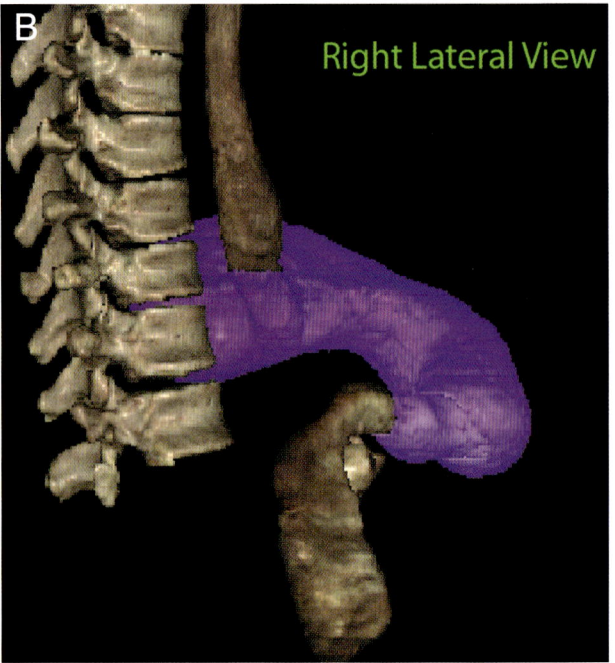

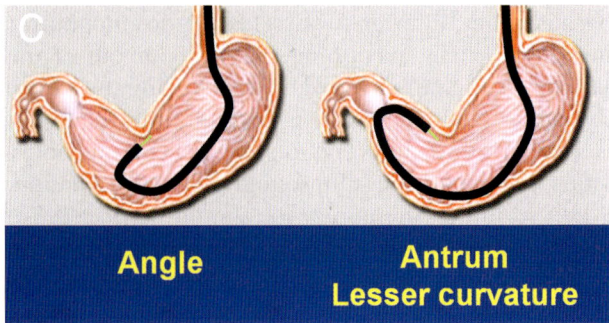

FIGURE 5–2. *A to C* To obtain good quality ultrasonic images and accurately assess a lesion located on the angle or lesser curvature of the antrum, the tip of the endoscope should be angled acutely.

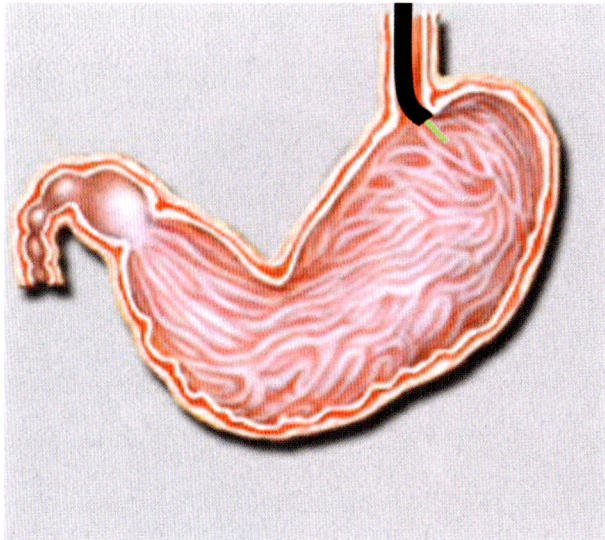

FIGURE 5–3. The posterior wall of the cardia can be scanned using a straight scope.

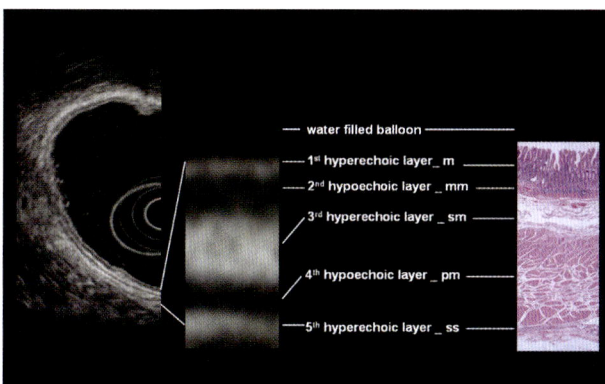

FIGURE 5–4. A 12-MHz endosonography image, showing the typical five-layer structure of the gastric wall compared to the microscopic findings.

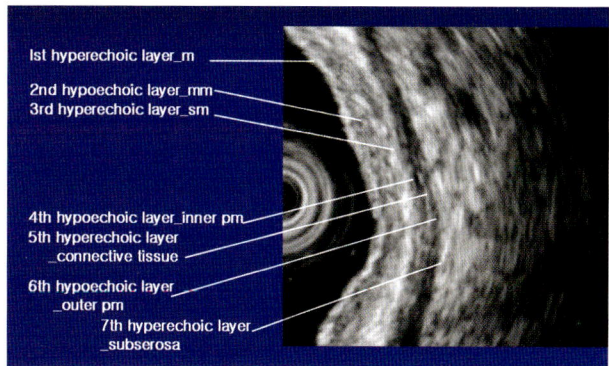

FIGURE 5–5. A 20 MHz miniprobe ultrasonography image showing the typical seven-layer ultrasonographic structure of the normal gastric wall. Hyperechoic first layer, interface with the mucosa; hypoechoic second layer, muscularis mucosa; hyperechoic third layer, submucosa; hypoechoic 4th layer, inner muscularis propria; hyperechoic fifth layer, connective tissue between the inner and outer layers of the muscularis propria; hypoechoic sixth layer, outer muscularis propria; hyperechoic seventh layer, subserosa.

visualized as a hypoechoic mass invading the first, second, and third layers of the stomach, resulting in disruption, thickening, and irregularity of the layers involved. The fourth and fifth layers are often intact (Figures 5–6, 5–10). Advanced gastric cancer is usually accompanied by disruption of the submucosa and muscularis propria and replacement of the normal structures by a hypoechoic mass as result of tumor invasion (Figure 5–11).

In 1986, Yasuda et al[6] reported the EUS criteria for diagnosing the depth of gastric carcinoma invasion for the first time. Subsequently, in 1988, they revised the criteria to include criteria for ulcerative lesions, with reference to the course of peptic ulcer healing (Figure 5–12).[7] The overall diagnostic accuracy of EUS for the depth of carcinoma invasion based on the revised criteria was 79.6% (79.5% m, 72.9% sm, 58.3% mp, and 91.6% deeper than ss).

From the perspective of the endoscopic types of gastric carcinoma, the accuracy was low for lesions with ulcerative change such as type IIc + III in which it is difficult to differentiate malignant fibrosis from benign fibrotic change (Figure 5–13) (type I 83.3%, IIa 86.2%, IIa + IIc 79.2%, IIc 76.6%, and IIc + III 72.3%). To improve the diagnostic accuracy, Kida et al.[8] suggested new EUS diagnostic criteria for the depressed types of early gastric cancer according to the stage of healing of the accompanying ulceration (Figure 5–14). The suggested diagnostic pattern of these criteria is that changes in the wall structure involve widening toward the outer portions of the wall in a fan shape if the ulcer is benign. In malignant ulcers, the changes involve widening toward the outer wall in an irregular arc shape. If the invasion involves the submucosa or deeper muscle layer, the stomach wall appears even thicker. Although, these criteria are effective for discriminating ulcers in the scarred or healing stages, they cannot be applied to lesions with active ulcers.

The accurate staging of gastric cancer is the most important prognostic factor for patient management, and EUS is the most reliable method in T- and N-staging of gastric cancer. The accuracy of EUS for gastric cancer from various studies ranges from 71 to 87.5% for T-staging and 68.6 to 90% for N-staging (Table 5–2). Together with other reports, these studies demonstrate that EUS is an accurate staging modality in most cases, although overstaging and understaging occur in a few exceptions.

Studies using conventional 7.5- or 12.0-MHz frequency EUS instruments were based on the

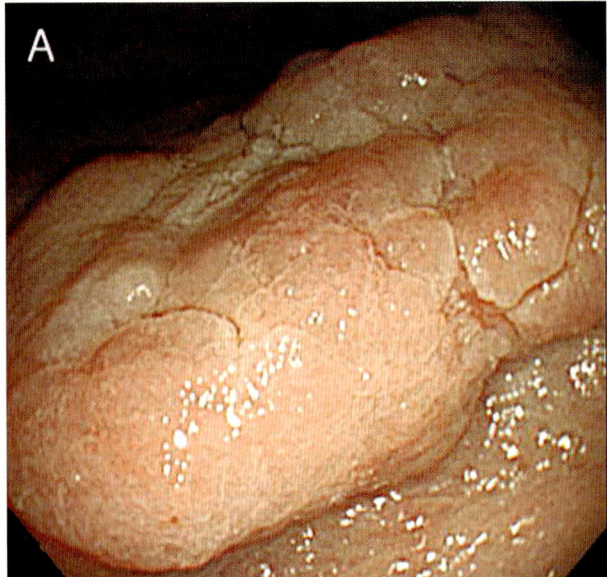
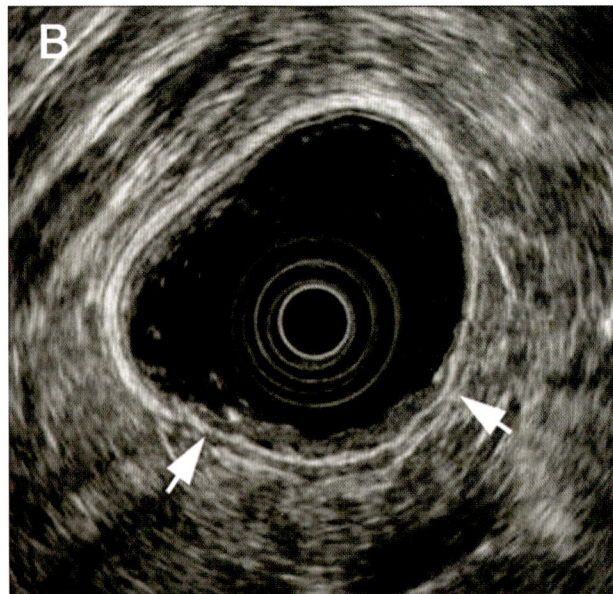

FIGURE 5–6. *A and B* Endoscopic and endoscopic ultrasonography (EUS) images of mucosal gastric cancer. (A) Gastroscopy shows a slightly elevated lesion on the gastric angle (early gastric cancer type IIa). (B) EUS shows elevation and thickening of the hyperechoic first and hypoechoic second layers suggestive of mucosal cancer. The hyperechoic third layer is intact (arrows).

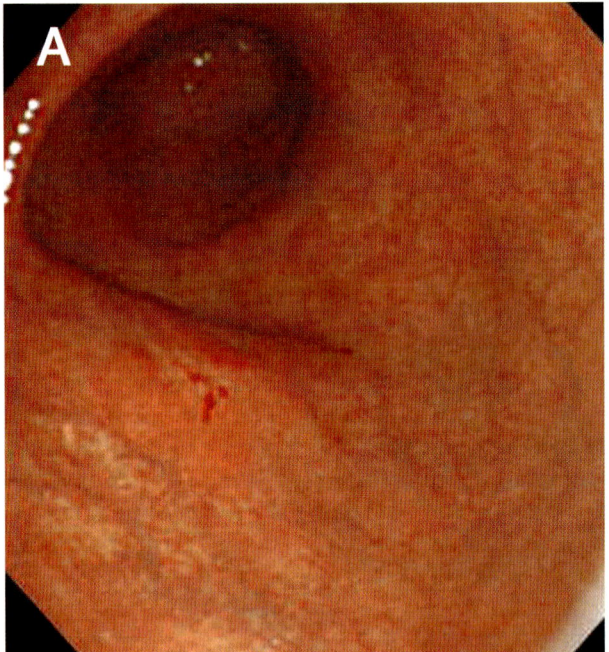
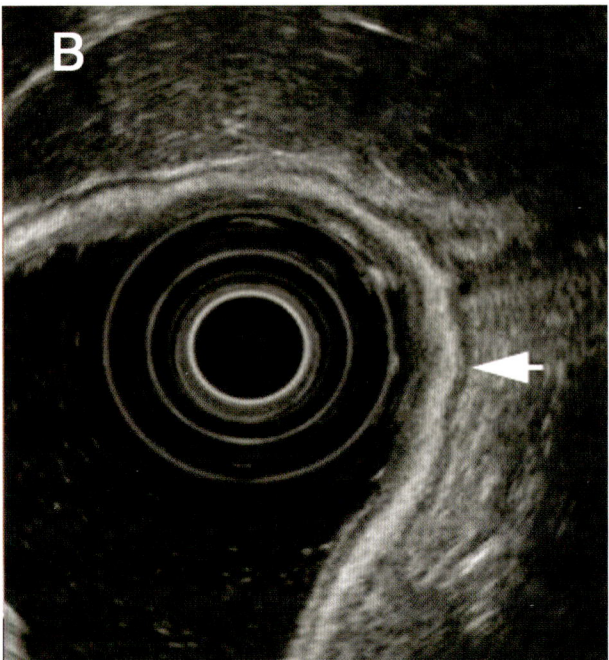

FIGURE 5–7. *A and B* Endoscopic and endoscopic ultrasonography (EUS) images of mucosal gastric cancer. (A) Gastroscopy shows discoloration and a tiny mucosal defect on the lower body of the greater curvature. (B) EUS shows a tiny defect (arrow) in the hyperechoic first layer. The hypoechoic second and hyperechoic third layers (submucosa) are intact.

TNM staging system, in which T1 includes both mucosal and submucosal cancer and does not distinguish between the two.[20-23] Some investigators have studied the accuracy of differentiating mucosal from submucosal early gastric cancer.[24-26] however, they did not analyze their data from a therapeutic perspective, considering endoscopic resection methods such as EMR and ESD. Therefore, the full clinical utility of EUS in early gastric cancer remains to be established.

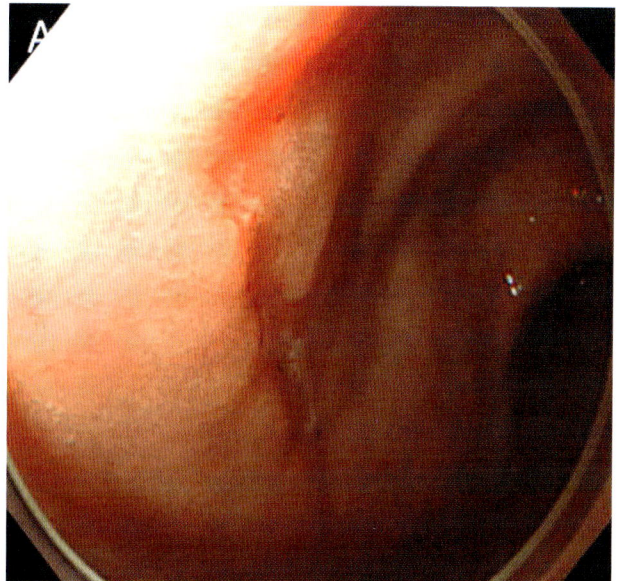
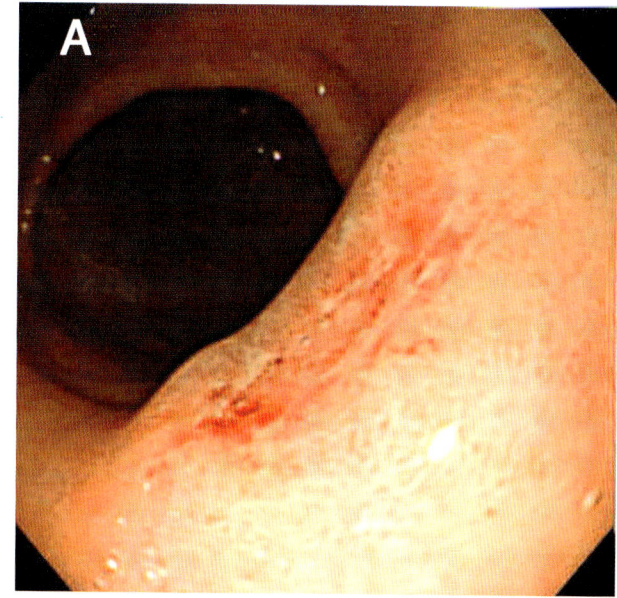
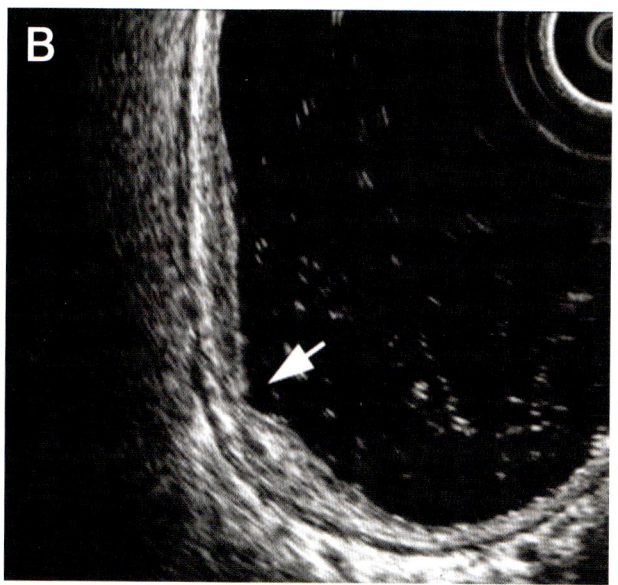
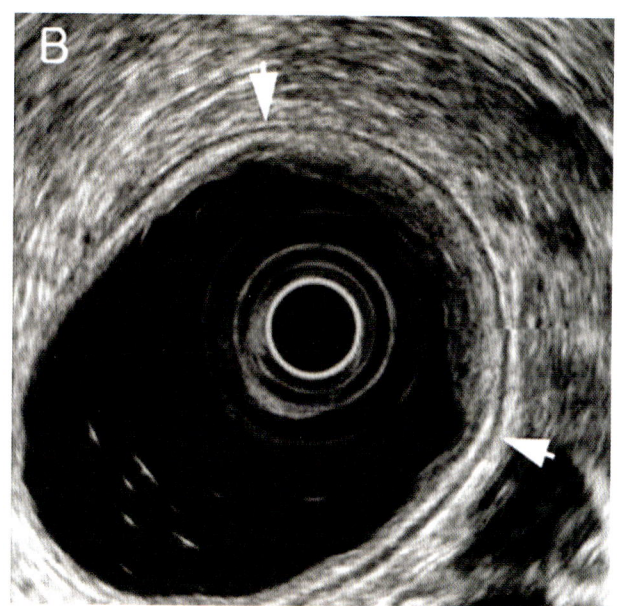
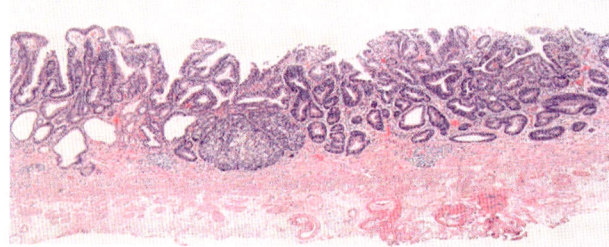

FIGURE 5–8. *A to C* Endoscopic and endoscopic ultrasonography (EUS) images of mucosal gastric cancer. (A) Gastroscopy shows a depressed lesion on the anterior wall of the gastric antrum. (B) EUS shows a small defect (arrow) in the hyperechoic first layer and thickening of the hypoechoic second layer. (C) Microscopic findings after endoscopic submucosal dissection show the proliferation of neoplastic glands confined to the mucosa.

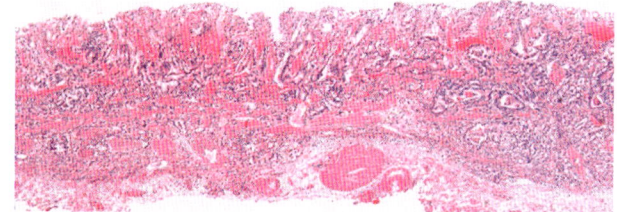

FIGURE 5–9. *A to C* Endoscopic and endoscopic ultrasonography (EUS) images of submucosal gastric cancer. (A) Gastroscopy shows a shallow ulcerated lesion on the lower body. (B) EUS shows a shallow depression in the hyperechoic first layer, a thickened hypoechoic second layer (arrows) and irregularity of the hyperechoic third layer, suggestive of cancer invasion limited to the submucosa. (C) Microscopic findings after endoscopic submucosal dissection show tumor glands spreading to the submucosa through the muscularis mucosa.

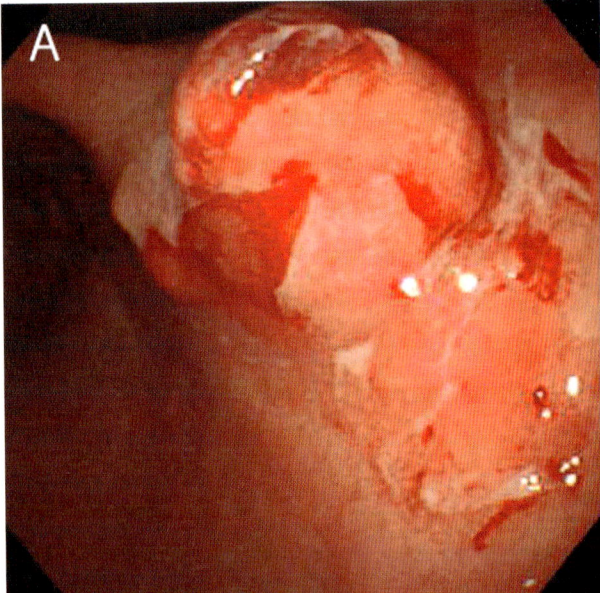
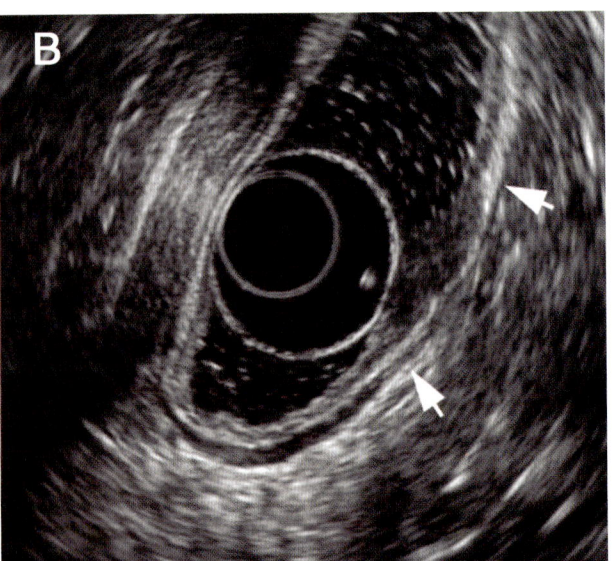

FIGURE 5-10. A and B Endoscopic and endoscopic ultrasonography (EUS) images of submucosal gastric cancer. (A) Gastroscopy shows an elevated lesion on the posterior wall of the gastric angle. (B) With the balloon slightly compressing the protruded lesion, EUS shows elevation of the hyperechoic first layer and irregularity and narrowing of the hyperechoic third layer (arrows).

A thin 20-MHz probe can visualize superficial or small early gastric cancer lesions. It has been reported that there are no statistically significant differences between endoscopy and EUS in terms of the accuracy of the measurement of the depth of invasion, but EUS tends to result in overstaging, whereas endoscopy tends to result in understaging.

Another study[27] used a 20-MHz linear ultrasound probe, which is useful for detailed imaging of the mucosa and submucosa, to evaluate the accuracy of differentiating mucosal and submucosal early gastric cancer. The accuracy was 72.3%. Overstaging resulting from various noncancerous changes in the third layer was a major problem with EUS. Edema, inflammation,

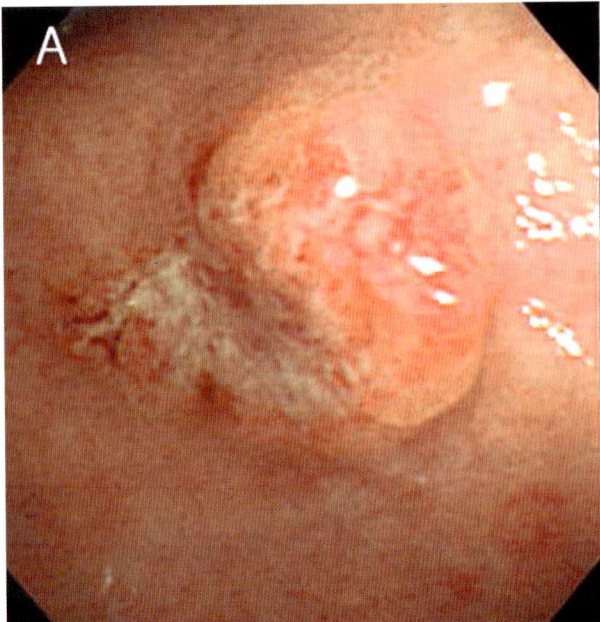
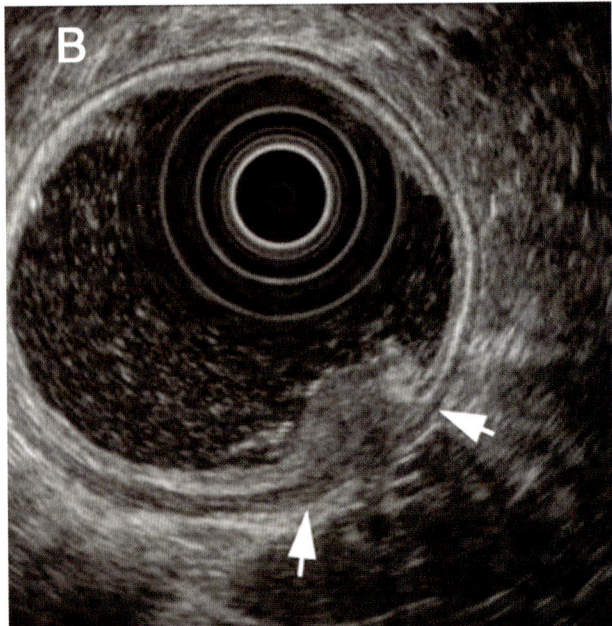

FIGURE 5-11. A and B. Endoscopy and endoscopic ultrasonography (EUS) images of advanced gastric cancer confined to the muscle proper. (A) Gastroscopy shows an elevated lesion with a shallow ulceration on the anterior wall of the gastric antrum. (B) EUS shows a hypoechoic protruding mass and abrupt interruption of the hyperechoic third layer (arrows).

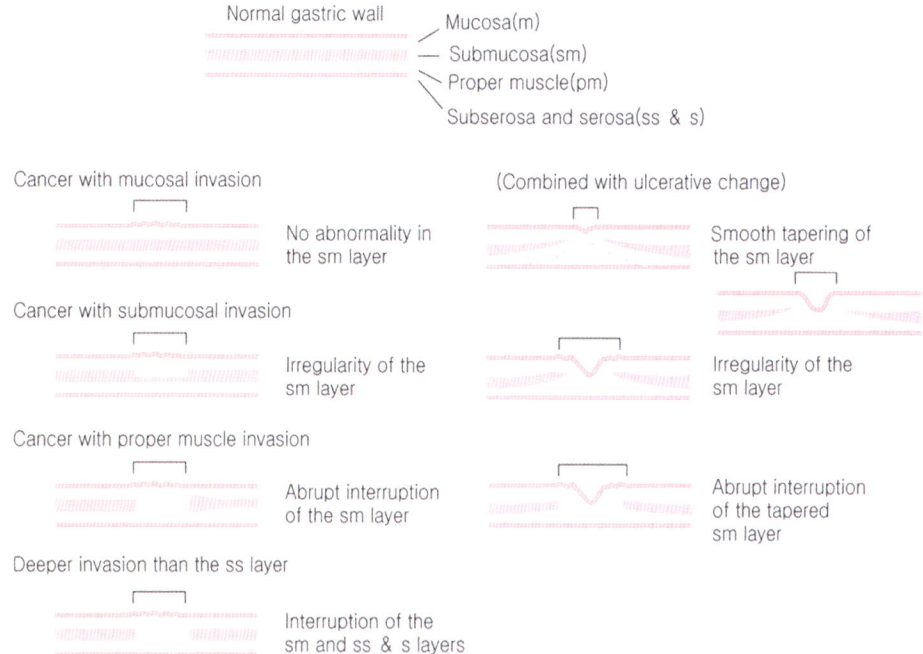

FIGURE 5–12. Revised endoscopic ultrasonography (EUS) diagnostic criteria of the depth of gastric carcinoma invasion, as reported by Yasuda et al. (Courtesy of Dr. K. Yasuda)

and fibrosis due to accompanying ulceration in early gastric cancer can induce changes in the third layer that may cause the endoscopist to overstage the lesion (Figures 5–15, 5–16). In addition, protruding lesions, necrotic masses, or gastric folds attenuate the high-frequency ultrasound beam (20 MHz), which produces unclear images of the gastric wall that ultimately result in improper interpretations of the wall structures, causing the lesion to be overstaged (Figures 5–17, 5–18). Other causes of staging errors are inadequate positioning of the EUS probes (Figure 5–19) and swelling of the submucosal layer after endoscopic biopsy. Therefore, this should be considered before endoscopic biopsy of a suspicious lesion.

A number of factors contribute to overstaging, including the misinterpretation of necrotic tissue overlaying the ulcer surface, scars, fibrosis, an inflammatory reaction in the peripheral structure of the cancer, and a thickened gastric wall. Conversely, microscopic cancer invasion causing focal destruction

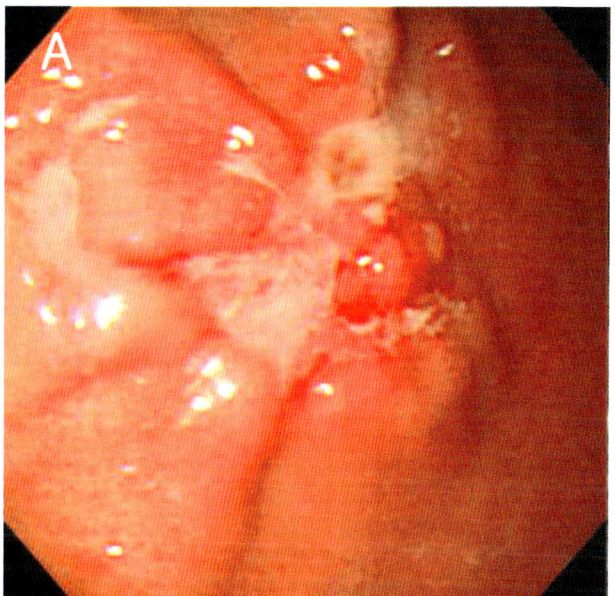
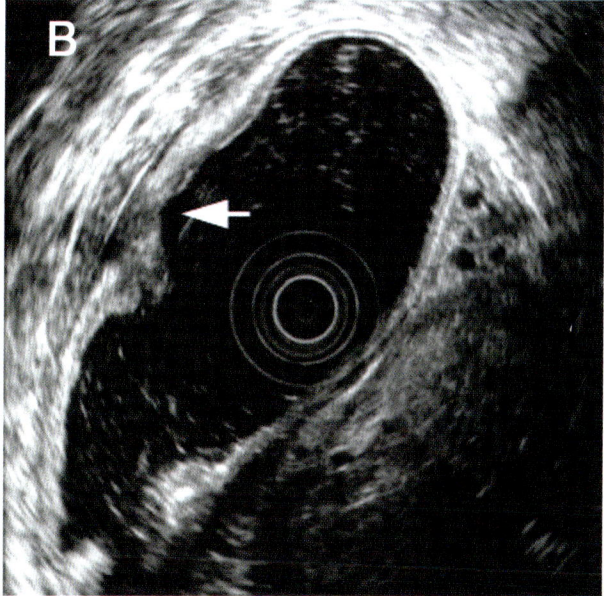

FIGURE 5–13. *A and B* Endoscopy and endoscopic ultrasonography (EUS) images of mucosal cancer overstaged as submucosal cancer. (A) Gastroscopy shows a geographic ulcer on the anterior wall of the gastric angle. (B) EUS shows an irregular, hyperechoic third layer.

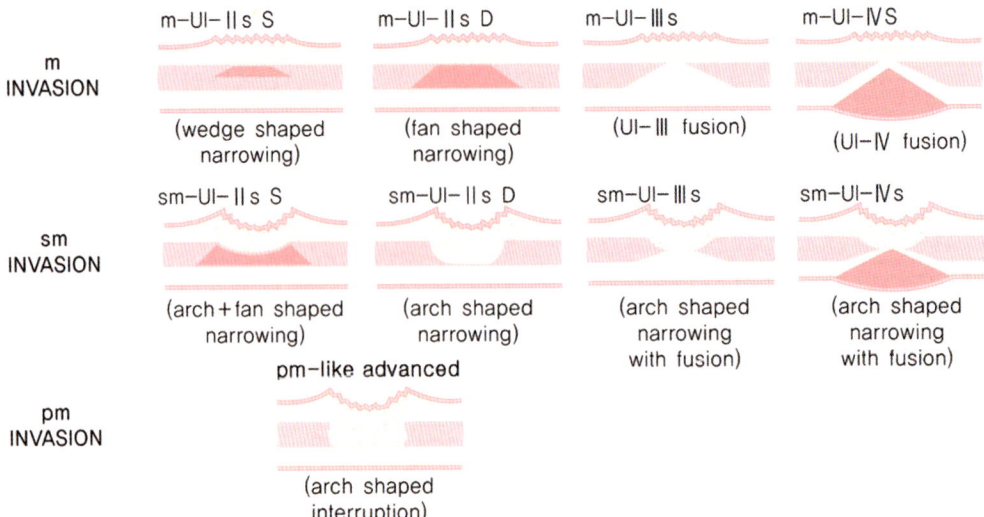

FIGURE 5–14. Endoscopic ultrasonography (EUS) diagnostic criteria for depressed types of early gastric cancer according to the healing stage of the accompanying ulceration by Kida et al. m; mucosa, sm; submucosa, pm; muscle proper, UI-II; ulcer depth to muscularis mucosa, UI-III; ulcer depth to submucosa, UI-IV; ulcer depth to muscle proper, s, S & D; scarred stage, shallow ulcer and deep ulcer, respectively. (Courtesy of Dr. M. Kida)

of a layer that is undetectable using lower-frequency ultrasound often results in understaging (Table 5–3). In general, the elevated type may be staged more readily than the ulcerated type with greater accuracy. To visualize the cancer best and improve the diagnostic accuracy, high-frequency probes (20 MHz) may be more suitable for early cancer, whereas low-frequency transducers (7.5 or 12 MHz) may be more suitable for advanced cancer.

The detection of regional lymph node metastasis and differentiating benign from malignant nodes is unsatisfactory with EUS in gastric carcinoma. Moreover, due to its limited depth of penetration, more distant lymph nodes such as the prepyloric and pericardia nodes may not be imaged at all. High-frequency EUS can be used to scan the left liver lobe, but only a small portion of the right lobe can be imaged and the evaluation of pulmonary metastasis and distant peritoneal metastasis is limited.

Several studies have focused on the accuracy of EUS for diagnosing lymph node metastasis. Lightdale[28] and Zuccaro et al[29] found that round lymph nodes with a clear margin and a hypo-echo pattern similar to that of the primary tumor were more likely to be malignant. The size of the imaged lymph nodes was found to be an unreliable criterion for malignancy. Malignant nodes as small as 3 mm could be imaged with EUS. Nevertheless, nodes larger than 10 mm were very suggestive of malignancy. Heintz et al.[30] reported that the sensitivity and specificity were 85% and 45–85%, respectively, using the following criteria for malignant nodes: nodes larger than 10 mm in diameter, with a heterogeneous echo pattern, and a sharp border.

Inaccuracy may result from the lack of a reliable standard for differentiating benign and malignant nodes. The diameter, location, and distance from the lymph node to the primary lesion and the

Table 5-2 Literature Summary of EUS Studies on Gastric Cancer

Authors	No. of patients	Accuracy (%) T-stage	Accuracy (%) N-stage
Yasuda et al. (1992)[9]	500	79	-
Guo et al. (1997)[10]	62	83.9	79
Kim JO et al. (1997)[11]	63	77.8	-
Hunerbein et al. (1998)[12]	30	82	80
Yanai et al. (1999)[13]	52	71	-
Kida et al. (1999)[14]	1428	79	-
Hizawa et al. (2002)[15]	234	78	-
Xi et al. (2003)[16]	32	80	68.6
Habermann et al. (2004)[17]	51	86	90
Shimoyama et al. (2004)[18]	45	71	80
Bhandari et al. (2004)[19]	63	87.5	79.1

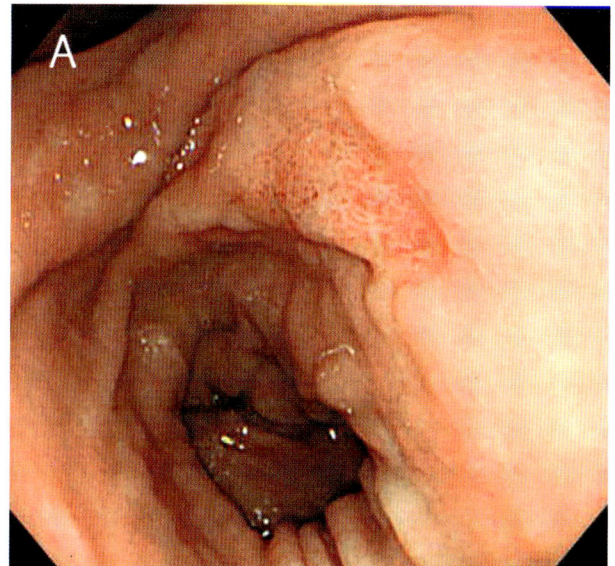

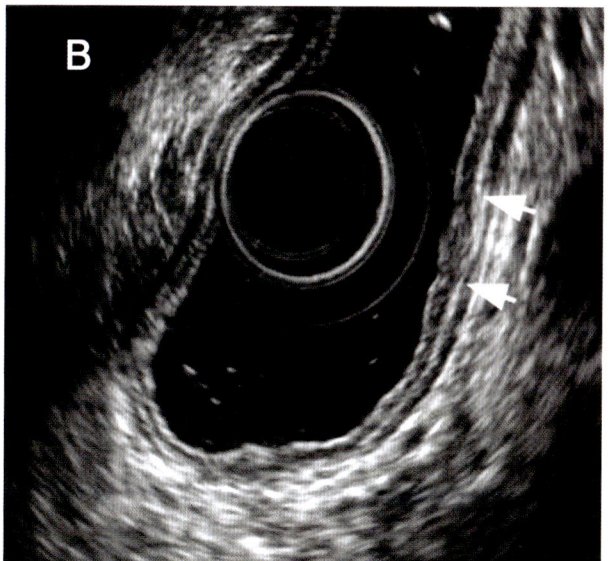

FIGURE 5–15. *A and B* Endoscopic and endoscopic ultrasonography (EUS) images of mucosal cancer overstaged as submucosal cancer. (A) Gastroscopy shows a depressed lesion on the posterior wall of the gastric antrum. (B) EUS shows a depressed hyperechoic first layer and an irregular hyperechoic third layer (arrows).

endoscopist's expertise are also important. Other factors affecting the accuracy include the frequency and penetration depth of the transducer used and intra-gastric substances.

To minimize inaccuracy, visualization of lymph nodes using EUS should start at the site of primary tumor, followed by gradual detection of each perigastric lymph node group. Lymph nodes can be differentiated from other perigastric structures such as vessels on EUS imaging by moving the probe forward and backward or by using EUS equipped with color Doppler. Recently, the electronic radial EUS

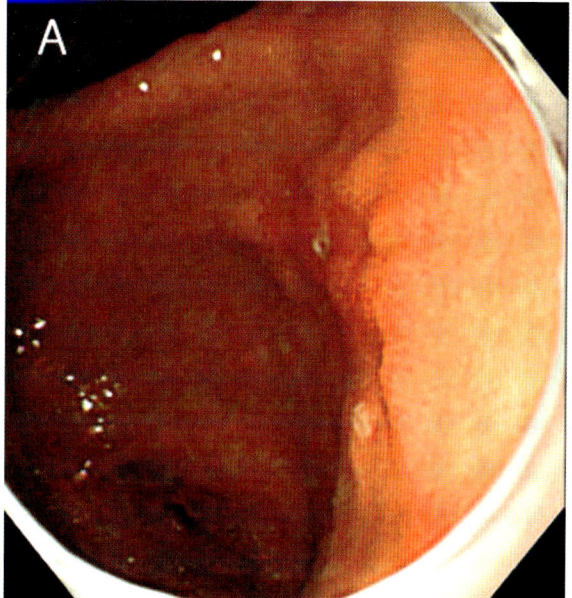

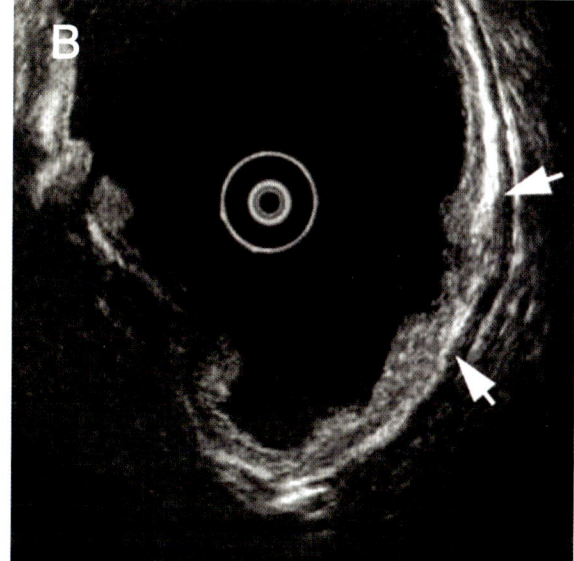

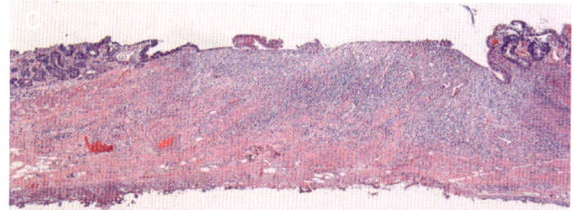

FIGURE 5–16. *A to C* Endoscopic and endoscopic ultrasonography (EUS) images of mucosal cancer overstaged as submucosal cancer. (A) Gastroscopy shows a shallow ulcer in the center of a depressed lesion on the posterior wall of the antrum. (B) EUS shows an irregular hyperechoic third layer (arrows). (C) Microscopic findings after endoscopic submucosal dissection show an ulcer base consisting of granulation tissue without malignant cells. Tumor cells are observed only in the mucosa at the margin of the ulcer.

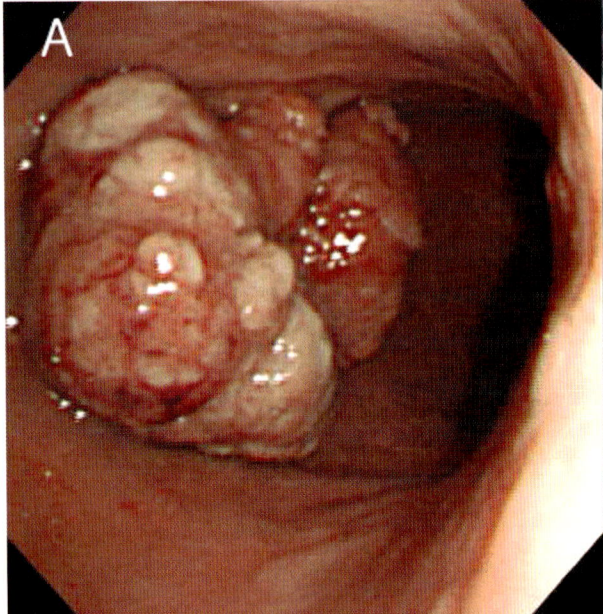
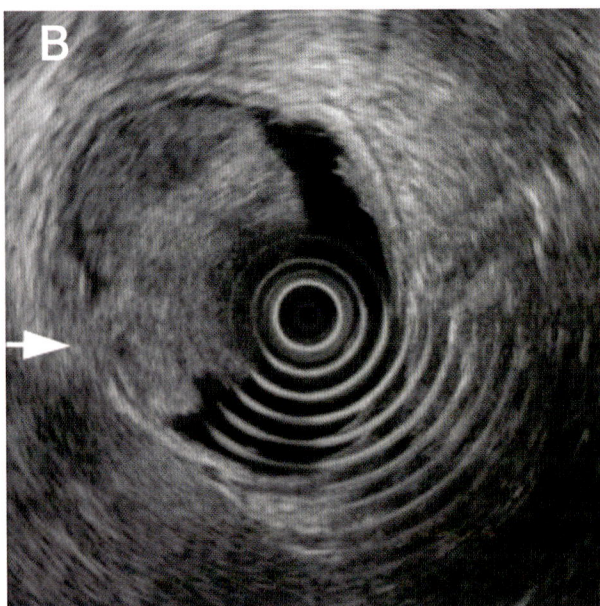

FIGURE 5–17. *A and B* Endoscopic and endoscopic ultrasonography (EUS) images of mucosal cancer overstaged as advanced gastric cancer. (A). Gastroscopy shows a huge polypoid mass on the greater curvature of the lower body. (B) EUS shows indistinct hyperechoic third, hypoechoic fourth, and hyperechoic fifth layers.

videoscope (Olympus GF-UE 260-AL5), which allows advanced imaging options such as color Doppler, has become available. Because many factors may influence the detection of nodes, a negative EUS does not reliably indicate the absolute absence of nodal involvement. Further assessment should be carried out to obtain a definite diagnosis. EUS-guided fine-needle aspiration (EUS-FNA) is now available clinically and has been accepted as obtaining the most reliable cytology for differentiation in this situation.[31]

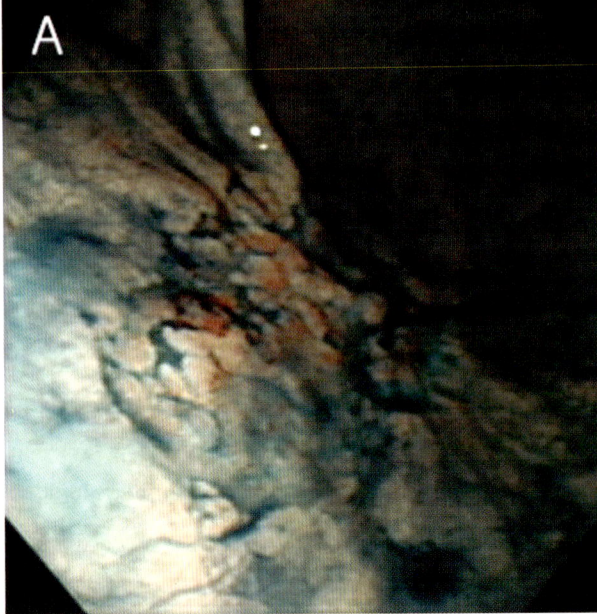
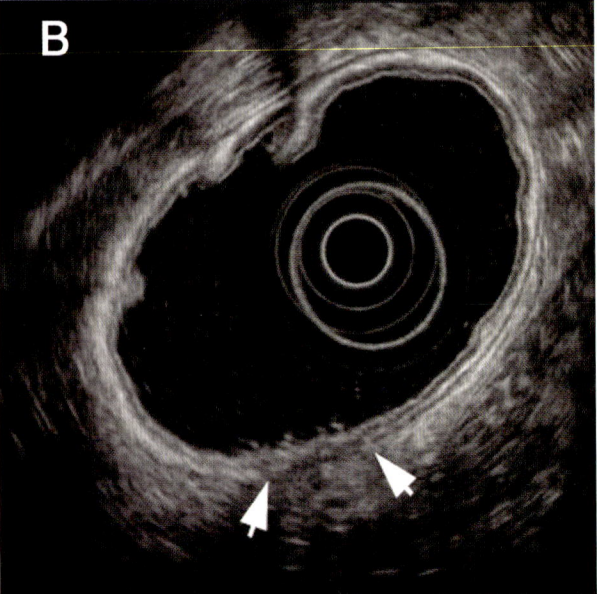

FIGURE 5–18. *A and B* Endoscopic and endoscopic ultrasonography (EUS) images of mucosal cancer (type IIc, early gastric cancer) overstaged as advanced gastric cancer. (A) Gastroscopy after indigocarmine dye spray shows a depressed lesion with convergence of the folds on the greater curvature of the lower body. (B) EUS shows an abrupt interruption of the hyperechoic third layer (arrows) and an indistinct hyperechoic fifth layer.

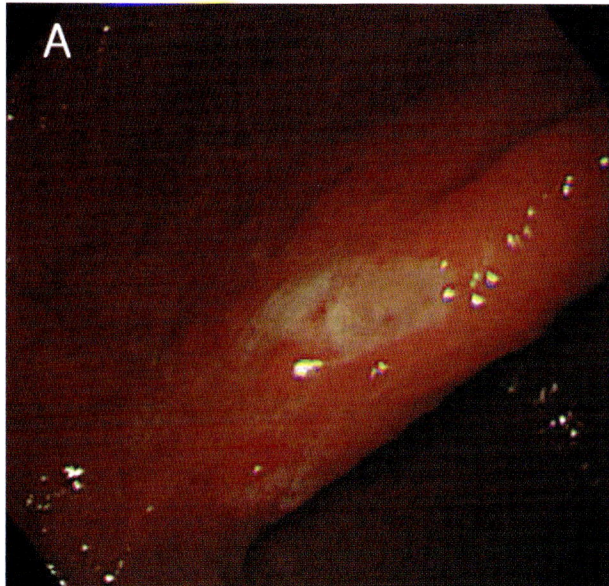 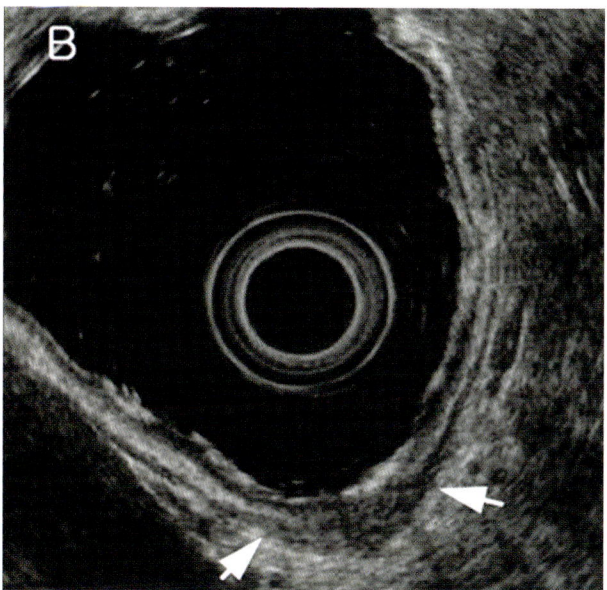

FIGURE 5–19. *A and B* Endoscopic and endoscopic ultrasonography (EUS) images of mucosal cancer overstaged as advanced gastric cancer due to an improper plane of the axis with respect to the lesion. (A) Gastroscopy shows a shallow ulcer on the gastric angle. (B) EUS shows abrupt interruption of the hyperechoic third layer (arrows) and an indistinct hyperechoic fifth layer.

 Future Perspectives of EUS

Lymph node metastasis is reported to occur in only 0–3% of cancer lesions limited to the mucosal layer, whereas approximately 20% of tumors invading the submucosa have been reported to show lymph node involvement.[3] Therefore, the selection of local endoscopic therapy as a curative treatment for early gastric cancer necessitates the precise discrimination of mucosal lesions from those infiltrating the submucosa. The muscularis mucosa is the clinical border at the lower margin of the mucosal layer and it is extremely useful to determine whether a tumor extends beyond it before treatment is decided. Unfortunately, most current EUS miniprobes do not allow precise visualization of the muscularis mucosa, particularly of the gastric wall, because their axial resolution is insufficient to visualize such a thin layer.

Recently, however, high-frequency instruments with sufficient axial resolution to distinguish wall layers with different acoustic impedances have been used. Yanai et al.[5] reported that the muscularis mucosa can be delineated in 50% of early gastric cancers scanned in vitro using a 20 MHz linear EUS probe. They found that the accuracy of estimating the tumor invasion depth is greater when such a layer can be delineated.

Table 5–3. Possible Causes of Staging Errors of Endosonography in Early Gastric Cancer

Overstaging	Neighboring ulcer or ulcer scar (especially type IIc + III)
	Misdiagnosis of lymph follicle as carcinoma
	Benign cyctic gland in the submucosa (especially type IIa)
	Unclear borderline echo between the second and third layers (especially Type I and Type IIa)
	Swelling of the submucosal layer by endoscopic biopsy
	Attenuated ultrasound beam
	Anomaly of the muscularis mucosa
Understaging	Dissemination of only a few malignant cells
	Submucosal microinvasion (especially IIa + IIc)
Indeterminant	Minute lesions (less than 5 mm)
	Attenuated ultrasound beam

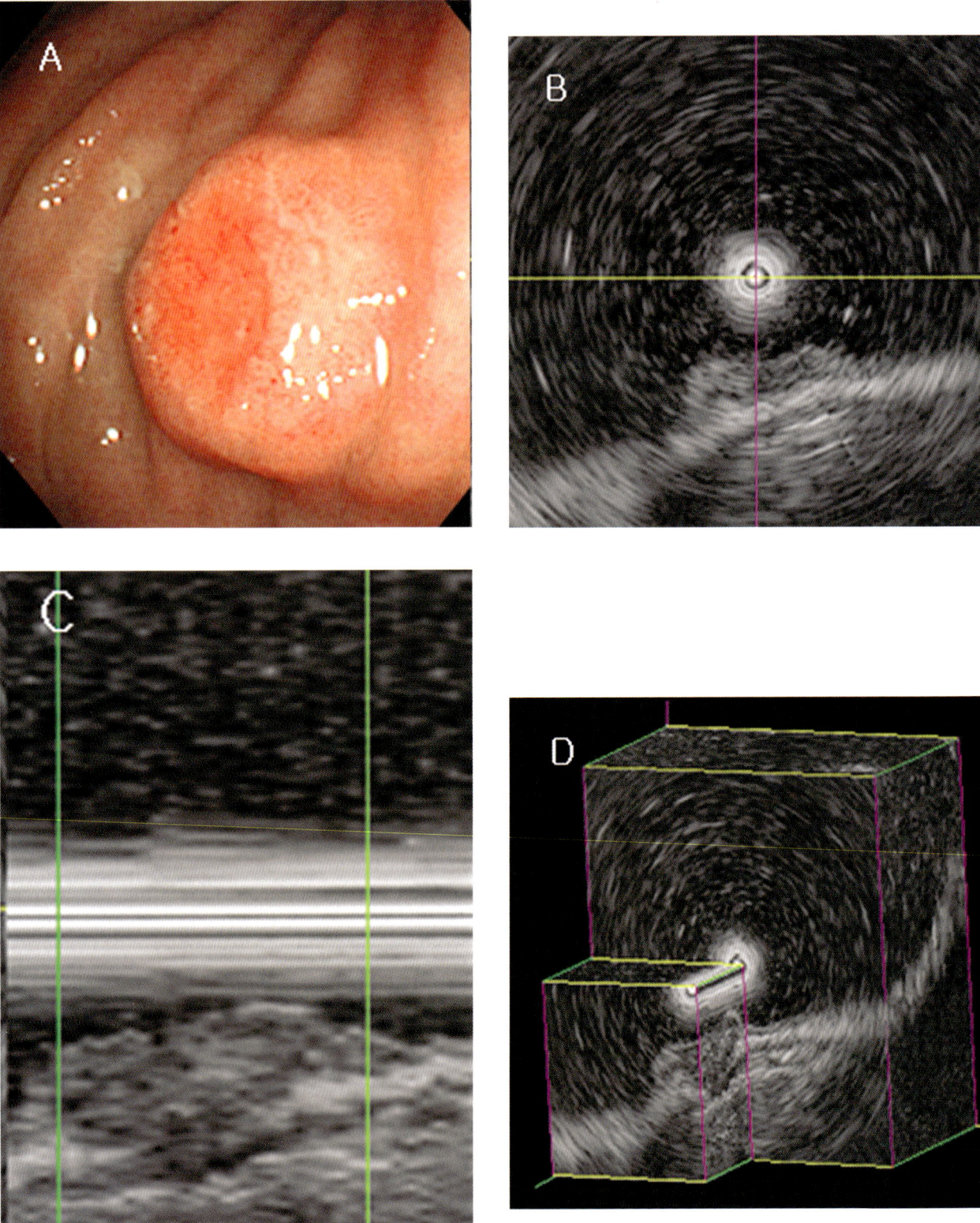

FIGURE 5–20. A to D Endoscopic and three-dimensional reconstructed images of cancer invading the submucosa. (A) Gastroscopy shows an elevated lesion on the greater curvature of the upper body. (B) Radial view shows an intact hyperechoic third layer. (C) Longitudinal view shows irregular narrowing of the hyperechoic third layer. (D) Three-dimensional reconstruction view.

Sabet et al.[32] used a 30-MHz miniprobe with an axial resolution of 102 μm and found it sufficient for visualizing the muscularis mucosa in all cases. The mucosa was visualized as four layers: the interface echo, an internal echo from the epithelial layer and gastric glands, another interface echo, and the muscularis mucosa. In addition, the submucosa was sometimes visualized as a multilayer structure. This might have been caused by reflection of the echo waves by collagen fibers, blood or lymphatic vessels with the mucosa. Although the muscularis mucosa was clearly delineated in all lesions, visualization of deeper layers in most cases was difficult and the echo waves were readily attenuated at the sites of deep ulcer fibrosis, preventing visualization of the tumor extent in lesions associated with an ulcer scar. This suggests that a 30-MHz probe is unlikely to provide useful information for the diagnosis of tumor infiltration depth in patients with ulceration at the tumor site. In addition, the focal distance of the 30 MHz probe was 5–10 mm, making it difficult to obtain a high-resolution image when the probe was further than 5 mm from the mucosal surface. In addition, because probe artifacts interfere with the imaging when the probe is closer to the mucosal surface, adequate positioning might be extremely difficult in clinical practice.

The recent introduction of three-dimensional (3D) imaging techniques that provide continuous scanning images might improve diagnostic accuracy. Using 3D-EUS, it is possible to diagnose submucosal invasion exceeding 500 μm with high accuracy. Recent data by Kida et al.[33,34] demonstrated that the diagnostic accuracy of 3D-EUS for diagnosing the depth of gastric cancer invasion was 96% in mucosal cancer, 74.6% in submucosal, 72% in muscularis mucosa, 76% in subserosal, and 81.8% in serosal cancer. The overall accuracy was 86.3%. Compared to conventional EUS and miniprobes, accurate detection of submucosal invasion exceeding 500 μm in lesions without ulcers or ulcer-induced fibrosis was significantly higher (77.8% vs. 70.8%). The authors also suggested that 3D-EUS was more useful to determine candidates for EMR or ESD. The main advantages of 3D-EUS are that it saves time compared to early gastric cancer staging with conventional EUS and minute lesions are more conveniently scanned (Figure 5–20).

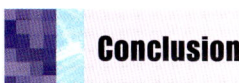

Conclusion

Early detection and early treatment comprise an essential part of the best therapeutic strategy for early gastric cancer. Because the rate of early gastric cancer is increasing, especially in Japan and Korea, endoscopic resection methods such as EMR or ESD are increasingly used for minimally invasive treatment. With the rise in demand for endoscopic curative resection of early gastric cancer, it has become imperative to assess the stage of the tumor accurately. Consequently, EUS has been and will continue to be extremely useful for accurate staging and the establishment of individualized therapy in patients with early gastric cancer. Although over- and understaging remain to be overcome, recent technological advances such as high-frequency EUS and 3D-EUS may provide answers in the future.

References

1. Ferlay, J., Bray, F., Pisani, P.: GLOBOCAN 2002: Cancer incidence, mortality and prevalence world-wide. Version 2.0. Lyon: IARC Press, 2004.
2. Yasud, K.: EUS in the detection of early gastric cancer. *Gastrointest Endosc* 2002; 56:S68–S75.
3. Sano, T., Kobori, O., Muto, T.: Lymph node metastasis from early gastric cancer : Endoscopic resection of tumor. Br J Surg 1992; 79:241–244.
4. Yanai, H., Matsumoto, Y., Harada, T., et al.: Endoscopic ultrasonography and endoscopy for staging depth of invasion in early gastric cancer: a pilot study. *Gastrointest Endosc* 1997; 46:212–216.
5. Yanai, H., Fujimura, H., Suzumi, M., et al.: Delineation of the gastric muscularis mucosa and assessment of depth of invasion of early gastric cancer using a 20-megahertz endoscopic ultrasound probe. *Gastrointest Endosc* 1993; 39:505–512.
6. Yasuda, K., Nakajima, M., Kawai, K.: Fundamentals of endoscopic laser therapy (ELT) for GI tumors: new aspects with endoscopic ultrasonography (EUS). *Endoscopy* 1987;19:S2–S6.
7. Yasuda, K., Nakajima, M., Kawai, K.: Endoscopic diagnosis and treatment of early gastric cancer using endoscopic ultrasonography (EUS). *Gastrointest Endosc Clin North Am* 1992;2:495–507.
8. Kida, M., Tanabe, S., Watanabe, M., et al.: Staging of gastric cancer with endoscopic ultrasonography and endoscopic mucosal resection. *Endoscopy* 1998; 30 Suppl 1:A64–A68.
9. Yasuda, K., Uno, K., Tanaka, S., et al.: Evaluation of the degree of gastric cancer invasion by endoscopic ultrasonography for endoscopic treatment. *Stomach Intestine* 1992;27:1167–1174.
10. Guo, W., Zhang, Y. L., Li, G. X., et al.: Comparison of preoperative staging of gastric carcinoma by endoscopic ultrasonography with CT examination. *China Natl J New Gastroenterol* 1997; 3:242–245.
11. Kim, J. O., Shim, C. S., Cho, Y. D., et al.: Comparison of Diagnostic Accuracy between Endoscopy and EUS for Depth of Invasion in Early Gastric Cancer. *Kor J Gastroenterol* 1997;29:742–750.
12. Hunerbein, M., Ghadimi, B. M., Haensch, W., Schlag, P. M.: Transendoscopic ultrasound of esophageal and gastric cancer using miniaturized ultrasound catheter probes. *Gastrointest Endosc* 1998;48:371–375.
13. Yanai, H., Matsumoto, Y., Harada, T., et al.: Endoscopic ultrasonography and endoscopy for staging depth of invasion in early gastric cancer: a pilot study. *Gastrointest Endosc* 1997; 46:212–216.

14. Kida, M., Kokutou, M., Watanbe, M., et al.: Accuracy of endoscopic ultrasonography for diagnosing the depth of early gastric cancer with or without ulcer. *Stomach Intestine* 1999;34:1095–1103.
15. Hizawa, K., Iwai, K., Esaki, M., et al.: Is Endoscopic Ultrasonography indispensable on assessing in the appropriateness of endoscopic resection of gastric cancer? *Endoscopy* 2002;34:973–979.
16. Xi, W. D., Zhao, C., Ren, G. S., Endoscopic ultrasonography in preoperative staging of gastric cancer: determination of tumor invasion depth, nodal involvement and surgical resectability. *World J Gastroenterol* 2003;9:254–257.
17. Habermann, C. R., Weiss, F., Riecken, R., et al. Preoperative staging of gastric adenocarcinoma: comparison of helical CT and endoscopic US. *Radiology* 2004; 230:465–471.
18. Shimoyama, S., Yasuda, H., Hashimoto, M., et al.: Accuracy of linear array EUS for preoperative staging of gastric cardia cancer. *Gastrointest Endosc* 2004;60:50–55.
19. Bhandari, S., Shim, C. S., Kim, J. H., et al.: Usefulness of three-dimensional, multidetector row CT (virtual gastroscopy and multiplanar reconstruction) in the evaluation of gastric cancer: a comparison with conventional endoscopy, EUS and histopathology. *Gastrointest Endosc* 2004;59:619–626.
20. Tio, T. l., Schouwink, M. H., Cikot, R. J. L. M., Tytgat, G. N. J.: Preoperative TNM classification of gastric carcinoma by endosonography in comparison with the pathological TNM system: a prospective study of 72 cases. *Hepatogastroenterology* 1989;36:51–56.
21. Akahoshi, K., Misawa, T., Fujishima, H., et al.: Preoperative evaluation of gastric cancer by endoscopic ultrasound. *Gut* 1991;32:479–482.
22. Dittler, H. J., Siewert, J. R., Role of endoscopic ultrasonography in gastric carcinoma. *Endoscopy* 1993;25: 162–166.
23. Grimm, H., Binmoeller, K. F., Hamper, K., et al.: Endosonography for preoperative locoregional staging of esophageal and gastric cancer. *Endoscopy* 1993; 25:224–230.
24. Nakazawa, S., Nakamura, T., Yoshino, J.: Endoscopic ultrasonography. In Oguro, Y., Takagi, K., eds.: Endoscopic approaches to cancer diagnosis and treatment. Tokyo: *Japan Scientific Societies press,* 1990:41–56.
25. Kimura, K., Yamanaka, T.: Endoscopic ultrasonography in the assessment of depth of invasion of gastric cancer. In Takemoto, T., Kawai, K., eds.: Recent topics of digestive endoscopy. Tokyo: *Excerpta Medica,* 1987:70–76.
26. Yasuda, K., Nakajima, M., Kawai, K.: Malignant lesions of the gastrointestinal tract. In Kawai, K., ed.: Endoscopic ultrasonography in gastroenterology. Tokyo: *Igaku-Shoin,* 1988:56–71.
27. Yanai, H., Tada, M., Karita, M., Okita, K.: Diagnostic utility of 20-megahertz linear endoscopic ultrasonography in early gastric cancer. *Gastrointest endosc* 1996;44;29–33.
28. Lightdale, C. J., Mierop, F. V.: Staging Gastric Cancer: The New York Experience. In Dam, J. V., Sivak, V. M., eds.: Gastrointestinal Endosonography. Chapter 18. W.B. *Saunders* 1999:185–192.
29. Zuccaro, G.: Diagnosis and staging of gastric carcinoma by endoscopic ultrasonography. Chapter 13. Neoplasms of the digestive tract. Imaging, staging and management. *New York: Lippincott Raven Publishers* 1998. pp. 137–142.
30. Heintz, A., Mildenberger, P., Georg, H., et al.: Endoscopic ultrasonography in the diagnosis of regional lymph nodes in esophageal and gastric cancer. Results of studies in vitro. *Endoscopy* 1993; 25:231–235.
31. Xi, W. D., Zhao, C., Ren, G. S.: Endoscopic ultrasonography in preoperative staging of gastric cancer : determination of tumor invasion depth, nodal involvement and surgical respectability. World J Gastroenterol 2003;9:254–257.
32. Sabet, E. A., Okai, T., Minamoto, T., et al.: Visualizing the gastric wall with a 30-MHz ultrasonic miniprobe: ex vivo imaging of normal gastric sites and sites of early gastric cancer. *Abdom Imaging* 2003;28:252–256.
33. Kida, M., Kikuchi, H., Araki, M., et al.: 3D-EUS for diagnosing the gastric cancer; especially concerning about the degree of submucosal invasion. *Stomach and Intestine* 2007;42:88–98.
34. Kida, M.: EUS in Gastric Cancer. Endosonography *Saunders* 2006. pp. 111–126.

CHAPTER 6

Advanced Gastric Cancer

Dr. Tony E. Yusuf
Dr. Michael J. Levy

Introduction

Since the introduction of endoscopic ultrasound (EUS) in 1980, this technology has become one of the most significant advances in the field of endoscopy. The first ultrasound endoscope (echoendoscope) incorporated an ultrasound probe into the tip of a side-viewing gastroscope (ACMI FX-5 and Olympus GF-B3 models respectively).[1,2] Use was limited due to the long and rigid tip and suboptimal image resolution. Technological advances over the past two decades have led to the routine use of EUS for evaluating a variety of gastrointestinal and nongastrointestinal disorders providing both diagnostic and therapeutic applications.[3-22] Use of EUS in these settings has been shown to enhance patient care and outcomes.[23] In this chapter, we will focus on the role of EUS for evaluating patients with advanced gastric cancer.

EUS and Gastric Cancer

Gastric cancer is the second-leading cause of cancer-related death worldwide.[24] In the United States, the incidence and mortality rates of gastric cancer are lower compared to those of other countries and have declined over the past several years. The incidence of distal gastric cancer is declining, while the incidence of proximal gastric cancer including gastric cardia is on the rise.[25-27] It is estimated that there were 21,260 new cases of gastric cancer and 11,210 deaths related to the disease in the United States in the year 2007.[24]

Current treatment protocols are guided by TNM staging as part of the American Joint Committee on Cancer (AJCC) staging criteria.[28] Accurate staging is necessary for predicting prognosis and for selection of the appropriate therapeutic strategy. A primary aim of EUS is to establish the tumor (T) stage, nodal (N) stage, and when possible to detect metastasis (M stage). TNM staging for gastric cancer is summarized as follows: T1, tumor invades lamina propria or submucosa; T2a, tumor invades muscularis propria; T2b, tumor invades subserosa; T3, tumor penetrates serosa (visceral peritoneum without invasion of adjacent structures); T4, tumor invades adjacent structures; N1, metastasis in 1-6 regional lymph nodes; N2, metastasis in 7-15 regional lymph nodes; N3, metastasis in more than 15 regional lymph nodes; M0, no evidence of distant metastasis and M1, when distant metastasis is present. Stage grouping reflects different degrees of tumor extent from stage I (early cancer) to stage IV (advanced and metastatic cancer).

The specific T-stage should be noted in the EUS report, and for patients with a T4 tumor, the report should specify which tissue is infiltrated that signifies this advanced stage. One should indicate whether the N-stage was determined by imaging characteristic alone or by onsite FNA results. It is necessary to document the exact location of nodal metastasis given the impact on prognosis and therapy.[29-32] Consider listing each nodal feature (size, echodensity, shape, and border).

In the context of advanced gastric cancer, it is essential to confirm or exclude a T4 tumor and/or presence of N2 or N3 disease. The finding of N1 disease has little impact on patient care, while presence of N2 or N3 disease has a more significant impact on care.[29] The ability to accurate counting the number of metastatic nodes with EUS has never been established. In fact, most centers make no effort to count the number of malignant nodes, rather only designate whether the patient has N0 or N1 disease. Similarly, distant (M stage) metastasis when present should be reported, including the sites examined to make this determination. Mention of ascites, omental thickening, and/or a pleural effusion should be included.

Gastric cancer prognosis strongly correlates with tumor stage, grade and lymph node metastasis.[29-31,33,34] In a study of 777 patients with advanced gastric cancer who underwent curative surgical resection, prognosis correlated well with the level and number of metastatic lymph nodes with 11 and more lymph node metastasis being most significant (p less than 0.0001).[30] Kim et al[32] analyzed 10,783 consecutive patients with gastric cancer of whom 84% had resection with a five-year survival of 64.8%. The ratio of involved to resected lymph nodes, depth of invasion and curative resection had prognostic value. Surgery may be curative in localized distal gastric cancer, however, most (80–90%) have advanced disease at presentation and a five-year prognosis of only 3-13%.[35] Radical surgery with curative intent is the cornerstone of therapy for advanced gastric cancer, but locoregional and peritoneal recurrence are common.[36] Surgical resection of adenocarcinoma of the stomach is curative in less than 40% of cases. Survival is not improved with chemotherapy or radiotherapy alone.[37-39] The effect of operative resection followed by adjuvant chemoradiation therapy was investigated by Macdonald et al[40] in 556 patients with resectable adenocarcinoma of the gastroesophageal junction. Patients were randomly assigned to surgery alone or surgery followed by adjuvant chemoradiation therapy and followed for a median of five years. The median overall survival in the surgery-alone group was 27 months, as compared with 36 months in the chemoradiation group; the hazard ratio for death was 1.35, P=0.005 and the hazard ratio for relapse was 1.52, P<0.001. These findings highlight the need for accurate preoperative staging, particularly when multimodal therapy is planned.[41,42]

EUS is the most accurate imaging modality for locoregional staging of gastric cancer. The overall accuracy of EUS for determination of the T-stage of gastric cancer is dependent on the particular T-stage with reported rate of 78–88%, 79–100%, 63–73.9%, 85.7–95%, and 72.7–100% for T1, T2, T3, and T4 tumors respectively.[4,43-45] The overall accuracy, sensitivity, and specificity of EUS in detecting lymph node metastasis has been reported in the range of 65–80%, 66.7–91%, and 73.7–84% respectively.[4,43-48] EUS has been shown to predict the necessary operative approach in 89% of patients, while tumor resectability was predicted with a sensitivity and specificity of 87.5–94% and 83–100% respectively.[4,44,45] In one study, EUS differentiated early from advanced gastric cancer with a concordance rate of 89%.[46] For the 11% of patients with incorrect staging, in 3% of cases the tumor extent was underestimated, versus 8% of cases where it was overestimated.[46]

Other imaging modalities used in gastric cancer staging include computed tomography (CT), magnetic resonance imaging (MRI) and positron emission tomography (PET).[49-52] In a comparative study of 51 consecutive patients with gastric cancer, T- and N-staging were correctly predicted by helical CT scan in 76% and 70%, respectively, as compared to histology. EUS was superior to helical CT with correct T- and N-staging in 86% and 96%, respectively, although statistical significance was not reached.[53] Data comparing MRI with EUS in the preoperative staging of gastric cancer are limited and a study of 17 patients found MRI to be superior to EUS in assessing overall depth of tumor invasion, while EUS was superior to MRI specifically for T1 tumors and nodal staging.[49] However, the limited sample size limits the strength of any conclusions one can draw from this study. The following are representative case presentations of advanced gastric cancer and endosonography. (Figures 6-1A-C, 6-2A-H, 6-3A and B, 6-4A and B).

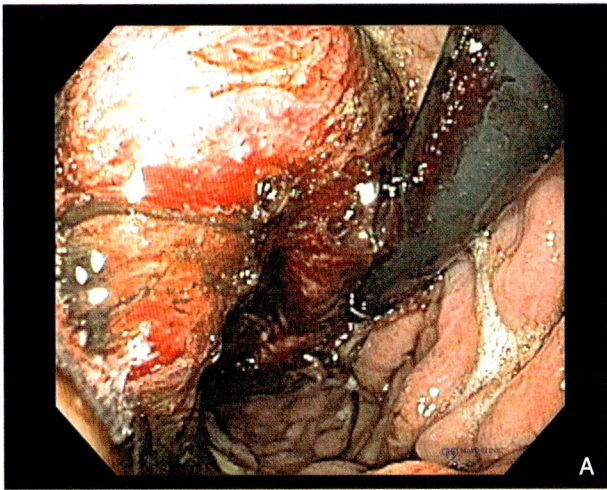

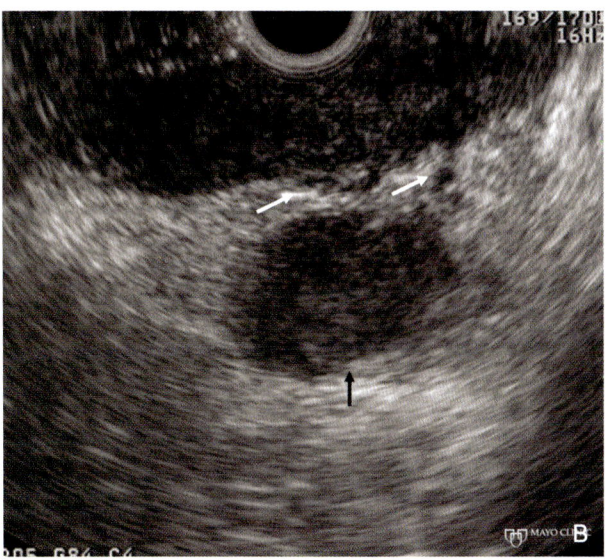

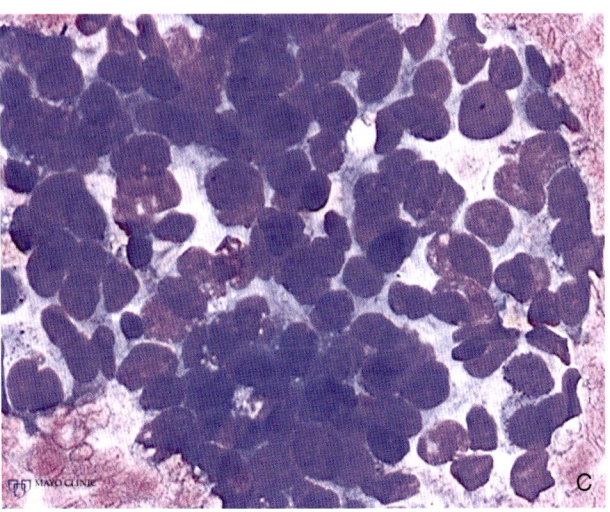

FIGURE 6–1. *A to C* This is the case of an elderly gentleman who presented with abdominal pain, weight loss, iron deficiency anemia, and occult gastrointestinal hemorrhage. On upper endoscopy, a large ulcerated and friable mass was seen in the proximal stomach (A). Biopsies revealed gastric adenocarcinoma. On radial EUS, the mass was hypoechoic and penetrated the serosa with pseudopodia-like extensions which classifies this tumor as T3 (Figure 6–1B, white arrows). A hypoechoic and round peritumoral lymph node with fairly smooth margins suspicious for metastatic involvement was also noted (B), black arrow). EUS-guided fine needle aspiration (EUS-FNA) of a nonperitumoral lymph node revealed metastatic cancer cells (C).

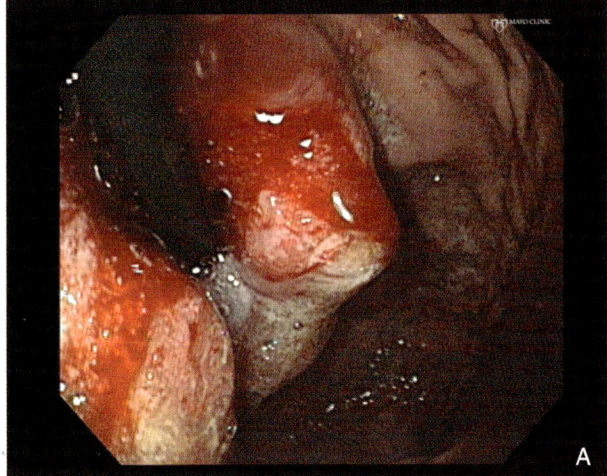
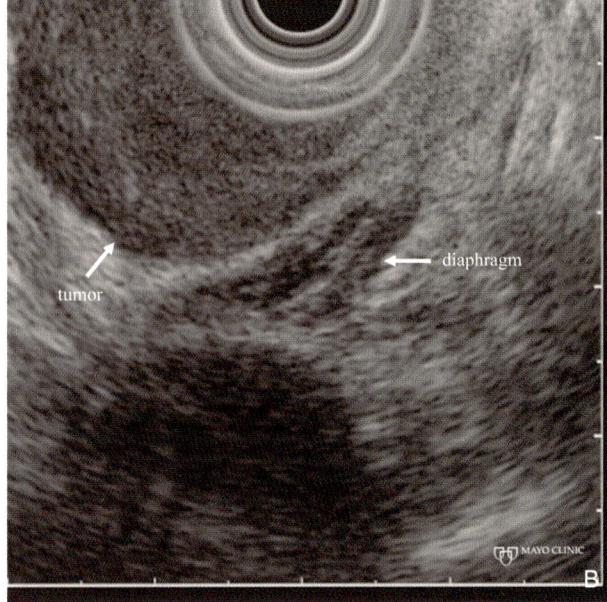
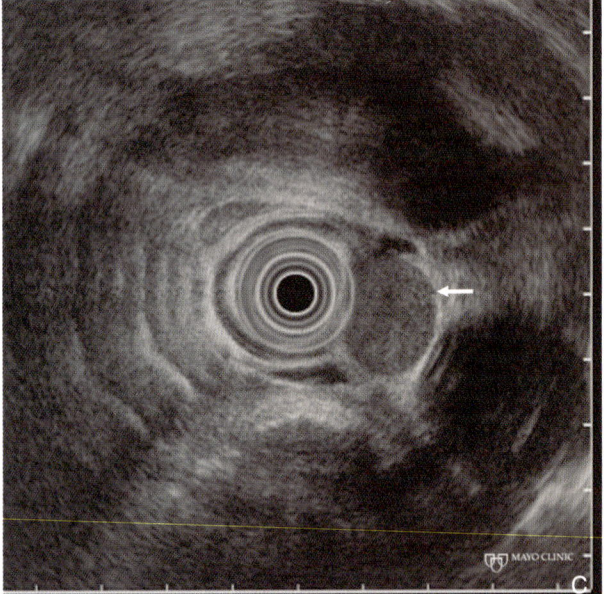
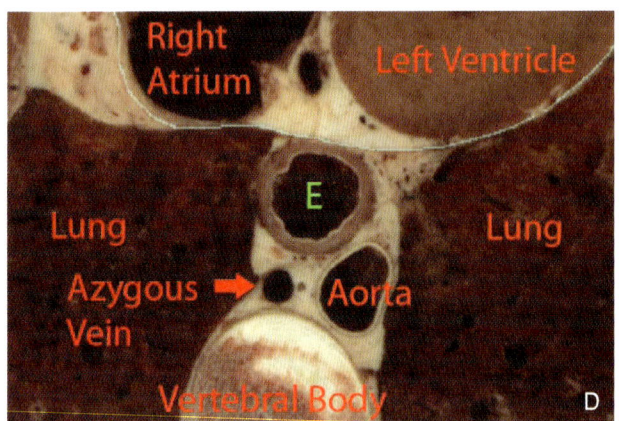
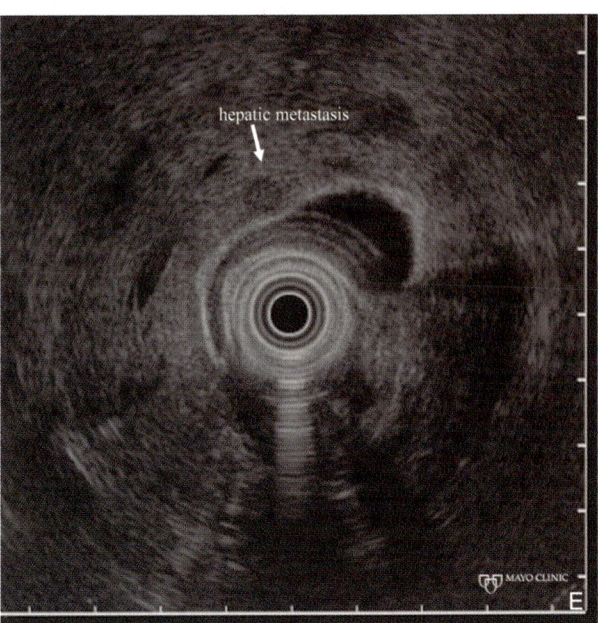

FIGURE 6–2. *A to H* (A) 66-year-old male patient presented to a hospital with dysphasia and abdominal pain. CT scan at the referring hospital identified an indeterminate hepatic mass (images not available). The patient was referred for EUS. Upper endoscopy revealed an ulcerated and friable mass at the cardia and fundus of the stomach (A). EUS showed a T3 hypoechoic tumor approaching but not invading the diaphragm (B) and malignant-appearing lymph nodes (C), mediastinal lymph node, white arrow). (D) Corresponding Visible Human Anatomy to C. Multiple lesions were also seen in the liver and spleen suspicious for metastasis (E). CT scan of the abdomen showed marked thickening of the proximal stomach and hepatic lesions suspicious for metastasis (F) Corresponding Visible Human Anatomy with localization within human model (G). PET scan revealed the primary tumor, hepatic metastasis, gastro-hepatic lymph nodes, and peri-esophageal lymph node (H).

Advanced Gastric Cancer 53

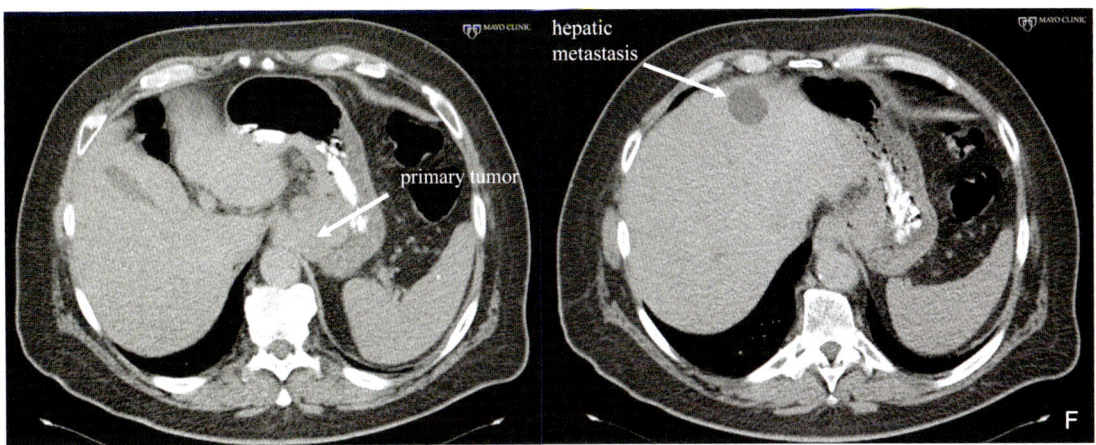

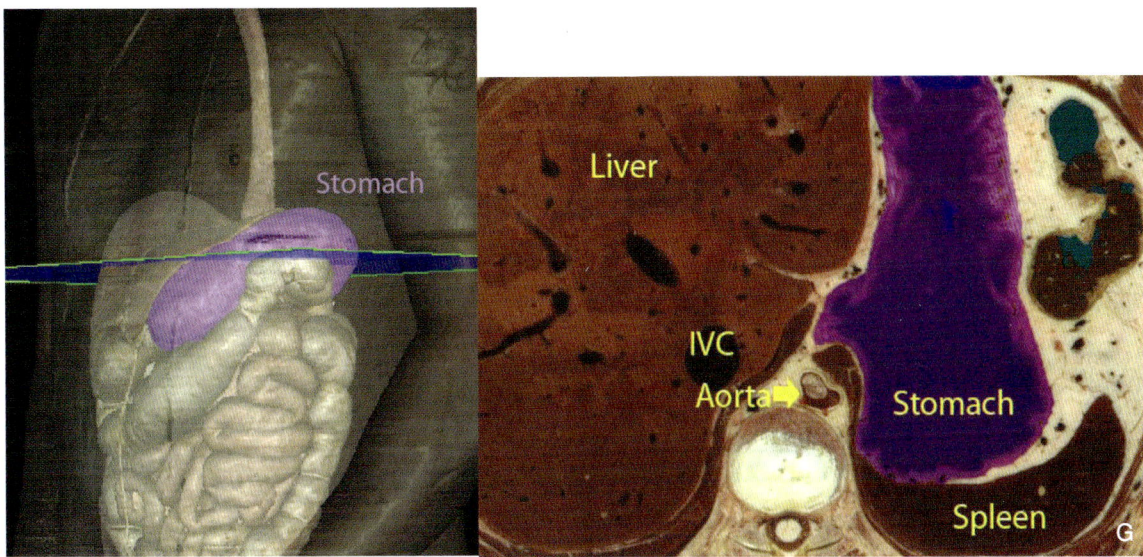

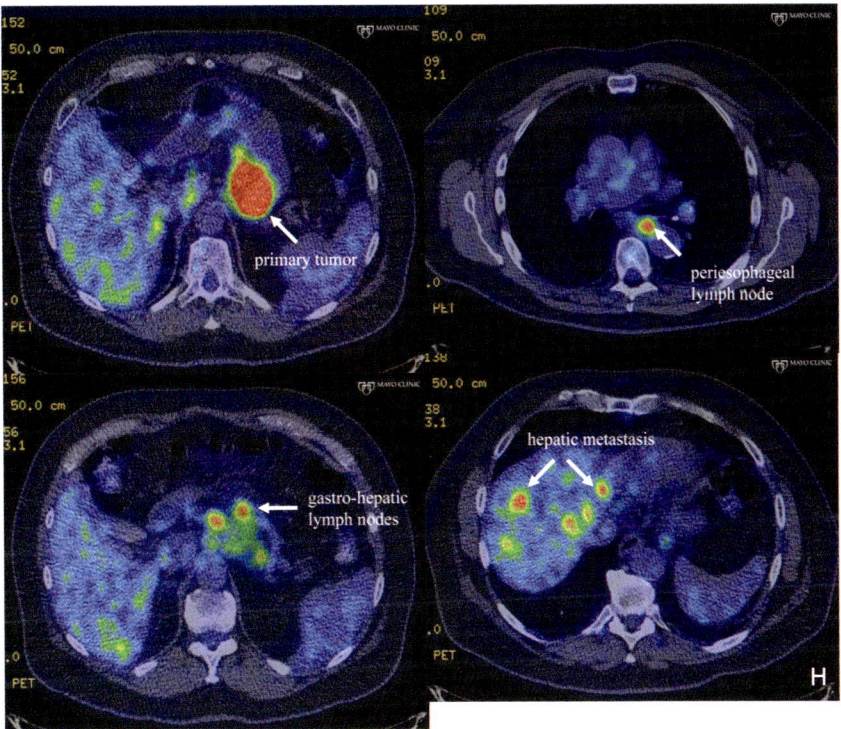

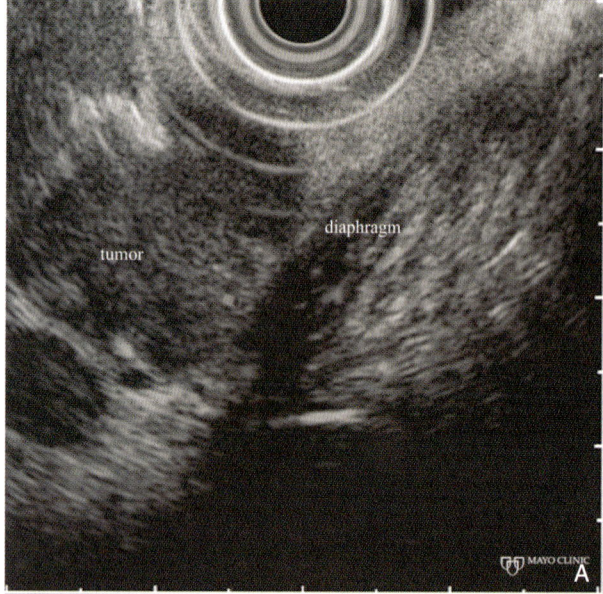 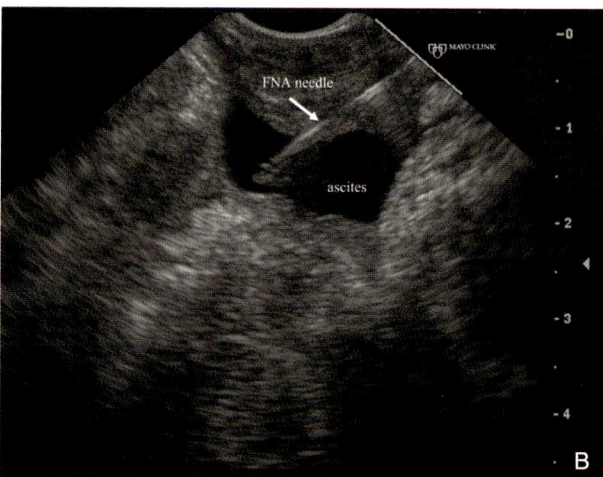

FIGURE 6–3. A and B. This figure illustrates a T4 gastric cancer with invasion into the diaphragm (A) and omental seeding with ascites (B).

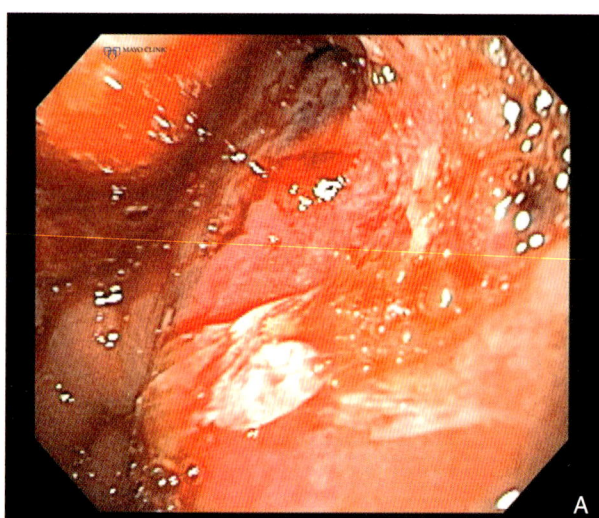 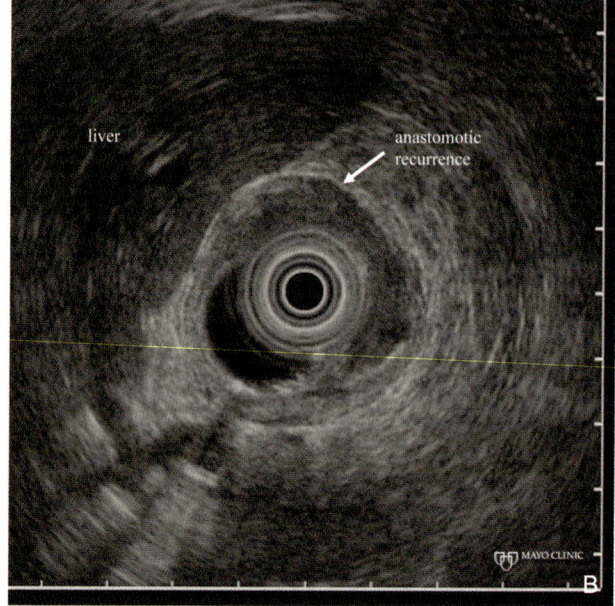

FIGURE 6–4. A and B This 66-year-old male patient with prior history of gastric cancer resected in 2003 presented with abdominal pain, weight loss, and early satiety. On upper endoscopy, there was an ulcerated and partially obstructing mass at the surgical anastomotic site (A). Endoscopic biopsies performed at the referring facility were nondiagnostic. EUS revealed hypoechoic thickening at the anastomosis abutting the liver and the presence of lymphadenopathy (B). EUS-guided FNA of the anastomosis and lymph nodes were positive for recurrent gastric cancer.

Summary

EUS is an accurate modality for staging patients with gastric cancer and has a prominent role in the decision-making process for selecting patient care.

When evaluating patients with potentially advanced gastric cancer, it is important to search for evidence of T4, N2/3, and M1 disease due to the impact on prognosis and therapy. Accurate detection of advanced disease requires use of noninvasive imaging and EUS, which should be considered complementary techniques in this setting.

References

1. DiMagno, E. P., Buxton, J. L., Regan, P. T., et al.: Ultrasonic endoscope. Lancet 1980;1:629–631.
2. Strohm, W. D., Phillip, J., Hagenmuller, F., Classen, M.: Ultrasonic tomography by means of an ultrasonic fiberendoscope. Endoscopy 1980;12:241–244.
3. Mariette, C., Balon, J. M., Maunoury, V., et al.: Value of endoscopic ultrasonography as a predictor of long-term survival in oesophageal carcinoma. Br J Surg 2003;90:1367–1372.
4. Xi, W. D., Zhao, C., Ren, G. S.: Endoscopic ultrasonography in preoperative staging of gastric cancer: determination of tumor invasion depth, nodal involvement and surgical resectability. World J Gastroenterol 2003;9:254–257.
5. Massari, M., De Simone, M., Cioffi, U., et al.: Value and limits of endorectal ultrasonography for preoperative staging of rectal carcinoma. Surg Laparosc Endosc 1998;8:438–444.
6. Midwinter, M. J., Beveridge, C. J., Wilsdon, J. B., et al.: Correlation between spiral computed tomography, endoscopic ultrasonography and findings at operation in pancreatic and ampullary tumors. Br J Surg 1999;86:189–193.
7. Yusuf, T. E., Bhutani, M. S.: Role of endoscopic ultrasonography in diseases of the extrahepatic biliary system. J Gastroenterol Hepatol 2004;19:243–250.
8. Chang, K. J., Nguyen, P., Erickson, R. A., Durbin, T. E., Katz, K. D.: The clinical utility of endoscopic ultrasound-guided fine-needle aspiration in the diagnosis and staging of pancreatic carcinoma. Gastrointest Endosc 1997;45:387–393.
9. Lindmark, G., Elvin, A., Pahlman, L., Glimelius, B.: The value of endosonography in preoperative staging of rectal cancer. Int J Colorectal Dis 1992;7:162–166.
10. Ziegler, K., Sanft, C., Zeitz, M., et al.: Evaluation of endosonography in TN staging of oesophageal cancer. Gut 1991;32:16–20.
11. Grimm, H., Binmoeller, K. F., Hamper, K., et al.: Endosonography for preoperative locoregional staging of esophageal and gastric cancer. Endoscopy 1993;25:224–230.
12. Yusuf, T. E., Bhutani, M. S.: Differentiating pancreatic cancer from pseudotumorous chronic pancreatitis. Curr Gastroenterol Rep 2002;4:135–139.
13. Frossard, J. L., Amouyal, P., Amouyal, G., et al.: Performance of endosonography-guided fine needle aspiration and biopsy in the diagnosis of pancreatic cystic lesions. Am J Gastroenterol 2003;98:1516–1524.
14. Awad, S. S., Fagan, S., Abudayyeh, S., et al.: Preoperative evaluation of hepatic lesions for the staging of hepatocellular and metastatic liver carcinoma using endoscopic ultrasonography. Am J Surg 2002;184:601–605
15. Gress, F. G., Savides, T. J., Sandler, A., et al.: Endoscopic ultrasonography, fine-needle aspiration biopsy guided by endoscopic ultrasonography, and computed tomography in the preoperative staging of non-small-cell lung cancer: a comparison study. Ann Intern Med 1997;127:604–612.
16. Larsen, S. S., Vilmann, P., Krasnik, M., et al.: Endoscopic ultrasound guided biopsy performed routinely in lung cancer staging spares futile thoracotomies: preliminary results from a randomised clinical trial. Lung Cancer 2005;49:377–385.
17. Larsen, S. S., Vilmann, P., Krasnik, M., et al.: Endoscopic ultrasound guided biopsy versus mediastinoscopy for analysis of paratracheal and subcarinal lymph nodes in lung cancer staging. Lung Cancer 2005;48:85–92.
18. Volmar, K. E., Vollmer, R. T., Jowell, P. S., Nelson, R. C., Xie, H. B.: Pancreatic FNA in 1000 cases: a comparison of imaging modalities. Gastrointest Endosc 2005;61:854–861.
19. Gress, F., Schmitt, C., Sherman, S., et al.: Endoscopic ultrasound-guided celiac plexus block for managing abdominal pain associated with chronic pancreatitis: a prospective single center experience. Am J Gastroenterol 2001;96:409–416.
20. Gunaratnam, N. T., Sarma, A. V., Norton, I. D., Wiersema, M. J.: A prospective study of EUS-guided celiac plexus neurolysis for pancreatic cancer pain. Gastrointest Endosc 2001;54:316–324.
21. Goldberg, S. N., Mallery, S., Gazelle, G. S., Brugge, W. R.: EUS-guided radiofrequency ablation in the pancreas: results in a porcine model. Gastrointest Endosc 1999;50:392–401.
22. Sun, S., Qingjie, L., Qiyong, G., et al.: EUS-guided interstitial brachytherapy of the pancreas: a feasibility study. Gastrointest Endosc 2005;62:775–779.
23. Shah, J. N., Ahmad, N. A., Beilstein, M. C., Ginsberg, G. G., Kochman, M. L.: Clinical impact of endoscopic ultrasonography on the management of malignancies. Clin Gastroenterol Hepatol 2004;2:1069–1073.
24. National Cancer Institute. Stomach (gastric) cancer. Available at: http://www.cancer.gov/cancertopics/types/stomach/, 2007.
25. Blot, W. J., Devesa, S. S., Kneller, R. W., Fraumeni, J. F., Jr.: Rising incidence of adenocarcinoma of the esophagus and gastric cardia. Jama 1991;265:1287–1289.
26. Craanen, M. E., Dekker, W., Blok, P., Ferwerda, J., Tytgat, G. N.: Time trends in gastric carcinoma: changing patterns of type and location. Am J Gastroenterol 1992;87:572–579.
27. Fuchs, C. S., Mayer, R. J.: Gastric carcinoma. N Engl J Med 1995;333:32–41.
28. AJCC Cancer Staging Manual (6th edition). New York: Springer, 2006.
29. Siewert, J. R., Bottcher, K., Stein, H. J., Roder, J. D.: Relevant prognostic factors in gastric cancer: ten-year results of the German Gastric Cancer Study. Ann Surg 1998;228:449–461.
30. Saito, H., Fukumoto, Y., Osaki, T., et al.: Prognostic Significance of Level and Number of Lymph Node Metastases in Patients with Gastric Cancer. Ann Surg Oncol 2007.
31. Adachi, Y., Shiraishi, N., Suematsu, T., et al.: Most important lymph node information in gastric cancer: multivariate prognostic study. Ann Surg Oncol 2000;7:503–507.
32. Kim, J. P., Lee, J. H., Kim, S. J., Yu, H. J., Yang, H. K.: Clinicopathologic characteristics and prognostic factors in 10 783 patients with gastric cancer. Gastric Cancer 1998;1:125–133.
33. Adachi, Y., Yasuda, K., Inomata, M., et al.: Pathology and prognosis of gastric carcinoma: well versus poorly differentiated type. Cancer 2000;89:1418–1424.
34. Nakamura, K., Ueyama, T., Yao, T., et al.: Pathology and prognosis of gastric carcinoma. Findings in 10,000 patients who underwent primary gastrectomy. Cancer 1992;70:1030–1037.
35. Wanebo, H. J., Kennedy, B. J., Chmiel, J., et al.: Cancer of the stomach. A patient care study by the

American College of Surgeons. Ann Surg 1993; 218:583–592.
36. Roukos, D. H.: Current status and future perspectives in gastric cancer management. Cancer Treat Rev 2000;26:243–255.
37. Chang, H. M., Jung, K. H., Kim, T. Y., et al.: A phase III randomized trial of 5-fluorouracil, doxorubicin, and mitomycin C versus 5-fluorouracil and mitomycin C versus 5-fluorouracil alone in curatively resected gastric cancer. Ann Oncol 2002;13:1779–1785.
38. Fenoglio-Preiser, C. M., Noffsinger, A. E., Belli, J., Stemmermann, G. N.: Pathologic and phenotypic features of gastric cancer. Semin Oncol 1996;23:292–306.
39. Scheiman, J. M., Cutler, A. F.: Helicobacter pylori and gastric cancer. Am J Med 1999;106:222–226.
40. Macdonald, J. S., Smalley, S. R., Benedetti, J., et al.: Chemoradiotherapy after surgery compared with surgery alone for adenocarcinoma of the stomach or gastroesophageal junction. N Engl J Med 2001;345: 725–730.
41. Takemoto, T., Tada, M., Dittler, H. J., Rosch, T., Siewert, J. R.: Impact of staging on treatment of gastric carcinoma. Endoscopy 1993;25:46–50.
42. Dittler, H. J., Siewert, J. R.: Role of endoscopic ultrasonography in gastric carcinoma. Endoscopy 1993;25: 162–166.
43. Chen, C. H., Yang, C. C., Yeh, Y. H.: Preoperative staging of gastric cancer by endoscopic ultrasound: the prognostic usefulness of ascites detected by endoscopic ultrasound. J Clin Gastroenterol 2002;35:321–327.
44. Ganpathi, I. S., So, J. B., Ho, K. Y.: Endoscopic ultrasonography for gastric cancer: does it influence treatment? Surg Endosc 2006;20:559–562.
45. Willis, S., Truong, S., Gribnitz, S., Fass, J., Schumpelick, V.: Endoscopic ultrasonography in the preoperative staging of gastric cancer: accuracy and impact on surgical therapy. Surg Endosc 2000;14:951–954.
46. Wang, J. Y., Hsieh, J. S., Huang, Y. S., et al.: Endoscopic ultrasonography for preoperative locoregional staging and assessment of resectability in gastric cancer. Clin Imaging 1998;22:355–359.
47. Tsendsuren, T., Jun, S. M., Mian, X.H.: Usefulness of endoscopic ultrasonography in preoperative TNM staging of gastric cancer. World J Gastroenterol 2006;12:43–47.
48. Shimoyama, S., Yasuda, H., Hashimoto, M., et al.: Accuracy of linear-array EUS for preoperative staging of gastric cardia cancer. Gastrointest Endosc 2004;60: 50–55.
49. Arocena, M. G., Barturen, A., Bujanda, L., et al.: MRI and endoscopic ultrasonography in the staging of gastric cancer. Rev Esp Enferm Dig 2006;98:582–590.
50. D'Elia, F., Zingarelli, A., Palli, D., Grani, M.: Hydrodynamic CT preoperative staging of gastric cancer: correlation with pathological findings. A prospective study of 107 cases. Eur Radiol 2000;10:1877–85.
51. Kim, A. Y., Kim, H. J., Ha, H. K.: Gastric cancer by multidetector row CT: preoperative staging. Abdom Imaging 2005;30:465–472.
52. Yun, M., Lim, J. S., Noh, S. H., et al.: Lymph node staging of gastric cancer using (18)F-FDG PET: a comparison study with CT. J Nucl Med 2005;46:1582–1588.
53. Habermann, C. R., Weiss, F., Riecken, R., et al.: Preoperative staging of gastric adenocarcinoma: comparison of helical CT and endoscopic US. Radiology 2004;230:465–471.

CHAPTER 7

Large Gastric Folds

Dr. Giancarlo Caletti
Dr. Pietro Fusaroli
Dr. Eugenio Giovannini
Dr. Antonino Grillo

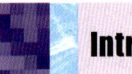

Introduction

A diagnosis of large gastric folds (LGF) is usually made if folds do not flatten at endoscopy (Figure 7–1), or if thickened folds are seen at barium upper gastrointestinal (UGI) series or CT scan[1-2] (Figure 7–2). EUS represents the best way to obtain in vivo images of the different layers of the gastric wall. At EUS, the normal gastric wall thickness range is assessed to be between 0.8 and 3.6 mm[3] (Figure 7–3). Diagnosis of gastric wall thickening and LGF is generally established

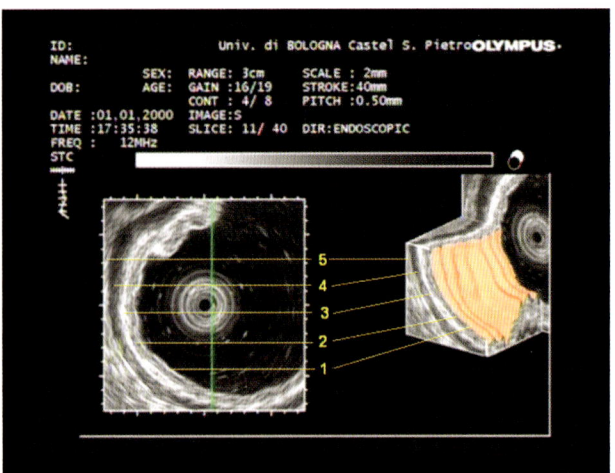

FIGURE 7–3. Normal gastric wall seen with a 3D miniature probe at 12 MHz. 1 = interface echo/mucosa; 2 = mucosa; 3 = submucosa; 4 = muscularis propria; 5 = serosa.

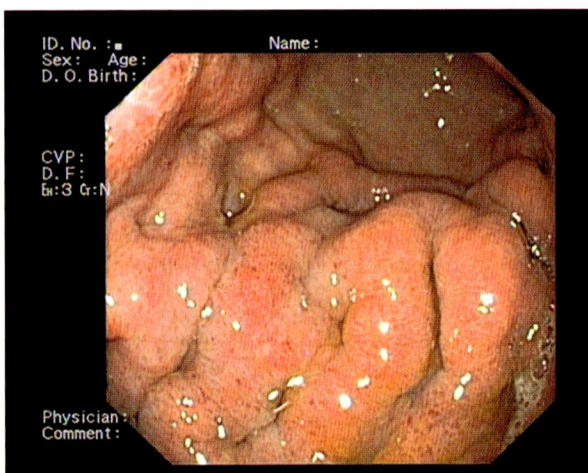

FIGURE 7–1. A typical endoscopic view of LGF in the gastric corpus. Folds do not flatten with air insufflation and appear indurated and infiltrated. Overlying mucosa looks edemathous, red, and inflamed. Differential diagnosis by sole means of endoscopy is almost impossible.

at EUS under routine clinical conditions, when the whole thickness of the five layers is greater than 4 mm.[4-5] This widening of the gastric folds is seen in a number of different benign and malignant conditions. Inflammatory and infectious diseases can be involved, including H. pylori infection;[6-11] vascular and infiltrating diseases may sometimes be present, although these do not appear to play a major etiological role.[12-13] Finally, malignant diseases, such as carcinoma and lymphoma, must always be considered[14-15] (Table 7-1). A differential diagnosis can be quite demanding; however, it is mandatory to

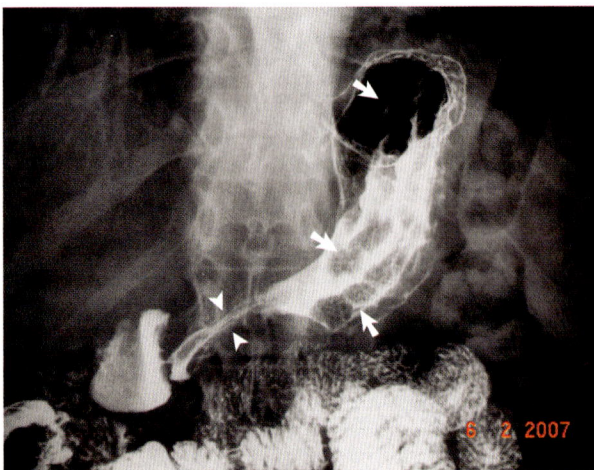

FIGURE 7–2. A typical aspect of LGF seen at barium UGI series. Contrast medium enhances the visualization of markedly thickened gastric folds (arrows). Stenosis of the lumen at the level of the antrum is also visible (arrowhead).

Table 7-1 — Etiology of Large Gastric Folds

Malignancies	Adenocarcinoma and linitis plastica; lymphoma; metastases
Infections	Secondary syphilis; tubercolosis; CMV; HSV; histoplasmosis; cryptococcosis; aspergillosis; H. pylori infection; anisakiasis
Infiltrative Diseases	Crohn's disease; sarcoidosis; amyloidosis; eosinophilic, granulomatous and lymphocytic gastritis
Vascular Diseases	Portal hypertensive gastropathy; gastric varices
Benign Conditions	Menetrier's disease; Zollinger-Ellison syndrome; gastritis; hyperrugosity; gastritis cystica profunda

establish the etiology of LGF correctly to assess the optimal treatment for these patients. EUS has been demonstrated to be an accurate technique for the differential diagnosis of LGF. Gastric lymphoma, linitis plastica, Menetrier's disease, inflammatory conditions, and gastric varices account for the most common etiologies that can be accurately identified by using EUS.

EUS for Differential Diagnosis

A differential diagnosis between gastric lymphoma, linitis plastica, and other forms of gastric wall infiltrative disease is fundamental for therapeutic purposes but may be challenging. Standard endoscopic mucosal biopsies are often unrevealing and have proven a limited diagnostic yield, as they contain only superficial mucosa and are unable to identify an involvement of the deep layers. In some series of infiltrative malignancies of the stomach, traditional biopsies were positive in only 50% of the cases.[16-20] Specimens obtained by large-valve biopsy forceps may increase diagnostic sensitivity only to a limited extent; diathermic snare can be used to obtain deeper samples, but at the cost of increased risk of hemorrhage or perforation.[21-22] For these reasons, even laparotomy was advocated to obtain a surgical, full-thickness, gastric biopsy specimen. Other authors have suggested and employed more refined techniques, such as EUS-guided fine-needle aspiration (FNA) (Figure 7–4) and the guillotine-needle biopsy.[23-26]

Nevertheless, the differential diagnosis can be very difficult by means of endoscopic appearance, X-ray

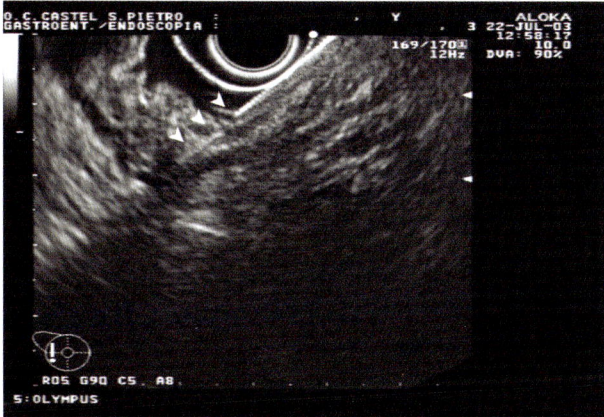

FIGURE 7–4. EUS-FNA of the gastric wall in a case of LGF. The needle (arrowhead) penetrating the deep layers of the wall (submucosa and muscularis propria) may allow for enhancement of the accuracy of malignancy detection.

Table 7–2. Layers Principally Involved According to Etiologies

Disease	Layers
H. pylori infection	2
Menetrier's disease	2
Gastritis, hyperrugosity	2
Anisakiasis	3
Gastritis cystica profunda	3
Gastric varices	3
Adenocarcinoma, linitis plastica	2, 2+3, 2+3+4
Gastric lymphoma	2, 2+3, 2+3+4

examination, and even biopsy, because widening of the gastric folds is seen in many benign and malignant conditions. Thus LGF may still escape a traditional combined endoscopic-histologic diagnostic approach. The advent of EUS has led to a marked improvement in diagnostic accuracy in this respect.[27] EUS, with its ability to visualize the different histological layers of the gastric wall, can correctly asses which layers are mainly thickened. Every disease presenting with LGF shows a different level of gastric wall infiltration, thus the spectrum of differential diagnosis can be limited (Table 7–2). A detailed discussion about the specific EUS appearance of different pathological entities appears in the paragraphs that follow.

Nevertheless, EUS must always be used in combination with endoscopic biopsy. EUS can help in determining where to perform biopsies in order to avoid false negative results, and in indicating the need of a large particle biopsy. Contraindication to perform biopsies can also emerge from EUS, for example when gastric varices are detected.

The ability of EUS to evaluate patients with LGF has been investigated in detail by a few authors. Mendis et al.[28] examined the utility of EUS in 28 patients with endoscopically or radiographically diagnosed LGF, for most of whom endoscopic biopsies were inconclusive for malignancy. EUS demonstrated gastric varices in four patients, and biopsy specimens were not taken. In three patients, biopsies were negative for malignancy. However, because of ultrasonographic findings of wall thickening involving layers three and four, they underwent laparotomy, which revealed primary gastric carcinoma. In the remaining patients, large-forceps endoscopic biopsy revealed acute or chronic inflammation in 16 patients (67%), malignancy in 4 patients (16%), and Menetrier's disease in 1 patient (4%). Malignancy did not develop in any of the patients with gastric wall thickening limited to layer two and negative bioptic results during a mean follow-up period of 35 months.

Songur et al.[29] analyzed the EUS features of 35 patients with LGF describing some findings useful to characterize each type of lesion. According to these authors, when the second layer alone is thickened, Menetrier's disease may be one of the possible pathologic entities. When the third layer alone is abnormally enlarged, anisakiasis might be suspected. Most patients with scirrhous carcinoma showed an abnormally enlarged third and fourth layer. Thus, the second and the third layer may be thickened in healthy subjects with simple hyperrugosity but also in patients with gastric lymphoma. The fourth layer was significantly thickened only in malignant conditions.

Maunoury et al.[30] stated that endosonographic aspects may be helpful in distinguishing Menetrier's disease from lymphocytic gastritis, although biopsies are necessary for final confirmation of diagnosis because some overlapping endosonographic aspects may exist.

A recent study from Ginès et al.[31] analyzed 61 patients evaluated with EUS after findings of LGF at endoscopy with biopsies negative for malignancy. Twenty-one patients with EUS findings suggestive of malignancies underwent surgery, macrobiopsy, or repeated follow-up endoscopies. Twenty patients (95%) had a final diagnosis of gastric cancer. Among the 40 patients without suspicious EUS findings, 4 had LGF due to histologically documented benign conditions. One case was affected by mucosa associated lymphoid tissue (MALT) lymphoma (2.5%). In the remaining 35 patients, followed for a median time of 43 months, no neoplastic conditions were reported. The enlargement of deep layers at EUS was the only independent predicting factor for malignancy. Other EUS factors suggestive of malignancy were thickened gastric wall, inability of water distension, nonpreserved wall layer structure, and presence of ascites or lymph nodes with suspicious features. In this study, overall EUS performance for a diagnosis of neoplasm was extremely good, with sensitivity and specificity of 95% and 97% respectively, and an accuracy value of 97%. Thus the authors described EUS as a reliable tool for assessment of the effective risk for malignancy in patients with LGF and negative biopsies.

In conclusion, when EUS abnormalities involve only the mucosal layer, endoscopic biopsies are often diagnostic, and a benign condition is often revealed. On the contrary, abnormalities involving the muscularis propria in the absence of ulceration strongly suggest malignancy and should be further investigated even if endoscopic biopsies are negative.

A final algorithm based on EUS findings can be suggested for patients with LGF of different etiologies.

When abnormalities involve the second layer, endoscopic biopsies are usually diagnostic; when abnormalities involve the second and third layers, large particle biopsy should be considered; when abnormalities involve the fourth layer, malignancy should be strongly suspected, and FNA or surgery are recommended even if standard biopsies are negative.

EUS for Staging of Malignancies

When a malignant condition is diagnosed, an accurate staging is essential to evaluate the patient's prognosis and to address the therapeutic choice between the available options. Both gastric carcinoma (linitis plastica, scirrhous carcinoma) and gastric lymphomas can present as LGF. At present, EUS is the most accurate imaging modality for evaluation and staging of these infiltrative gastric lesions, as shown by the number of papers dealing with this subject, which has progressively increased in recent years.[32]

For gastric carcinoma, the tumor, lymph nodes, and metastasis (TNM) system is commonly used and has a proven superior prognostic value in respect to previous systems.[33] The most recent update of the TNM classification for gastric cancer[34] is shown in Table 7-3. An accuracy of about 80% has been reported in the T staging of gastric cancer,[35,36] with a slight tendency of EUS to overestimate between T2 and T3 stages.[37,38] However, EUS is 90% to 99% accurate in distinguishing between stage T1 and stage T2,[39,40] which is the basic criterion for the diagnosis between early and advanced gastric cancer. These results indicate EUS as the more accurate technique for the T staging, superior to helical CT.[41]

EUS is an extremely reliable technique also for the diagnosis and staging of gastric lymphoma and in particular of mucosa associated lymphoid tissue (MALT) lymphoma, which is the most relevant cause of LGF.[42] Accuracy of EUS for staging gastric lymphoma, both before and after therapy, has been demonstrated by several authors.[43-47] Our group reported 89% sensitivity, 97% specificity, and 95% overall accuracy of EUS evaluation of lymphoma depth of invasion.[42] However, Fischbach et al.[48] have raised a word of caution in this respect. They performed a multicenter study evaluating the accuracy of EUS in the staging of gastric lymphoma at 34 different centers. Data from preoperative EUS procedures were compared with the histopathologic stage of resection specimens in 70 patients with newly diagnosed primary gastric lymphoma. They found that EUS correctly classified the lymphoma in only 37 of 70

Table 7-3 TNM Staging System for Gastric Cancer

TX	Tumor extent not specified
T0	No evidence of tumor
Tis	Intraepithelial tumor without lamina propria invasion
T1	Tumor confined to the mucosa/submucosa
T2	Tumor involving muscularis propria or subserosa
T3	Tumor which penetrates serosa (visceral peritoneum) without invasion of adjacent structures
T4	Tumor which invades adjacent structures or organs
NX	Involvement of lymph nodes not assessed
N0	No evidence of lymph node involvement
N1	Involvement of 1 to 6 regional* lymph nodes
N2	Involvement of 7 to 15 regional lymph nodes
N3	Involvement of more than 15 regional lymph nodes
MX	Metastatic dissemination not assessed
M0	No evidence of metastatic dissemination
M1	Presence of distant metastases

* Perigastric lymph nodes and those located along the ramifications of the coeliac artery (left gastric artery, common hepatic artery, splenic artery).

patients (53%). However, the authors found an explanation for the relative lack of accuracy, due to a high number of participating centers performing few EUS procedures. Nevertheless, this study underlines the importance of the presence of highly experienced operators in large-volume EUS centers in order to maximize the accuracy and diagnostic yield of the technique.

We believe, as stated before by Shimodaira et al.,[49] that the TNM rather than the modified Ann Arbor or Lugano classifications should be adopted to stage gastric lymphoma. TNM classification allows a detailed assessment of lymphoproliferative disease as it differentiates the degree of mural involvement layer by layer, while other classifications contemplate only few stages of mural involvement.[50-51] As shown by different studies, an accurate EUS assessment of infiltration of every single layer is fundamental for predicting prognosis and establishing the appropriate therapy. Ruskone-Fourmestraux et al.[52] tend to agree upon the opportunity of adopting the TNM system for EUS purposes of staging. However, as the TNM was created for staging carcinomas rather than lymphomas, they suggested a modified staging system, termed as the Paris classification, centered upon the previously mentioned TNM, but with some slight modifications. This new staging system adequately records depth of tumor infiltration, extent of nodal involvement, and specific lymphoma spreading (Table 7–4). It is adjusted to the gastrointestinal origin of the lymphoma, considering histopathological characteristics of extranodal B- and T-cell lymphomas. According to the authors, the use of this system in future studies will permit accurate comparison of the reported cohorts and should allow rapid accumulation of good data for proper stratification of patients for risk assessment and treatment options.

Regarding perigastric lymph nodes, EUS can detect nodes as small as 3-4 mm in diameter (Figure 7–5). However, for the differential diagnosis between benign and malignant lymph nodes, relying only on EUS features can be problematic. One of the most comprehensive series on this subject came from Catalano et al.[53] who suggested that rounded, sharply demarcated, homogeneous, hypoechoic lymph nodes of less than 1 cm indicate malignancy, whereas elongated, heterogeneous, hyperechoic lymph nodes with indistinct borders are more likely to be benign. However, the assessment of these features is operator-dependent and micrometastases can not be identified.

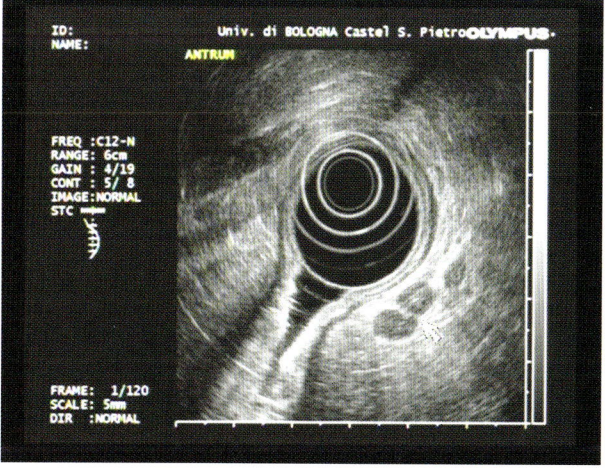

FIGURE 7–5. Small perigastric lymph nodes (arrow) can be reliably detected by EUS. These lymph nodes are round, hypoechoic, and sharply demarcated. This patient was affected by gastric MALT lymphoma (stage T1sm N1).

Table 7-4 Paris Staging System for Primary Gastrointestinal Lymphomas *

TX	Lymphoma extent not specified
T0	No evidence of lymphoma
T1	Lymphoma confined to the mucosa/submucosa
T1m	Lymphoma confined to mucosa
T1sm	Lymphoma confined to submucosa
T2	Lymphoma infiltrates muscularis propria or subserosa
T3	Lymphoma penetrates serosa (visceral peritoneum) without invasion of adjacent structures
T4	Lymphoma invades adjacent structures or organs
NX	Involvement of lymph nodes not assessed
N0	No evidence of lymph node involvement
N1**	Involvement of regional lymph nodes
N2	Involvement of intra-abdominal lymph nodes beyond the regional area
N3	Spread to extra-abdominal lymph nodes
MX	Dissemination of lymphoma not assessed
M0	No evidence of extranodal dissemination
M1	Non-continuous involvement of separate site in gastrointestinal tract (eg, stomach and rectum)
M2	Noncontinuous involvement of other tissues (eg, peritoneum, pleura) or organs (eg, tonsils, parotid gland, ocular adnexa, lung, liver, spleen, kidney, breast etc.)
BX	Involvement of bone marrow not assessed
B0	No evidence of bone marrow involvement
B1	Lymphomatous infiltration of bone marrow
TNM	Clinical staging: status of tumor, node, metastasis, bone marrow
PTNMB	Histopathological staging: status of tumor, node, metastasis, bone marrow
PN	The histological examination will ordinarily include six or more lymph nodes.

*Valid for lymphomas originating from the gastro-oesophageal junction to the anus (as defined by identical histomorphological structure). In case of more than one visible lesion synchronously originating in the gastrointestinal tract, give the characteristics of the more advanced lesion.

**Anatomical designation of lymph nodes as "regional" according to site:
(a) stomach: perigastric nodes and those located along the ramifications of the coeliac artery (that is, left gastric artery, common hepatic artery, splenic artery) in accordance with compartments I and II of the Japanese Research Society for Gastric Cancer (1995);
(b) duodenum: pancreaticoduodenal, pyloric, hepatic, and superior mesenteric nodes;
(c) jejunum/ileum: mesenteric nodes and, for the terminal ileum only, the ileocolic as well as the posterior caecal nodes;
(d) colorectum: pericolic and perirectal nodes and those located along the ileocolic, right, middle, and left colic, inferior mesenteric, superior rectal, and internal iliac arteries.

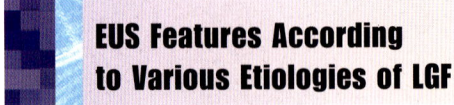

EUS Features According to Various Etiologies of LGF

Lymphoma

The gastrointestinal tract is the most common extranodal site of non-Hodgkin's lymphomas (NHLs), gastric localization being the most common one. In case of endoscopic diagnosis of LGF, a lymphoma is the malignant cause more commonly involved. The stomach can harbor a primary NHL or be involved secondarily by a disseminated nodal disease. Primary gastric NHL is very often the unique localization of the disease in which EUS plays a central role for diagnosis and staging. Large B-cell lymphoma and mucosa-associated lymphoid tissue (MALT) lymphoma represent the more common etiologies, accounting for more than 80% of cases. Less commonly, primary gastric mantle cell (Figure 7–6) or T-cell lymphomas have been described.[54-55] Cases of synchronous or metachronous occurrence of gastric lymphoma and gastric adenocarcinoma have also been reported (56). In particular, after conservative treatment for MALT lymphoma, both rapid progression of precancerous lesions (57) and occurrence of gastric carcinoma de novo (Figure 7–7a - 7–7c)[58-59] can happen.

Signs and symptoms in case of primary gastric lymphoma are generally extremely unspecific, making a clinical diagnosis almost impossible. Sometimes CT scan or abdominal ultrasound can identify an enlarged gastric wall, but usually an endoscopic examination

Large Gastric Folds 63

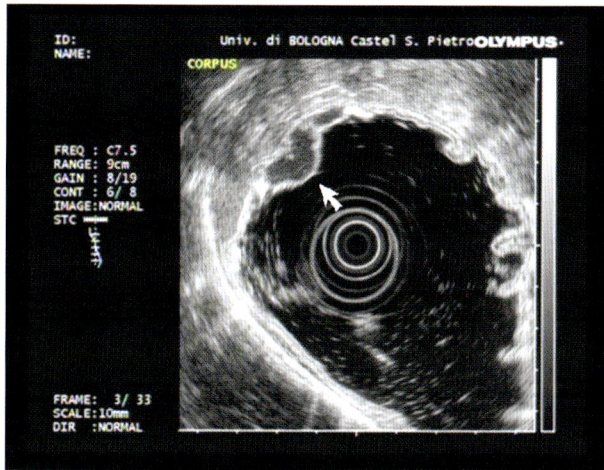

FIGURE 7–6. Mantle cell lymphoma of the stomach. A focal thickening (arrow) of the second layer (mucosa) is visible; the underlying layers appear normal. This finding is compatible with a T1m stage.

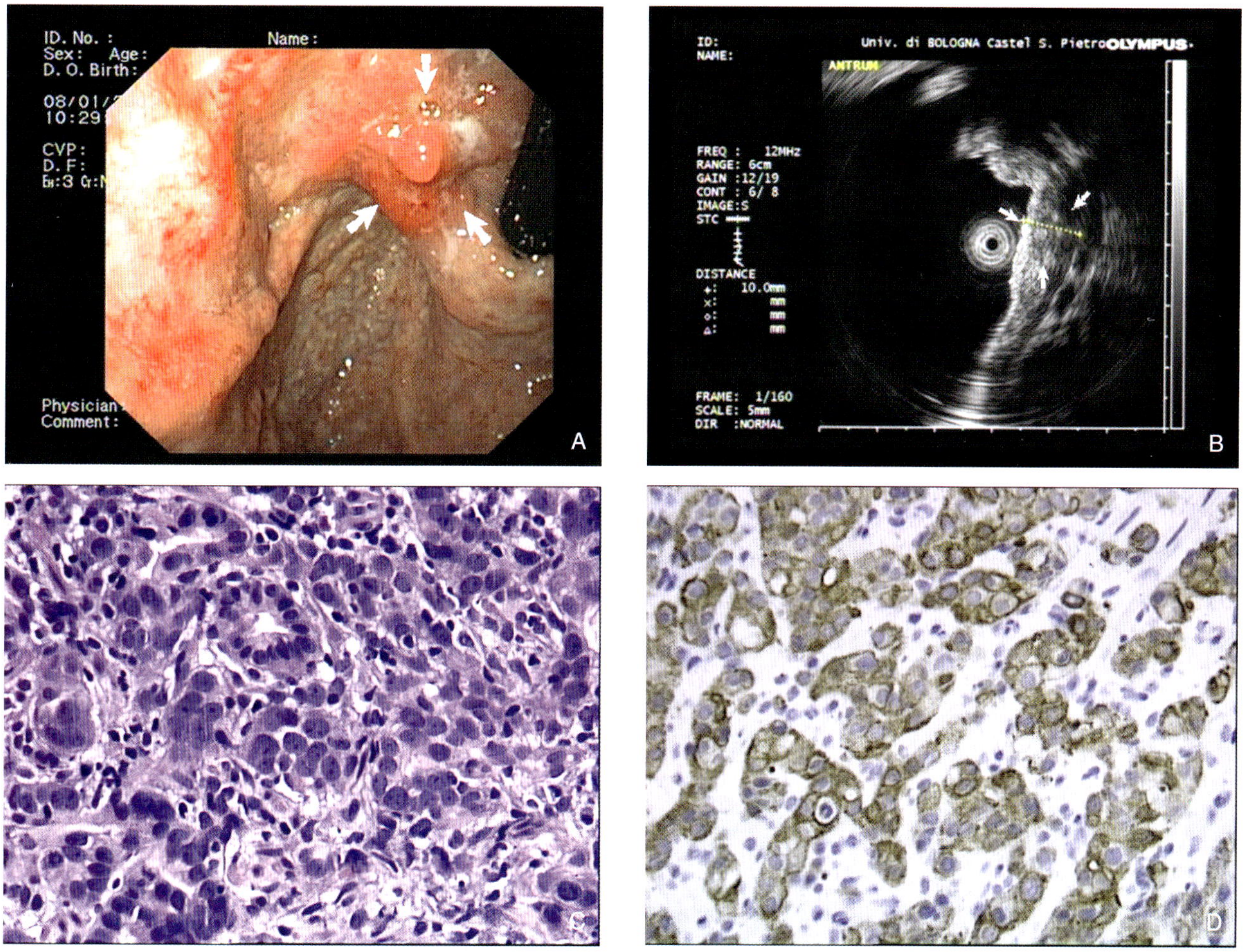

FIGURE 7–7 *A to D* (A) A case of gastric carcinoma arisen on a gastric high grade lymphoma. The mucosa of the fundus appears markedly inflamed and dystrophic, with cobblestone aspect and diffuse fragility. Under the cardia, a small ulcerated and elevated lesion is visible (arrows). This lesion turned out to be positive for carcinoma at histology. (B) EUS scanning with a 12 MHz miniprobe at the level of the cardia. A hypoechoic nodule is shown (arrows) corresponding to the carcinoma detected histologically. The gastric wall is thickened, and the layers are not distinguishable anymore. The level of infiltration seems to be reaching the fourth layer (muscularis propria). The neoplasm is staged T2. (C) A histological specimen of this lesion shows irregular aggregates of epithelial cells spreading over a diffuse lymphoid infiltrate. The normal glandular structure is poorly recognizable. (D) The epithelial origin of carcinomatous cells, with enlarged and irregular nuclei, is shown by positive staining for AE1 and AE3 cytokeratins (Courtesy of Dr. Roberto Nannini, Dept. of Pathology, AUSL of Imola, Italy).

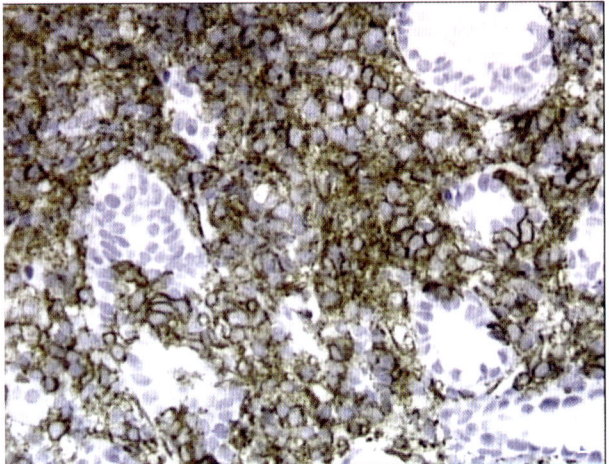

FIGURE 7–7. E (E) At immunohistochemistry, a positive staining for the B cell-associated antigen CD20 confirms the lymphomatous infiltration (Courtesy of Dr. Roberto Nannini, Dept. of Pathology, AUSL of Imola, Italy).

with gastric biopsies, combined with EUS, is the only way to reach a definitive diagnosis (Figure 7–8a - 7–8c).

MALT lymphomas, first differentiated from low-grade nodal B-cell lymphomas in 1983 by Isaacson and Wright,[60] are of particular interest for the endosonographer. In this pathology, an accurate EUS staging can address the choice among completely different therapeutic approaches. The impact of EUS on clinical outcome is consistent for these patients, as EUS can predict MALT remission after the simple eradication therapy of H. pylori.[61-6263] In fact, early stage disease infiltrating only the mucosa and/or submucosa, without involvement of lymph nodes, showed up to 80% response rate (64-6566). These results suggest that more aggressive therapies, such as chemotherapy and surgery, can now be avoided in the majority of patients affected from low-grade MALT lymphoma, and can be reserved only for those with advanced disease or with no response to antibiotic treatment.

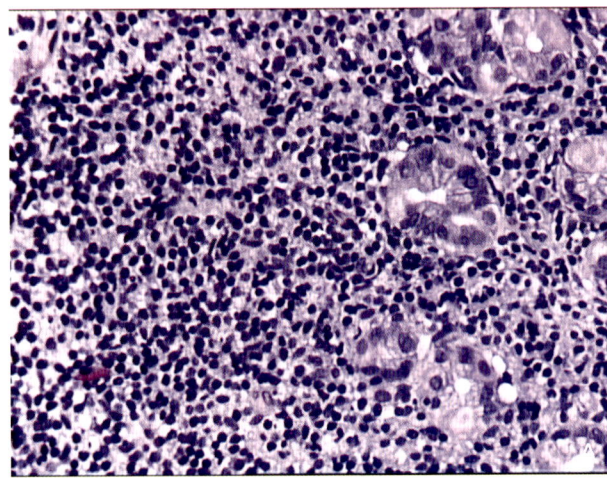

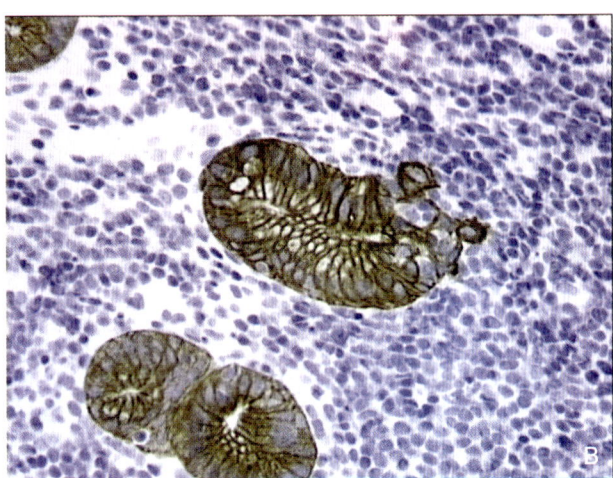

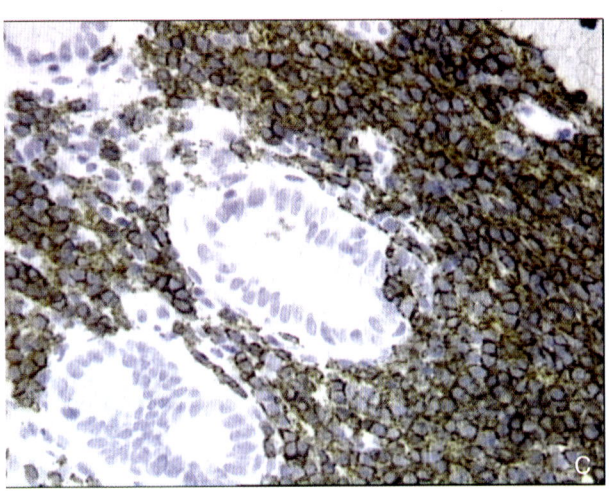

FIGURE 7–8. A to C Typical histological picture of a gastric low-grade MALT lymphoma. (A) diffuse lymphocitic infiltrate covers a large part of the slide. Some epithelial glandular structures, distorted and partially infiltrated (Lymphoepithelial lesions) are detectable. (B) Staining for cytokeratins AE1 and AE3, in this case positive for normal epithelial cells, clearly highlights a lymphoepitelial lesion. The glandular shape is still recognizable although partially disrupted by small cytokeratin-negative lymphocytes (C) A staining of the same lesion shown in 4-8b for B cell-associated antigen CD20 brings into view the lymphomatous infiltration, providing a "negative" image of the previous slide. (Courtesy of Dr. Roberto Nannini, Dept. of Pathology, AUSL of Imola, Italy).

The importance of EUS lies not only in its ability to stage MALT lymphoma before treatment but also in follow up. EUS may determine response to therapy and detect early relapse. On one hand, EUS may show restoration of normal gastric wall layers prior to evident histological remission. On the other hand, recurrent wall thickening or disruption may be seen in individuals who were previously in remission. For patients who persist to have a thickened gastric wall on EUS despite antibiotic therapy, other treatment modalities should be considered, even if endoscopic biopsies are negative. In fact, as shown by Levy et al.,[67] these patients are likely to have persistent lymphoma.

It should be underlined that EUS is an operator-dependent technique. Suboptimal interobserver agreement has been reported with staging of gastric lymphoma.[68] As a consequence, it should be kept in mind that high operator's experience and careful examination technique are always warranted to maintain the high levels of accuracy reported in the literature.

Finally, Lugering et al.[69] confirmed previous findings on the use of miniprobes for staging and follow-up of gastric lymphoma, providing a more accurate staging compared to dedicated echoendoscopes. The use of miniprobes in clinical practice is also recommended because the examination can be performed as a single-step procedure during diagnostic endoscopy.

Several studies on gastric cancer and lymphoma demonstrated specific EUS features that allow correct diagnosis and staging of lymphoma in the majority of patients.[42,44] While infiltrative carcinoma tends to show a vertical growth in the gastric wall, with transmural involvement, lymphoma tends to show mainly a horizontal extension.

In an early stage, lymphoma may be seen at EUS as a thickening of the second layer alone, or of the second and third layer, preserved as different layers. Interestingly, these alterations of the gastric wall can be found not only within and around the lesions observed at endoscopy, but also in areas where the mucosa appears normal[70-71]

In particular T1m lymphoma is usually seen as a hypoechoic thickening of the second layer (mucosa) of variable extension or even with a multifocal involvement, but still with a clearly identifiable and normal third layer (submucosa) all around the gastric wall. (Figures 7–9a - 7–9c)

When the thickening involves both the second and third layer (mucosa and submucosa) or, in correspondence of the lesion, a clear boundary between these two layers is no more visible, a T1sm stage is diagnosed if all the remaining layers (muscularis propria and sierosa) are of normal appearance (Figures 7–10a - 7–10b).

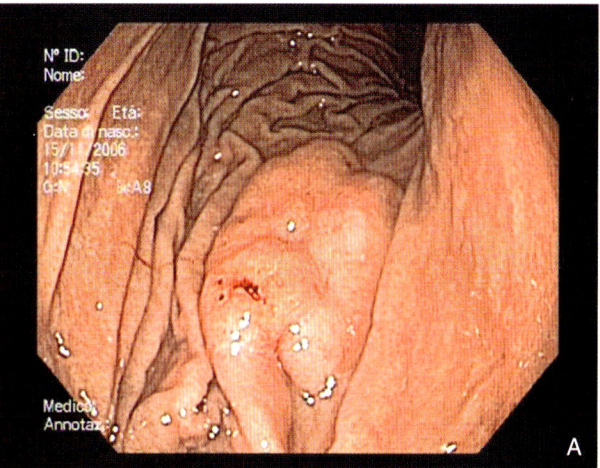
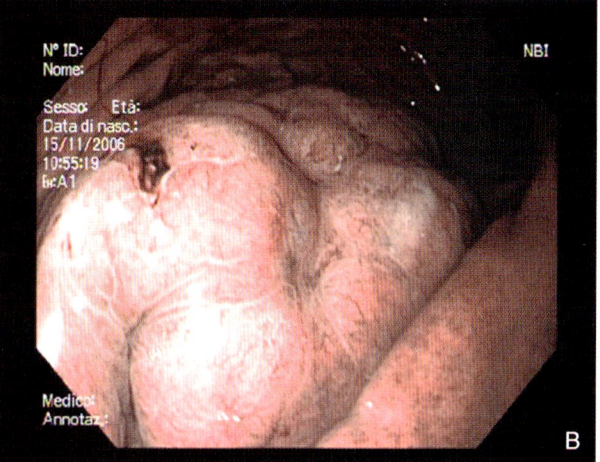
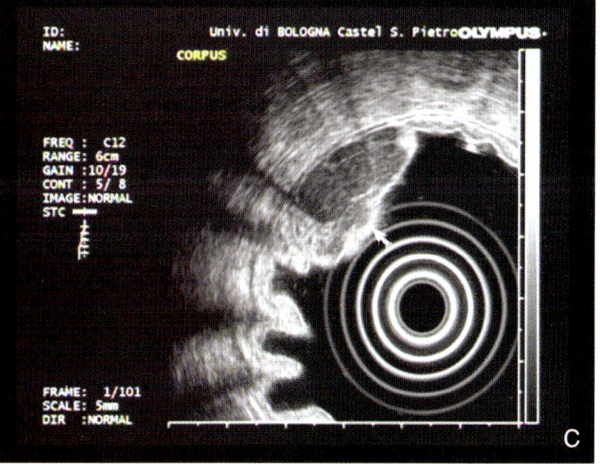

FIGURE 7–9. *A to C* (A) Low-grade gastric MALT lymphoma. Endoscopic view shows a large vegetating lesion of the greater curve in the gastric corpus. (B) Endoscopic view of the lesion shown in 7-9a, using Narrow Band Imaging. Mucosal surface visualization is enhanced; in particular, disruption of microvessels suggestive of malignant behaviour is detectable. (C) EUS radial scanning at 12 MHz. The lesion is now visualized as a large hypoechoic mass (arrow) originating from the second layer (mucosa); the underlying layers are normal. The stage is T1m.

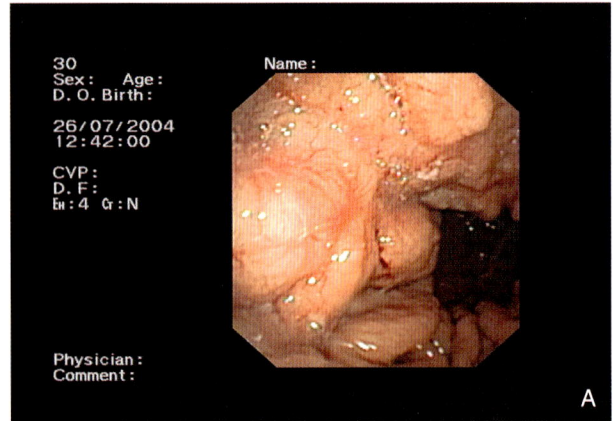 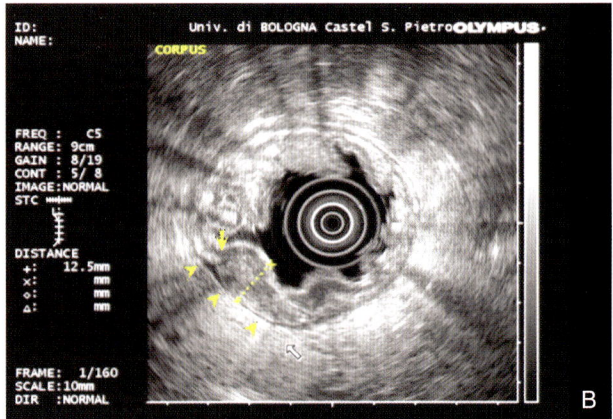

FIGURE 7–10. *A and B* (A) LGF on the anterior face of the gastric corpus in a case of low grade MALT lymphoma. Overlying mucosa presents erosions, neoangiogenesis and scar retraction. EUS radial scanning at 5 MHz. A hypoechoic thickening is visible in the second and third layers (mucosa and submucosa). In particular, infiltration of the submucosa is clearly detected as a neat interruption of the third layer (arrow). The fourth layer (muscularis propria) is preserved (arrowheads). The stage is T1sm.

At more advanced stages, lymphoma shows an ultrasonographic pattern of diffuse hypoechoic thickening with fusion of the layers. A T2 lesion is diagnosed when the second, third, and fourth layers are fused together and thickened, but the fifth hyperechoic layer (serosa) is not interrupted (Figures 7–11a – 7–11b, 7–12a - 7–12c).

When the lesion involves the entire gastric wall and interrupts the serosa at least in one point, the stage is T3, if no involvement of adjacent extra-gastric structures is seen (Figures 7–13a – 7–13b).

Finally a T4 lymphoma is characterized by a hypoechoic mass that crosses all layers of the gastric wall and continues into adjacent organs (i.e. the liver) (Figure 7–14).

Linitis Plastica

Although a focal mass is a more common presentation, gastric cancer can manifest a diffuse growth of malignant cells in the deep layers of the gastric wall. This situation is commonly defined as "linitis plastica." Both primary gastric cancer and metastases, especially from breast carcinoma (72, 73), have been described as possible causes of linitis.

The most common endoscopic appearance is a rigid, poorly distensible gastric wall, either with loss of the gastric folds and a tunnel-like appearance or with abnormally enlarged gastric folds (Figure 7–15).

Typical EUS findings are a thickened gastric wall, with significantly enlarged third and fourth layers

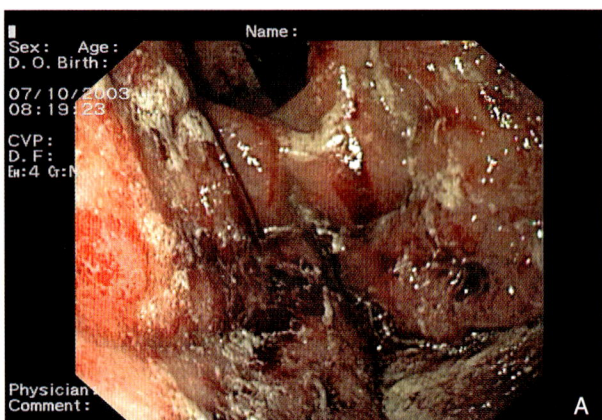 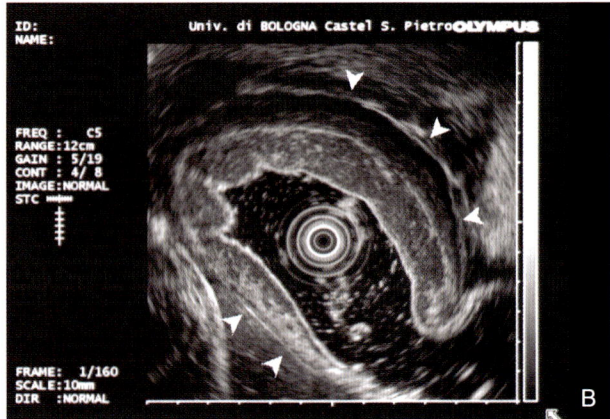

FIGURE 7–11. *A and B* (A) High-grade gastric MALT lymphoma. The fundus of the stomach presents diffuse LGF; overlying mucosa is markedly inflamed, fragile and spontaneously bleeding. (B) EUS scanning at 5 MHz. Gastric wall is markedly thickened circumferentially; the second (mucosa), third (submucosa), and fourth (muscularis propria) layers are all infiltrated. The fifth layer (serosa) is still intact (arrowheads). The stage is T2.

Large Gastric Folds 67

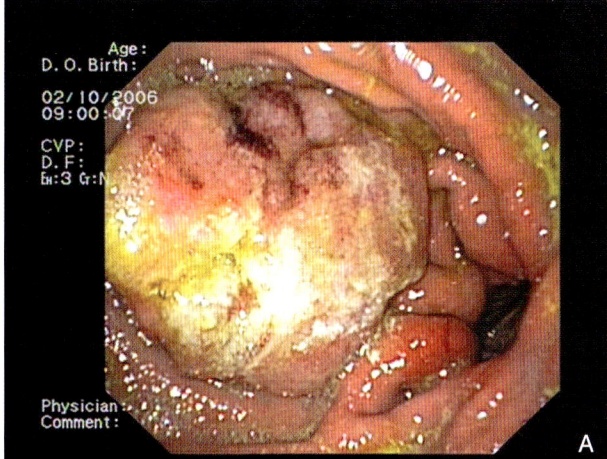

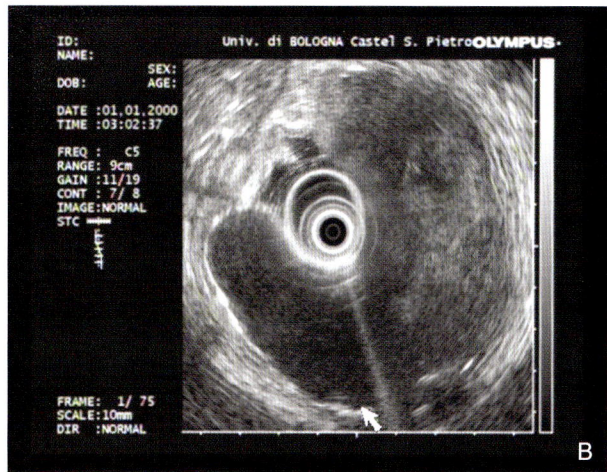

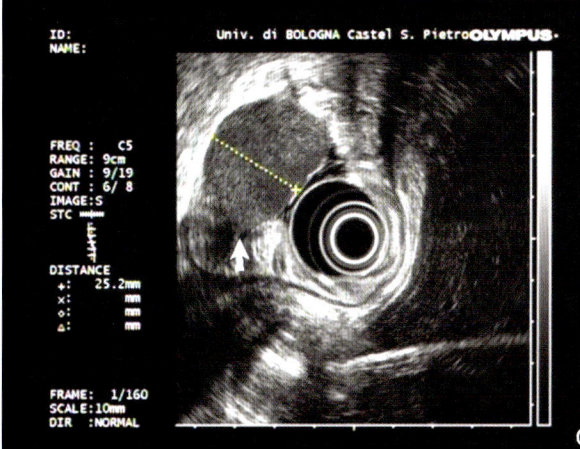

FIGURE 7–12. *A to C* (A) Recurrence of high-grade lymphoma in a gastric stump. This patient had undergone partial gastrectomy four years before for the same disease. A large vegetating irregular mass is visible. Surgery has been almost abandoned as a sole form of therapy for gastric lymphoma; however, it should be emphasized that partial gastrectomy is never indicated, as this disease has often multiple locations in the stomach. (B) EUS scanning at 5 MHz at the level of the mass. A huge hypoechoic lesion is shown, infiltrating the stomach up to the fourth layer (muscularis propria). The EUS normal stratification is completely disrupted. The stage is T2. (C) EUS scanning in the same patient, after eight cycles of chemotherapy. The mass (arrow) is significantly reduced in size. However, the stage is still T2.

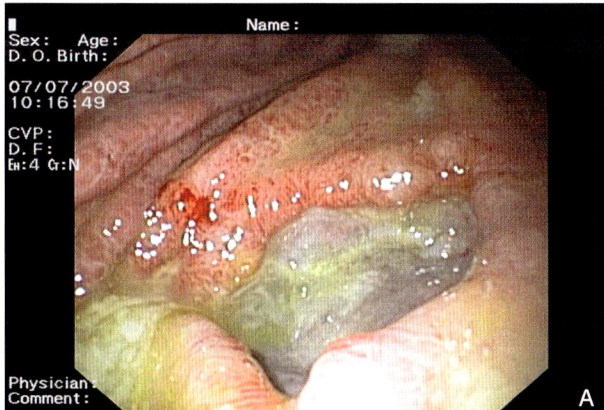

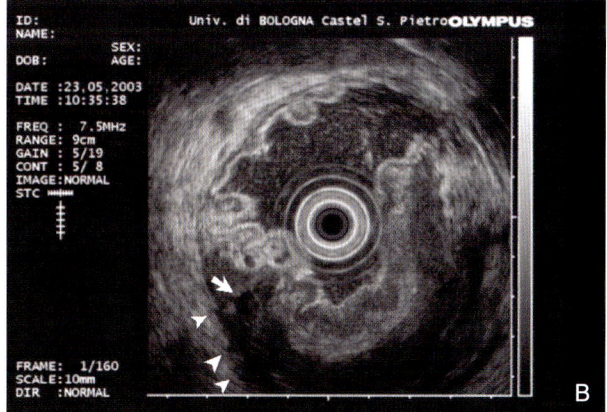

FIGURE 7–13. *A and B* (A) High grade gastric MALT lymphoma. Endoscopic view of a deep ulcer of the greater curve of the gastric corpus; it is possible to see the muscularis propria at the bottom of the lesion. The ulcer is surrounded by LGF covered by erythematous and fragile mucosa. (B) EUS scanning at 7.5 MHz. The gastric wall shows a huge thickening; the layers are completely disrupted. In particular, interruptions of the fifth layer (serosa) are visible as pseudopodia (arrowheads). Moreover, an anechoic lacuna compatible with necrosis is visible (arrow). The stage is T3.

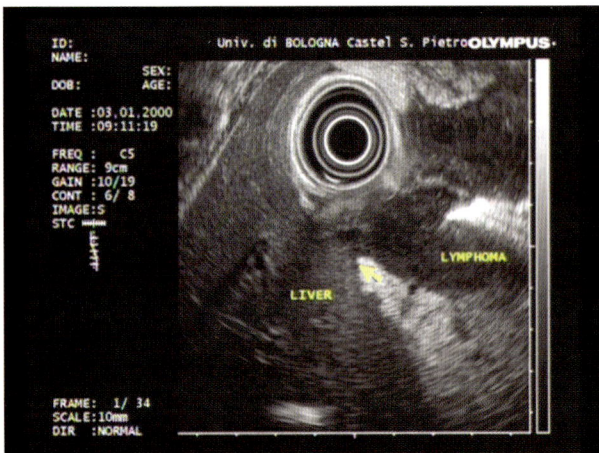

FIGURE 7–14. High-grade gastric lymphoma. The tumor has extended well outside the stomach invading the perigastric fat and the left lobe of the liver. In fact, no cleavage is seen between lymphoma and the hepatic parenchyma (arrow). The stage is T4.

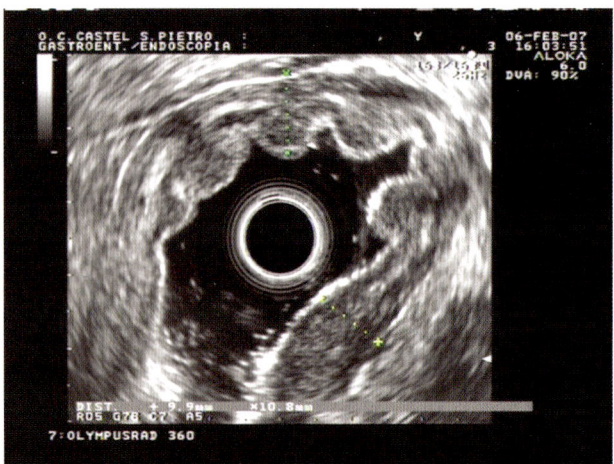

FIGURE 7–16. EUS scanning at 6 MHz with an electronic radial echoendoscope. Gastric wall is markedly thickened. The second, third, and fourth layers (mucosa, submucosa, and muscularis propria) are thickened and severely disrupted; nevertheless the endosonographer can still detect some glimpse of the original stratification.

(submucosa and muscolaris propria). The second layer (mucosa) is enlarged too and slightly more echogenic than the fourth.[73] However, the layers are still distinguishable as separate entities, particularly in the body and fundus (Figures 7–16 – 7–17). Sometimes perigastric ascites is also detected and is generally indicative of a metastatic spread (Figure 7–18a-7–18b).

Again, EUS features can help in the differential diagnosis, especially with lymphoma or gastritis. In case of lymphoma, usually the five-layered stratification is completely lost at advanced stages (Figure 7–19), while in the initial stages the lesions are mainly limited to the second (mucosal) or the third (submucosal) layers. Benign conditions (gastritis) never present with a marked involvement of the deep layers.[31]

As the neoplastic infiltration affects mainly deep layers, standard endoscopic biopsies are often unrevealing. EUS-guided fine needle aspiration (FNA) has been employed in some occasions as an efficacious method to obtain a diagnostic cytological sample in case of linitis.[24,74]

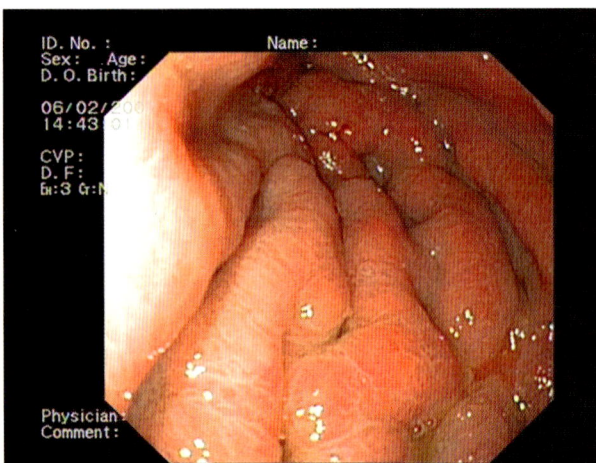

FIGURE 7–15. Gastric linitis plastica. LGF are seen that do not flatten with air insufflation and appear indurated and infiltrated. Endoscopic biopsies are very often unrevealing.

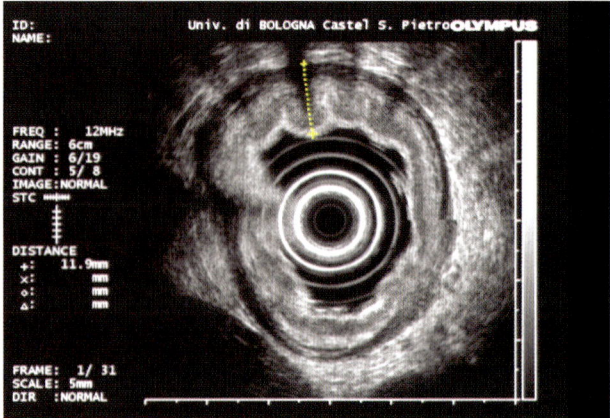

FIGURE 7–17. EUS scanning at 12 MHz with a mechanic radial echoendoscope. Gastric wall is markedly thickened. Unlike gastric lymphoma, in the present case normal stratification is preserved to a certain extent.

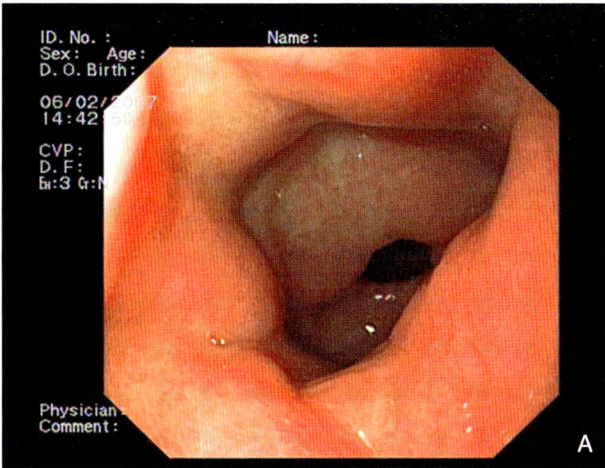 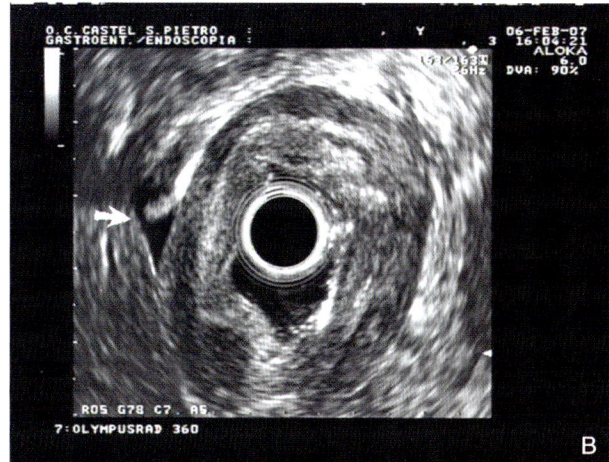

FIGURE 7–18. *A and B* (A) Gastric linitis plastica. The antrum shows a circumferential infiltration by the tumor resulting in partial stenosis of the lumen. (B) EUS scanning at the same level. Gastric wall is markedly thickened in its whole circumference. All the layers are thickened and severely disrupted but still recognizable. A small perigastric fluid collection is clearly visible (arrow).

Menetrier's Disease

Menetrier was the first to describe the presence of giant gastric folds in patients with hypertrophic gastritis, and Menetrier's disease has been the most commonly used eponym since then.[75] LGF in Menetrier's disease are due to foveolar cell hyperplasia, edema, and variable degrees of inflammation. This condition is typically associated with increased mucus secretion, protein-losing gastropathy, and hypochlorhydria, but also a hypersecretory variant has been described. The mechanism responsible for the disease is still unclear. CMV or H. pylori infections have been proposed as possible etiologies.[76] Also genetic factors have recently been suggested.[77]

Patients may present with weight loss, epigastric pain, vomiting, anorexia, dyspepsia, hematemesis, or positive fecal occult blood test. At endoscopy, the typical mucosal appearance of Menetrier's disease demonstrates irregular hypertrophic folds that involve the whole body, with a swollen, spongy appearance signed by creases, creating a picture similar to cerebral convolutions.

The differential diagnosis of malignant causes of LGF is mandatory for a correct management but is not always immediate, even with EUS. In particular, EUS differential diagnosis between early lymphoma and Menetrier's disease may be challenging. These lesions almost show a similar echo pattern, which is displayed as an extended thickening of the second and sometimes third layer, with preservation of the layers as distinct structures. Nevertheless, because the differential diagnosis among these pathologies is very important due to their different prognosis, it is possible to find some peculiar differences. While a lymphoma is usually of hypoechoic appearance and can reach the third layer also in initial stages, Menetrier's disease is displayed as a more localized thickening, which is hyperechoic rather than hypoechoic and involves mainly the second layer,[78] sometimes with an intra-mucosal cystic component[79] (Figures 7–20a - 7–20b). Menetrier's disease is never associated with involvement of the deep layers or loss of the gastric wall stratification, thus a differential diagnosis with advanced malignancies is usually possible.

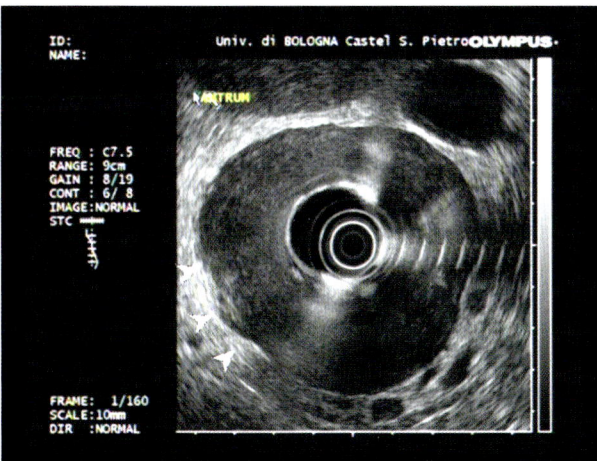

FIGURE 7–19. EUS scanning at level of gastric antrum in a case of lymphoma. As in the case shown in Figure 18b, the gastric wall is markedly thickened in its whole circumference. However, there is clear evidence that in this case the stratification is completely lost and the individual layers are not recognizable anymore. Initial infiltration of the perigastric tissue is shown (arrows). The stage is T3.

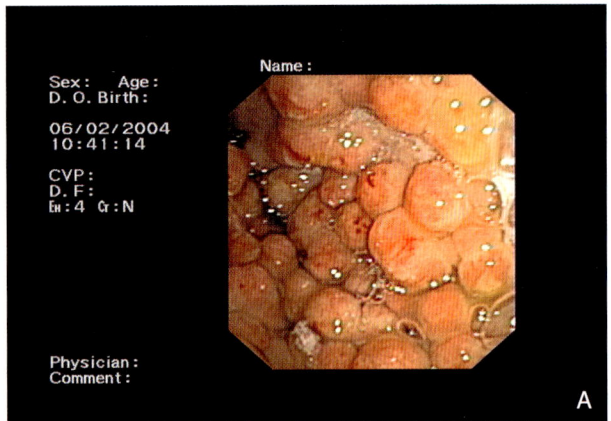 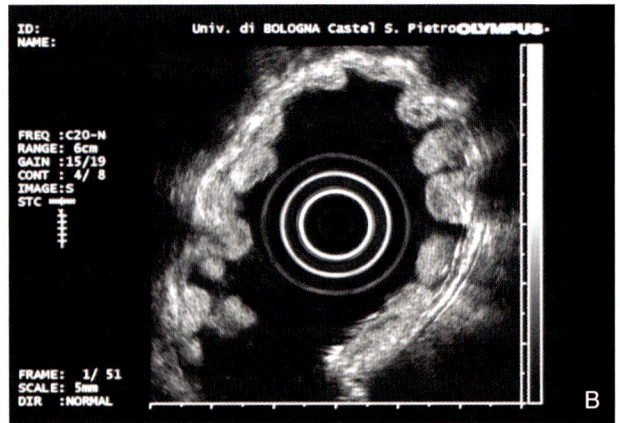

FIGURE 7–20. A and B (A) A case of Menetrier's disease. LGF are covered by irregular mucosa with coarse cobblestone aspect. This female patient had hypoalbuminemia, anemia, and diarrhea. (B) EUS scanning at 20 MHz. A hyperechoic diffuse thickening of the second layer is visible. Moreover, some small anechoic lacunae, compatible with cystic spaces, are present inside the 2nd layer itself. The underlying layers are normal. This finding is highly suggestive of Menetrier's disease. After antibiotic treatment for H. pylori the patient experienced a complete and stable normalization of her symptoms and signs.

The ideal treatment is not well defined yet. Sometimes spontaneous resolution may occur but the association with gastric carcinoma has also been described. Ganciclovir has been successfully used in children with Menetrier's disease and CMV gastritis (80). When H. pylori is present, the treatment of the infection can resolve the entire syndrome.[81] Some patients have improved after administration of antisecretory drugs, corticosteroids, octreotide, or even monoclonal antibodies.[82] Surgery is usually reserved for severe complications, like recurrent bleeding, severe hypoprotidemia, or cancer development.

Zollinger-Ellison Syndrome

Zollinger-Ellison syndrome (ZES), firstly described in 1955, is a clinical syndrome characterized by excessive gastric acid secretion due to ectopic production of gastrin.[83] Pancreatic or duodenal gastrinomas are generally responsible for this situation. Recurrent or complicated peptic ulcer disease, gastroesophageal reflux disease, or diarrhea represent the most common clinical manifestations. All of these symptoms regress when gastric secretion is controlled medically, with antisecretory drugs, or surgically, with the removal of the gastrinoma.

Laboratory tests usually show a markedly increased fasting gastrinemia with a positive response to secretin stimulation (increase >200 pg/ml).

High serum gastrin levels stimulate the growth of the gastric mucosa, resulting in parietal cell hyperplasia and proliferation of gastric enterochromaffin-like cells (ECL cells), which secrete histamine.[84-85] Consequent ECL cells hyperplasia can lead to the development of gastric carcinoid like tumors, especially in patients with MEN 1 syndrome.[85]

At endoscopy, ZES can show a diffuse mucosal hyperplasia with enlargement of the gastric folds, involving mainly the body, or the fundus, of the stomach. Erosions or ulcerations can often be seen in the gastric or in the duodenal mucosa, but these signs are not always reported. In these cases, a differential diagnosis with other causes of LGF is not always immediate.

At EUS, a thickening of the second layer (mucosa) with nonhomogenous echogenicity is identifiable (Figures 7–21a - 7–21c). As in Menetrier's disease and in other benign causes of LGF, in ZES too, the deep layers of the gastric wall show normal stratification and thickness. Once a diagnosis of ZES is established, it is of paramount importance to correctly localize the primary lesion for two reasons. First, a gastrinoma should be regarded as potentially malignant tumor. Second, a complete resection of the lesion leads to a definitive healing from ZES. An exact identification of the gastrinoma site, most commonly localized in the pancreas or in the duodenum, is not always easy with conventional imaging techniques. EUS, with its ability to obtain high-frequency scans of the pancreatic gland, can also be helpful in this field. EUS, which could be performed also as an intraoperatory exam,[86] can identify even small pancreatic lesions missed by other techniques[87] or exclude with great accuracy the pancreatic localization of the gastrinoma.[88-89,90] On the other hand, identification of duodenal gastrinoma is always very problematic, even by EUS;. they are usually detected only at surgery, using transillumination of the duodenal wall.[91]

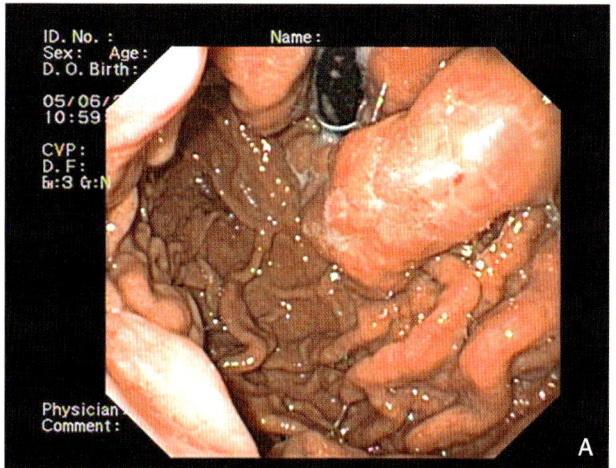
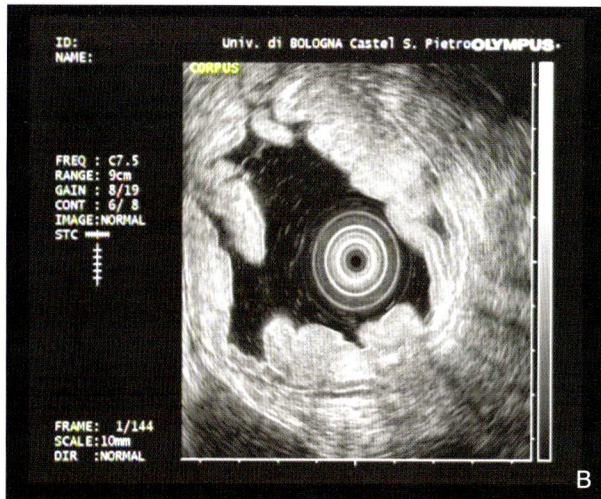
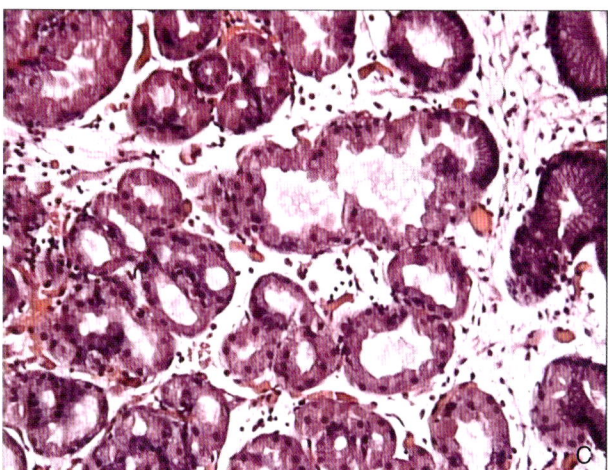

FIGURE 7–21. *A to C* (A) A case of Zollinger-Ellison syndrome. LGF covered by mucosa with marked accentuation of areolar pattern in the gastric fundus. This patient had a recent history of duodenal ulcer perforation. Differential diagnosis can be very problematic on the sole basis of endoscopy, and biopsies should not be taken before having ruled out the presence of varices. (B) EUS radial scanning at 7.5 MHz. A marked thickening of the second layer is shown; its echogenicity is slightly inhomogeneous. The underlying layers are normal. In view of the clinical presentation and of the rest of diagnostic work up data, this finding was thought to be consistent with the diagnosis of Zollinger-Ellison syndrome. (C) Large particle biopsy performed by cap-assisted mucosectomy. Histology shows multiple cystic dilatations inside the mucosa. This finding is compatible with Zollinger-Ellison syndrome (Courtesy of Dr. Roberto Nannini, Dept. of Pathology, AUSL of Imola, Italy).

Gastric Varices

Gastric varices are classically found in association with cirrhosis and portal hypertension, often together with esophageal varices as a consequence of the portosystemic shunts. However, abnormal vessels in the gastric wall can also be found on rare occasions in patients without known liver disease. The most widely used classification for gastric varices is the Sarin classification (Table 7-5).[92] Varices involving the fundus (GOV2 and IGV1) are thought to be at an increased risk for bleeding.

A diagnosis of gastric varices is often possible at standard endoscopy when a typical vascular aspect is clearly identifiable, especially in high-risk patients with known cirrhosis or other signs of portal hypertension. However, gastric varices tend to be larger in diameter than esophageal varices, can present as isolated lesions, and are sometimes covered by normally appearing gastric mucosa. In these cases, it is possible to misjudge a gastric varix as a hypertrophic gastric fold and to take bioptic samples that could potentially lead to massive bleeding.

EUS examination of the suspicious lesion can clearly identify the typical anechoic aspect of a vascular structure, which is usually localized in the third layer (submucosa) (Figures 7–22A - 7–22B). If an electronic scanning instrument is used, the presence of a Doppler signal inside the anechoic areas can remove any doubt (Figures 7–23A - 7–23C)

As a consequence, we recommend always performing EUS before taking biopsies in all uncertain lesions, thus avoiding the potential risks of bleeding from gastric varices.[28]

Table 7-5	Sarin Classification of Gastric Varices
Gastroesophageal varices (GOV)	
Type 1 (GOV1)	Varices extended 2 to 5 cm below the gastroesophageal junction in continuity with esophageal varices.
Type 2 (GOV2)	Varices that reach the fundus of the stomach in continuity with esophageal varices
Isolated gastric varices (IGV)	
Type 1 (IGV1)	Varices that occur in the fundus of the stomach in absence of esophageal varices
Type 2 (IGV2).	Varices that occur in the body, antrum, or pylorus in absence of esophageal varices.

Other Causes of LGF

Some other benign conditions, mainly of infective or inflammatory origin, can manifest as LGF. One common case is H. pylori infection presenting as hypertrophic gastritis.[10] In this case, a hypoechoic thickening is mainly localized to the second layer. All of the remaining layers are well defined and of normal appearance (Figure 7–24). Usually a normal gastric wall thickness is restored after antibiotic eradication of the bacteria.

Other infections, as CMV[93] or even secondary syphilis[8] or gastric tuberculosis,[94] have been described as rare causes of LGF. Also infection with roundworms can be implied: acute gastric Anisakiasis, contracted eating raw fish containing nematode larvae of the gender Anisakis,[11] is another possible cause of LGF. Many cases occurred in Japan, but the disease has also been reported in the United States and Europe. Usually endoscopy is diagnostic because the larva can be detected, but in some cases LGF represent the only finding. A typical EUS feature is a thickening of the third layer with irregular hypoechoic pattern.[29,95] An anechoic lacuna in the second layer can sometimes be visible around the site of penetration. Microscopically, sections of the stomach at the site of infection show a marked eosinophilic granulomatous inflammatory process with intramural abscess and granulation tissue. This eosinophilic abscess can contain a small worm measuring about 0.3 mm.

Okada et al.[96] described another rare condition: two patients suffering from gastritis cystica profunda, a rare condition where multiple small cysts in the mucosa and submucosa of the stomach are detected, presenting as LGF at endoscopy (Figure 7–25). In these cases the diagnosis was based on EUS and mucosectomy findings.

Inflammatory polyps can sometimes grow to giant dimensions and mimic LGF; in this case, the lesion is usually localized mainly in the mucosal layer. Nevertheless, the final diagnosis is obtained only by histology (Figures 7–26a - 7–26c).

It should be noted that all of these conditions show at EUS an involvement of the second or third layer, while the deep layers are always spared and clearly delimited. In all of the studies[28-29,31] about LGF, the

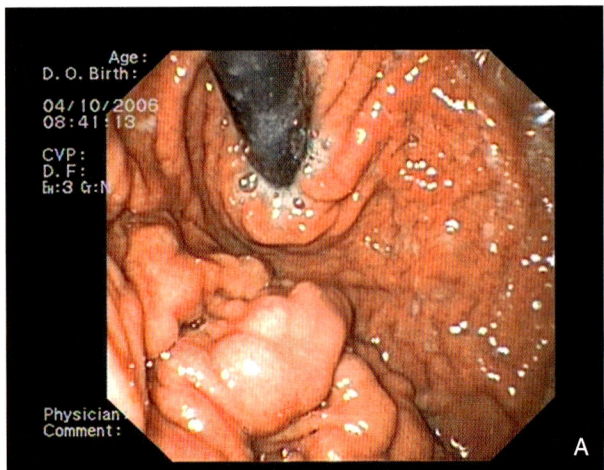 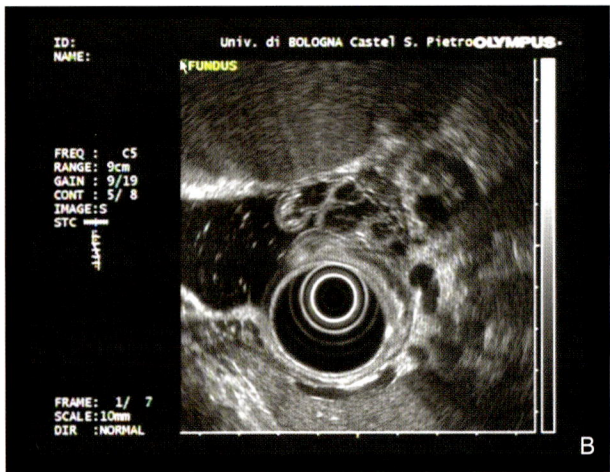

FIGURE 7–22. *A and B* (A) Gastric fundal varices. LGF covered with normal mucosa are seen. In cases like this differential diagnosis on the sole basis of endoscopy may be impossible. For this reason, endoscopic biopsies should never be taken without a prior EUS to rule out the presence of varices. (B) EUS scanning at 5 MHz at the same level. Large anechoic lacunae, compatible with varices, are seen inside the third layer (submucosa). EUS diagnosis avoided endoscopic biopsies, which may have caused a massive bleeding.

Large Gastric Folds 73

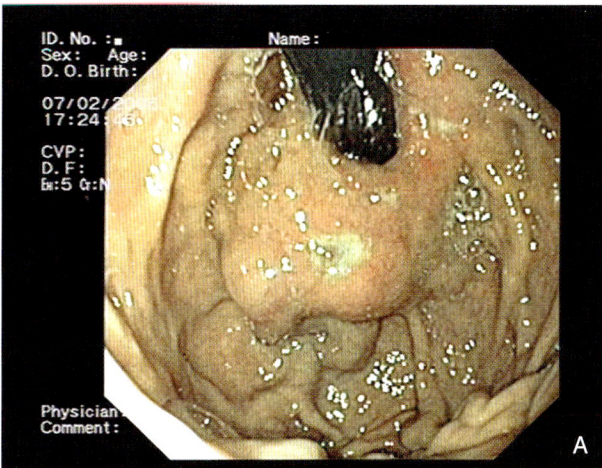

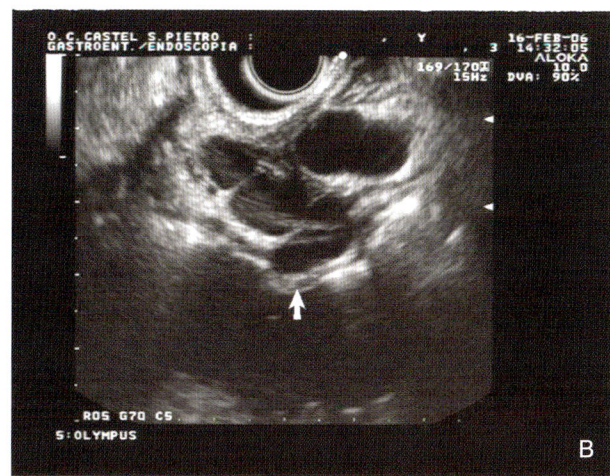

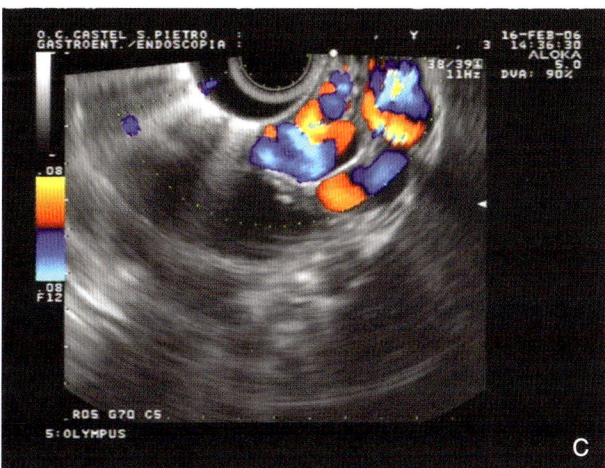

FIGURE 7–23. *A to C* (A) Another case of gastric fundal varices. The ulceration of the overlying mucosa is a stigmata of recent bleeding. Again, differential diagnosis based on endoscopy alone is very difficult, and biopsies should never be taken without a prior EUS. (B) EUS with an electronic sector scanning echoendoscope at 10 MHz. Large anechoic lacunae, compatible with varices, are seen inside the third layer (submucosa). A large afferent vessel is also visible (arrow). (C) Color Doppler definitely confirms the diagnosis of gastric varices.

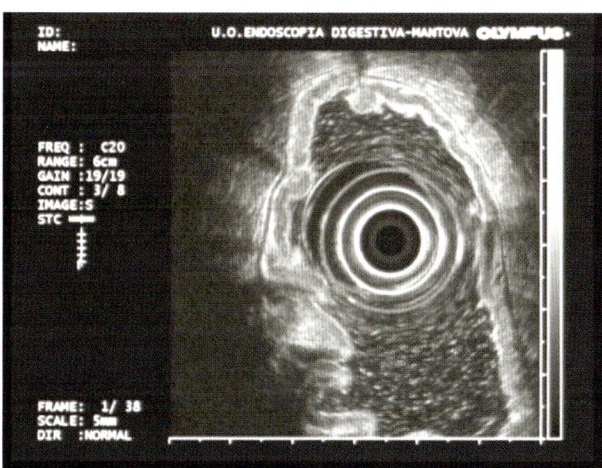

FIGURE 7–24. H. pylori gastritis. Circumferential mild thickening of the second layer is seen with a homogeneous echogenicity. The underlying layers are normal. (Courtesy of Dr. Thomas Togliani, Dept. of Gastroenterology, AUSL of Mantova, Italy).

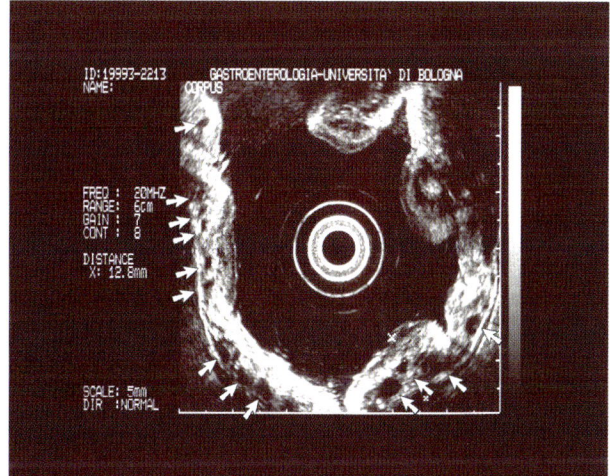

FIGURE 7–25. Gastritis cystica profunda. LGF were detected at endoscopy. EUS scanning at 20 MHz shows multiple anechoic lacunae compatible with cysts in the third layer (submucosa). The underlying layers are normal.

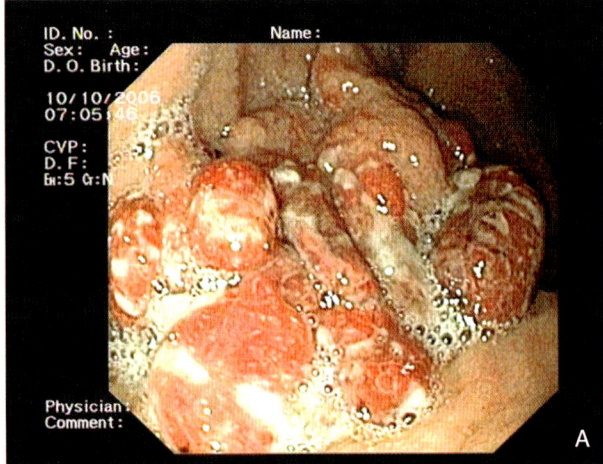

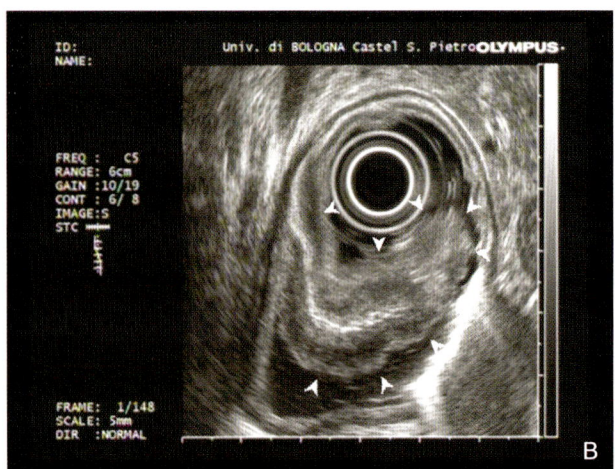

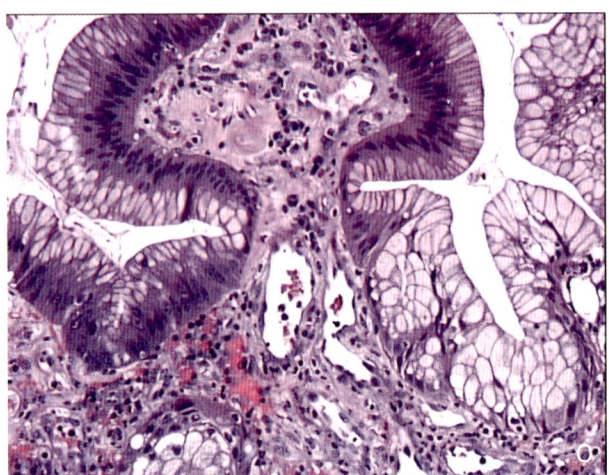

FIGURE 7–26. *A to C* (A) A large vegetating mass is detected in the greater curvature/anterior face of the gastric corpus. Biopsies were performed that revealed a hyperplastic polyp. However, further investigation was deemed necessary to rule out malignancy. (B) EUS scanning at the level of the mass at 5 MHz. A diffuse thickening of the second layer (mucosa) is visible, protruding in the lumen with a polypoid-like appearance (arrowheads). Also the third layer (submucosa) is clearly visible inside the mass. The fourth layer (muscularis propria) appears intact. On these basis, polipectomy was felt to be feasible for further diagnosis and/or therapy. (C) After polipectomy a complete histological analysis confirmed the inflammatory and benign nature of this lesion (Courtesy of Dr. Roberto Nannini, Dept. of Pathology, AUSL of Imola, Italy).

fourth ultrasound layer was significantly enlarged only in patients with gastric malignancies (i.e. gastric cancer or lymphoma).

Acknowledgments:

We thank Fondazione CARISBO for fundamental financial support to our research activities.

References

1. Bjork, J. T., Geenen, J. E., Soergel, K.H., et al. : Endoscopic evaluation of large gastric folds: A comparison of biopsy techniques. Gastrointest Endosc 1977; 24: 22–23.
2. Vilardell, F. : Gastritis. In Berk J. E., ed. Gastroenterology. 4th ed. Philadelphia: WB Saunders, 1985: 941–974.
3. Kimmey M.B., Martin, R.W., Hagitt, R.C., et al. : Histologic correlates of gastrointestinal ultrasound images. Gastroenterology 1989; 96:433–441.
4. Gordon S. J., Rifkin, M. D., Goldberg, B. B. : Endosonographic evaluation of mural abnormalities of the upper gastrointestinal tract. Gastrointest Endosc 1986; 32:193–198.
5. Botet, J.F., Lightdale, C.J. : Endoscopic sonography of the gastrointestinal tract. AJR Am J Roentgenol 1991; 156:63–68.
6. Reeder, M. M., Olmstead, W.W., Cooper, P. H. : Large gastric folds, local or widespread. JAMA 1974; 230:273–274.
7. Fisher, J. R., Sanowski, R. A. : Disseminated histoplasmosis producing hypertrophic gastric folds. American Journal of Digestive Diseases 1978; 23:282–285.
8. Morin, M. E., Tan, A. : Diffuse enlargement of gastric folds as a manifestation of secondary syphilis. Am J Gastroenterol 1980; 74:170–172.
9. Kusuhura, T., Watanabe, K., Fukuda, M. : Radiographic studies of acute gastric anisakiasis. Gastrointest Radiol 1984; 9:305–309.
10. Avunduk, C., Navab, F., Hampf, F., et al. : Prevalence of Helicobacter pylori infection in patients with large gastric folds: evaluation and follow-up with endoscopic ultrasound before and after antimicrobial therapy. Am J Gastroenterol 1995; 90:1969–1973.
11. Sakanari, J. A., McKerrow, J. H., Anisakiasis. : Clin Microbiol Rev 1989; 2:278–284.
12. Caletti, G. C., Brocchi, E., Ferrari, A., et al. : Value of endoscopic ultrasonography in the management of portal hypertension. Endoscopy 1992; 24 Suppl 1:342–346.
13. Gandolfi, L., Colecchia, A., Leo, P., et al. : Endoscopic ultrasonography in the diagnosis of gastrointestinal

amyloid deposits: clinical case report. Endoscopy 1995; 27:132–134.
14. Levine, M. S., Kong, V., Rubeswin, S. E, et al. : Scirrhous carcinoma of the stomach: radiologic and endoscopic diagnosis. Radiology 1990; 175:151–154.
15. Nelson, R.S., Lanza. F. L. : The endoscopic diagnosis of gastric lymphoma. Gross characteristics and histology. Gastrointest Endosc 1974; 21:66–68.
16. Winawer, S. J., Posner, G., Lightdale, C. J., et al. Endoscopic diagnosis of advanced gastric cancer. Gastroenterology 1975; 69:1183–1187.
17. Andriulli, A., Recchia, A., De Angelis, C., et al.: Endoscopic ultrasonographic evaluation of patients with biopsy negative gastric linitis plastica. Gastrointest Endosc 1990; 36:611–615.
18. Fork F. T., Haglund, U., Hogstrom, H., et al.: Primary gastric lymphoma v. gastric cancer. An endoscopic and radiographic study of differential diagnostic possibilities. Endoscopy 1985; 17:5–7.
19. Caletti, G., Fusaroli, P., Bocus, P.: Endoscopic ultrasonography in large gastric folds. Endoscopy 1998; 30Suppl1:72–75.
20. Meuwissen, S. G., Ridwan, B. U., Hasper, H. J., Innemee, G.: Hypertrophic protein-losing gastropathy: A retrospective analysis of 40 cases in The Netherlands. The Dutch Menetrier Study Group. Scand J Gastroenterol Suppl. 1992;194:1–7.
21. Komorowski, R. A., Caya, J. G., Geenen, J. E.: The morphologic spectrum of large gastric folds: utility of the snare biopsy. Gastrointest Endosc 1986; 32:190–192.
22. Martin, T.R., Onstad, G. R., Silvis, S. E., et al. : Lift and cut biopsy technique for submucosal sampling. Gastrointest Endosc 1976; 23:29.
23. Tio, T. L. : Large gastric folds evaluated by endoscopic ultrasonography. Gastrointest Endosc Clin N Am 1995; 5:683–691.
24. Vander Noot, M. R., 3rd, Eloubeidi, M. A., Chen, V. K., et al.: Diagnosis of gastrointestinal tract lesions by endoscopic ultrasound-guided fine-needle aspiration biopsy. Cancer 2004; 102:157–163.
25. Caletti, G.C., Brocchi, E., Ferrari, A., et al.: Guillotine needle biopsy as a supplement to endosonography in the diagnosis of gastric submucosal tumors. Endoscopy 1991; 23:251–254.
26. Feng, J., Al-Abbadi, M., Kodali, U., et al.: Cytologic diagnosis of gastric linitis plastica by endoscopic ultrasound guided fine-needle aspiration. Diagn Cytopathol 2006; 34: 177–179.
27. Caletti, G. C., Ferrari, A., Bocus, P., et al.: Endoscopic ultrasonography in gastric lymphoma. Schweiz Med Wochenschr 1996; 126:819–825.
28. Mendis, R.E., Gerdes, H., Lightdale, C. J., et al. : Large gastric folds: a diagnostic approach using endoscopic ultrasonography. Gastrointest Endosc 1994; 40:437–441.
29. Songur, Y., Takashi, O., Watanabe, H., et al. : Endosonographic evaluation of giant gastric folds. Gastrointest Endosc 1995; 41:468–474.
30. Maunoury, V., Klein O, Houcke ML, et al. : Endoscopic ultrasonography in the diagnosis of hypertrophic gastropathy. Gastroenterology 1994; 106:820.
31. Ginès, A., Pellisé, M, Fernandez-Esparrach, G., et al. : Endoscopic ultrasonography in patients with large gastric folds at endoscopy and biopsies negative for malignancy: predictors of malignant disease and clinical impact. Am J Gastroenterol 2006; 101:64–69.
32. Fusaroli, P., Vallar, R., Togliani, T., et al.: Scientific publications in endoscopic ultrasonography: a 20-year global survey of the literature. Endoscopy 2002; 34: 451–456.
33. Sobin, L., Wittekind, C.: International union against cancer. TNM classifications of malignant tumors.: New York, John Wiley, 1997.
34. Greene, Frederick L., et. al., eds.: AJCC cancer staging manual. 6th ed. / New York: Springer Verlag, 2002.
35. Tio, T., Schouwinck, M., Cikot, R., et al.: Preoperative TNM classification of gastric carcinoma by endosonography in comparison with the pathological TNM system: a prospective case of 172 patients. Hepatogastroenterology 1989; 36:51–56.
36. Sano, T., Okuyama, Y., Kobeori, O., et al.: Early gastric cancer: endoscopic diagnosis of depth of invasion. Dig Dis Sci 1990; 35:1340–1344.
37. Yanhai, H., Noguchi, T., Mizumachi, S., et al.: a blind comparison of the effectiveness of endoscopic ultrasonography and endoscopy in staging early gastric cancer. Gut 1999; 44:361–365.
38. Kuntz, C., Herfarth, C.: Imaging diagnosis for staging of gastric cancer. Semin Surg Oncol 1999; 17: 96–102.
39. Botel, J. C., Lightdale, C., Zauber, A., et al.: Preoperative staging of gastric cancer: comparison of endocopic US and dynamic CT. Radiology 1991; 181:426–432.
40. Okai, T., Yamakawa, O., Matsuda, N., et al.: Analysis of gastric carcinoma growth by endoscopic ultrasonography. Endoscopy 1991; 23:121–125.
41. Polkowsky, M., Palucki, J., Wronska, E., et al.: Endosonography versus helical computed tomography for locoregional staging of gastric cancer. Endoscopy 2004; 36:617–623.
42. Caletti, G., Ferrari, A., Brocchi, E., Barbara, L.: Accuracy of endoscopic ultrasonography in the diagnosis and staging of gastric cancer and lymphoma. Surgery 1993;113:14–27.
43. Suekane, H., Iida, M., Yao, T., et al. : Endoscopic ultrasonography in primary gastric lymphoma: correlation with endoscopic and histologic findings. Gastrointest Endosc 1993; 39:139–145.
44. Palazzo, L., Roseau, G., Ruskone-Fourmestraux, A., et al. : Endoscopic ultrasonography in the local staging of primary gastric lymphoma. Endoscopy 1993; 25: 502–508.
45. Van Dam, J.: The role of endoscopic ultrasonography in monitoring treatment: response to chemotherapy in lymphoma. Endoscopy 1994; 26:772–773.
46. Hordijk, M. L.: Restaging after radiotherapy and chemotherapy: value of endoscopic ultrasonography. Gastrointest Endosc Clin N Am 1995; 5:601–608.
47. Caletti, G., Fusaroli, P., Togliani, T., et al.: Endosonography in gastric lymphoma and large gastric folds. Eur J Ultrasound 2000; 11:32–40.
48. Fischbach, W., Goebeler-Kolve, M. E., Greiner, A. : Diagnostic accuracy of EUS in the local staging of primary gastric lymphoma: results of a prospective, multicenter study comparing EUS with histopathologic stage. Gastrointest Endosc 2002; 56:696–700.
49. Shimodaira, M., Tsukamoto, Y., Niwa, Y., et al. : A proposed staging system for primary gastric lymphoma. Cancer 1994; 73:2709–2715.
50. Musshoff, K., Schmidt-Vollmer, H.: Prognosis of non Hodgkin's lymphomas with special emphasis on staging classification. Z Krebsforschung 1975; 83:323–328.
51. Rohatiner, A., D'Amore, F., Coiffier, B., et al.: Report on a workshop convened to discuss the pathological

and staging classifications of gastrointestinal tract lymphoma. Ann Oncol 1994; 5:397–400.
52. Ruskoné-Fourmestraux, A., Dragosics, B., Morgner, A., et al. : Paris staging system for primary gastrointestinal lymphomas. Gut 2003; 52:912–913.
53. Catalano, M. F., Sivak, M. V., Rice, T. et al. : Endosonographic features predictive of lymph node metastasis. Gastrointest Endosc 1994; 40:442–446.
54. Murata, T., Nakamura, S., Oka, K., et al. : Granzyme B positive primary gastric T-cell lymphoma:gastric T-cell lymphoma with the possibility of extrathymic T-cell origin. Pathol Int 2000; 50: 853.
55. Niitsu, N., Nakamine, H, Kohri, M., et al.: Primary gastric T-cell lymphoma not associated with human T-lymphotrophic virus type 1: a case report and a review of the literature. Ann Hematol 2003 ; 82:197.
56. Nakamura, S., Aoyagi, K., Iwanaga, S., et al.: Synchronous and metachronous primary gastric lymphoma and adenocarcinoma: a clinicopathological study of 12 patients. Cancer. 1997; 79:1077–1085.
57. Lamarque, D., Levy, M., Chaumette, M. T., et al. : Frequent and rapid progression of atrophy and intestinal metaplasia in gastric mucosa of patients with MALT lymphoma. Am J Gastroenterol. 2006;101: 1886–1893.
58. Suenaga, M., Ohta, K., Toguchi, M., et al.: Colliding gastric and intestinal phenotype well-differentiated adenocarcinoma of the stomach developing in an area of MALT-type lymphoma. Gastric Cancer. 2003; 6: 270–276.
59. Hamaloglu, E., Topaloglu, S., Ozdemir, A.: Synchronous and metachronous occurrence of gastric adenocarcinoma and gastric lymphoma: A review of the literature. World J Gastroenterol. 2006; 12: 3564–74.
60. Isaacson, P., Wright, D. H.: Extranodal malignant lymphoma arising from the mucosa-associated lymphoid tissue. Cancer 1984; 53:2515–2524.
61. Ruskonè-Fourmestraux, A., Lavergne, A., Aegerter, P.H., Megraud, F., Palazzo, L., de Mascarel, A., et al.: Predictive factors for regression of gastric MALT lymphoma after anti-Helicobacter pylori treatment. Gut 2001;48:297–303.
62. Caletti, G., Zinzani, P. L., Fusaroli, P., Buscarini, E., Parente, F., Federici, T., et al.: The importance of endoscopic ultrasonography in the management of low-grade gastric mucosa-associated lymphoid tissue lymphoma. Aliment Pharmacol Ther 2002;16:1715–1722.
63. Sackmann, M., Morgner, A., Rudolph, B., et al. : A MALT lymphoma study group. Regression of gastric MALT lymphoma after eradication of Helicobacter pylori is predicted by endosonographic staging. Gastroenterology 1997; 113:1087–1090
64. Levy, M., Copie-Bergman, C., Traulle, C, et al. : Conservative treatment of primary gastric low-grade B-cell lymphoma of mucosa-associated lymphoid tissue: predictive factors of response and outcome. Am J Gastroenterol 2002; 97:292–297.
65. Nakamura, S., Matsumoto, T., Suekane, H., et al. : Predictive value of endoscopic ultrasonography for regression of gastric low grade and high grade MALT lymphomas after eradication of Helicobacter pylori. Gut 2001; 48:454–460.
66. El-Zahabi, M., Jamal, F., El-Hajj, I., et al.: The value of EUS in predicting the response of gastric mucosa-associated lymphoid tissue lymphoma to Helycobacter pylori eradication. Gastrointestinal Endoscopy 2007; 65: 89–96.
67. Levy, M., Hammel, P., Lamarque, D., et al. : Endoscopic ultrasonography for the initial staging and follow-up in patients with low-grade gastric lymphoma of mucosa-associated lymphoid tissue treated medically. Gastrointest Endosc 1997; 46:328–333.
68. Fusaroli, P., Buscarini, E., Peyre, S., Federici, T., Parente, F., De Angelis, C., Bonanno, G., Meroni, E., Napolitano, V., Pisani, A., Sottili, S., Togliani, T., Caletti, G. : Interobserver agreement in staging gastric lymphoma by endoscopic ultrasonography. Gastrointest Endosc 2002;55:662–668.
69. Lugering, N., Menzel, J., Kucharzik, T., et al.: Impact of miniprobes compared to conventional endosonography in the staging of low-grade gastric malt lymphoma. Endoscopy 2001; 33:832–837.
70. Bolondi, L., Casanova, P., Caletti, G. C., et al. : Primary gastric lymphoma versus gastric carcinoma: endoscopic US evaluation. Radiology 1987; 165:821–826.
71. Caletti, G.C., Zani, L., Bolondi, L., et al. : Impact of endoscopic ultrasonography on diagnosis and treatment of primary gastric lymphoma. Surgery 1988, 103:315–320.
72. Whitty, L. A., Crawford, D. L., Woodland, J.H. et al.: Metastatic breast cancer presenting as linitis plastica of the stomach. Gastric Cancer 2005;8:193–197.
73. Lorimier, G., Binelli, C., Burtin, P., et al.: Metastatic gastric cancer arising from breast carcinoma: endoscopic ultrasonographic aspects. Endoscopy. 1998; 30: 800–804.
74. Feng, J., Al-Abbadi, M., Kodali, U., et al.: Cytologic diagnosis of gastric linitis plastica by endoscopic ultrasound guided fine-needle aspiration. Diagn Cytopatol 2006; 34: 177–179.
75. Menetrier, P.: Des polyadenomes gastriques et leurs rapports avec le cancer de stomach. Arch Physiol Norm Path 1888; 1:32–35, 236–262.
76. Badov, D., Lambert, Jr., Finlay, M., et al. : Helicobacter pylori as a pathogenic factor in Menetrier's disease. Am J Gastroenterol. 1998; 93: 1976–1979.
77. Ibarrola, C., Rodriguez-Pinilla, M., Valino, C., et al.: An unusal expression of hyperplastic gastropathy (Menetrier type) in twins. Eur J Gastroenterol Hepatol 2003; 15: 441–445.
78. Hizawa, K., Kawasaki, M., Yao, T., et al. : Endoscopic ultrasound features of protein-losing gastropathy with hypertrophic gastric folds. Endoscopy 2000; 32: 394–397.
79. Hizawa, K., Kawasaki, M., Yao, T., et al.: Endoscopic ultrasound features of protein-losing gastropathy with hypertrophic gastric folds. Endoscopy. 2000; 32: 394–397.
80. Hoffer, V., Finkelstein, Y., Balter, J. et al.: Ganciclovir treatment in Menetrier's disease. Acta Paediatr 2003; 92:983–985.
81. Di Vita, G., Patti, R., Aragona, F. et al.: Resolution of Menetrier's disease after Helicobacter pylori eradicating treatment. Dig Dis 2001; 19:179–183.
82. Burdick, J., Chung, E., Tanner, G., et al.: Treatment of Menetrier's disease with a monoclonal antibody against the epidermal gross factor receptor. N Engl J Med 2000; 344: 1697–1701.
83. Zollinger, R. M., Ellison, E. H.: Primary peptic ulcerations of the jejunum associated with islet cells tumors of the pancreas. Ann Surg 1955; 142: 709–723.

84. Polacek, M. A., Ellison, E. H.: Parietal cell mass and gastric acid secretion in the Zollinger-Ellison sindrome. Surgery 1966; 60:606–614.
85. Peghini, P.L., Annibale, B., Azioni, C., et al.: Effect of cronic hypergastrinemia on human enterocromaffine-like cells: insights from patients with sporadic gastrinomas. Gastroenterology 2002; 123:68–85.
86. Bhutani, M. S., Dexter, D., McKellar, D. P., et al. : Intraoperative endoscopic ultrasonography in Zollinger-Ellison syndrome. Endoscopy. 1997; 29:754–756.
87. Bloomfeld, R., Bornstein, J., Jowell, P. A.: report of a gastrinoma localized preoperatively by endoscopic ultrasound only and a review of the approach to imaging in Zollinger-Ellison syndrome. Dig Dis 1999;17: 316–318.
88. Thompson, N. W., Czako, P.F., Fritts, L. L. et al.: Role of endoscopic ultrasonography in the localization of insulinomas and gastrinomas.Surgery 1994; 116:1131–1138.
89. Palazzo, L., Roseau, G., Salmeron, M.: Endoscopic ultrasonography in the preoperative localization of pancreatic endocrine tumors. Endoscopy 1992; 24 Suppl 1: 350–353.
90. Ruszniewski, P., Amouyal, P., Amouyal, G., et al.: Localization of gastrinomas by endoscopic ultrasonography in patients with Zollinger-Ellison syndrome.Surgery. 1995; 117:629–635.
91. Frucht, H., Norton, J. A., London, J. F., et al.: Detection of duodenal gastrinomas by operative endoscopic transillumination. A prospective study. Gastroenterology. 1990; 99:1622–1627.
92. Sarin, S. K., Lahoti D, Saxena SP et al. Relevance, classification and natural history of gastric varices: a long term-follow-up study in 568 portal hypertension patients. Hepatology 1992; 16:1343–1349.
93. Xiao, S.Y., Hart, J.: Marked gastric foveolar hyperplasia associated with active cytomegalovirus infection. Am J Gastroenterol 2001; 96:223–226.
94. Talukdar, R, Khanna, S., Saikia, N., et al.: Gastric tuberculosis presenting as linitis plastica: a case report and review of the literature. Eur J Gastroenterol Hepatol. 2006; 18:299–303.
95. Okai, T., Mouri, I., Yamaguchi, Y., et al. : Acute gastric anisakiasis: observations with endoscopic ultrasonography. Gastrointest Endosc 1993; 39:450–452.
96. Okada, M., Lizuka, Y., Oh, K., et al. : Gastritis cystica profunda presenting as giant gastric mucosal folds: the role of endoscopic ultrasonography and mucosectomy in the diagnostic work-up. Gastrointest Endosc 1994; 40:640–644.

CHAPTER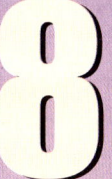

Subepithelial Lesions of the Upper GI Tract

Dr. Joo Ha Hwang
Dr. Stephen J. Rulyak

Introduction

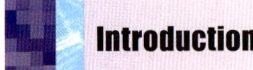

The endoscopic appearance of a subepithelial lesion in the gastrointestinal tract is that of a mass, bulge, or impression visible within the lumen, which is covered by normal-appearing mucosa. Subepithelial lesions in the upper GI tract are relatively common findings in patients undergoing upper gastrointestinal endoscopy. While such masses are often referred to as "submucosal," these lesions are more correctly termed **subepithelial** because they may arise from layers of the gastrointestinal wall other than the submucosa or from extrinsic compression by a number of normal or abnormal intra-abdominal structures. The prevalence of subepithelial lesions on routine endoscopies is uncertain although one retrospective study reported that subepithelial gastric lesions were identified in 0.36% of upper endoscopies performed between 1976 and 1984.[1]

Diagnostic Techniques

Endoscopy

Features of subepithelial lesions that can be assessed during endoscopy include an estimate of the size, shape, mobility, consistency (pillow sign, firm, cystic), pulsation, color, and mucosal appearance. Typically, subepithelial lesions have normal-appearing mucosa overlying the lesion, although reactive mucosal changes can occur with subepithlial lesions. Furthermore, subepithelial lesions usually appear smooth with tapered margins along the edge of the lesion. However, it can be difficult to differentiate an intramural lesion from extramural compression with endoscopy alone. Two prospective studies have demonstrated that the sensitivity and specificity of endoscopy to correctly differentiate an intramural lesion from extramural compression was between 89 and 98%, and 29 and 64%, respectively.[2,3]

A subepithelial lesion identified during endsocopy should be probed with closed biopsy forceps to determine its consistency. The consistency of the mass can occasionally suggest a diagnosis. For example, a mobile mass that is soft and indents when depressed using biopsy forceps (the so-called "pillow sign") is highly suggestive of a lipoma, although a subepithelial cyst can have a similar finding.[4] Lesions that are firm when probed with a biopsy forceps are not typically a cyst or lipoma and require further evaluation with endoscopic ultrasound (EUS).

Endosonography

Endoscopic ultrasound examination can reliably differentiate intramural lesions from extrinsic compression. Furthermore, EUS will often result in a specific diagnosis, particularly if the lesion is due to extrinsic compression. An example of extrinsic compression of the gastric lumen from an enlarged gallbladder is shown in Figure 8–1. If an intramural lesion is identified, EUS can be used to determine the size, layer of origin, and additional imaging features

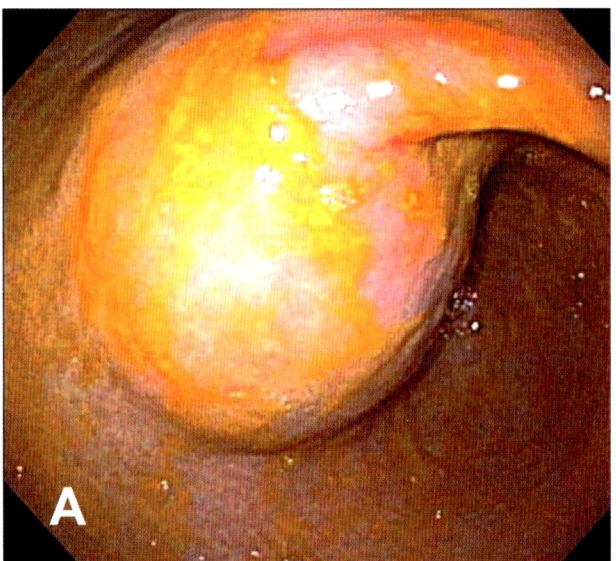

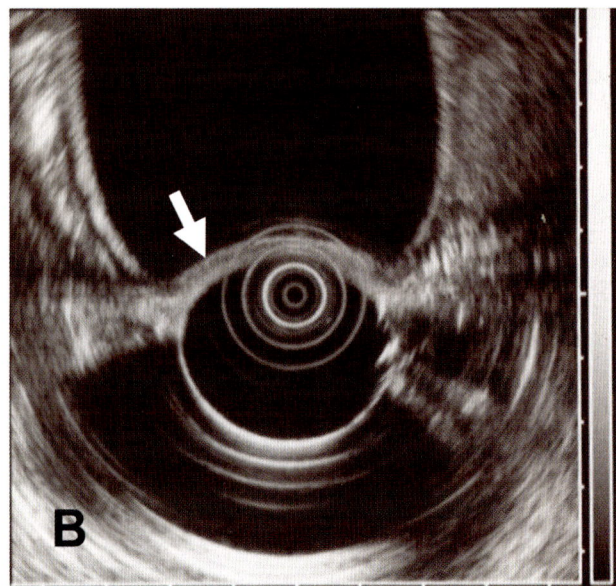

FIGURE 8–1. *A and B* Extrinsic compression from an enlarged gallbladder. (A) Endoscopic view of a subepithelial lesions resulting from extrinsic compression of an enlarged gallbladder. (B) EUS image of the subepithelial lesion demonstrating a normal gastric wall (white arrow) and an enlarged gallbladder.

Table 8–1. The Five-Layered Gastrointestinal Wall on EUS Imaging

EUS layer	Corresponding histologic structure
1	superficial mucosa
2	deep mucosa
3	submucosa **plus** acoustic interface between submucosa and muscularis propria
4	muscularis propria **minus** acoustic interface between submucosa and muscularis propria
5	serosa and subserosal fat

that can suggest a diagnosis. On EUS, imaging lesions can be either homogeneous or heterogeneous and can be hyperechoic, hypoechoic, isoechoic, or anechoic. Anechoic lesions can also be interrogated with Doppler to assess for blood flow if using an imaging transducer with this capability. EUS imaging can also be used to assess the margins of lesions to determine if they are smooth or have an irregular contour. In addition, EUS imaging can be used to assess if lesions are invading adjacent structures. Small, well-circumscribed lesions are typically benign, whereas lesions with irregular margins that extend into other layers or adjacent structures are more likely to represent a malignant process.[5,6] The features identified on EUS can then be used to determine if surgery or further tests such as endoscopic resection, fine-needle aspiration (FNA), or core biopsies are required.

EUS imaging of the GI tract wall typically exhibits five distinct layers but can also exhibit seven or nine layers, depending on the region of the GI tract being examined and the frequency of the ultrasound (US) transducer. The histological correlation to the five layers seen on EUS imaging (usually seen when imaging at 5 or 7.5 MHz) is given in Table 8-1.[7] Most intramural subepithlial lesions in the upper GI tract are identified in the deep mucosa (layer two), submucosa (layer three), or the muscularis propria (layer four).

Tissue Diagnosis

Imaging of subepithelial lesions with EUS helps identify those lesions where tissue diagnosis may be necessary. If a subepithelial lesion is found to be a hypoechoic mass in the third or fourth EUS layer, then tissue sampling should be strongly considered in order to establish the diagnosis, because malignant or premalignant lesions are included in the differential diagnosis. EUS imaging findings alone have been shown to be inadequate to correctly establish the diagnosis in such lesions.[8] However, preoperative tissue diagnosis may not be necessary in patients who will require surgery irrespective of histology.

EUS-Guided Fine Needle Aspiration

EUS-guided fine needle aspiration (EUS-FNA) can be used to obtain a specimen for cytologic examination, and occasionally core tissue specimens, by directing the needle into the area of interest under direct ultrasound guidance.[7,8] Complications from EUS-FNA are rare but include perforation, infection, or hemorrhage.[7,9-13] For EUS-FNA of cysts, infection has been reported in up to 15% of cases, justifying the use of preprocedural antibiotic prophylaxis.[14,15] In reports where prophylactic antibiotics were administered prior to aspiration of cysts, fewer infectious complications have been reported.[11,16]

Cytology can distinguish benign from malignant lesions, but is less useful for determining the type of benign lesion present. Thus, the reported sensitivity, specificity, and accuracy of cytologic evaluation for intramural lesions is low.[8,9,17] The yield of EUS-FNA in the diagnosis of hypoechoic fourth layer masses, such as gastrointestinal stromal tumors (GISTs), may be improved with the application of immunohistochemical analysis when sufficient tissue for staining can be obtained.[8,18,19] Common markers used to evaluate hypoechoic intramural masses are CD-117 (C-KIT), CD-34, smooth muscle actin (SMA), and S-100.[19,20] The C-KIT protein is a transmembrane receptor with tyrosine kinase activity that is highly sensitive and specific for GISTs. CD-34 is also expressed in approximately 80% of GISTs. Positive staining for smooth muscle actin suggests the presence of a leiomyoma or glomus tumor, and the presence of S-100 suggests a neural origin or Schwannoma.

EUS-Guided Core Needle Biopsy

EUS-guided core needle biopsy using a 19-gauge Trucut needle (QuickCore, Wilson-Cook, Inc., Winston-Salem, NC) can obtain sufficient tissue for histologic evaluation.[21,22] The Trucut needle provides a core of tissue that can be examined histologically, as opposed to cytologically, for changes in tissue architecture in addition to evaluating cellular morphology. Initial experience using the Trucut biopsy needle in intramural lesions yielded the correct diagnosis in four of five cases compared to one of five cases using EUS-FNA.[21]

Stacked Forceps Biopsy

Standard biopsy forceps are designed to sample primarily the mucosa, although the submucosa is sometimes sampled in mucosal biopsy specimens. By taking multiple biopsies of the same site using a jumbo forceps (interchangeably referred to as "stacked", "bite-on-bite", or "tunneled" biopsies), tissue from deeper layers of the gastric wall can potentially be obtained. This technique appears to be safe with a relatively low risk of bleeding, although the diagnostic yield also appears to be limited. In one study, the diagnostic yield of stacked biopsies was 42% (15 of 36 lesions) and the complication rate was 2.8% (1 in 36 cases complicated by bleeding).[23] In another study, the yield of stacked forceps biopsy in evaluating subepithelial lesions limited to the submucosa was only 17% (4 of 23 cases).[24]

Endoscopic Submucosal Resection (ESMR) and Dissection (ESD)

The use of ESMR or ESD to resect submucosal lesions is another technique to obtain tissue specimens for accurate histologic diagnosis.[23-28] This technique provides greater yield than stacked biopsies. EUS evaluation prior to attempting ESMR or ESD is essential. These techniques are usually reserved for lesions that are confined to the submucosal or deep mucosal layers due to the increased risk of perforation associated with endoscopic resection of lesions from the muscularis propria. Intraprocedural and delayed bleeding and perforations can occur with ESMR and ESD as with all endoscopic resection techniques, but both are relatively infrequent when the procedures are performed by experienced endoscopists.

Differential Diagnosis

The initial distinction that needs to be made regarding an upper GI subepithelial mass is whether the lesion represents compression from a normal or abnormal structure adjacent to the gastric wall, or if it originates from the wall itself. This differentiation is accurately made by performing EUS imaging. When an intramural subepithelial lesion is identified, additional findings on EUS imaging, including the histologic layer of origin and echogenicity, can help to narrow the differential diagnosis.[29] The differential diagnoses for intramural causes of upper GI subepithelial lesions are given in Table 8-2. Table 8-3 provides a summary of additional lesions that can be seen within specific regions of the upper GI tract (i.e., esophagus, stomach, or duodenum).

Table 8–2. Differential Diagnosis of Upper GI Tract Intramural Subepithelial Masses Based on EUS Features

Subepithelial Lesion	EUS Layer*	Echogenicity
Malignant or potentially malignant lesions		
GIST	4 (rarely 2)	hypoechoic
Lymphoma	2, 3 or 4	hypoechoic
Glomus tumor	3 or 4	hypoechoic
Metastatic carcinoma	any	hypoechoic
Benign lesions		
Leiomyoma	2 or 4	hypoechoic
Fibroma	3	hyperechoic
Neurofibroma	3 or 4	hyperechoic
Osteochondroma	3	hyperechoic
Lipoma	3	intensely hyperechoic
Lymphangioma	3 or 4	hypoechoic
Fibrovascular polyp	3 or 4	hyperechoic
Duplication cyst	any or extramural	anechoic
Varices	2 or 3	anechoic

*Refer to Table 5-1 for histological structure corresponding to EUS layer. (Adapted from Hwang and Kimmey[29]).

Table 8-3 Additional Intramural Subepithelial Masses Based on EUS Features and Location in the Upper GI Tract

Subepithelial Lesion	EUS Layer*	Echogenicity
Esophagus:		
Granular cell tumor	2 or 3	hypoechoic
Bronchogenic cyst	extramural	anechoic
Stomach:		
Carcinoid	2 or 3	hypoechoic
Pancreatic rest	2 or 3	hypoechoic
Glomus tumor	any	hypoechoic
Duodenum:		
Carcinoid	2 or 3	hypoechoic
Brunner's gland hyperplasia	2 or 3	hypoechoic
Pancreatic rest	2 or 3	hypoechoic

*Refer to Table 5-1 for histological structure corresponding to EUS layer.

Extramural Lesions

The most common cause of extraluminal compression seen in the stomach on endoscopoy is from the spleen and splenic vessels.[2,3,30] Other sources of extraluminal compression include normal abdominal structures, such as the left lobe of the liver, gallbladder (Figure 8–1), colon, and pancreas. In addition, pathologic lesions—such as tumors, abscesses, pancreatic pseudocysts, renal cysts, aneurysms, and enlarged lymph nodes—can sometimes be identified as gastric subepithelial lesions at endoscopy.

Intramural Lesions

The differential diagnosis for intramural gastric subepithelial masses can be divided into benign lesions or lesions that are malignant or premalignant (Table 8-2).

Benign Intramural Lesions

Lipomas

Lipomas are frequently encountered subepithelial masses in the upper GI tract.[31] Lipomas are benign and generally slow-growing lesions; however, they can cause significant clinical symptoms, such as bleeding due to ulceration, obstruction from intussusception of the lesion into the pylorus or duodenal bulb, and abdominal pain.[31-33] Lipomas typically present as solitary lesions; however, multiple lipomas of the stomach and duodenum have been reported.[34] On endoscopy, lipomas can have a yellow hue, often exhibit a pillow sign when probed with closed biopsy forceps, and may also exhibit some mobility. A recent study demonstrated that the pillow sign had 98% specificity, but only 40% sensitivity in identifying lipomas.[2] Based on this study, a yellow-appearing subepithelial lesion with a pillow sign is very likely to be lipoma and may not require confirmation with EUS, although this question requires prospective evaluation. The finding of an intensely hyperechoic well-circumscribed mass arising from the submucosal wall layer on EUS examination is essentially diagnostic for a lipoma, and no further evaluation is needed in such cases (Figures 8–2 and 8–3).

Leiomyomas

Leiomyomas are smooth muscle tumors that arise from either the muscularis mucosae or muscularis propria within the wall of the GI tract. These are benign tumors composed of well-differentiated smooth muscle cells. True leiomyomas are rarely found in the stomach, although case reports are abundant in the older literature because GISTs were often misclassified as leiomyomas or leiomyosarcomas in the past. With new immunohistochemical methods, it is clear that tumors of smooth muscle origin, as identified by positive staining for alpha-smooth muscle actin (SMA) and desmin and negative staining for CD117, CD34, and S100 protein, are rare in the stomach.[35] However, true leiomyomas are relatively commonly in the esophagus. Leiomyomas appear as hypoechoic, well- circumscribed masses arising from the muscularis propria or the muscularis mucosae on EUS examination, although tissue sampling is necessary to confirm this diagnosis.

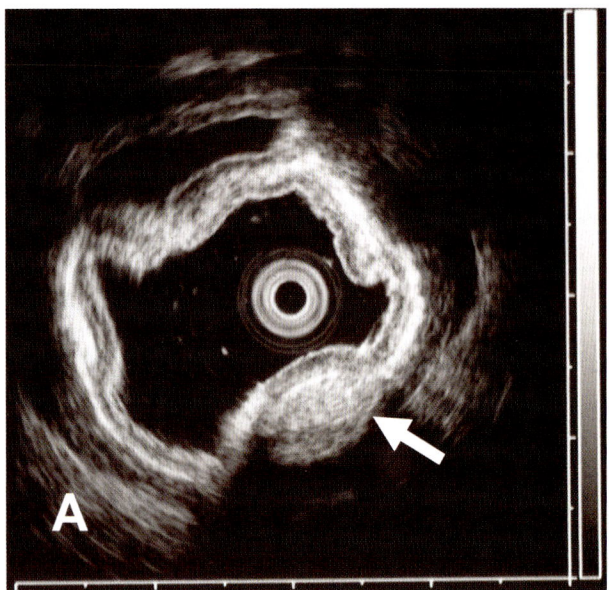
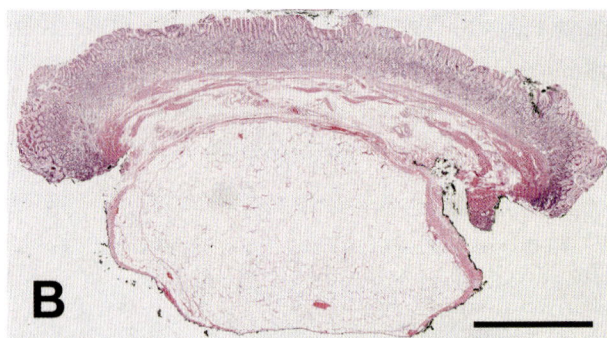

FIGURE 8–2. *A and B* Lipoma. (A) EUS image using a 20 MHz catheter probe demonstrating a well-circumscribed intensely hyperechoic lesion (white arrow) in the third EUS layer of the gastric wall corresponding to the submucosa. (B) EMR specimen of a lipoma (H&E, original magnification 20x, scale bar = 2 mm).

Varices

Gastric varices can have the appearance of a subepithelial mass or large gastric fold on endoscopy.[36] Gastric varices should be suspected in patients with portal hypertension (end-stage liver disease, Budd-Chiari syndrome, and portal vein thrombosis) and in patients with splenic vein thrombosis, typically due to pancreatitis, which can result in isolated gastric varices. Endoscopic examination may also reveal the presence of portal hypertensive gastropathy. Probing with closed biopsy forceps may reveal a soft consistency to the lesion. EUS examination will demonstrate a round or tubular hypoechoic or anechoic structure located in the submucosa (third layer), and Doppler examination will demonstrate venous flow within the structure.

Pancreatic Rests

A pancreatic rest, also known as heterotopic pancreatic tissue, is the presence of ectopic pancreatic tissue within the wall of the stomach. Pancreatic rests are typically found in the gastric antrum, and usually within the submucosal layer (third EUS layer).[37] Although they generally do not cause symptoms, pancreatic rests have been reported to present with nausea, epigastric pain, weight loss, hematemesis, and gastric outlet obstruction.[37,38] In addition, there are rare case reports of heterotopic pancreatic tissue that have undergone malignant change.[39-43] On endoscopy, a pancreatic rest commonly exhibits an umbilication on the surface of the nodule (Fig. 8-4A), although the specificity of this finding is not known. On EUS examination, a pancreatic rest will appear hypoechoic relative to the surrounding submucosal layer and will often have a heterogeneous echotexture (Fig. 8-4B). Because the differential diagnosis for hypoechoic third layer lesions includes potentially malignant lesions, tissue sampling to establish the

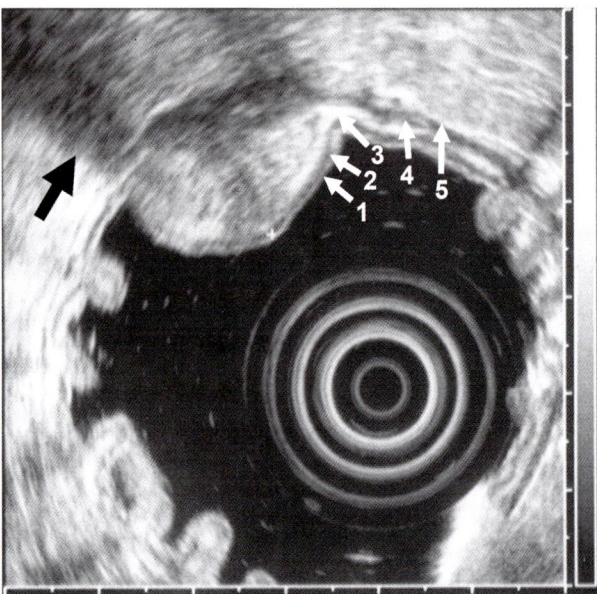

FIGURE 8–3. EUS image of a lipoma imaged at 5 MHz. The lesion is in the third EUS layer and is hyperechoic. Note that larger lipomas may appear heterogeneous. In addition, the size and shape of this lesion is causing refraction artifact (hypoechoic shadows identified by black arrow). The numbered white arrows correspond to the EUS layers as described in Table 5-1. (Courtesy of Dr. Michael Saunders)

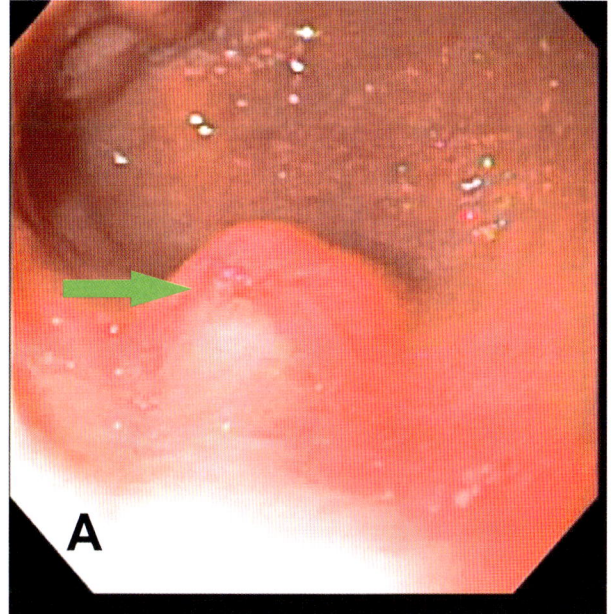
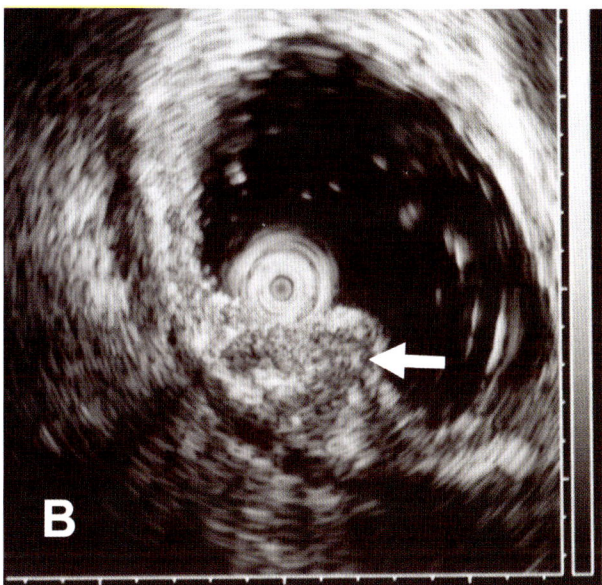
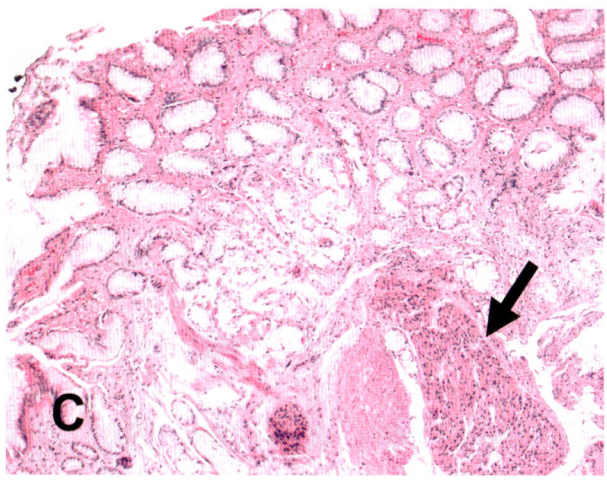

FIGURE 8–4. *A to C* Heterotopic pancreas. (A) Endoscopic image of an umbilicated (green arrow), subepithelial mass in the gastric antrum. (B) EUS image of a hypoechoic, heterogeneous mass in the second and third EUS layers (white arrow) as imaged using a 12 MHz catheter probe. (C) Histology from an EMR performed on the lesion in (A) demonstrating a focus of pancreatic tissue (black arrow) underlying normal gastric mucosa (H&E, original magnification 100x).

diagnosis is necessary. Cap-assisted ESMR has been reported as an effective endoscopic method of obtaining an adequate histological sample to diagnose a pancreatic rest (Fig. 8-4C).[44]

Benign Cystic Lesions Including Duplication Cysts

Gastrointestinal cysts can be acquired or developmental, and include simple mucosal and submucosal cysts, retention cysts, and duplication cysts. Duplication cysts are benign lesions that result from an error in the embryonic development of the foregut. They are often diagnosed in the pediatric population, but are also identified throughout adulthood.[45,46] The cysts can be located either within or adjacent to the wall of the gastrointestinal tract and are lined with gastrointestinal epithelium.[47] Because duplication cysts generally do not communicate with the gastrointestinal lumen, they can occasionally enlarge resulting in mass effect, rupture, or bleeding.[45,48,49] The diagnosis of a gastric duplication cyst can easily be made using EUS, which will demonstrate an anechoic, smooth, spherical, or tubular structure with a well-defined wall and increased through transmission (Figure 8–5).[50,51]

Inflammatory Fibroid Polyps

Gastric inflammatory fibroid polyps (IFP) are rare benign lesions in the stomach that are characterized histologically by fibrous tissue that is not encapsulated. In addition there are commonly many small blood vessels and an eosinophilic inflammatory infiltrate.[52,53] On EUS imaging, the polyps are located in the deep mucosal or submucosal layers without involvement of the muscularis propria (Figure 8–6).[52] They are typically hypoechoic with a homogenous echotexture and indistinct margins. Occasionally they will appear slightly hyperechoic, which corresponds histologically with multiple small penetrating vessels within the fibrous stroma of the polyp.[52] Given similar EUS findings as other lesions, tissue sampling is necessary to correctly establish this diagnosis.

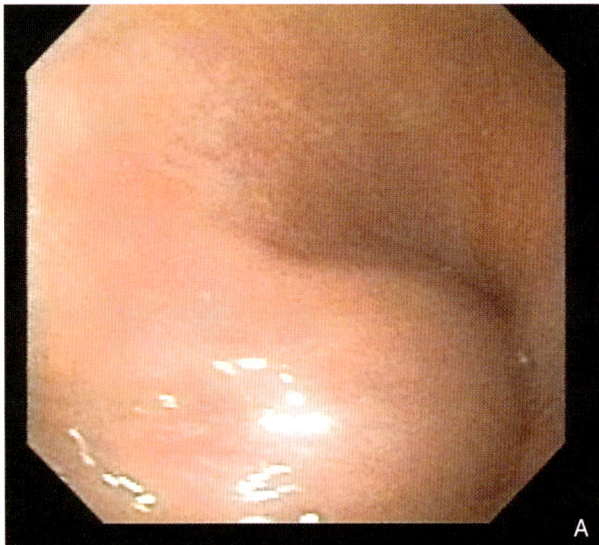
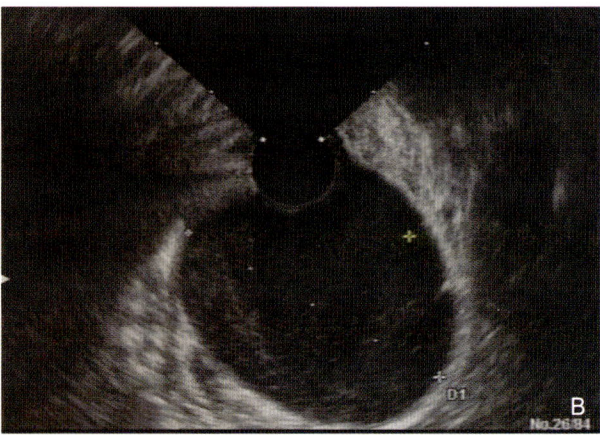

FIGURE 8–5. *A and B* Duplication cyst. (A) Endoscopic image of a duplication cyst at the gastroesophageal junction. (B) EUS image demonstrating an anechoic structure with increased echogenicity beyond the cyst (through transmission).

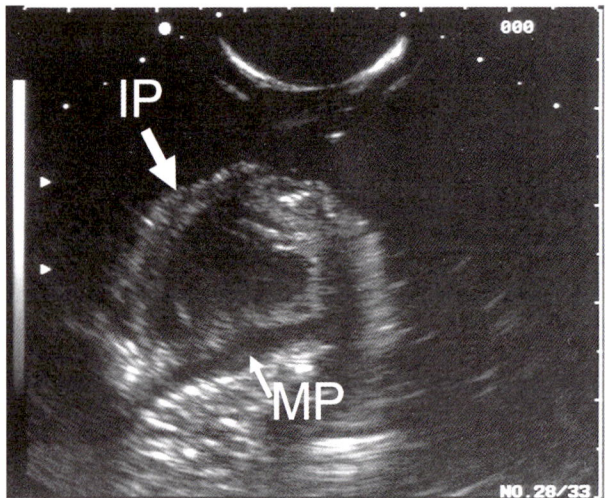

FIGURE 8–6. Gastric inflammatory polyp. The inflammatory polyp (IP) has a hypoechoic core with normal overlying mucosa. The muscularis propria (MP) is also identified.

Malignant and Potentially Malignant Intramural Lesions

Gastrointestinal Stromal Tumors

GISTs are the most commonly identified intramural subepithelial masses in the upper GI tract, and some controversy exists regarding the diagnosis and management of these tumors. It is believed that 5,000 to 6,000 new cases of GIST are diagnosed each year with 10 to 30% being malignant at the time of diagnosis.[54] It should be noted that all GISTs are thought to have malignant potential, although their natural history is incompletely understood, and many GISTs will never metastasize. The most common location of GISTs is the stomach.[20,54] GISTs were once thought to represent smooth muscle tumors (leiomyomas and leiomyosarcomas); however, they are now believed to arise from the interstitial cells of Cajal and can be identified using immunohistochemistry for expression of CD-117, which is also known as C-KIT protein (a cell membrane receptor with tyrosine kinase activity). A study of archived histological slides of masses previously classified as smooth muscle tumors demonstrated that most were actually GISTs—with the exception of masses in the esophagus, where true leiomyomas were more common.[35]

GISTs most commonly arise from the muscularis propria, but also rarely from the muscularis mucosa. GISTs are usually asymptomatic until the tumor becomes large or ulcerated, which can result in bleeding. EUS examination of a GIST demonstrates a hypoechoic mass with a homogeneous echotexture that is continuous with the muscularis propria (fourth EUS layer, Figure 8–7). Findings on EUS of a mass diameter greater than 3 cm, irregular extraluminal border, cystic spaces, echogenic foci (heterogenous echotexture), and adjacent malignant-appearing lymph nodes are features that can suggest malignancy,[4,5] however, even small GISTs have malignant potential and have been reported to metastasize.[55-57] Unfortunately, EUS findings do not accurately predict the malignant potential of a small GIST, and histologic examination is necessary. Suspected GIST lesions can be sampled using EUS-FNA or core needle biopsies that may be helpful in determining the malignant potential of a GIST without having to perform surgical resection; however, studies examining their clinical utility in large numbers of patients have yet to be reported.[7,58,59] Examples of EUS-FNA and

Subepithelial Lesions of the Upper GI Tract

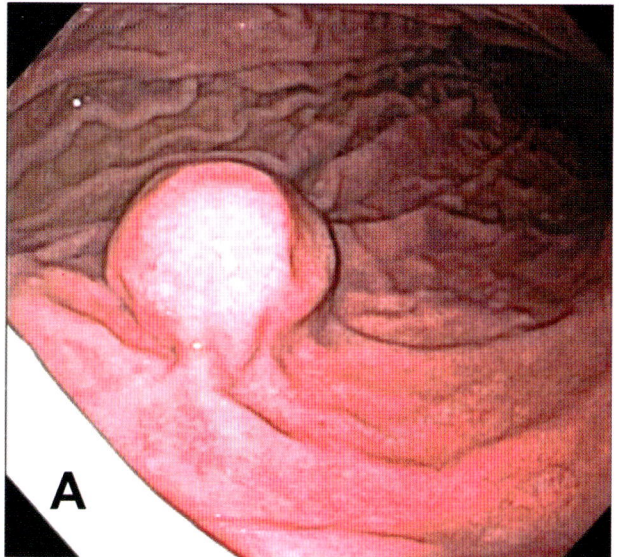
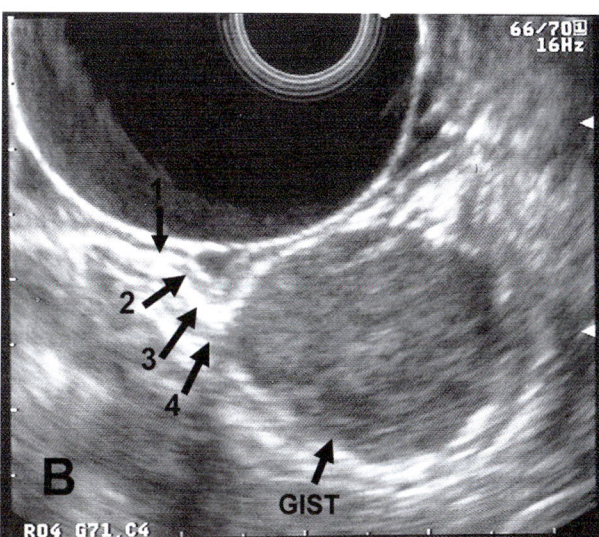

FIGURE 8–7. A and B Gastrointestinal stromal tumor (GIST). (A) Endoscopic image of a GIST located in the gastric body. (B) EUS image demonstrating a hypoechoic lesion arising from the fourth EUS layer (imaging frequency was 7.5 MHz). The numbered arrows correspond to EUS layers as described in Table 5-1.

EUS-guided core biopsies samples of GIST lesions are shown in Figures 8–8 and 8–9.

Carcinoid tumors

Gastric carcinoid tumors are neuroendocrine tumors that originate from enterochromaffin-like (ECL) cells located in the gastric mucosa. Carcinoid tumors can be solitary or multiple, the latter usually occurring in the setting of hypergastrinemia due to gastrinoma or autoimmune atrophic gastritis. Carcinoid tumors originate in the mucosal layer, but can also invade into deeper structures of the gastrointestinal tract wall and present as predominately subepithelial masses.[60] The biologic behavior appears to differ between solitary gastric carcinoids and multiple gastric carcinoids due

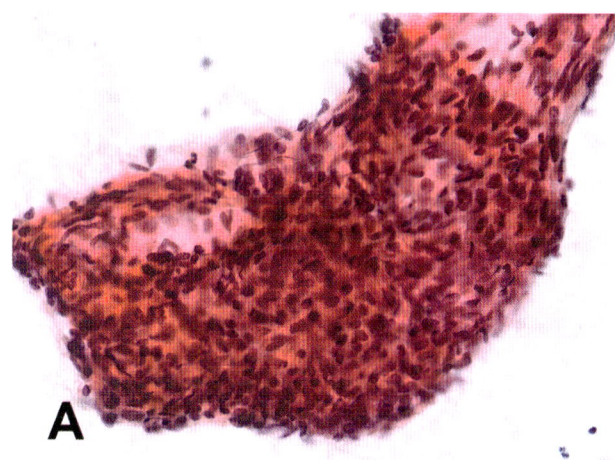
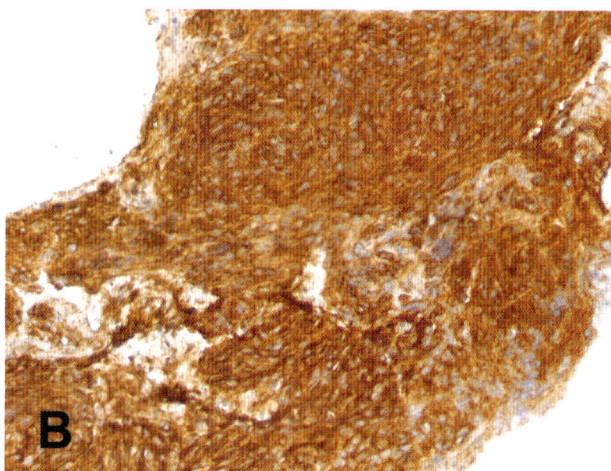
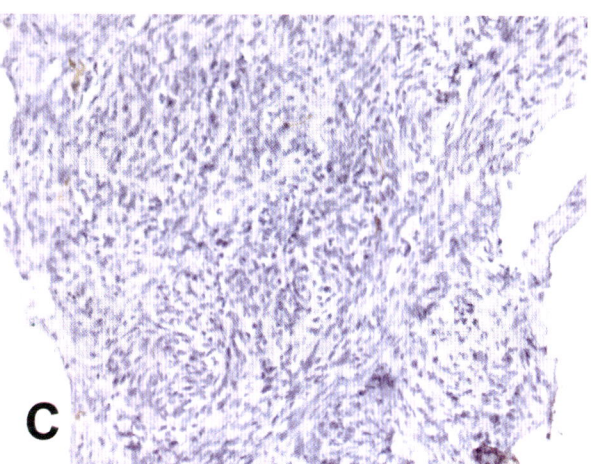

FIGURE 8–8. A to C Tissue specimen obtained from EUS-FNA of a GIST. (A) Papanicolaou stained smear (original magnification 400x) showing crowded, disorganized cluster of spindled cells. (B) Positive immunohistochemical staining for C-KIT (CD117). (C) Negative immunohistochemical staining for smooth muscle actin. (Courtesy of Dr. Verena Greco)

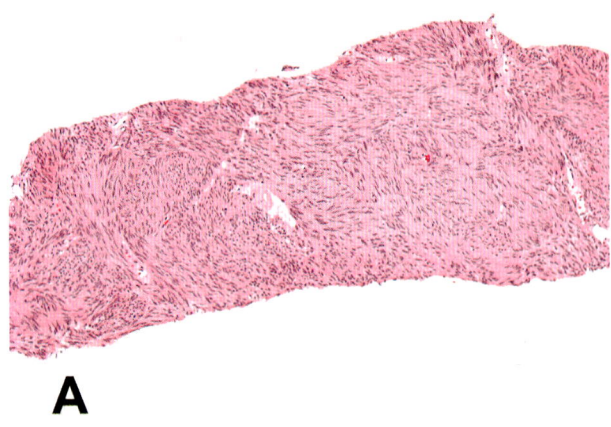
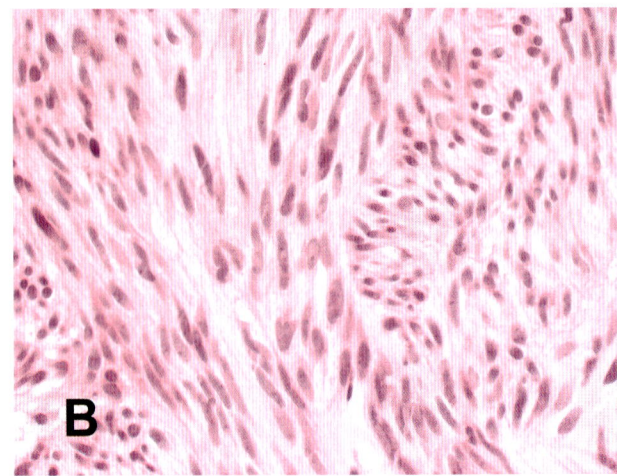
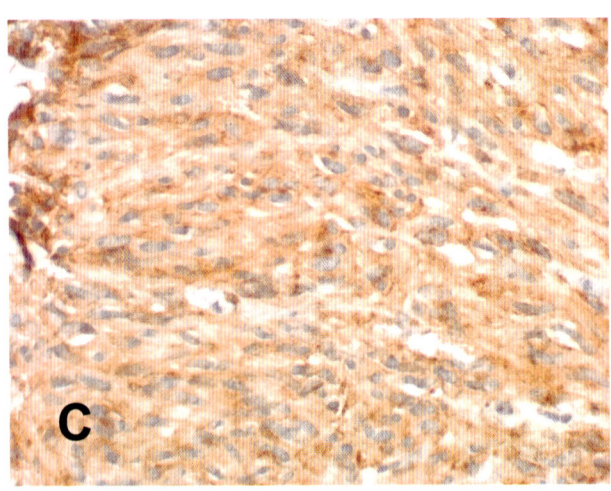

FIGURE 8–9. *A to C* Tissue specimen obtained from EUS-guided core biopsy of a GIST. (A) Photomicrograph of a core biopsy (H&E, original magnification 100x). (B) Photomicrograph demonstrating spindle cell morphology with uniform cigar-shaped cells and elongated nuclei (H&E, original magnification 400x). (C) Photomicrograph demonstrating positive immunohistochemical staining for C-KIT (original magnification 400x). (Courtesy of Dr. Melissa Upton)

to hypergastrinemia; solitary gastric carcinoids exhibit a much greater potential for malignancy and metastasis to local lymph nodes and the liver.[61-63] On endoscopy, carcinoids typically appear as polypoid lesions with normal-appearing overlying mucosa (Figure 8–10 A).[64] EUS examination of a carcinoid tumor will demonstrate a hypoechoic lesion, typically originating from the deep mucosa or submucosa (second or third EUS layer), and can be useful in identifying the depth of invasion of the carcinoid tumor (Figure 8–10 B).[65] Furthermore, EUS can be used to asses for possible local lymph node metastasis, and to facilitate tissue sampling to establish the diagnosis.

Lymphomas

Primary gastric lymphomas are typically either diffuse large B-cell lymphomas or low-grade B-cell mucosa-associated lymphoid tissue (MALT) lymphomas.[66,67] In addition, disseminated nodal disease can secondarily involve the gastrointestinal tract.[68] Endoscopically, a gastric lymphoma can present as an ulcerated polypoid mass, thickened gastric folds, or a subepithelial mass. Since gastric lymphomas typically involve the deep mucosa, standard biopsies usually provide sufficient tissue to make the diagnosis, although FNA or core biopsy is occasionally needed to establish the diagnosis. EUS of primary gastric lymphoma typically demonstrates a hypoechoic lesion that can be localized to the second and third layers of the gastric wall or extend through the entire wall (Figure 8–11).[69] EUS can also be used to assess for local lymph node involvement, and EUS-FNA can be used to obtain tissue for flow cytometry to establish the diagnosis.[70,71]

Glomus Tumors

Glomus tumors originate from modified vascular smooth muscle cells and usually occur in peripheral soft tissue, but can also occur in the gastrointestinal tract, typically the stomach.[72,73] These lesions are usually benign, but they have potential for malignant behavior and can also present with ulceration and hemorrhage. A retrospective study of 31 gastric glomus tumors showed that all but one tumor exhibited

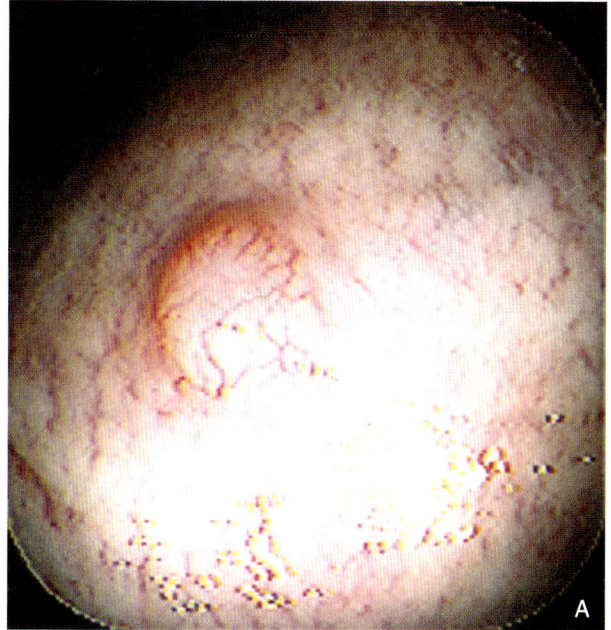
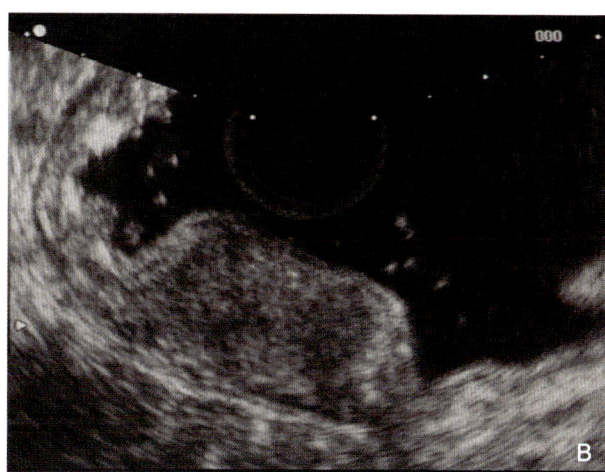

FIGURE 8–10. *A and B* Carcinoid tumor. (A) Endoscopic appearance of a gastric carcinoid tumor. (B) EUS image of a carcinoid tumor. The tumor is hypoechoic and located in the third EUS layer (submucosa).

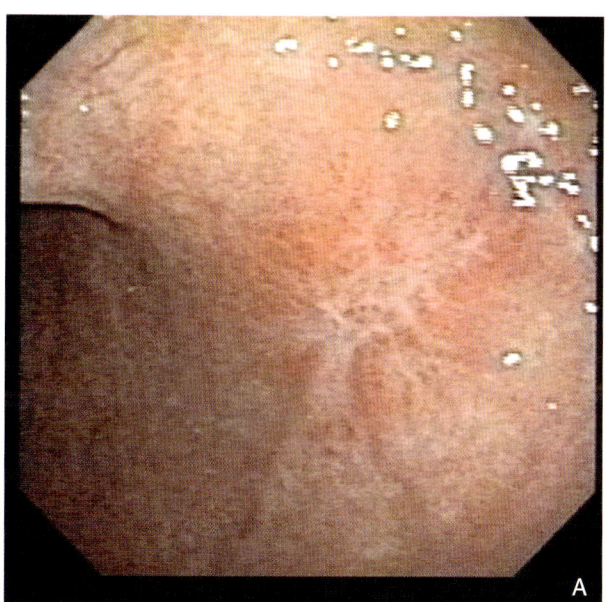
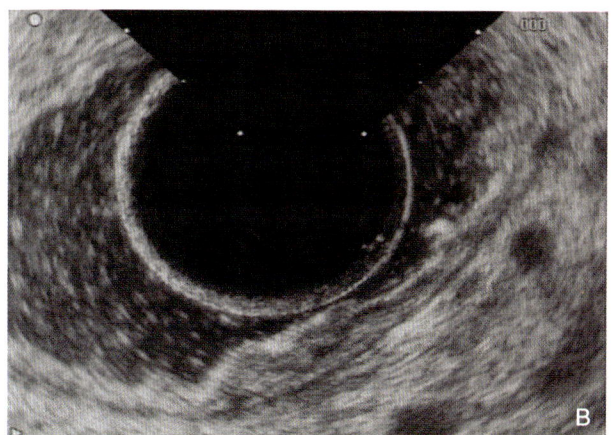

FIGURE 8–11. *A and B* Mucosa associated lymphoid tissue (MALT) lymphoma. (A) Endoscopic appearance of a gastric MALT lymphoma. (B) EUS image of the same MALT lymphoma as shown in (A) demonstrating a hypoechoic lesion expanding the second EUS layer (deep mucosa).

benign behavior; however, one patient died due to liver metastases of the glomus tumor.[72] On EUS examination, glomus tumors will be located in the third and/or fourth EUS layer and appear hypoechoic and well-circumscribed; however, EUS findings are insufficient to establish the diagnosis and cannot be used to predict the malignant potential of the tumor.[74]

EUS-guided FNA has been reported to successfully diagnose glomus tumors using cytologic and immunohistochemical analysis. Immunohistochemical staining will demonstrate positivity for smooth muscle actin and vimentin, while being negative for CD117 (C-KIT), which helps to differentiate these lesions from GISTs.[72,75]

Table 8-4	Immunohistochemical (IHC) Analysis of GI Mesenchymal Tumors
Tumor	Positive IHC Staining
GIST	CD-117 (C-KIT), CD-34
Smooth muscle tumor	Smooth muscle actin, Desmin
Schwannoma	S-100
Glomus tumor	Smooth muscle actin, Vimentin

Granular Cell Tumors

Granular cells tumors are relatively rare tumors that are thought to arise from Schwann cells. They are most commonly identified in the oropharynx or skin and subcutaneous tissues, although they are also found in the gastrointestinal tract. In the upper GI tract, they are most often identified in the esophagus. Granular cell tumors are usually asymptomatic, although on rare occasions they can present with bleeding, obstructive symptoms, or dysphagia. Most granular cell tumors are benign, although malignant granular cell tumors have been reported.[76] They are usually firm when probed with a biopsy forceps, and on EUS imaging they are typically hypoechoic lesions involving the deep mucosa or submucosa (EUS layers two or three, respectively; Figure 8–12). Given the similarity to other intramural lesions on EUS imaging, tissue diagnosis should be established using FNA or ESMR.[77] Immunohistochemistry can also be helpful, because granular cell tumors stain positive for s-100.

Metastasis

Metastatic spread of malignancies to the esophageal or gastric wall is extremely rare; however, various malignancies have potential to metastasize to the gastric wall, including malignant melanoma as well as carcinomas of the breast, lung, kidney, and ovaries.[78-83] EUS examination of most metastatic lesions will demonstrate a hypoechoic lesion that can occur in any layer of the esophageal or gastric wall (Figure 8–13). EUS-guided FNA can be performed to obtain tissue to establish the diagnosis of metastasis to the gastric wall.[82]

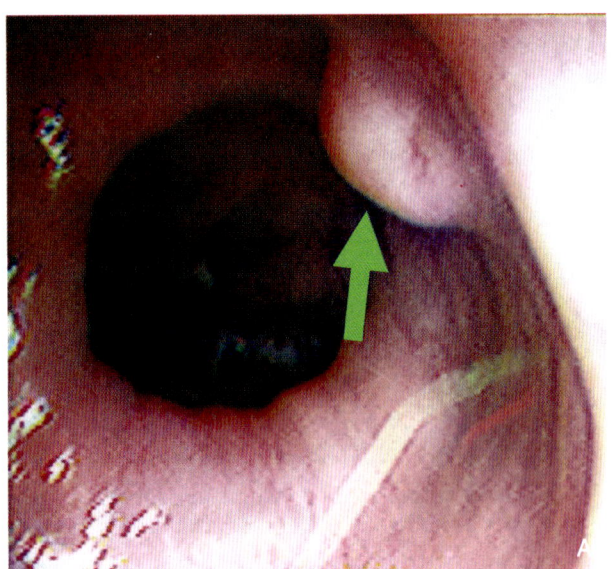
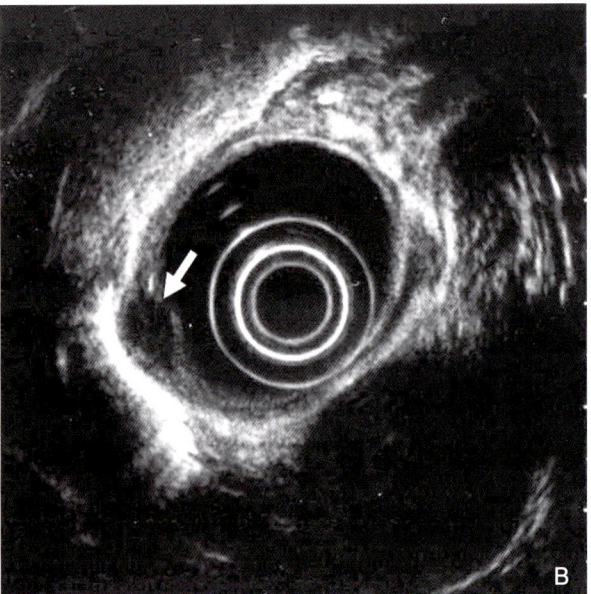

FIGURE 8–12. *A and B* Granular cell tumor. (A) Endoscopic of a granular cell tumor in the distal esophagus (green arrow). (B) EUS image of a granular cell tumor (white arrow). The lesion appears hypoechoic and is located in the second EUS layer (deep mucosa).

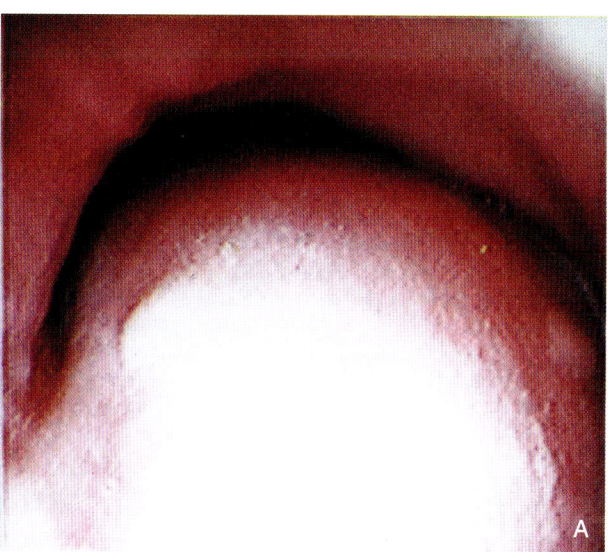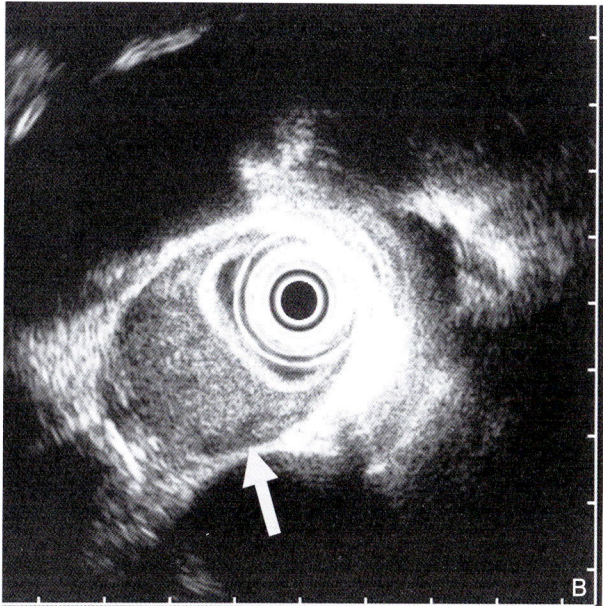

FIGURE 8–13. *A and B* Metastasis to the esophageal wall. (A) Endoscopic image of a large subepithelial mass in the distal esophagus. (B) EUS image of the lesion demonstrates a hypoechoic lesion in fourth EUS layer (muscularis propria). FNA demonstrated this lesion to be squamous cell carcinoma. The primary origin was not from the esophagus.

Conclusions

Identifying a subepithelial mass during endoscopy is common, and evaluation with EUS allows for improved characterization of subepithelial lesions, aiding the clinician in narrowing the differential diagnosis. Although the specificity of EUS in diagnosing the etiology of subepithelial lesions is low, it remains the best test for determining the need for further evaluation and can often direct management. Obtaining tissue using EUS-FNA, core biopsy, or endoscopic submucosal resection is often necessary to establish the diagnosis and direct further patient management.

References

1. Hedenbro, J. L., Ekelund, M., Wetterberg, P.: Endoscopic diagnosis of submucosal gastric lesions. The results after routine endoscopy. Surg Endosc 1991;5: 20–23.
2. Hwang, J. H., Saunders, M. D., Rulyak, S.J., et al.: A prospective study comparing endoscopy and EUS in the evaluation of GI subepithelial masses. Gastrointest Endosc 2005:62:202–208.
3. Rösch, T., Kapfer, B., Will, U., et al.: Accuracy of endoscopic ultrasonography in upper gastrointestinal submucosal lesions: a prospective multicenter study. Scand J Gastroenterol 2002;37:856–862.
4. Hwang, Saunders, Rulyak, et al.: A pospective study comparing endoscopy and EUS in the evaluation of GI subepithelial masses
5. Chak, A., Canto, M. I., Rösch, T., et al.: Endosonographic differentiation of benign and malignant stromal cell tumors. Gastrointest Endosc 1997;45: 468–472.
6. Hwang, Saunders, Rulyak, et al.: A pospective study comparing endoscopy and EUS in the evaluation of GI subepithelial masses
7. Ibid.
8. Ibid
9. Palazzo, L., Landi, B., Cellier, C., et al.: Endosonographic features predictive of benign and malignant gastrointestinal stromal cell tumors. Gut 2000;46: 88–92.
10. Kimmey, M. B., Martin, R. W., Haggitt, R.C., et al.: Histologic correlates of gastrointestinal ultrasound images. Gastroenterology 1989;96:433–441.
11. Matsui, M., Goto, H., Niwa, Y., et al.: Preliminary results of the needle aspiration biopsy histology in upper gastrointestinal submucosal tumors. Endoscopy 1998; 30:750–755.
12. Gu, M., Ghafari, S., Nguyen, P.T., Lin, F.: Cytologic diagnosis of gastrointestinal stromal tumors of the stomach by endoscopic ultrasound-guided fine-needle aspiration biopsy: cytomorphologic and immunohistochemical study of 12 cases. Diagn Cytopathol 2001;25:343–350.
13. Williams, D. B., Sahai, A. V., Aabakken L., et al.: Endoscopic ultrasound guided fine needle aspiration biopsy: a large single centre experience. Gut 1999; 44:720–726.
14. Affi, A., Vazquez-Sequeiros, E., Norton, ID, et al.: Acute extraluminal hemorrhage associated with EUS-guided

fine needle aspiration: frequency and clinical significance. Gastrointest Endosc 2001;53:221–225.
15. O'Toole, D., Palazzo, L., Arotcarena, R., Dancour, A., et al.: Assessment of complications of EUS-guided fine-needle aspiration. Gastrointest Endosc 2001;53: 470–474.
16. Barawi, M., Gottlieb, K., Cunha, B., et al.: A prospective evaluation of the incidence of bacteremia associated with EUS-guided fine-needle aspiration. Gastrointest Endosc 2001;53:189–192.
17. Levy, M. J., Norton, I. D., Wiersema, M. J., et al.: Prospective risk assessment of bacteremia and other infectious complications in patients undergoing EUS-guided FNA. Gastrointest Endosc 2003;57:672–678.
18. Wildi, S. M., Hoda RS, Fickling W, et al.: Diagnosis of benign cysts of the mediastinum: the role and risks of EUS and FNA. Gastrointest Endosc 2003;58:362–368.
19. Wiersema, M. J., Vilmann, P., Giovannini, M., et al.: Endosonography-guided fine-needle aspiration biopsy: diagnostic accuracy and complication assessment. Gastroenterology 1997;112:1087–1095.
20. Lee, L. S., Saltzman, J. R., Bounds, B. C., et al.: EUS-guided fine needle aspiration of pancreatic cysts: a retrospective analysis of complications and their predictors. Clin Gastroenterol Hepatol 2005;3:231–236.
21. Wiersema, M. J., Wiersema, L. M., Khusro, Q., et al.: Combined endosonography and fine-needle aspiration cytology in the evaluation of gastrointestinal lesions. Gastrointest Endosc 1994;40:199–206.
22. Hunt, G. C., Rader, A.E., Faigel, D. O.: A comparison of EUS features between CD-117 positive GI stromal tumors and CD-117 negative GI spindle cell tumors. Gastrointest Endosc 2003;57:469–474.
23. Stelow, E.B., Stanley, M. W., Mallery, S., et al.: Endoscopic ultrasound-guided fine-needle aspiration findings of gastrointestinal leiomyomas and gastrointestinal stromal tumors. Am J Clin Pathol 2003;119: 703–708.
24. Fletcher, C. D., Berman, J. J., Corless, C., et al.: Diagnosis of gastrointestinal stromal tumors: A consensus approach. Hum Pathol 2002;33:459–465.
25. Levy, M. J., Jondal, M. L., Clain, J., Wiersema, M. J.: Preliminary experience with an EUS-guided trucut biopsy needle compared with EUS-guided FNA. Gastrointest Endosc 2003;57:101–106.
26. Wiersema, M. J., Levy, M. J., Harewood, G. C., et al.: Initial experience with EUS-guided trucut needle biopsies of perigastric organs. Gastrointest Endosc 2002;56:275–278.
27. Hunt, G. C., Smith, P.P., Faigel, D. O..: Yield of tissue sampling for submucosal lesions evaluated by EUS. Gastrointest Endosc 2003;57:68–72.
28. Cantor, M. J., Davila, R.E., Faigel, D.O.: Yield of tissue sampling for subepithelial lesions evaluated by EUS: a comparison between forceps biopsies and endoscopic mucosal resection. Gastrointest Endosc 2006;64:29–34.
29. Hyun, J. H., Jeen, Y.T., Chun, H.J., et al.: Endoscopic resection of submucosal tumor of the esophagus: results in 62 patients. Endoscopy 1997;29:165–170.
30. Kojima, T., Takahashi, H,, Parra-Blanco, A., et al.: Diagnosis of submucosal tumor of the upper GI tract by endoscopic resection. Gastrointest Endosc 1999;50: 516–522.
31. Waxman, I., Saitoh, Y., Raju, G. S., et al.: High-frequency probe EUS-assisted endoscopic mucosal resection: a therapeutic strategy for submucosal tumors of the GI tract. Gastrointest Endosc 2002;55:44–49.
32. Sun, S., Wang, M., Sun, S.: Use of endoscopic ultrasound-guided injection in endoscopic resection of solid submucosal tumors. Endoscopy 2002;34:82–85.
33. Hwang, J. H., Kimmey, M. B.: The incidental upper gastrointestinal subepithelial mass. Gastroenterology 2004;126:301–307.
34. Motoo, Y., Okai, T., Ohta, H., et al.: Endoscopic ultrasonography in the diagnosis of extraluminal compressions mimicking gastric submucosal tumors. Endoscopy 1994;26:239–242.
35. Fernandez, M.J., Davis, R.P., Nora, P.F..: Gastrointestinal lipomas. Arch Surg 1983;118:1081–1083.
36. Thompson, W. M., Kende, A. L., Levy, A. D..: Imaging characteristics of gastric lipomas in 16 adult and pediatric patients. AJR Am J Roentgenol 2003;181:981–985.
37. Maderal, F., Hunter, F., Fuselier, G., et al.: Gastric lipomas—an update of clinical presentation, diagnosis, and treatment. Am J Gastroenterol 1984;79:964–967.
38. Deeths, T. M., Madden, P. N., Dodds, W. J.: Multiple lipomas of the stomach and duodenum. Am J Dig Dis 1975;20:771–774.
39. Miettinen, M., Sobin, L. H., Sarlomo-Rikala, M.: Immunohistochemical spectrum of GISTs at different sites and their differential diagnosis with a reference to CD117 (KIT). Mod Pathol 2000;13:1134–1142.
40. Mendis, R. E., Gerdes, H., Lightdale, C. J., Botet, J.F.: Large gastric folds: a diagnostic approach using endoscopic ultrasonography. Gastrointest Endosc 1994;40:437–441.
41. Thoeni, R. F., Gedgaudas, R. K.: Ectopic pancreas: usual and unusual features. Gastrointest Radiol 1980;5:37–42.
42. Lai, E. C., Tompkins, R. K.: Heterotopic pancreas. Review of a 26 year experience. Am J Surg 1986; 151:697–700.
43. Goldfarb, W. B., Bennett, D., Monafo, W.: Carcinoma in a heterotopic gastric pancreas. Ann Surg 1963;158: 56–58.
44. Tanimura, A., Yamamoto, H., Shibata, H., Sano, E.: Carcinoma in heterotopic gastric pancreas. Acta Path Jap 1979;29:251–257.
45. Hickman, D. M., Frey, C. F., Carson, J. W.: Adenocarcinoma arising in gastric heterotopic pancreas. West J Med 1981;135:57–62.
46. Jeng, K. S., Yang, K. C., Kuo, S. H.: Malignant degeneration of heterotopic pancreas. Gastrointest Endosc 1991;37:196–198.
47. Ura, H., Denno, R., Hirata, K., et al.: Carcinoma arising from ectopic pancreas in the stomach: endosonographic detection of malignant change. J Clin Ultrasound 1998;26:265–268.
48. Faigel, D.O., Gopal, D., Weeks, D. A., Corless, C.: Cap-assisted endoscopic submucosal resection of a pancreatic rest. Gastrointest Endosc 2001;54:782–784.
49. Lamont, A. C., Starinsky, R., Cremin, B. J.: Ultrasonic diagnosis of duplication cysts in children. Br J Radiol 1984;57:463–467.
50. Hulnick, D. H., Balthazar, E. J.: Gastric duplication cyst: GI series and CT correlation. Gastrointest Radiol 1987;12:106–108.
51. Mathur, M., Gupta, S. D., Bajpai, M., Rohatagi, M.: Histochemical pattern in alimentary tract duplications of children. Am J Gastroenterol 1991;86:1419–1423.
52. Ott, D. J., Wolfman, N. T., Wu, W. C., et al.: Endoscopic ultrasonography of benign esophageal cyst simulating leiomyoma. J Clin Gastroenterol 1992;15:85–87.
53. Stringer, M. D., Dinwiddie, R., Hall, C. M., Spitz, L.: Foregut duplication cysts: a diagnostic challenge. J R Soc Med 1993;86:174–175.

54. Geller, A., Wang, K. K., DiMagno, E. P.: Diagnosis of foregut duplication cysts by endoscopic ultrasonography. Gastroenterology 1995;109:838–842.
55. Faigel, D. O., Burke, A., Ginsberg, G. G., et al.: The role of endoscopic ultrasound in the evaluation and management of foregut duplications. Gastrointest Endosc 1997;45:99–103.
56. Kim, Y, I., Kim, W. H.: Inflammatory fibroid polyps of gastrointestinal tract. Evolution of histologic patterns. Am J Clin Pathol 1988;89:721–727.
57. Matsushita, M., Hajiro, K, Okazaki, K., Takakuwa, H.: Gastric inflammatory fibroid polyps: endoscopic ultrasonographic analysis in comparison with the histology. Gastrointest Endosc 1997;46:53–57.
58. Miettinen, M., Sarlomo-Rikala, M., Lasota, J.: Gastrointestinal stromal tumors: recent advances in understanding of their biology. Hum Pathol 1999;30:1213–1220.
59. Meesters, B., Pauwels, P. A. A, Pijnenburg, A. M., et al.: Metastasis in a 'benign' duodenal stromal tumor. Eur J Surg Oncol 1998;24:334–335.
60. Trupiano, J. K., Stewart, R. E., Misick, C., et al.: Gastric stromal tumors: a clinicopathologic study of 77 cases with correlation of features with nonaggressive and aggressive clinical behaviors. Am J Surg Pathol 2002;26:705–714.
61. Evans, H. L.: Smooth muscle tumors of the gastrointestinal tract. A study of 56 cases followed for a minimum of 10 years. Cancer 1985;56:2242–2250.
62. Levy, A. D., Remotti, H. E., Thompson, W. M., et al. Gastrointestinal stromal tumors: radiologic features with pathologic correction. Radiographics 2003;23:283–304.
63. Ando, N., Goto, H., Niwa, Y., et al.: The diagnosis of GI stromal tumors with EUS-guided fine needle aspiration with immunohistochemical analysis. Gastrointest Endosc 2002;55:37–43.
64. Soga, J.: Early-stage carcinoids of the gastrointestinal tract: an analysis of 1914 reported cases. Cancer 2005;103:1587–1595.
65. Rindi, G., Azzoni, C., La Rosa, S., et al.: ECL cell tumor and poorly differentiated endocrine carcinoma of the stomach: prognostic evaluation by pathological analysis. Gastroenterology 1999;116:532–542.
66. Rindi, G., Luinetti, O., Cornaggia, M., et al.: Three subtypes of gastric argyrophil carcinoid and the gastric neuroendocrine carcinoma: a clinicopathologic study. Gastroenterology 1993;104:994–1006.
67. Soga, J.: Gastric carcinoids: a statistical evaluation of 1,094 cases collected from the literature. Surg Today 1997;27:892–901.
68. Nakamura, S., Lida, M., Yao, T., Fujishima, M.: Endoscopic features of gastric carcinoids. Gastrointest Endosc 1991;37:535–538.
69. Matsumoto, T., Lida, M., Suekane, H., et al.: Endoscopic ultrasonography in rectal carcinoid tumors: contribution to selection of therapy. Gastrointest Endosc 1991;37:539–542.
70. Brooks, J. J., Enterline, H. T.. Primary gastric lymphomas. A clinicopathologic study of 58 cases with long-term follow-up and literature review. Cancer 1983;51:701–711.
71. Lewin, K.J., Ranchod, M., Dorfman, R. F.: Lymphomas of the gastrointestinal tract: a study of 117 cases presenting with gastrointestinal disease. Cancer 1978;42:693–707.
72. Kolve, M., Fischbach, W., Greiner, A., Wilms, K.: Differences in endoscopic and clinicopathological features of primary and secondary gastric non-Hodgkin's lymphoma. German Gastrointestinal Lymphoma Study Group. Gastrointest Endosc 1999;49:307–315.
73. Bolondi, L., Casanova, P., Caletti, G. C., et al.: Primary gastric lymphoma versus gastric carcinoma: endoscopic US evaluation. Radiology 1987;165:821–826.
74. Tio, T. L., den Hartog Jager, F. C., Tijtgat, G. N.: Endoscopic ultrasonography of non-Hodgkin lymphoma of the stomach. Gastroenterology 1986;91:401–408.
75. Vander Noot, M. R., 3rd, Eloubeidi, M. A., Chen, V. K., et al.: Diagnosis of gastrointestinal tract lesions by endoscopic ultrasound-guided fine-needle aspiration biopsy. Cancer 2004;102:157–163.
76. Miettinen, M., Paal, E., Lasota, J., Sobin, L. H..: Gastrointestinal glomus tumors: a clinicopathologic, immunohistochemical, and molecular genetic study of 32 cases. Am J Surg Pathol 2002;26:301–311.
77. Tsuneyoshi, M., Enjoji, M.: Glomus tumor: a clinicopathologic and electron microscopic study. Cancer 1982;50:1601–1607.
78. Imamura, A., Tochihara, M., Natsui, K., et al.: Glomus tumor of the stomach: endoscopic ultrasonographic findings. Am J Gastroenterol 1994;89:272–272.
79. Debol, S. M., Stanley, M. W., Mallery, S., et al.: Glomus tumor of the stomach: cytologic diagnosis by endoscopic ultrasound-guided fine-needle aspiration. Diagn Cytopathol 2003;28:316–321.
80. Yoshizawa, A., Ota, H., Sakaguchi, N., et al.: Malignant granular cell tumor of the esophagus. Virchows Arch. 2004;444:304–306.
81. Prematilleke, I. V., Piris, J., Shah, K. A..: Fine needle aspiration cytology of a granular cell tumor of the oesophagus. Cytopathology. 2004;15:120–121
82. Panagiotou, I., Brountzos, E. N., Bafaloukos, D., et al.: Malignant melanoma metastatic to the gastrointestinal tract. Melanoma Res 2002;12:169–173.
83. Kadakia, S. C., Parker, A., Canales, L.: Metastatic tumors to the upper gastrointestinal tract: endoscopic experience. Am J Gastroenterol 1992;87:1418–1423.
84. Saunders, N. J.: Haematemesis due to gastric involvement by metastatic ovarian carcinoma 30 years after removal of the primary tumor. Br J Clin Pract 1986;40:298–299.
85. Taylor, R. R., Phillips, W. S., O'Connor, D. M., Harrison, C. R.: Unusual intramural gastric metastasis of recurrent epithelial ovarian carcinoma. Gynecol Oncol 1994;55:152-155.
86. Sangha S, Gergeos F, Freter P, et al. Diagnosis of ovarian cancer metastatic to the stomach by EUS-guided FNA. Gastrointest Endosc 2003;58:933–935.
87. Taal, B. G., Peterse, H., Boot, H.: Clinical presentation, endoscopic features, and treatment of gastric metastases from breast carcinoma. Cancer 2000;89:2214–2221.

CHAPTER 9

Esophageal and Gastric Varices

Dr. Atsushi Irisawa
Dr. Tadayuki Takagi
Dr. Goro Shibukawa
Dr. Katsutoshi Obara
Dr. Hiromasa Ohira
Dr. Manoop S. Bhutani

Introduction

In patients with esophageal varices accompanied by complicating portal hypertension, a large network of portal-systemic collateral veins develops. Frequent and significant pathways of collaterals consist of gastro-esophageal varices and veins outside the esophageal/gastric wall extending from the left and short gastric veins.[1,2,3] Endoscopic ultrasonography is able to clearly visualize the veins inside and outside the esophageal/gastric wall. In general, an ultrasonic miniprobe (UMP) is used because the higher ultrasound frequency of the catheter-based miniature transducer provides better resolution than conventional EUS systems.

Ideally, treatment of varices should lead to a successful outcome with no recurrence. Especially in cases of esophageal varices, EUS provide useful management information.

Observational Method[4]

For detection of the detailed structure of vessels inside and outside the esophageal wall, a 20-MHz ultrasound mini-probe (UMP) passed through the biopsy channel of the video endoscope is used. This system enables a 360-degree radial scan. Before examination, the esophagus is filled with deaerated water through a water supply tube attached to the endoscope. For detection of the gastric varices in detail, a 20MHz UMP is also used. Especially for veins outside the gastric wall, a conventional EUS scope (7.5MHz) is useful. Before examination, the gastric lumen (especially the fundus) is filled by about 400-500 ml of deaerated water. In addition, color Doppler endoscopic ultrasonography (CDEUS) may obviate the need for EUS to confirm gastric varices when the upper GI endoscopy diagnosis is uncertain. Doppler is also useful for confirming the direction of blood flow.

Vascular Anatomy

Familiarity with the pertinent vascular anatomy is useful for those who are performing EUS to assess and manage varices. Models of the venous structures derived from Visible Human anatomy are shown. Figures 9–1 A-F show the anterior view of the portal

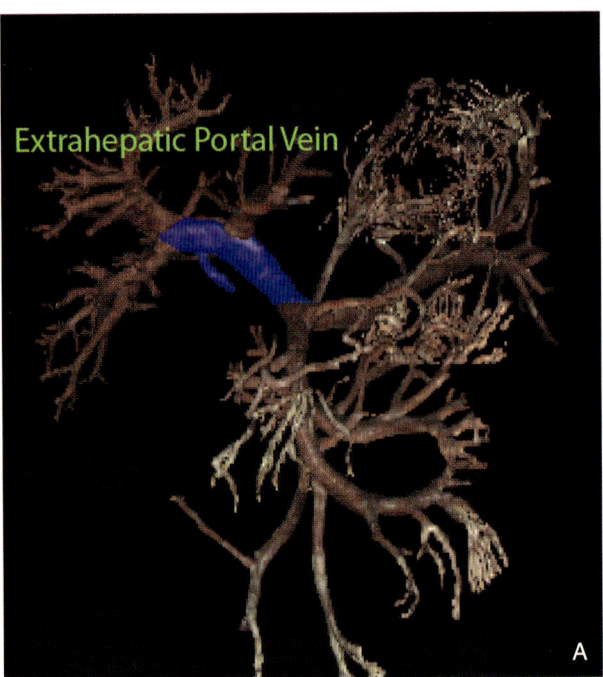
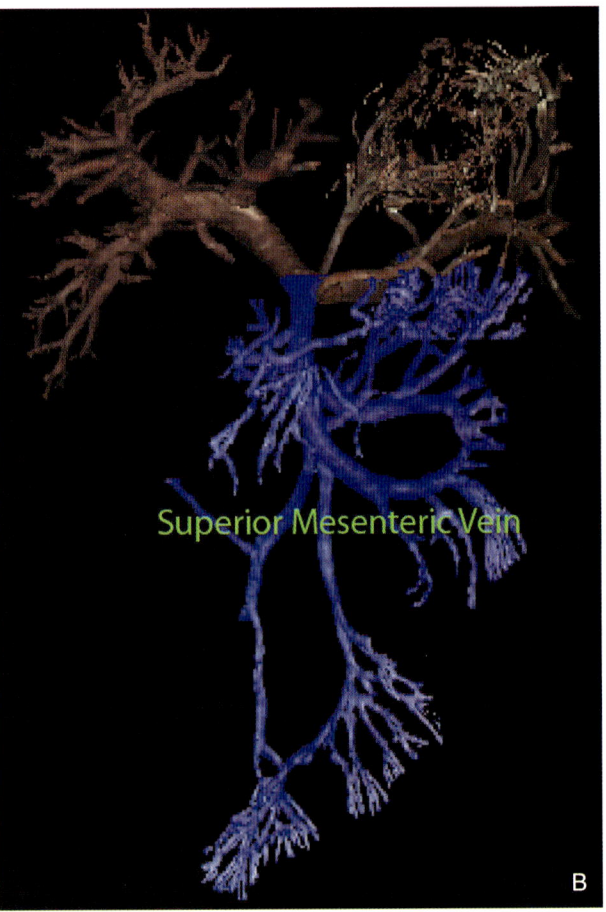

FIGURE 9–1. *A and B* (A) Visible Human anatomy of the portal venous system from the anterior viewpoint. Specific veins are highlighted in blue. A. Extrahepatic portal vein (B). Superior mesenteric vein

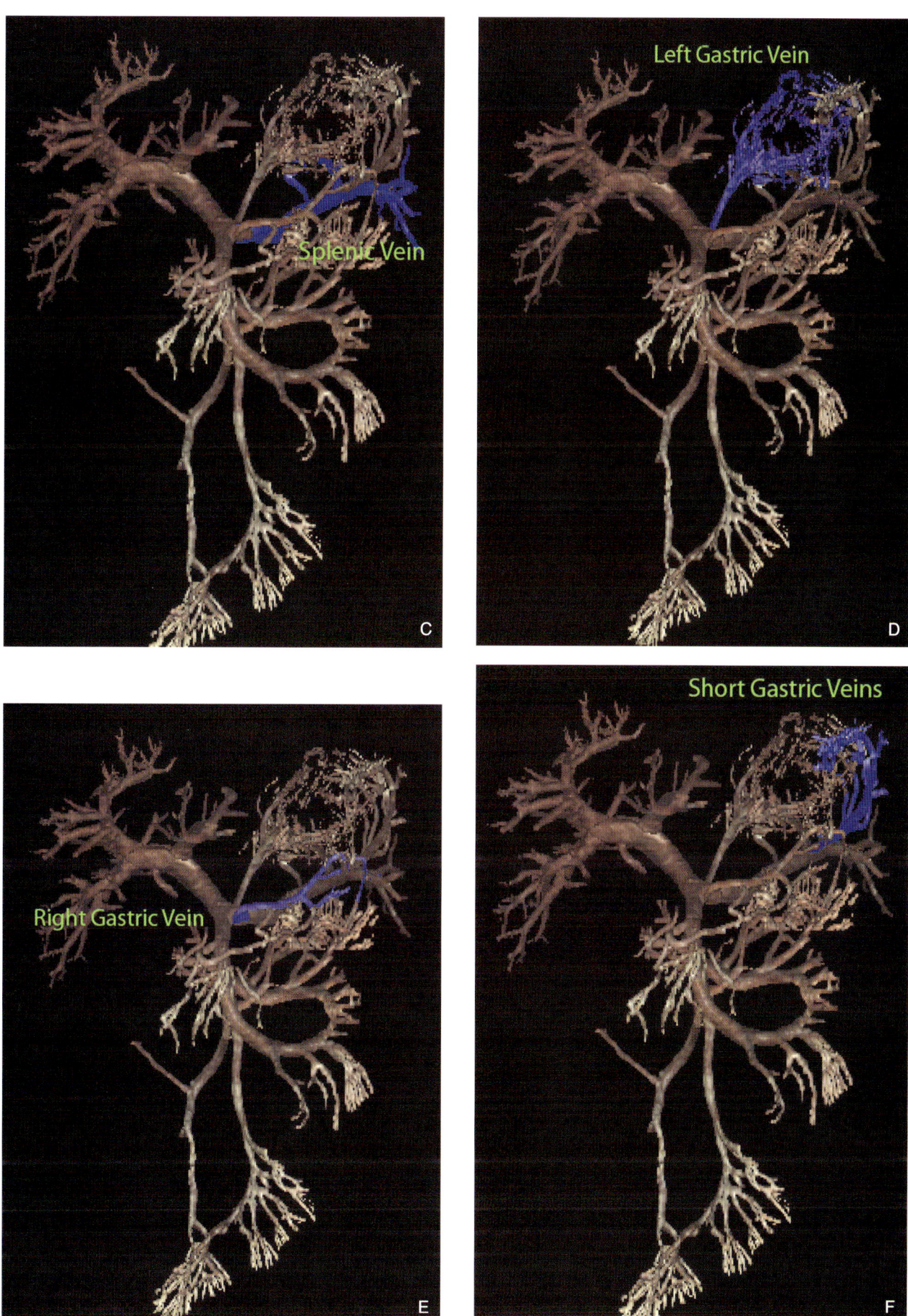

FIGURE 9–1. *C to F* (Continued) (C) Splenic Vein (D) Left gastric vein (E) Right gastric vein (F) Short gastric veins

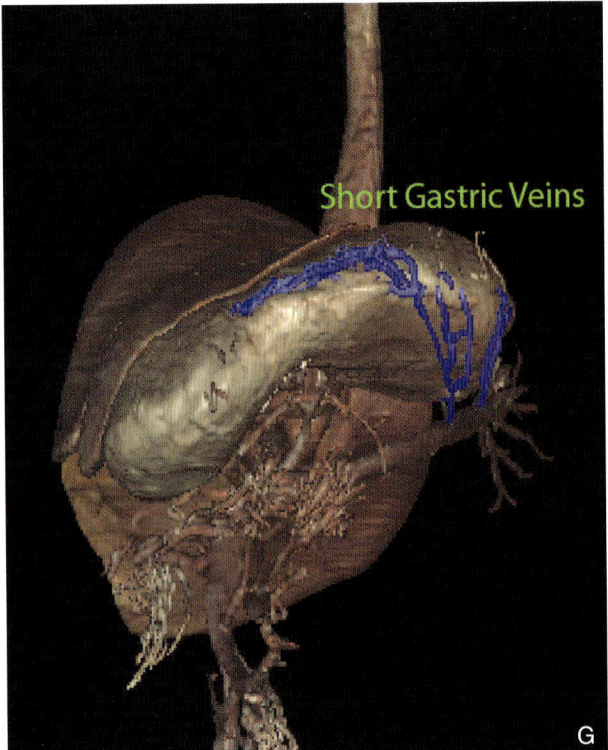
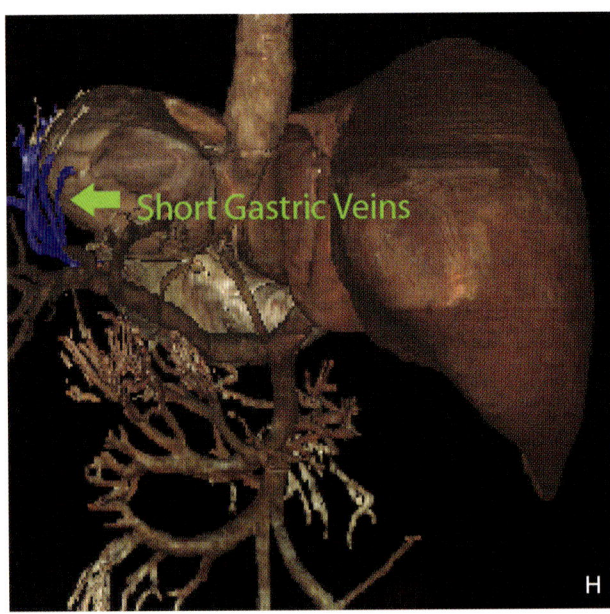

FIGURE 9–1. *G and H* (Continued) (G) Short gastric veins from the lateral view with stomach, esophagus and liver (H) Short gastric veins from the posterior view with stomach, esophagus and liver.

venous system. Each figure highlights (in blue) specific entities, including A) the extrahepatic portal vein, B) the superior mesenteric vein, C) the splenic vein, D) the left gastric vein, E) the right gastric vein, and F) the short gastric veins. Lateral and posterior views of the short gastric veins are shown in Figures 9–1 G and H. Simple figures of the vascular system in a patient with portal hypertension are shown as Figures 9–2 A-D. In portal hypertension, there are several variceal feeders from the portal venous system (portal vein and splenic vein; left gastric vein, post gastric vein, and short gastric vein), which supply to esophageal and gastric varices. These feeders provide blood flow to esophageal and gastric varices not only inside but also outside the esophageal or gastric wall. In many esophageal variceal cases, esophageal varices are supplied by blood flow via palisade and/or bar-type veins at the esophago-gastric junction from previously mentioned feeders. Moreover, the feeders supply to collateral outside the esophageal wall. There are two kinds of collateral outside esophageal varices, peri- and para-esophageal collateral veins. Some esophageal varices connect with the collaterals outside the esophageal wall, via the perforating vein. On the other hand, gastric varices consist of the vessels that break into the gastric wall from feeders. The blood flow of collaterals inside and outside the esophageal wall drain into the superior vena cava via the azygos/hemiazygos vein (Normal Visible Human anatomy shown in Figure 9–2 E), and gastric variceal flow discharges into the inferior vena cava via a major porto-systemic shunt (so-called gastro-renal shunt and/or gastro-subphrenic shunt) in many cases. Normal Visible Human anatomy of the renal vein is shown in Figure 9–2 F.

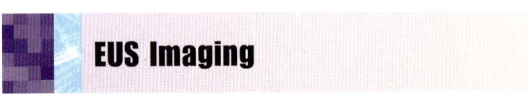

EUS Imaging

An understanding of EUS abnormalities based on the hemodynamics around the esophagus/stomach is thought to be important for management of esophageal and gastric varices in patients with portal hypertension. Schematic representation of EUS images of esophageal and gastric varices are shown in[4] Figure 9–3 and Figure 9–4.

Esophagus [4,5,6]

Esophageal Varices

Esophageal varices are visualized as hypoechoic or anechoic lumens in the esophageal wall (almost in the submucosal layer) by high-resolution ultrasound (20MHz) (Figures 9–5 A, B). In many cases of high

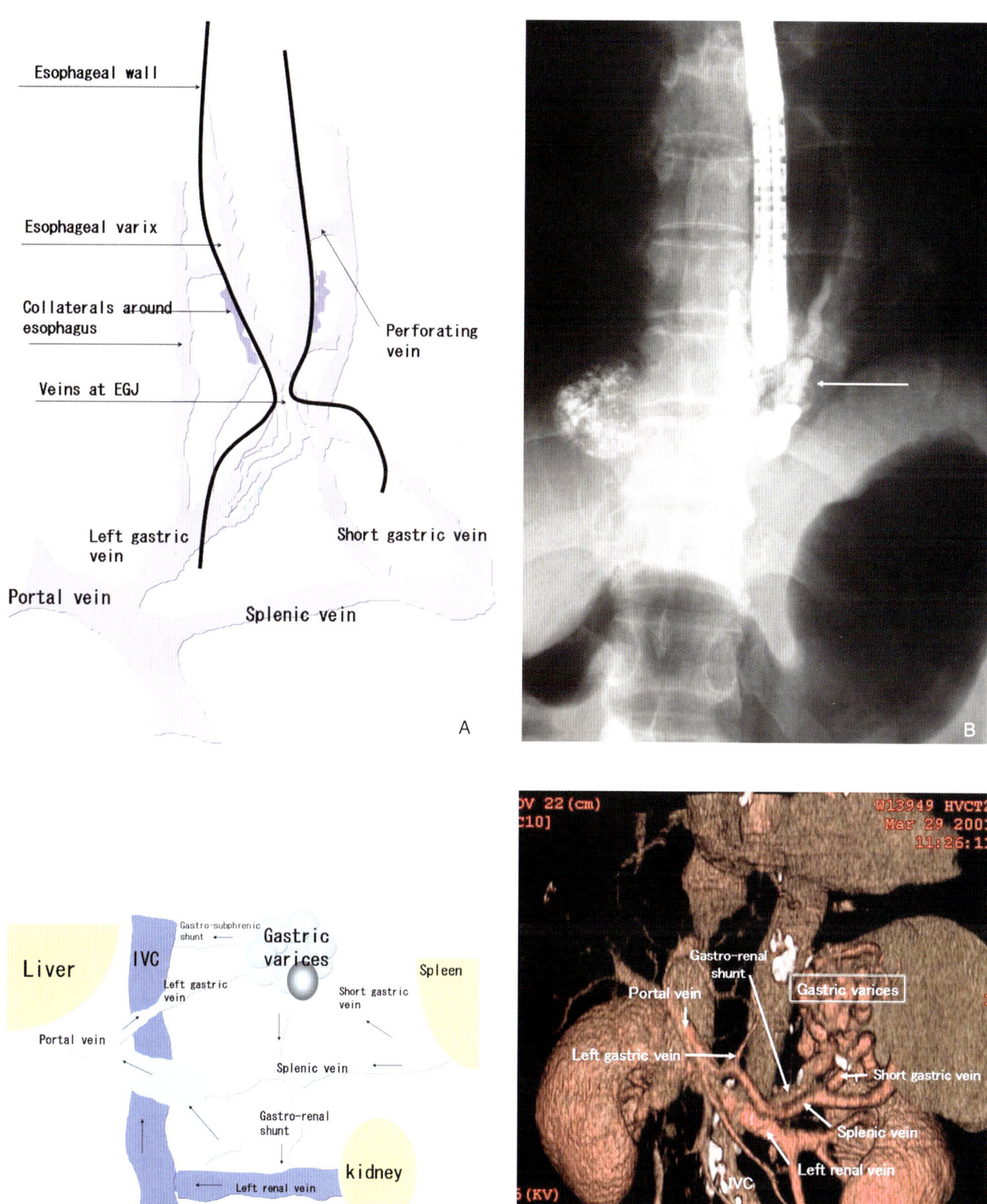

FIGURE 9–2. *A to D* (A) Schema of esophageal variceal hemodynamics. (B) Endoscopic varicealography during injection sclerotherapy. Esophageal varices and its feeders are identified (long arrow: varices and collaterals around esophagus, short arrow: left gastric vein as a feeder for varices) (C) Schema of gastric variceal hemodynamics. Arrows indicate the direction of blood flow. (D) Three-dimensional CT scan imaging of gastric varices and portal venous system.

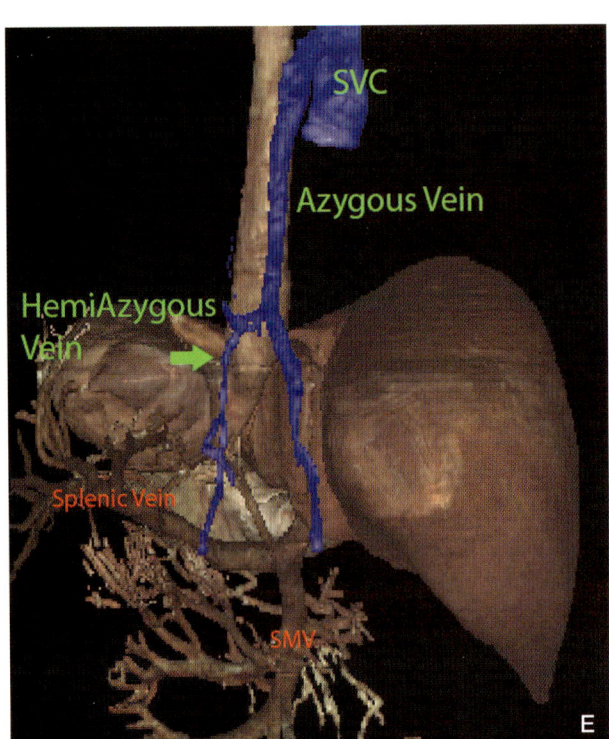
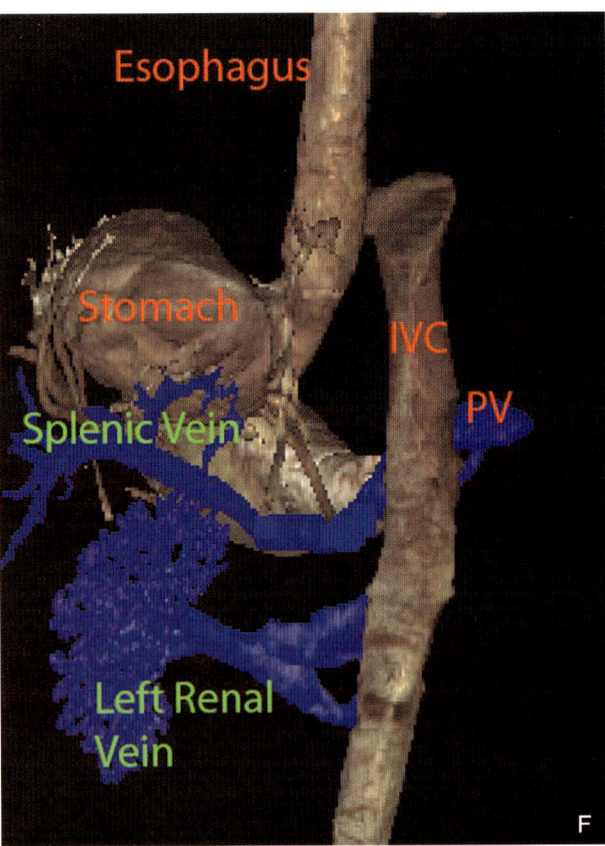

FIGURE 9–2. *E and F* (Continued) (E) Posterior view of Visible Human anatomy showing azygous, hemiazygous, superior mesenteric (SMV), and splenic veins. The superior vena cava (SVC) is also shown. (F) Posterior view of Visible Human anatomy showing splenic vein and left renal vein. The stomach, esophagus, portal vein (PV), and inferior vena cava (IVC) are also shown.

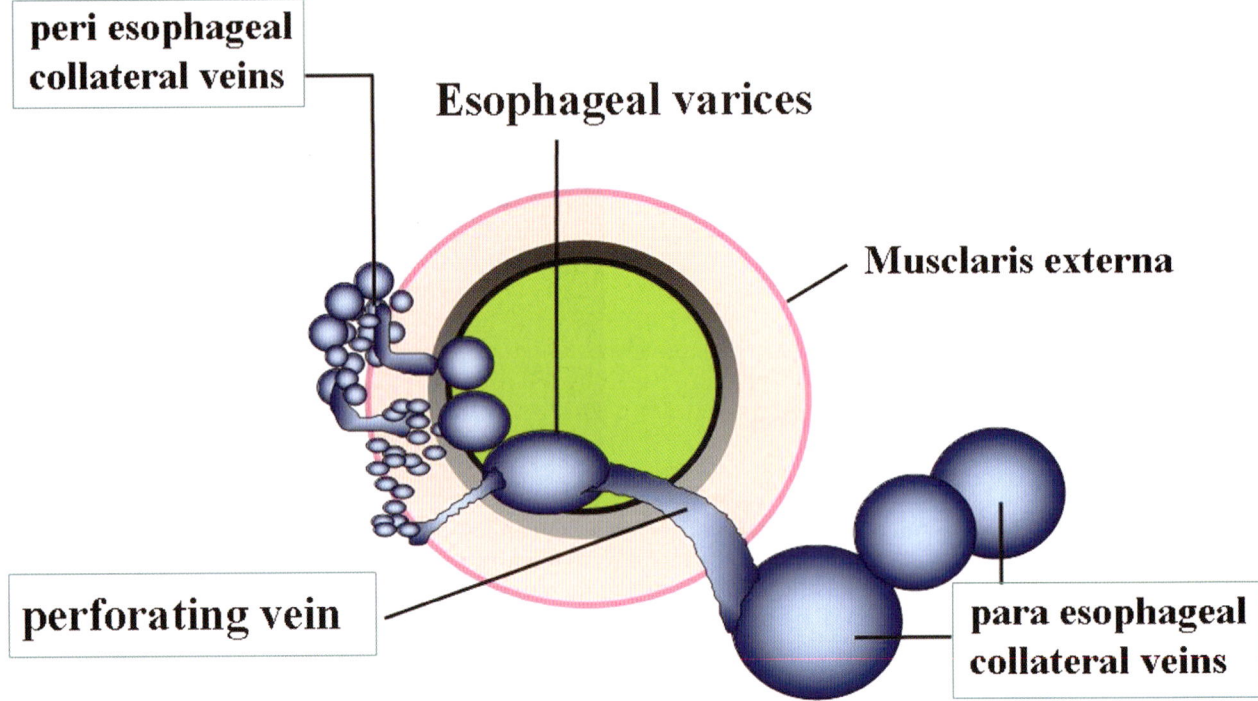

FIGURE 9–3. Schema of EUS findings in a case of esophageal varices

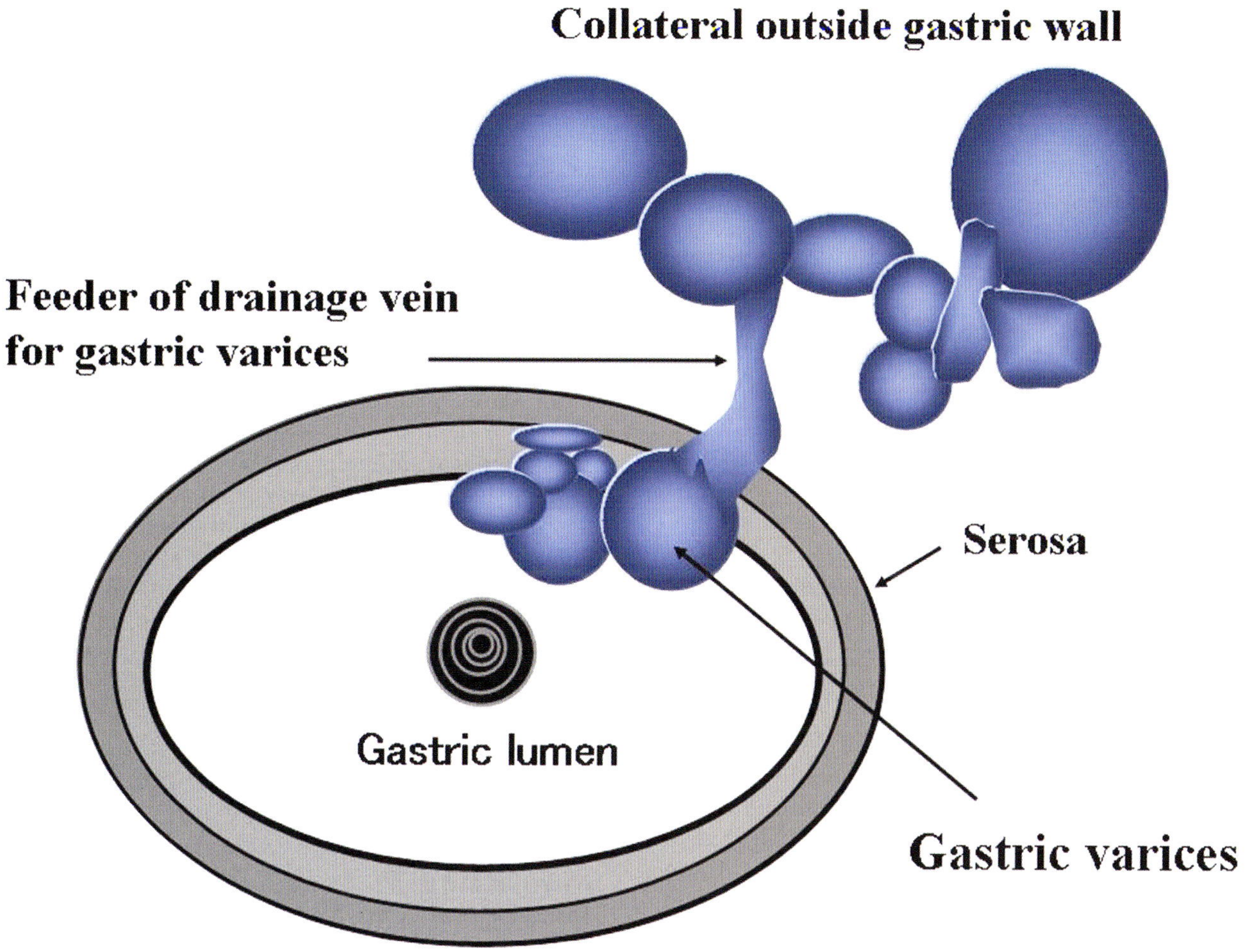

FIGURE 9–4. Schema of EUS findings in a case of gastric varices

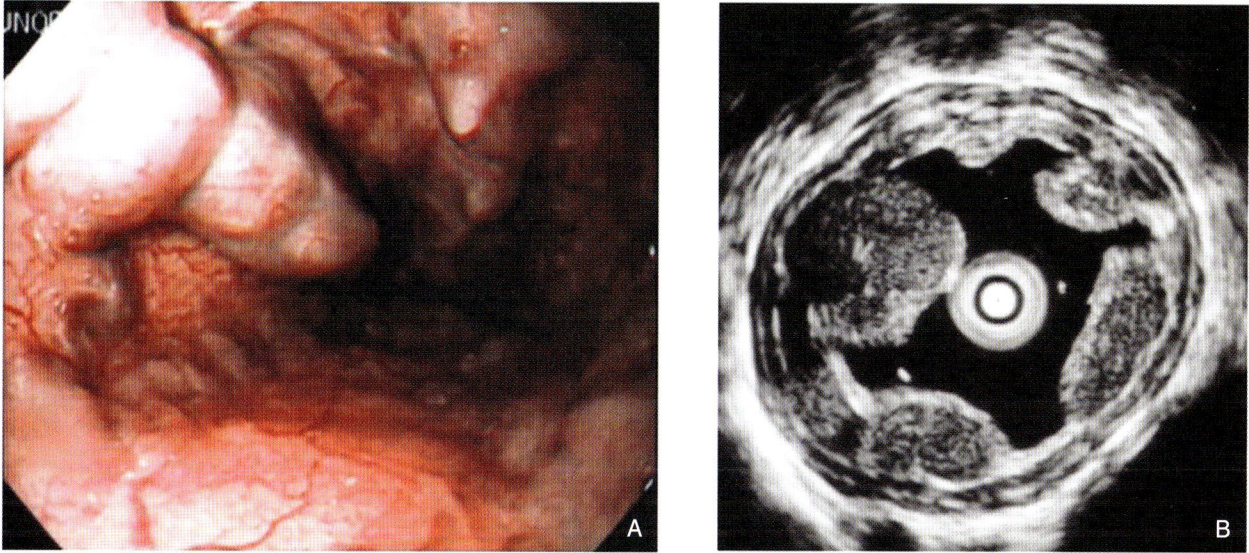

FIGURE 9–5. *A and B* (A) Esophageal varices on endoscopy (B) Esophageal varices on EUS. Hypoechoic lumens are visible mainly in the submucosal layer.

resolution EUS images of varices, since variceal blood flow tends to be turbulent and at low velocity, high resolution ultrasound images the blood corpuscles as hypoechoic within the variceal lumen instead of anechoic.

Veins at Esophageal-Gastric Junction

At the esophageal-gastric junction, two types of vessels are visualized on EUS. One is palisade-type vessels, and the other is bar-type vessels (Figures 9–6 A, B). Esophageal varices are connected with the feeders (left gastric vein/short gastric vein) via these veins at the esophageal-gastric junction. In addition, CDEUS is useful for detecting these feeders.[7]

Peri- and Para-esophageal Collateral Veins

The collaterals around the esophagus in patients with portal hypertension are divided into two groups: 1) Peri-esophageal collateral veins (peri-ECVs) are small vessels lateral to the muscularis propria, or veins within the adventitia (adjacent to the muscularis externa of the esophagus), and 2) para-esophageal collateral veins (para-ECVs) are larg vessels lateral and separate from the muscularis propria of the esophagus (distal to the esophageal wall without contact with the muscularis externa) (Figure 9–7). Peri- and para-ECVs are scored as mild or severe, according to the stage of development (Figures 9–8 A, B). At endoscopy, the variceal form is significantly larger in patients with severe peri-ECVs than in patients with mild peri-ECVs. In contrast, the variceal form does not differ significantly among patients with mild and severe para-ECVs. The presence of severe peri-ECVs strongly correlates with occurrence and recurrence of esophageal varices in patients with portal hypertension. In addition, it is difficult to distinguish between the azygos vein and para-ECVs in the case of severe para-ECVs.

Perforating Veins

The perforating veins connecting the submucosal and subepithelial veins to peri-esophageal veins contain valves that draw the blood flow away from the esophageal lumen. EUS can easily detect the perforating veins (Figure 9–9 A). On EUS, perforating veins have penetrated the esophageal wall and have connected with either peri-ECVs or para-ECVs. The prevalence of perforating veins increases according to the varix form. Color Doppler endoscopic ultrasonography (CDEUS) indeed confirms that almost all perforating veins serve as afferent veins to esophageal varices (Figure 9–9 B). Therefore, perforating veins play an important role in the development of esophageal varices by acting as the feeder from the veins around the esophagus. Moreover, perforating veins are highly associated with variceal recurrence after treatment, even if perforating veins are independent.

Correlating EUS Image with Histological Findings [8]

The authors of this chapter material compared radial EUS images of collaterals around the esophagus with histological findings in five autopsy cases of patients who had undergone endoscopic treatment

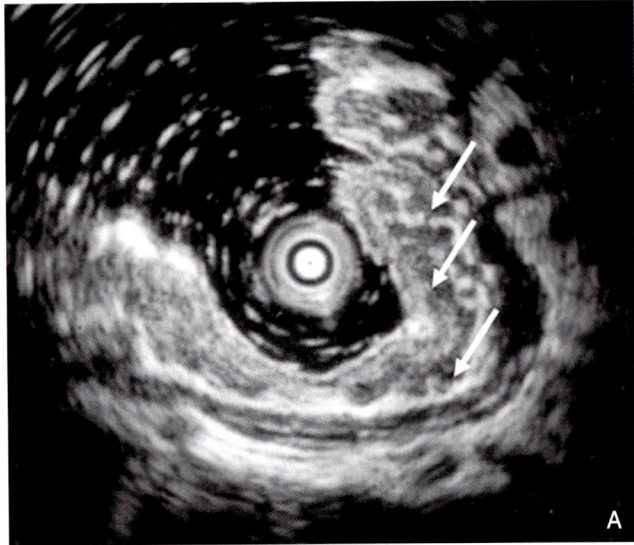
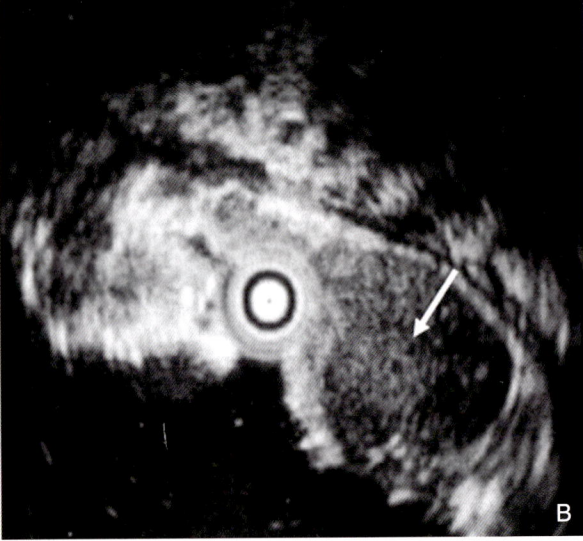

FIGURE 9–6. *A and B* (A) Many small vessels can be seen in the gastro-esophageal wall at the esophago-gastric junction. These vessels are feeders for esophageal varices, so-called palisade-type veins (arrows). (B) A large vein can be seen in the gastro-esophageal wall at the esophageal gastric junction.

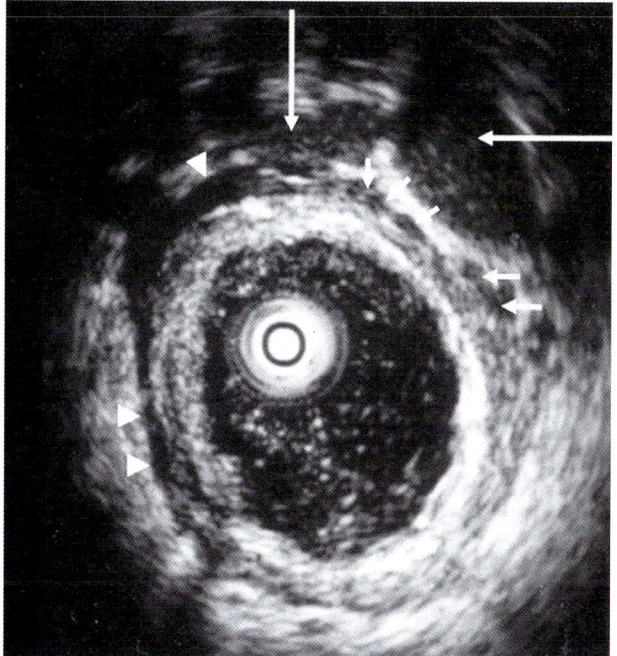

FIGURE 9–7. EUS shows two types of collaterals outside the esophagus, 1) peri-esophageal collateral veins (short arrows) are smaller vessels lateral to the muscularis propria, or veins within the adventitia (adjacent to the muscularis externa of the esophagus), and 2;) para-esophageal collateral veins (long arrows) are larger vessels lateral and separate from the muscularis propria of the esophagus (distal to the esophageal wall without contact with the muscularis externa). Musclaris externa is indicated by arrow heads.

for esophageal varices. Radial EUS after EIS showed peri-ECVs and perforating veins in all cases, and para-ECVs in three cases. Based on histological findings, veins associating the esophageal wall were divided into three groups: veins adjacent to the muscularis propria of the esophagus, veins distal to the esophageal wall without contact with the muscularis propria, and veins perforating the muscularis propria (Figures 9–10 A, B). These veins were observed in all cases. These three kinds of veins, which were identified by histological examination, were considered to correspond to the peri-ECVs, para-ECVs, and perforating veins observed in EUS images, respectively. This study revealed that the collaterals shown in radial EUS images corresponded to histological findings. Therefore, EUS is useful for assessment of vascular anatomy around the esophageal wall in patients with portal hypertension.

Stomach

Gastric Varices

Gastric varices are visualized as hypoechoic or anechoic lumens in the gastric wall (in the submucosal layer) by high resolution ultrasound (20MHz) (Figure 9–11). When the CDEUS is used, turbulent signals are visualized in the varices. Measurement of the short diameter of gastric varices is helpful for estimating the variceal blood flow volume.[9]

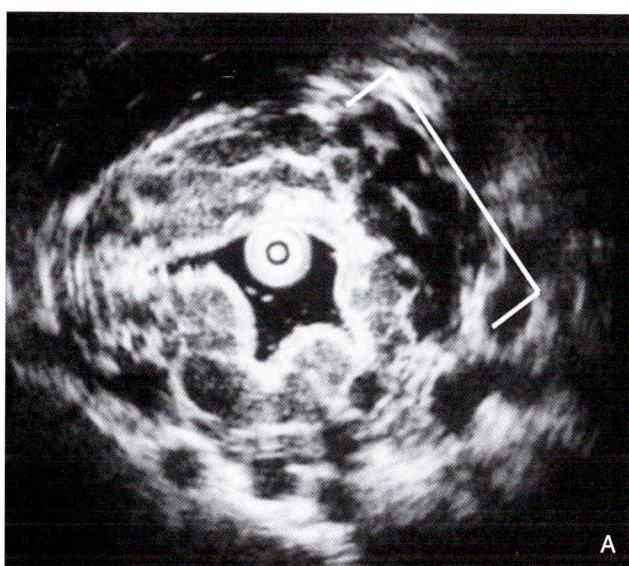 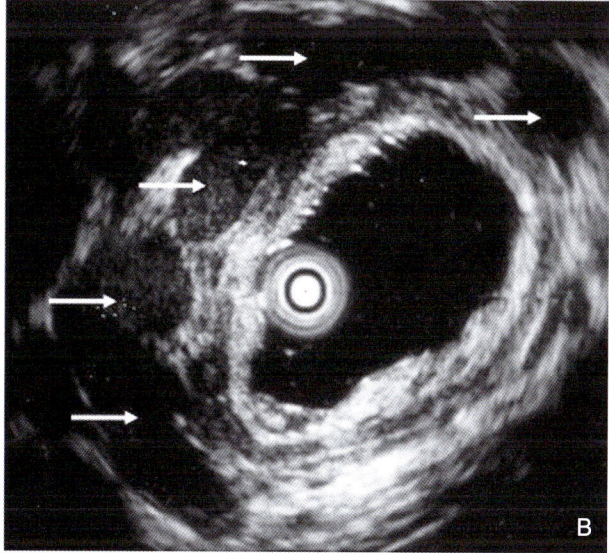

FIGURE 9–8. *A and B* (A) EUS revealed severe peri-ECVs. Severe peri-ECVs is defined as five or more small vessels adjacent to the esophageal wall. (B) EUS revealed severe peri-ECVs. Severe para-ECVs (arrows) are defined as vessels with diameters of more than 5 mm and away from the esophageal wall.

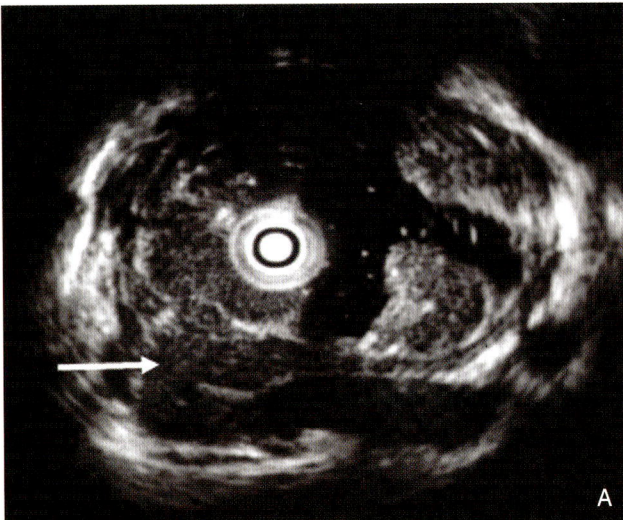
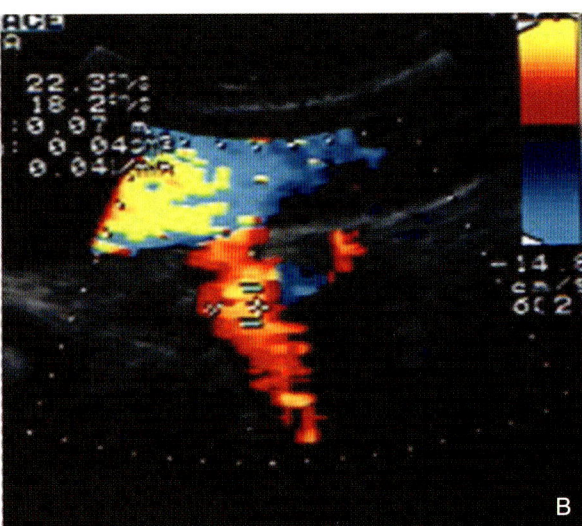

FIGURE 9–9. *A and B* (A) Perforating vein (arrow) (which is a vessel connecting the esophageal varices and the para-ECVs through the muscularis propria) is visualized on EUS image. (B) CDEUS shows the flow direction of the perforating vein as afferent veins to esophageal varices (arrow).

Collaterals Outside Gastric Wall

In patients with portal hypertension, many vessels are visualized outside the gastric wall by EUS. These vessels contain two kinds of vessels: 1) vessels feeding gastric varices and 2) draining vein of gastric varices (Figure 9–12). It is difficult to distinguish among the two types using conventional EUS. However, CDEUS may be helpful for judgment of the direction of blood flow.

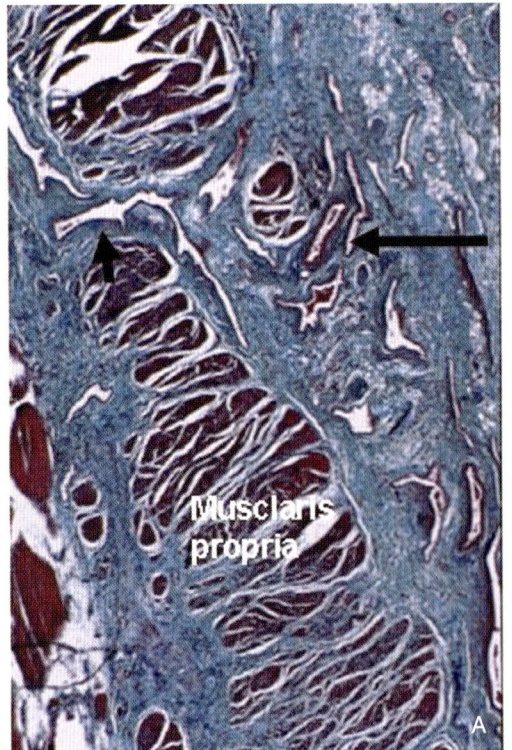
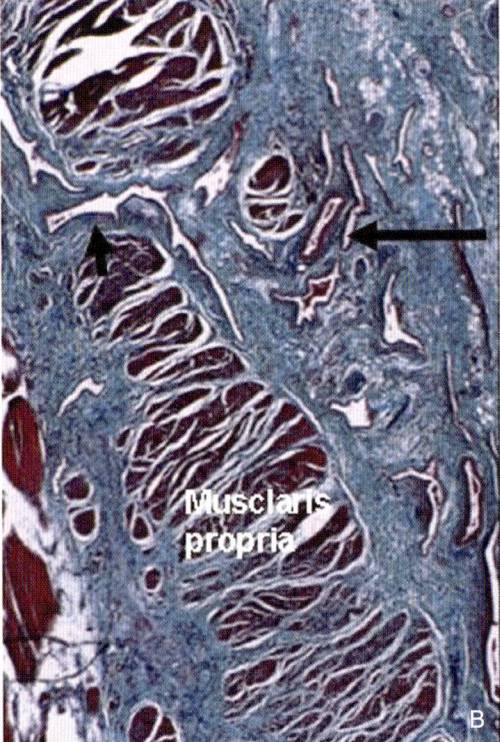

FIGURE 9–10. *A and B* Histological findings of collaterals around the esophagus in patient with portal hypertension. (A) A perforating vein (short arrow) and peri-ECVs (long arrow) were observed. (B) Peri-ECVs (long arrow) and para-ECVs (short arrow) were observed.

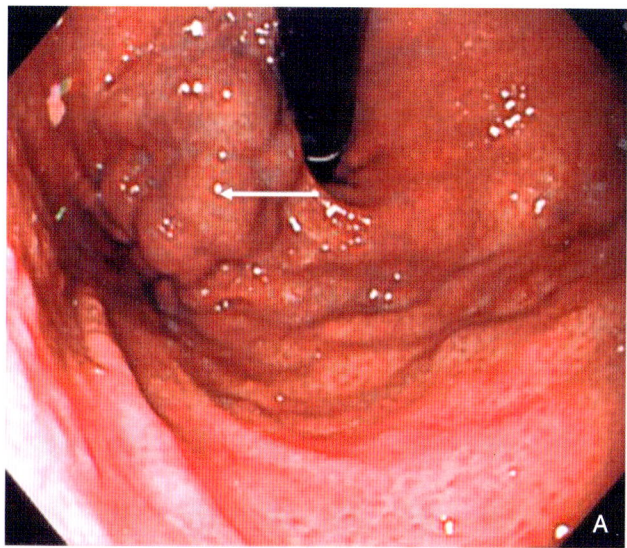
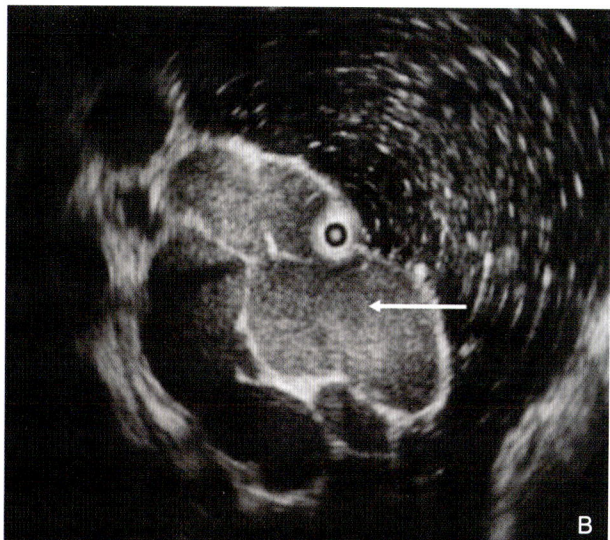

FIGURE 9–11. *A and B* (A) Gastric varices (fundal type) are seen on endoscopic view. (B) Gastric varices are visualized as hypoechoic lesion on EUS image (arrow).

Feeders of Gastric Varices: Left, Post and Short Gastric Veins

EUS (especially linear array echoendoscope) reveals that some vessels are arising from (or connecting to) the portal vein or splenic vein. These vessels are feeders of gastric varices.

Drainage Vein of Gastric Varices: Gastro-renal Shunt

In some cases, the vessel that is connecting gastric varices with the left renal vein is identified. This vessel is the so-called gastro-renal shunt, which is a major collateral between the portal venous system and systemic circulation, to reduce high portal pressure.

Conclusion

An understanding of EUS abnormalities based on the hemodynamics around the esophagus and stomach is important for management of esophageal gastric varices in patients with portal hypertension—whether or not EUS is employed in patients with portal hypertension.

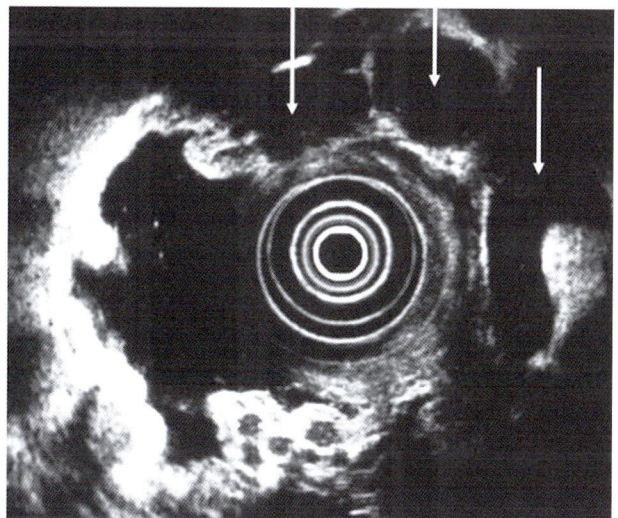

FIGURE 9–12. Many large vessels (arrows) are visualized outside the gastric wall by EUS. These vessels contain two kinds of vessels, 1) feeding vessels of gastric varices and 2) draining vein of gastric varices.

References

1. Widrich, W. C., Srinivasan, M., Semine, M.C., et al.: Collateral pathways of the left gastric vein in portal hypertension. Am J Roenterol. 1984; 142, 375–382.
2. Hashizume, M., Kitano, S., Sugimachi, K., et al.: Three-dimensional view of the vascular structure of the lower esophagus in clinical portal hypertension. Hepatology. 1988; 8, 1482–1487.
3. Frederick, H. M., Clements, J. L., Colvin, R. S.: Retrocardiac densities due to paraesophageal varices: Roentgenographic detection. Southern medical journal. 1985; 78, 1371–1372.
4. Irisawa, A, Obara, K, Sato, Y., et al.: An endoscopic analysis of collateral veins inside and outside the esophageal wall in portal hypertension. Gastrointest Endosc. 1999; 50, 374–380.
5. Irisawa, A., Saito, A., Shibukawa, G., et al.: Endoscopic recurrence of esophageal varices is associated with the specific EUS abnormalities; severe peri-esophageal

collateral veins and large perforating veins. Gastrointest Endosc. 2001; 53, 77–84.
6. Irisawa, A., Obara, K., Bhutani, M. S., et al.: Role of para-esophageal collateral veins in patients with portal hypertension based on the results of endoscopic ultrasonography and liver scintigraphy analysis. J Gastroenterol Hepatol. 2003; 18, 309–314.
7. Hino, S., Kakutani, H., Ikeda, K., et al.: Hemodynamic assessment of the left gastric vein in patients with esophageal varices with color Doppler EUS: factors affecting development of esophageal varices. Gastrointest Endosc. 2002; 55, 512–517.
8. Irisawa, A., Shibukawa, G., Obara, K., et al.: Collaterals around the esophageal wall among patients with portal hypertension: comparison of endoscopic ultrasound imaging and microscopic findings on autopsy. Gastrointest Endosc. 2002; 54, 249–253.
9. Irisawa, A., Obara, K., Sato, Y., et al.: Adherence of cyanoacrylate which leaked from gastric varices to the left renal vein during injection sclerotherapy: a histopathologic study. Endoscopy. 2000; 32, 804–806.

CHAPTER 10

Vascular Anomolies

Dr. John C. Deutsch

EUS is generally not a primary modality employed for assessing vascular structures. Nonetheless, EUS commonly identifies previously unidentified vascular abnormalities and anomalies. In some instances, as shown below, EUS can uncover a vascular etiology for GI symptoms, or discover a vascular process for which the management takes precedent over the gastrointestinal indication that lead to the EUS examination.

A good working knowledge of normal arterial vascular anatomy seen during an EUS examination (Figure 10–1) is necessary if one is to identify vascular anomalies or acquired vascular diseases. This chapter will demonstrate some common arterial abnormalities that can be seen during EUS examinations. Other vascular problems (venous thrombosis, varicies) will be covered in detail in other chapters.

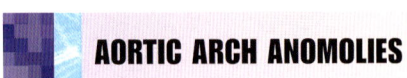

AORTIC ARCH ANOMOLIES

Aortic Arch anomalies are uncommon and occur in a small proportion—1 out of 500 people, or 1 in every 3 people among the general population. Abnormalities include :

- Aberrant right common carotid artery arising directly from the aortic arch. The right subclavian artery (R SCA) arises from the arch distal to the left subclavian artery. The R SCA passes posteriorly to the trachea and esophagus.
- An accessory aorta located anterior to the esophagus and trachea, with the true aorta remaining in its usual posterior location.
- A right-sided aortic arch.

Anomalies here can form symptomatic vascular rings leading to "dysphagia lusoria" or can be found incidentally. A model of a normal aortic arch viewed posteriorly is shown in Figure 10–2. Normal trans-axial cross-sections above the aortic arch and at the aortic arch are shown in Figures 10–3 and 10–4. The most common aortic arch anomaly (posterior right subclavian artery, R SCA) is shown schematically in Figures 10–5 and 10–6. Figures 10–7 A, B, and C show this anomaly at various levels, as seen during a radial array EUS examination. A radial array EUS video shows a normal aortic arch followed by an EUS exam in a patient with an anamalous right subclavian artery (Video 10–1).

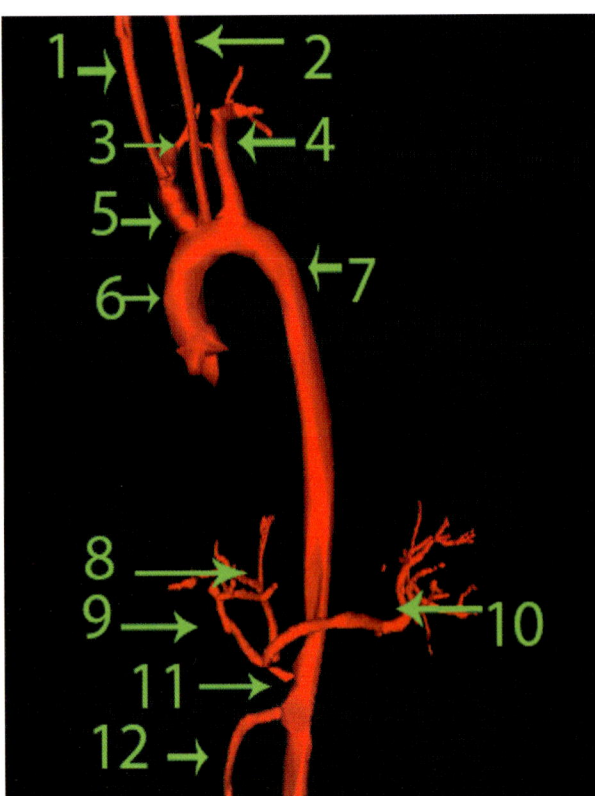

FIGURE 10–1. Arterial tree visualized during EUS examinations. 1) right carotid artery, 2) left carotid artery 3) right subclavian artery 4) left subclavian artery 5) brachiocephalic artery 6) ascending aorta 7) descending aorta 8) left gastric artery 9) common hepatic artery 10) splenic artery 11) celiac artery 12) superior mesenteric artery

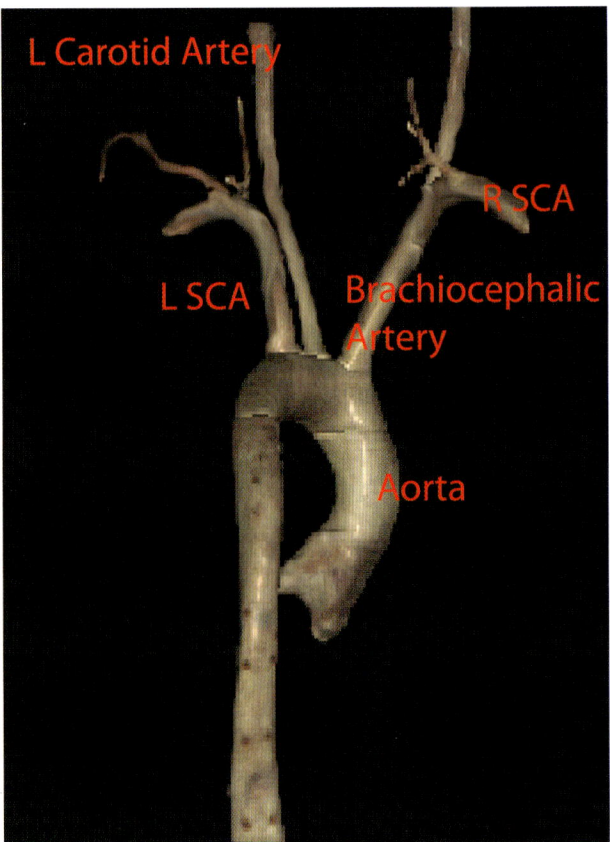

FIGURE 10–2. Three-dimensional aortic arch and associated vessels. L = left R= Right SCA = subclavian artery

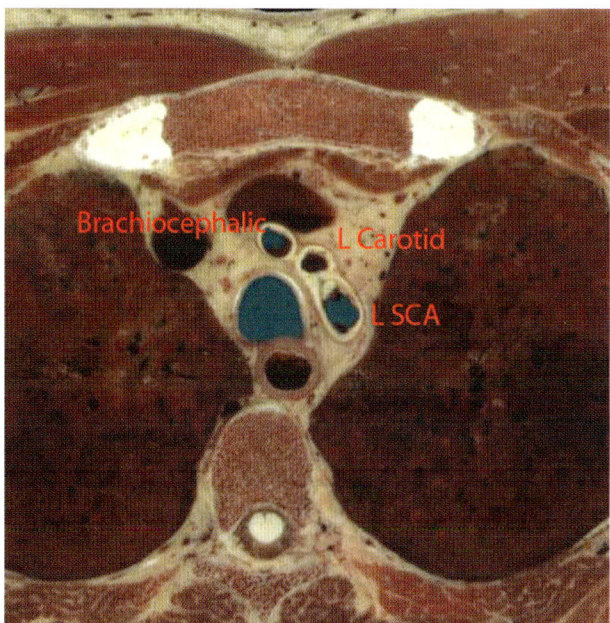

FIGURE 10-3. Transaxial cross-section just above the aortic arch. L = left SCA = subclavian artery

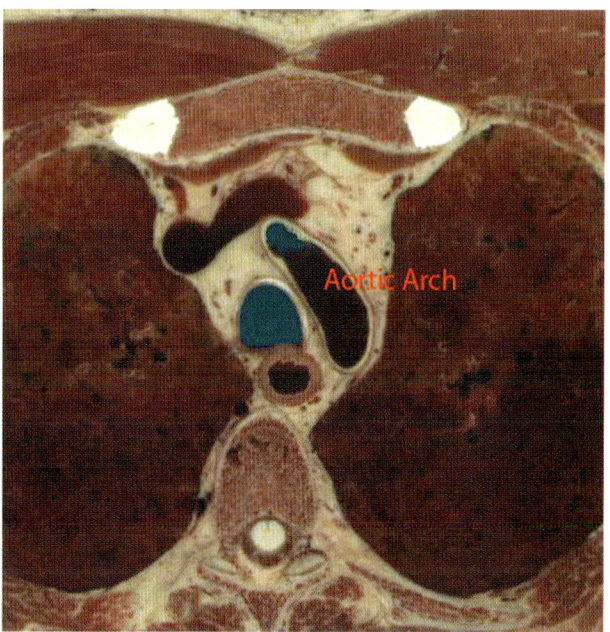

FIGURE 10-4. Transaxial cross-section at level of the aortic arch.

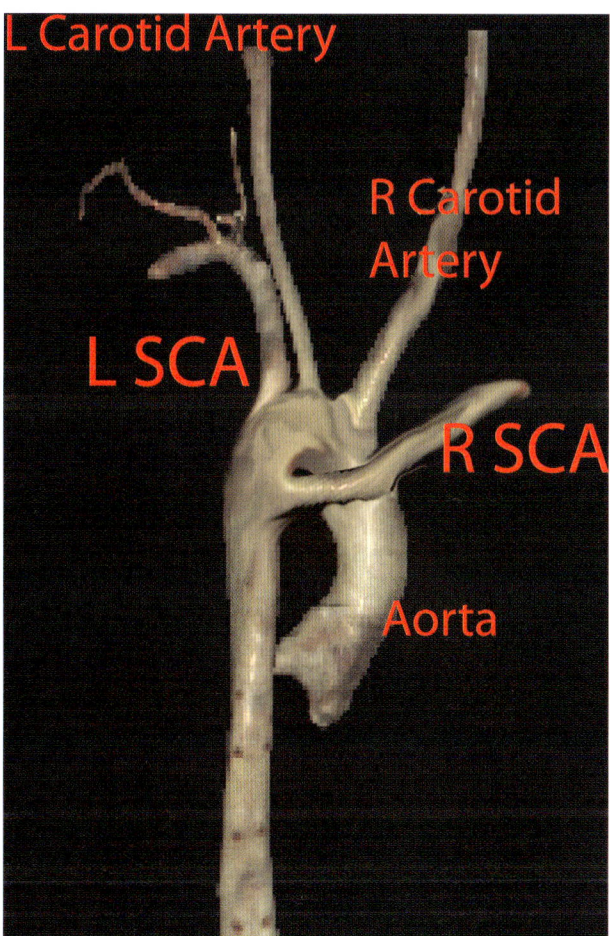

FIGURE 10-5. Modified three-dimensional model of the aortic arch showing an anaomolous right subclavian artery. L = left R= Right SCA= subclavian artery

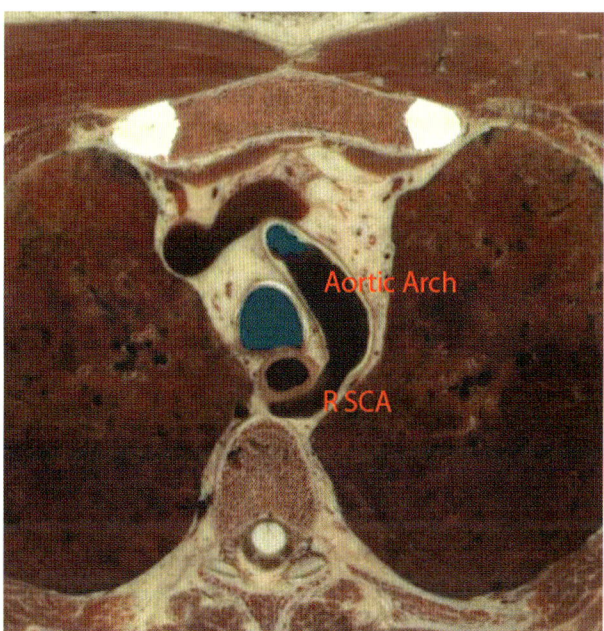

FIGURE 10-6. Modified transaxial cross-section showing anomalous right subclavian artery between esophagus and spine. R = Right SCA = subclavian artery

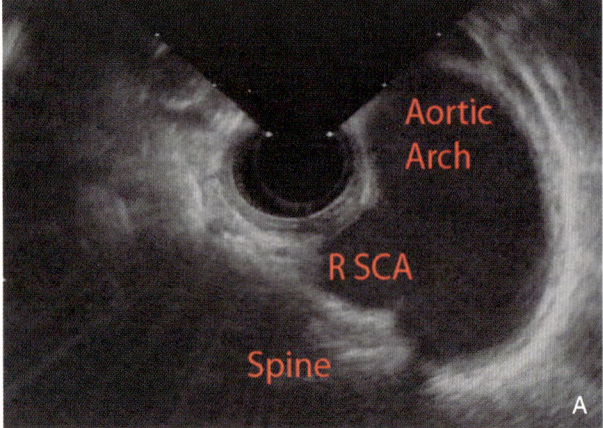
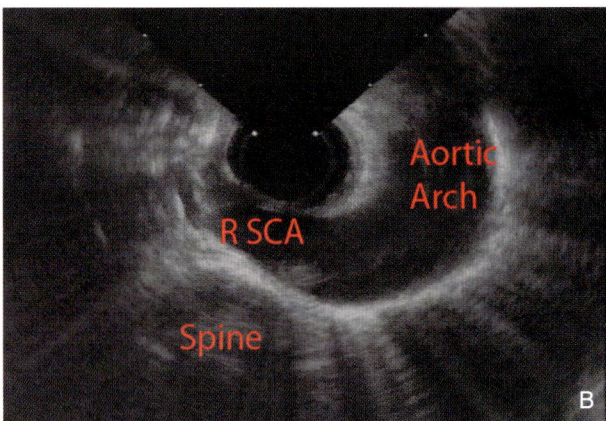
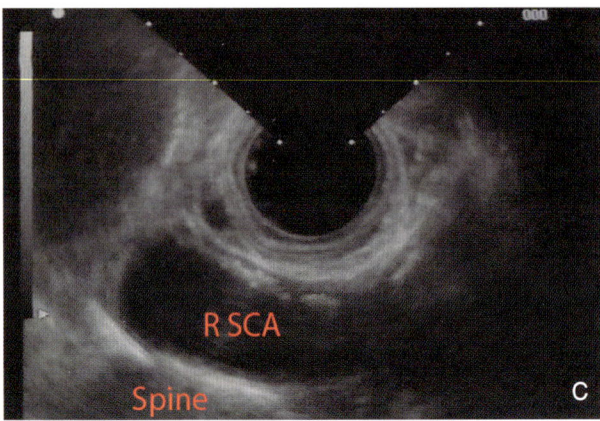

FIGURE 10–7. *A to C* A to C, Radial array EUS images that correspond to the modified transaxial cross-section in Figure 10-6 showing anomalous right subclavian artery between the esophagus and the spine. R = Right SCA = subclavian artery

Although less common, a right-sided aortic arch can also present with dysphagia, sometimes with concomitant anomalous left subclavian artery (3). When making a diagnosis of a right-sided aortic arch, it is important to make sure the EUS image isn't inadvertently transposed on the EUS processor. The relation of the aorta to other structures in the chest is useful to confirm the right-sided location of the aberrant aorta. Figure 10–8 A shows a radial array EUS image of a right-sided aortic arch. Figure 10–8 B shows an EUS image at the level of the left atrium in this same patient. Figure 10–9 shows a Visible Human image of the normal anatomy at the level of the left atrium.

EUS imaging can sometimes falsely suggest aortic arch anomalies. CT or MRI can confirm or disprove these EUS findings. Two examples are shown in Figures 10–10 through 10–12. The first is from a patient in which the azygous arch crosses the midline just below the aortic arch (Figure 10–10). If one is not

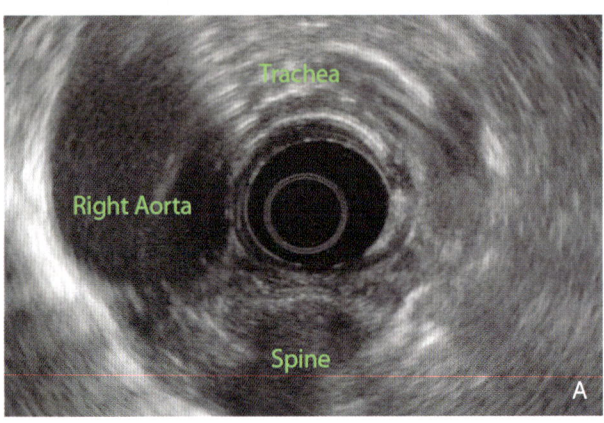
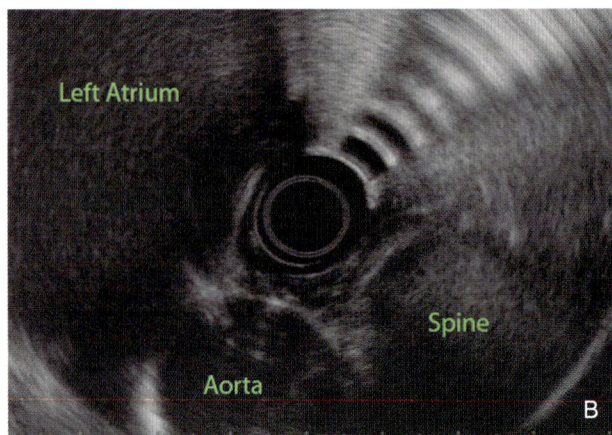

FIGURE 10–8. *A and B* (A) A radial EUS showing a right-sided aortic arch. (B) A radial EUS image of a right-sided descending aorta t the level of the left atrium.

Vascular Anomalies

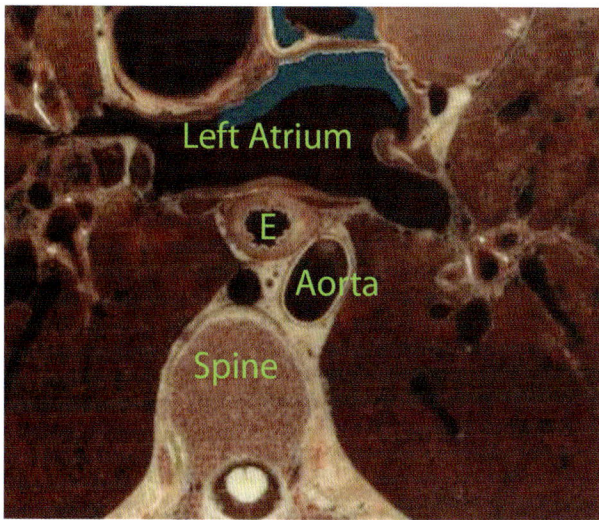

FIGURE 10–9. Visible Human Data Set image showing a normal left-sided aortic arch at the level of the left atrium.

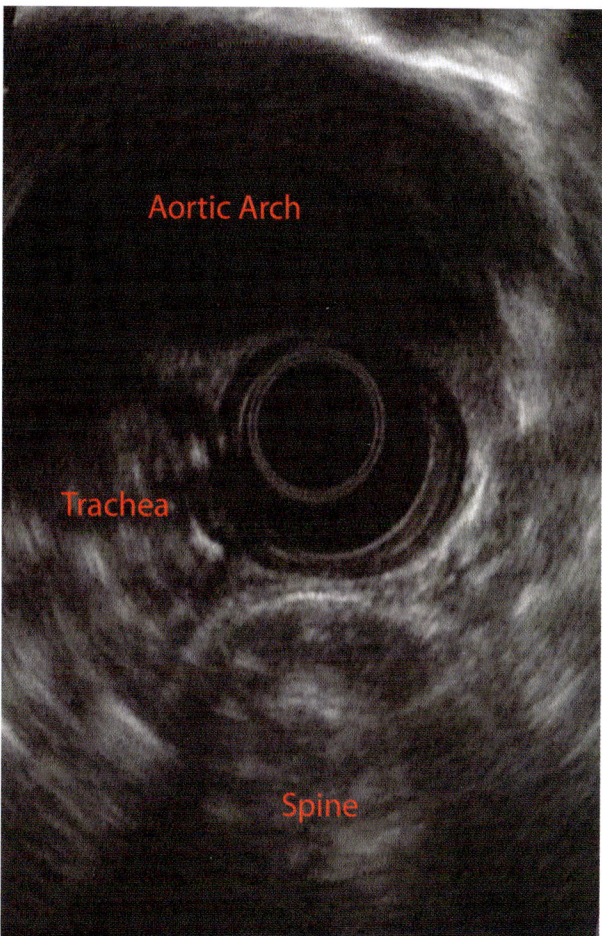

FIGURE 10–11. A radial array EUS image that is suspicious for an aortic arch developmental anomaly in a 20-year-old immigrant. The trachea appears displaced to the right chest by an abnormal right-sided aortic arch.

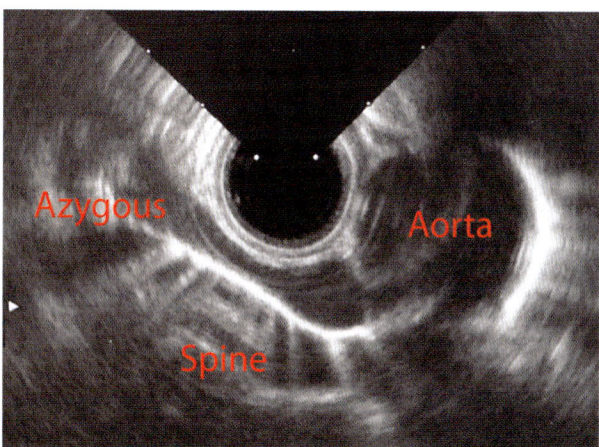

FIGURE 10–10. A radial array EUS image showing the azygous vein crossing to the left chest. This could be mistaken for an anomalous right subclavian artery between the esophagus and the spine.

careful to trace vessels, the azygous vein shown here could be mistaken for an anomolous right subclavian artery. The second example is from a young adult patient with dysphagia in whom a right-sided aortic arch was suspected on the basis of EUS (Figure 10–11). CT imaging revealed chronic fibrotic pleural changes with volume loss of the left lung, which caused the esophagus to be moved to the left (Figure 10–12).

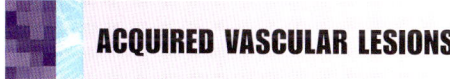

ACQUIRED VASCULAR LESIONS

Atherosclerosis and plaques are commonly seen in the descending aorta as shown in Figure 10–13. Sometimes dense calcification and shadowing is noted (Figure 10–14). During live EUS examinations, some plaques can be seen moving within the vascular lumen during arterial pulsation.

Thoracic aortic aneurisms are easily seen during EUS. They can appear relatively bland or quite dramatic, as shown in two different patients (Figures 10–15 and 10–16). In both of these patients there was apparent disruption of the wall of the aorta. An EUS video from the patient illustrated in Figure 10–16 is also provided (Video 10–2).

Calcifications and obstruction of the celiac and superior mesenteric artery origins can lead to gastrointestinal ischemia. Figure 10–17 shows an EGD from a severely malnourished patient referred with weight loss and abdominal pain felt to be pancreatic in origin.

112 EUS Pathology with Digital Anatomy Correlation

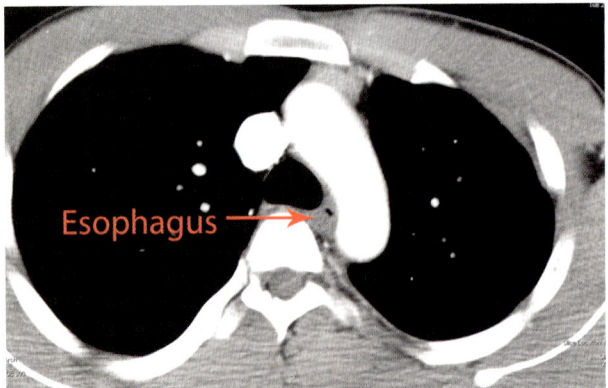

FIGURE 10–12. A CT scan from the patient illustrated by EUS in Figure 7–11 shows displacement of the esophagus to the left by a chronic fibrotic process in the left pleura, which likely occurred in early childhood. The right lung is larger than the left lung, and mediastinal structures are pulled to the left.

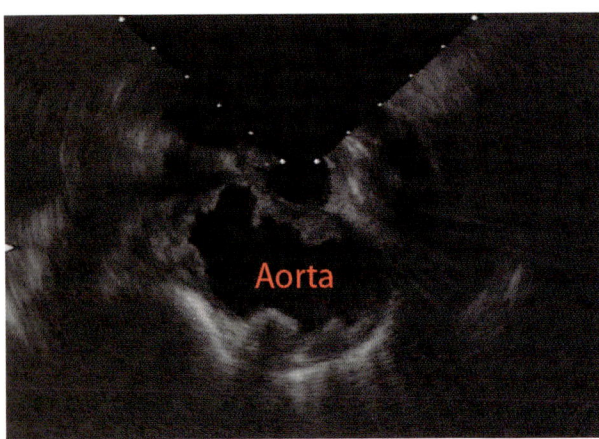

FIGURE 10–13. Atherosclerosis in the descending aorta

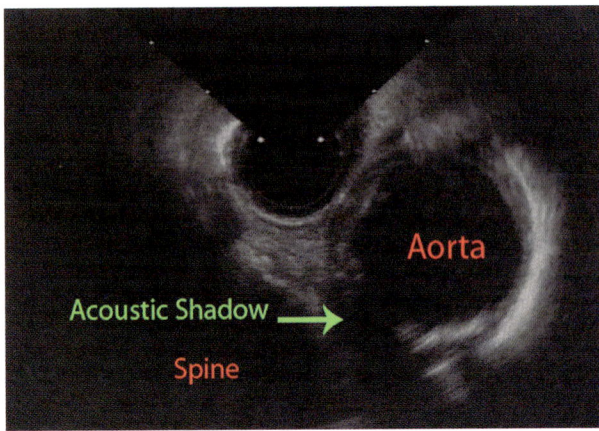

FIGURE 10–14. Calcification of the aorta with acoustic shadowing

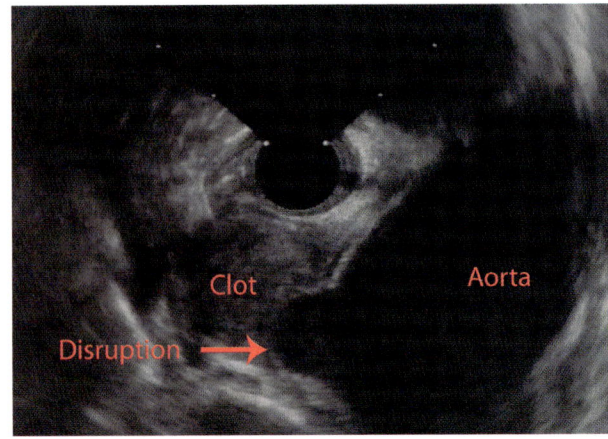

FIGURE 10–15. Aortic aneurysm with disruption and clot

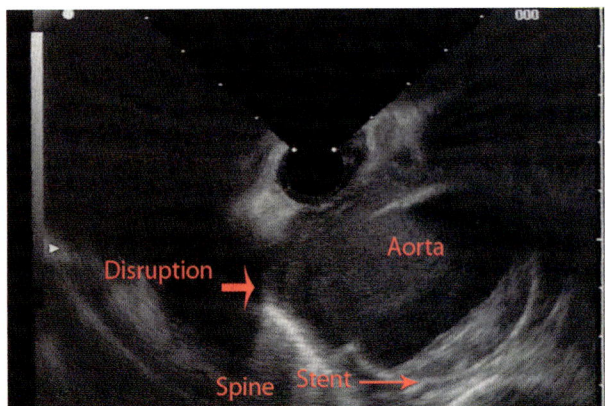

FIGURE 10–16. Aortic disruption below an aortic stent placed for an aneurysm

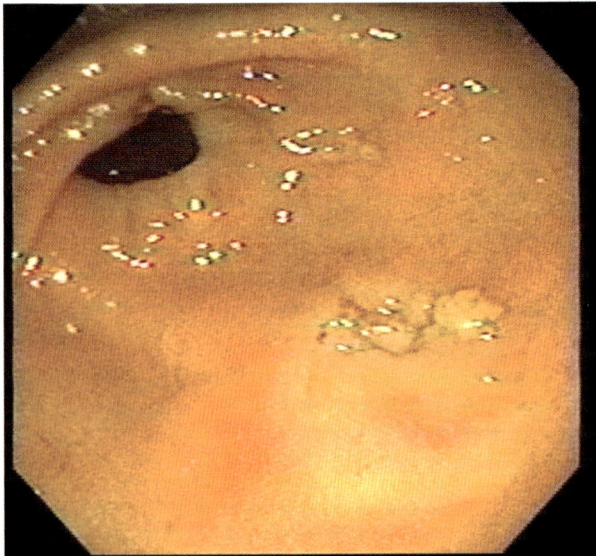

FIGURE 10–17. Endoscopic picture of an ischemic stomach. Biopsy produced no appreciable bleeding.

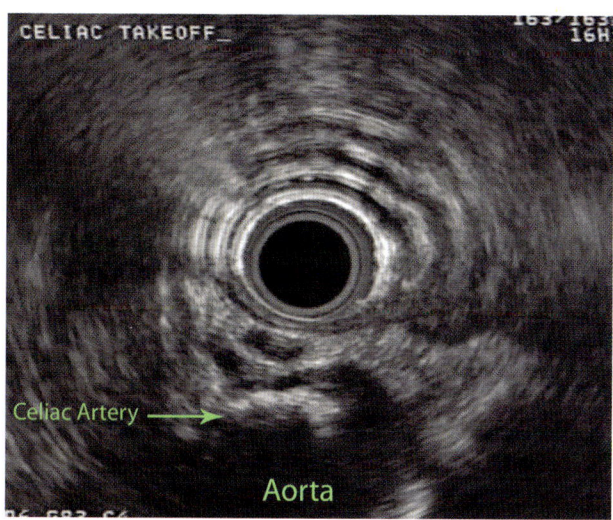

FIGURE 10–18. Celiac artery obstruction by radial array EUS on the patient shown in Figure 10–16

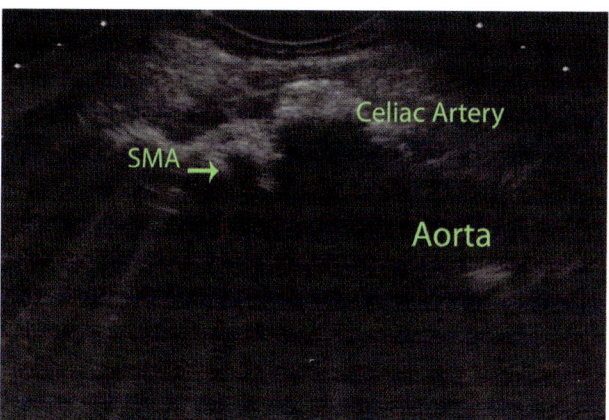

FIGURE 10–19. Linear array EUS showing obstruction of the celiac and superior mesenteric arteries (SMA) on the patient shown in Figure 7–16.

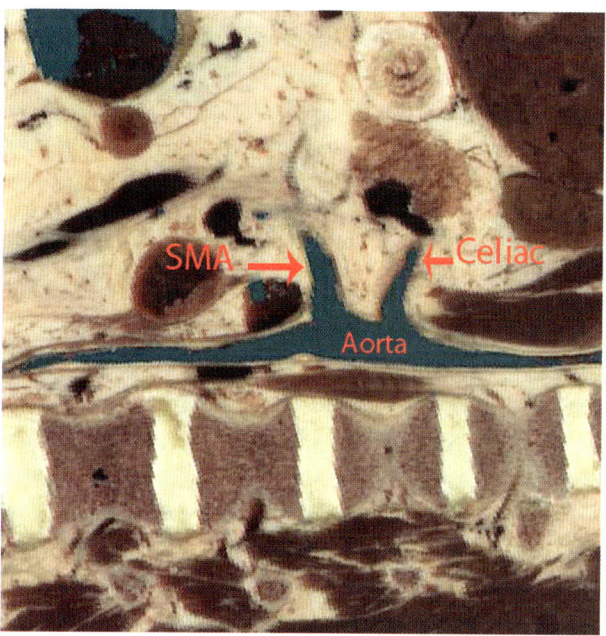

FIGURE 10–20. An image from the Visible Human Data Set showing a sagittal view of the aorta at the level of the celiac and superior mesenteric arteries (SMA) arising from the aorta.

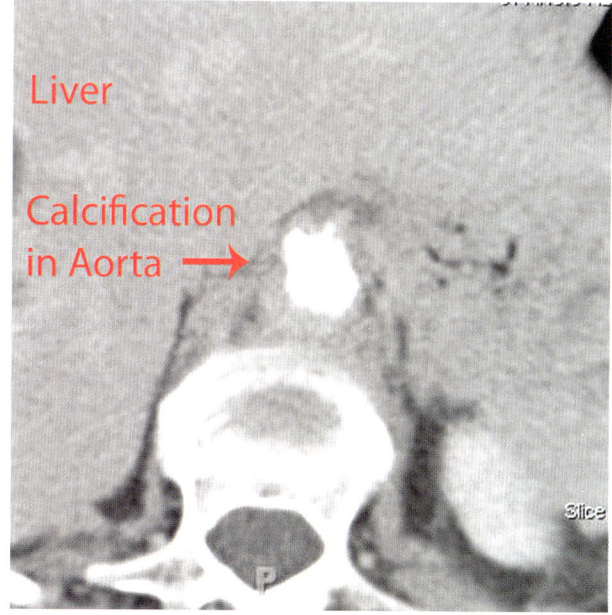

FIGURE 10–21. CT scan showing dense calcification at the celiac artery origin

An EGD at the time of EUS revealed gastric ulcers, and pale mucosa that didn't bleed during biopsy. Radial EUS (Figure 10–18) revealed dense calcification at the superior mesenteric artery (SMA) and celiac artery origins, with acoustic shadowing obscuring the aorta. Linear array examination (Figure 10–19) showed abrupt truncation of the celiac and SMA origins on the aorta. Corresponding normal anatomy from the Visible Human Data Set (Figure 10–20) is shown. Conventional CT scanning (Figure 10–21) and CT vascular reconstruction (Figure 10–22) confirmed the findings of calcification and obliteration of both the celiac and SMA origins. The patient underwent urgent vascular grafting with improvement in abdominal pain and severe malnutrition.

Aneurysms of the celiac artery and its branches are often the result of atherosclerosis. Figure 10–23 shows a radial array EUS examination in which a celiac artery aneurysm was discovered. The normal transaxial cross-section Visible Human anatomy is shown in Figure 10–24, and the patient's CT scan is shown in Figure 10–25.

Splenic artery aneurysms can sometimes be seen endoscopically, as submucosal projections in the stomach. The patient illustrated in Figure 10–26 was referred for EUS evaluation of a submucosal gastric

114   EUS Pathology with Digital Anatomy Correlation

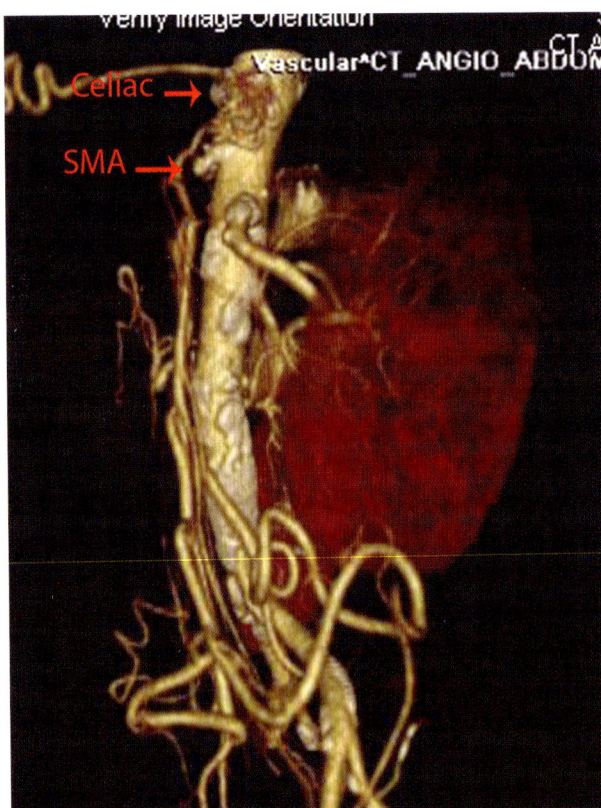

FIGURE 10–22. CT angiogram with reconstruction showing lack of flow in celiac and superior mesenteric arteries (SMA)

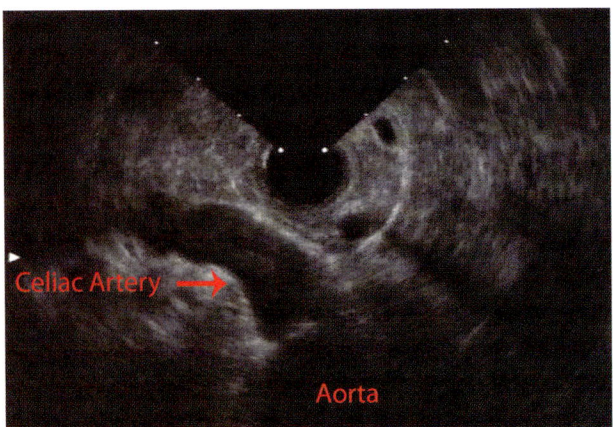

FIGURE 10–23. Celiac artery aneurysm by radial array EUS

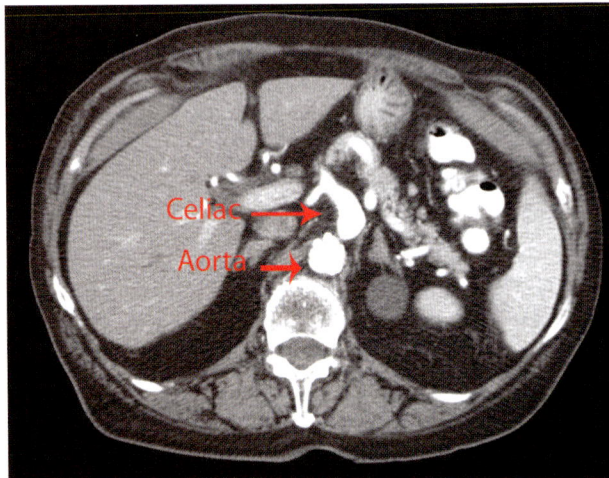

FIGURE 10–25. CT scan showing celiac artery aneurysm observed during EUS

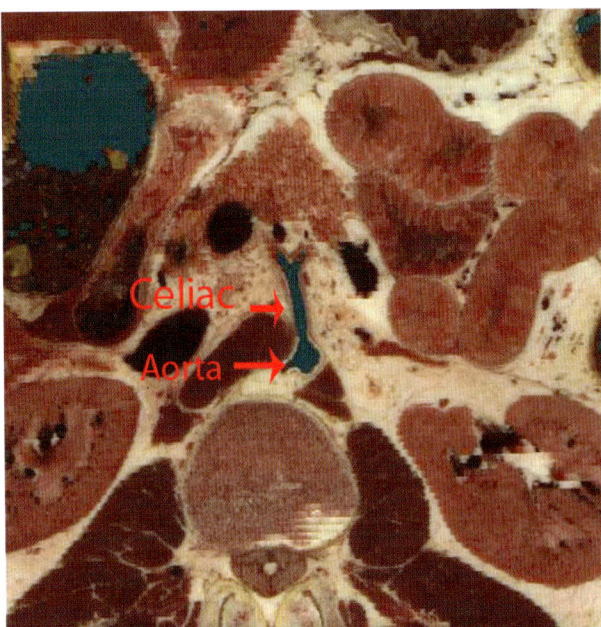

FIGURE 10–24. An image from the Visible Human Data Set showing an axial cross-section of the aorta at the level of the celiac artery.

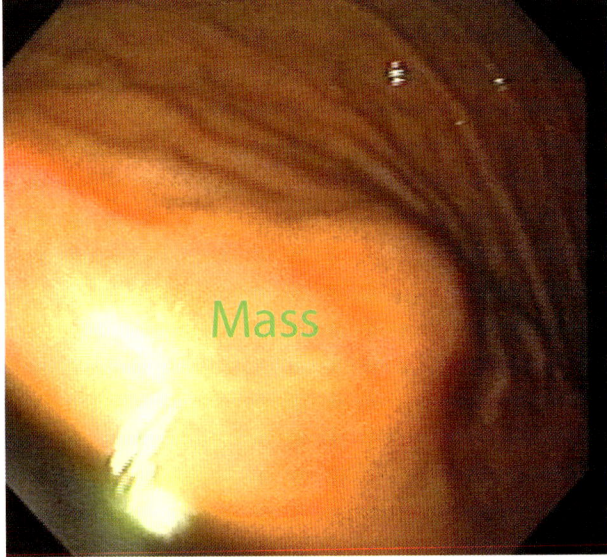

FIGURE 10–26. Endoscopic view of extrinsic gastric mass referred in for EUS. Previous biopsies were nondiagnostic.

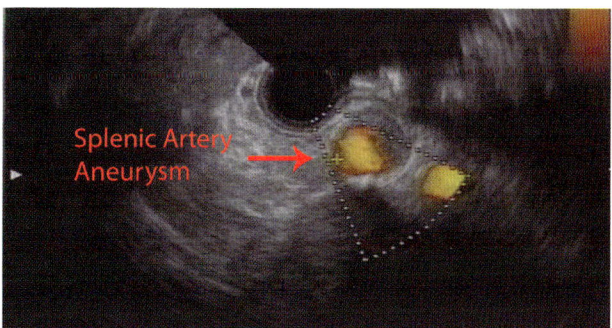

FIGURE 10–27. Radial EUS with color Doppler showing splenic artery aneurysm with thrombus

mass. This patient had a nondiagnostic biopsy of this protrusion by an outside endoscopist. Radial EUS with color Doppler revealed a splenic artery aneurysm with nonocclusive thrombosis (Figure 10–27).

Pseudoaneurysm of the splenic artery can occur following pancreatitis (4) and is more likely to be the diagnosis when luminal dilation of the splenic artery is found, a history of pancreatitis is obtained, and atherosclerosis is not prominent. The patient illustrated in Figure 10–28 had gallstone pancreatitis several months earlier and had persistent abdominal pain. A pseudoaneurysm of the splenic artery was found by EUS (Figure 10–28). Pulsatile flow was seen by Doppler flow (Figure 10–29). This pseudoaneurysm was subsequently managed with endovascular stenting.

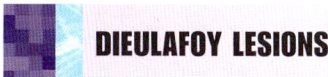

DIEULAFOY LESIONS

Dieulafoy lesions can be located throughout the gastrointestinal tract. Histologically, they are submucosal arterioloes, which can bleed profusely. An example of a histological section of a small bowel Dieulafoy artery is shown in Figure 10–30. Dieulafoy lesions can occasionally come to medical attention before bleeding. Figure 10–31 shows an endoscopic image taken of

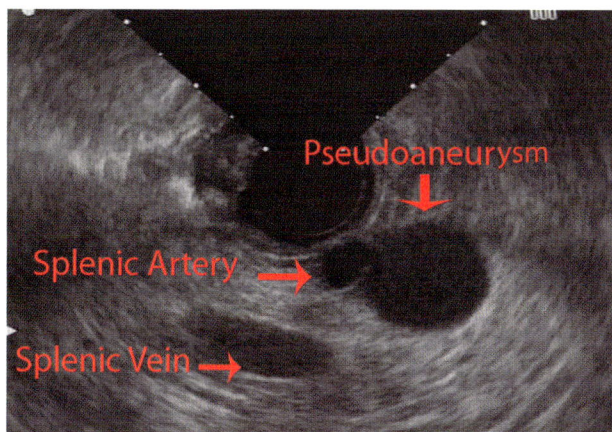

FIGURE 10–28. Splenic artery pseudoaneurysm, which was discovered six months after a bout of gallstone pancreatitis

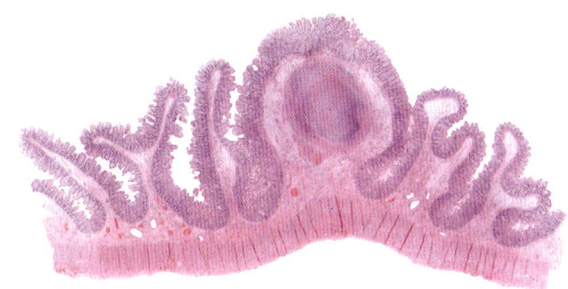

FIGURE 10–30. Histology of a Dieulafol lesion (Permission granted from Visible Human Journal of Endoscopy, www.vhjoe.com)

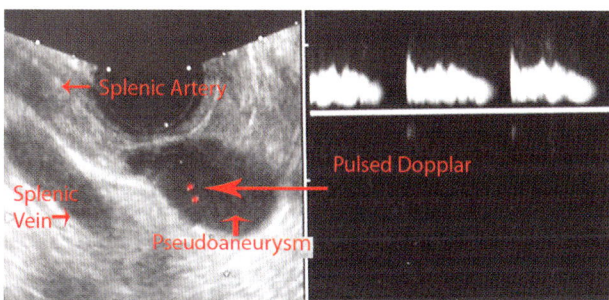

FIGURE 10–29. Radial EUS with pulsed Doppler of the splenic artery pseudoaneurysm

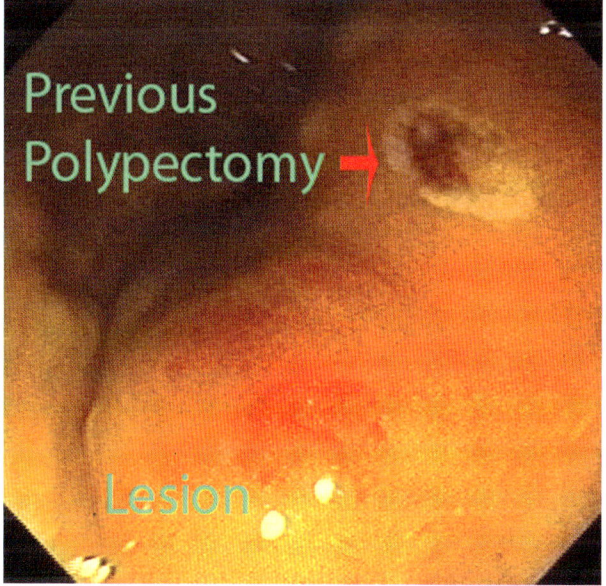

FIGURE 10–31. Endoscopic image of a pulsatile rectal lesion that was found adjacent to a polypectomy site

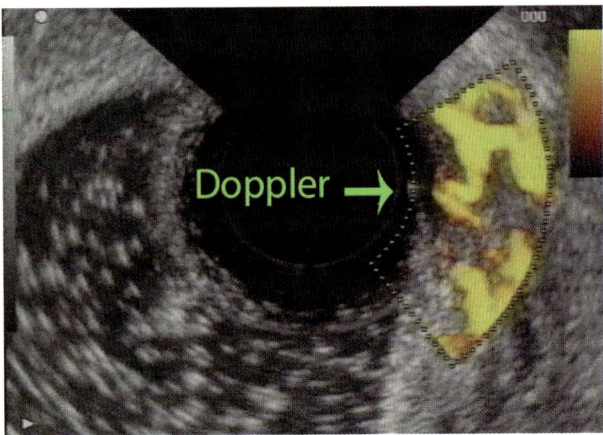

FIGURE 10–32. Color Doppler image of the vessel in the submucosa. Pulsed Doppler demonstrated pulsatile flow.

a patient referred with a pulsatile area detected in the rectum during colonoscopy with polypectomy. EUS revealed a large submucosal vascular channel best appreciated by color Doppler (Figure 10–32). Pulsed Doppler confirmed the arterial nature of this lesion.

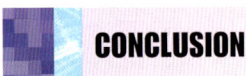 **CONCLUSION**

Vascular abnormalities, particularly acquired ones such as atherosclerosis, are commonly seen during EUS examinations. They are often incidental, but can sometimes become the key finding that significantly alters patient management. Comfort with vascular anatomy is useful and improves the quality of EUS evaluations.

Videos: Available at www.pmph-usa.com/bhutani

Video 10–1: A Visible Human transaxial film clip of the normal region around the aortic arch. Normally there are no vessels between the spinal column and the esophagus. This is followed by a radial EUS film clip from a patient with an aberrant right subclavian artery, which passes between the esophagus and the spinal column.

Video 10–2: An EUS video of a thoracic aortic aneurysm, which had previously been stented and now appears to be expanding toward the stomach. This unexpected finding was observed during EUS evaluation of a small gastric cancer.

References

1. De Luca, L, Bergman, J. J., Tytgat, G. N., Fockens P.: EUS imaging of the arteria lusoria: case series and and review. Gastrointest Endosc. 2000 Nov;52(5):670–673.
2. Parasher, V. K.: EUS in the diagnosis of aberrant subclavian artery. Gastrointest Endosc. 2001 Feb;53(2): 244–247.
3. McNally, P. R., Rak, K. M.: Dysphagia lusoria caused by persistent right aortic arch with aberrant left subclavian artery and diverticulum of Kommerell. Dig Dis Sci. 1992 Jan;37(1):144–149.
4. Argibay Filgueira, A. B., Maure Noia, B., Lamas Dominguez, P., Martinez-Vazquez, C.: Thrombosis of splenic artery pseudoaneurysm complicating pancreatitis. Gut. 1993 Sep;34(9):1271–1273.

CHAPTER 11

EUS for Mediastinal Lymph Nodes and Masses

Dr. Thomas J. Savides

Transesophageal endoscopic ultrasound-guided fine needle aspiration (EUS FNA) offers a safe and effective technique for sampling posterior mediastinal lymph nodes and masses. This technique is complementary, and often superior, to other methods of biopsying these lesions, such as mediastinoscopy or bronchoscopy with transbronchial FNA. Additionally, EUS without FNA can be very important for identifying mediastinal lesions, which should not undergo FNA biopsy, such as mediastinal cysts.

Posterior mediastinal lesions generally are either lymph nodes with a peripheral lung mass, lymph nodes alone, or a central lung/mediastinal mass. Lymph nodes with a peripheral lung mass are likely metastatic lung cancer. In these cases, EUS FNA is an important tool for providing diagnosis and nodal staging for lung cancer (especially for non-small-cell lung cancer). Patients with non-small-cell lung cancer and metastatic lymph nodes on the contralateral side as the primary mass, or with bulky subcarinal adenopathy, are generally considered to either be nonsurgical candidates, or possibly candidates for neoadjuvant therapy prior to possible surgery. The differential diagnosis of diffuse mediastinal adenopathy includes lymphoma, lung cancer, infections, and reactive lymph nodes. Isolated posterior mediastinal masses may be lung cancer, metastatic disease, infections, or cysts. Transesophageal EUS FNA is highly accurate for diagnosing a variety of benign and malignant mediastinal lesions. (Table 11–1)

EUS Technique

Generally an abnormal CT finding prompts referral for a transesophageal EUS of a mediastinal lesion. Given that the anatomic landmarks from the CT scan can be used to guide localization of the lesion, many endosonographers will use a linear EUS scope as the only scope to evaluate the lesion and obtain an FNA. However some endosonographers will prefer to use a radial EUS scope first to completely survey the entire posterior mediastinum and determine the best lesion to biopsy. When a patient is suspected to have non-small-cell lung cancer, an evaluation of distant metastatic sites should be performed, including the left adrenal gland and the liver.

The anatomy of the mediastinum readily lends itself to EUS and FNA.

The Visible Human anatomy of the subcarinal space is shown in Figures 11–1 A-C. Transaxial cross-sections (Figures 11–1 A, B) are similar to what is obtained using radial array EUS. The sagittal image (Figure 11–1 C) is similar to what is obtained with linear array EUS.

Table 11–1 Posterior Mediastinal Lesions That can be Diagnosed with EUS/FNA

Primary pulmonary cancer
Non-small cell lung cancer
Small Cell Lung Cancer
Metastatic cancer from extra-thoracic malignancy
Lymphoma
Reactive lymph nodes
Granulomatous disease
    Sarcoid
    Histoplasmosis
    Tuberculosis
Duplication cysts
Neurogenic tumors
Infections
    Mediastinal abscess
    Mediastinitis
    Cryptococcus

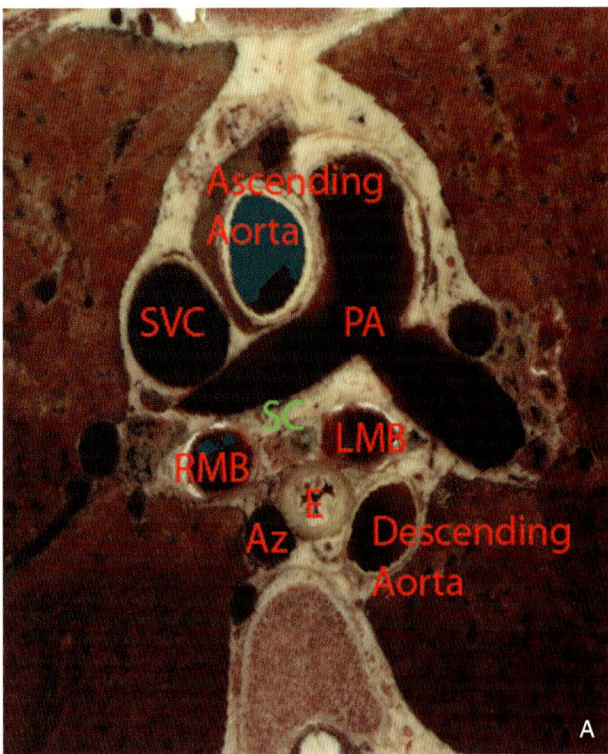

FIGURE 11–1. *A* (A) Visible Human transaxial image of the subcarinal space just below the carina similar to radial EUS.

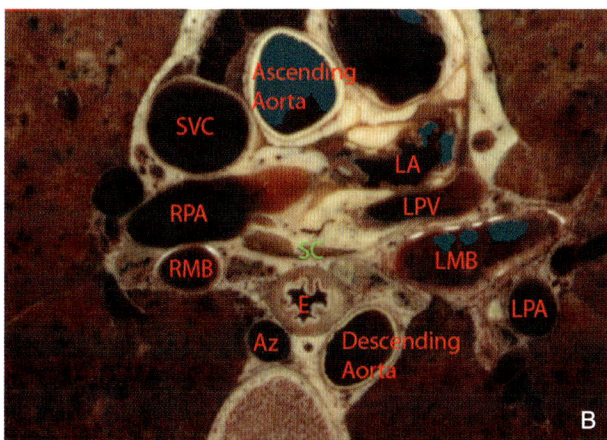 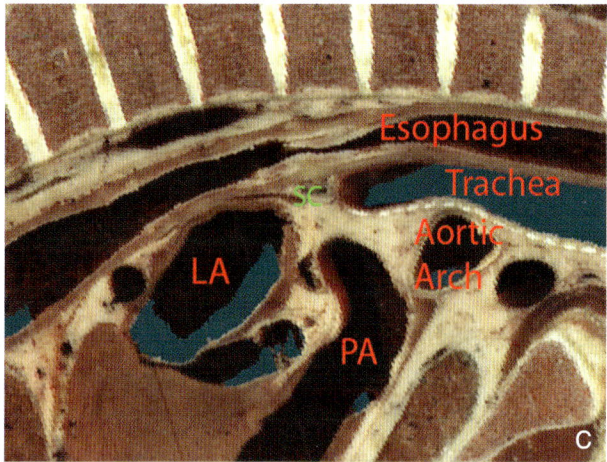

FIGURE 11–1. *B and C* (Continued) (B) Visible Human transaxial image made in the caudal portion of the subcarinal space similar to radial EUS. Figure 11–1 (C) Visible Human sagittal image of the subcarinal space, similar to linear EUS. Az=azygous vein, E=esophagus, LA=left atrium, LPV=left pulmonary vein, LMB=left mainstem bronchus, RMB=right mainstem bronchus, PA=pulmonary artery, RPA=right pulmonary artery, LPA=left pulmonary artery, SVC=superior vena cava, SC=subcarinal space (Courtesy Dr John Deutsch).

The process of transesophageal EUS FNA is the same as in other parts of the peri-gastrointestinal tract. The only difference is that immediate cytological evaluation may be even more important, as the differential diagnosis not uncommonly will include lymphoma versus infection. By having a preliminary cytologic evaluation of the material during the procedure, one can determine if material also needs to be sent for microbiology cultures for infection, flow cytometry, or immunostains. Tru-Cut core needle biopsy can also be performed to obtain tissue cores for histological evaluation. This usually is not needed, and may lead to increased risk of mediastinitis, but can sometimes be helpful in making a diagnosis of lymphoma.[1]

Benign Posterior Mediastinal Lymph Nodes and Masses

EUS Appearance of Normal Benign Reactive Posterior Mediastinal Lymph Nodes

Benign mediastinal lymph nodes are commonly encountered during EUS for nonthoracic indications. These often have a triangular or crescent shape (Figure 11–2). An echogenic center may be visualized, representing the hilum of the lymph node. These may be normal, or may be reactive lymph nodes from prior infections or inhaled irritants. Cytologically they show a polymorphous population of lymphoid elements.

Granulomatous Lymph Nodes

The differential diagnosis includes sarcoid, histoplasmosis, tuberculosis, and coccidiomycosis. The EUS appearance of granulomatous lymph nodes is usually single or multiple enlarged lymph nodes. The cytology

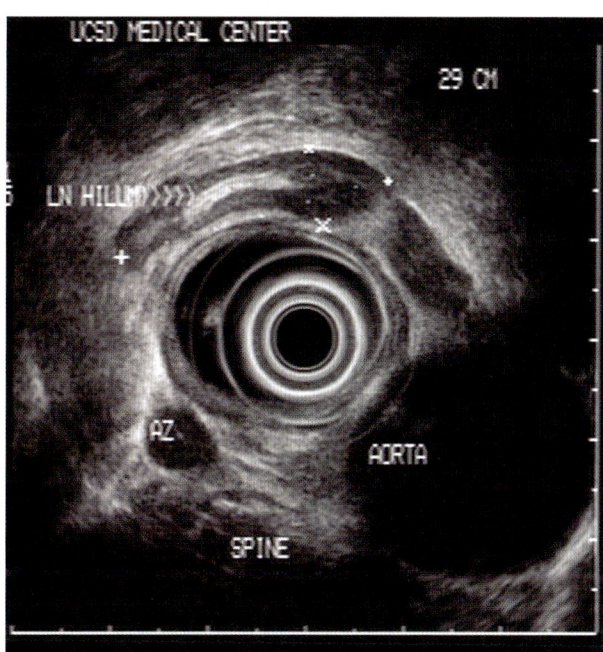

FIGURE 11–2. Benign posterior mediastinal lymph node. Note the draping, triangular shape, and hyperechoic central stripe of the lymph node hilum.

reveals collections of palisaded histiocytes in a background of lymphocytes. Necrosis (caseation) may be observed in any granulomatous lymph node. If granulomas are noted during immediate cytologic evaluation, material should be sent for fungal and mycobacterial stains.

Sarcoid

Sarcoid is a multisystem granulomatous disease of unknown etiology. The EUS appearance of mediastinal sarcoid lymphadenopathy is generally several enlarged benign appearing lymph nodes (Figures 11–3 A-D). This is a clinical diagnosis that is supported by non-necrotic granulomatous lymph nodes, and elevated serum angiotensin converting enzyme levels. EUS/FNA can obtain granulomatous material with high accuracy.[2-4] One retrospective study found the sensitivity and specificity of EUS/FNA for diagnosing granulomas in suspected sarcoid to be 89%

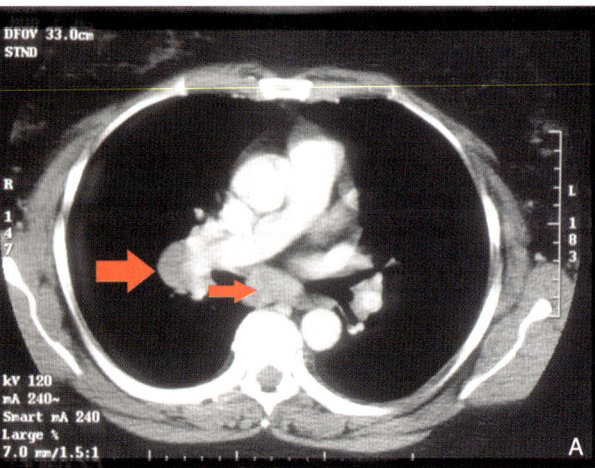
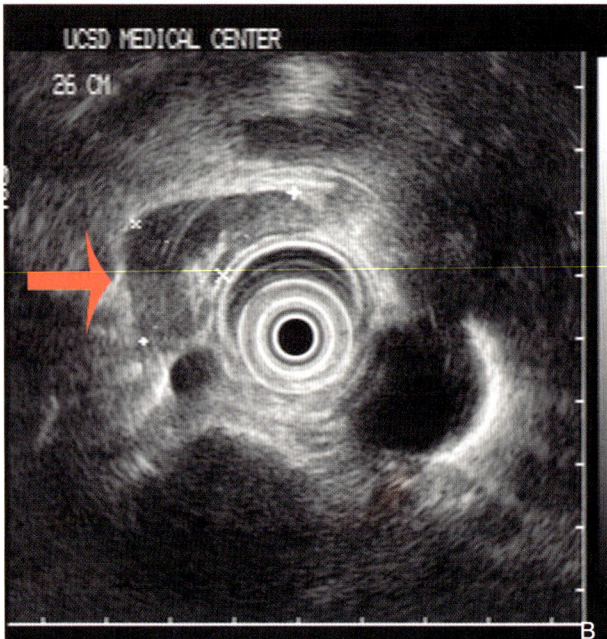
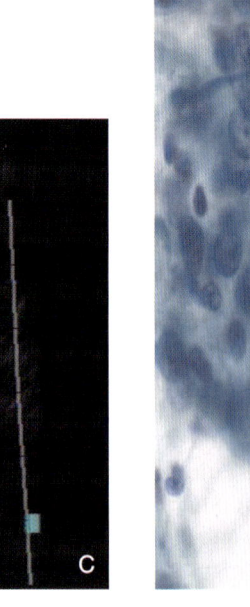
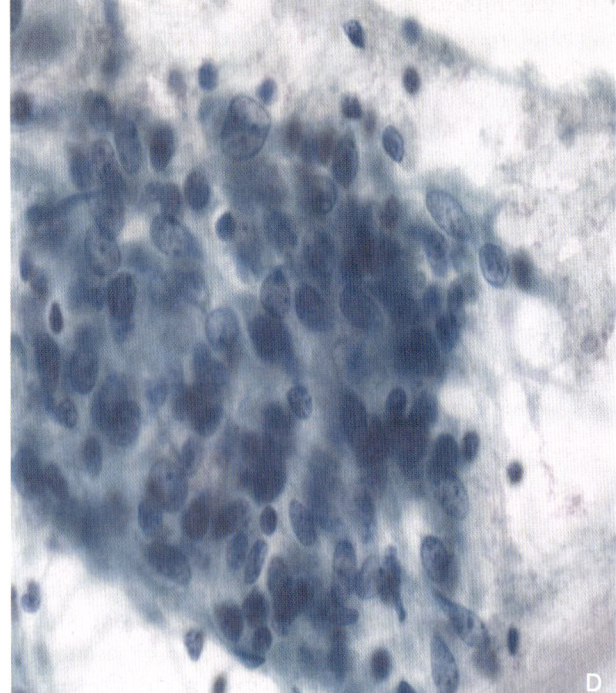

FIGURE 11–3. *A to D* (A) CT scan of enlarged subcarinal lymph node in a patient with sarcoidosis. (B) Radial EUS image of enlarged subcarinal lymph node in a patient with sarcoidosis. (C) Linear EUS FNA of enlarged subcarinal lymph node in a patient with sarcoidosis. (D) EUS FNA cytology of sarcoid lymph node. (Courtesy of Cynthia Behling, M.D., Ph.D.)

and 96%, respectively.[5] Another EUS/FNA study demonstrated noncaseating granulomas in 41 of 50 patients (82%) with a final clinical diagnosis of sarcoidosis.[4]

Fungal Infections

Fungal infections such as histoplasmosis or blastomycosis are usually suspected in patients from endemic areas with pulmonary symptoms or because of incidentally found posterior mediastinal adenopathy. The diagnosis is made by histopathology, serologic testing, and/or antigen testing. The EUS appearance varies, but includes bland enlarged benign-appearing lymph nodes or irregular nodes, which may be matted together and calcified (Figures 11–4 A, B). EUS/FNA can also identify granulomas in patients with suspected fungal infections.[6,7]

Tuberculosis

Mycobacterium tuberculosis can cause enlarged mediastinal lymph nodes or a nodal mass. EUS/FNA can obtain material for *M. tuberculosis* culture.[3,8-11] The addition of polymerase chain reaction testing for mycobacterium tuberculosis in EUS/FNA- obtained samples may increase the diagnostic yield compared to cytology and culture in patients suspected to have tuberculosis.

Mediastinal Cysts

Mediastinal cysts can be mistaken for lymph nodes or masses on CT scans. Congenital foregut cysts are most common, and probably arise as a result of aberrant development of the primitive foregut. They are categorized on the basis of embryonic origin into bronchogenic or neuroenteric (esophageal duplication cysts and neuroenteric cysts). Esophageal duplication cysts are adherent to the esophagus, while those away from the esophageal wall suggest bronchogenic cysts. The pathologic evaluation of duplication cysts reveals them to be typically lined by columnar epithelia.

Most patients with posterior mediastinal cysts are asymptomatic; cysts are incidentally found during other imaging studies. Rare symptomatic cysts may be considered for surgical resection. Because the malignant potential is considered to be extremely rare, incidentally found lesions can be followed clinically.

The EUS appearance of a mediastinal cyst is usually a round or tubular anechoic structure with acoustic enhancement[12-15] (Figures 11–5 A, B). Some cysts appear to be a mass lesion or lymph node because of a more hypoechoic (rather than anechoic) echotexture and minimal acoustic enhancement. These cysts usually consist of a thick, gelatinous cyst material.[15-18]

Cysts can be aspirated with EUS/FNA, but usually only when the EUS is not highly compatible with a cyst, and instead appears to be a possible mass.[12,15,17-20] There have been reports of patients developing mediastinitis and/or cyst infection after undergoing EUS/FNA, including several with the use of Tru-Cut needle biopsy.[16,17,20-23] These patients required treatment with antibiotics, surgery, and/or endoscopic cyst drainage. Of note, most of these cases reported no antibiotic prophylaxis. A more recent series that used antibiotics around the time of the FNA reported no complications.[18]

Because most posterior mediastinal cysts are benign, and mediastinitis is a recognized complication, obvious posterior mediastinal duplication cysts should not be aspirated with EUS/FNA. If it is unclear whether the lesion is a cyst or a malignancy, then the safest next diagnostic test might be thoracic MRI or

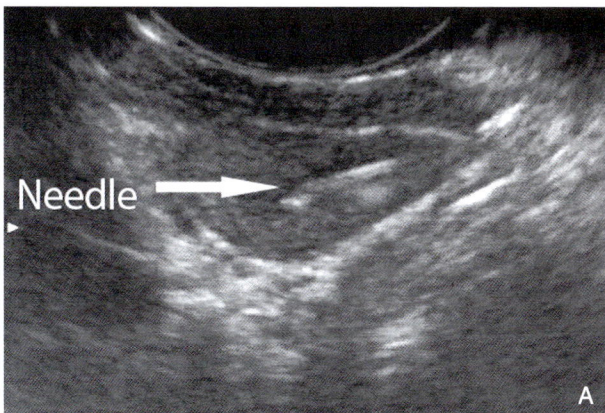 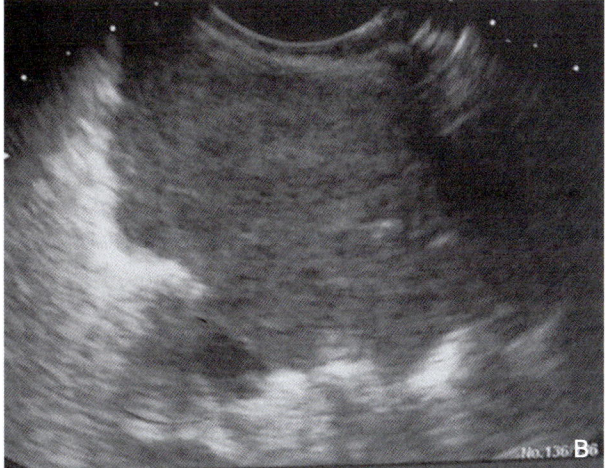

FIGURE 11–4. *A and B* (A) EUS appearance of mediastinal lymph node in which enlargement was due to histoplasmosis. (B) Irregular mediastinal lymph node due to blastomycosis (Courtesy Dr John Deutsch).

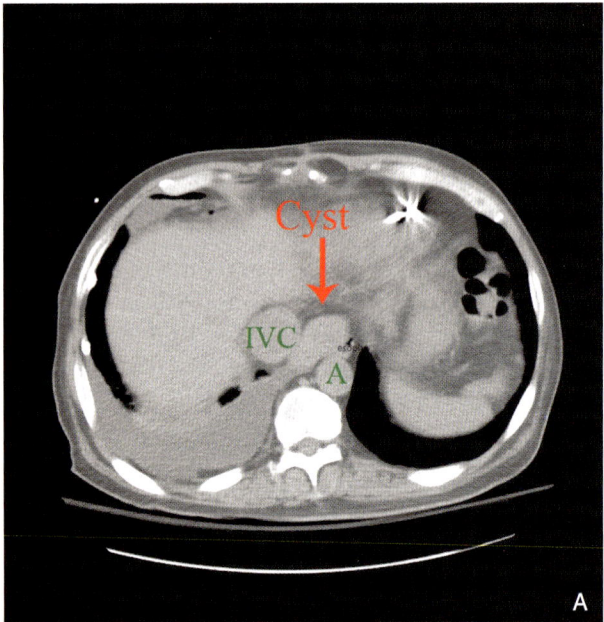 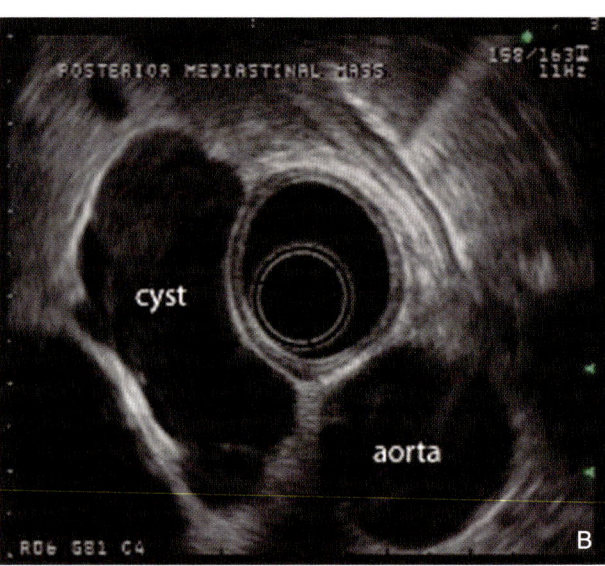

FIGURE 11–5. *A and B* (A) Duplication cyst located in the right para-esophageal space. A=aorta, IVC=inferior vena cava. (B) EUS of peri-esophageal duplication cyst. Note the acoustic enhancement and the debris and septum within the cyst.

CT to confirm the presence of a cyst.[17] If EUS/FNA is performed on a lesion that turns out to be a cyst rather than a solid mass, then the cyst should be completely drained if possible (although usually this is not possible due to the thick nature of the cyst material), and prophylactic antibiotics should be administered, such as intravenous antibiotics during the procedure and oral antibiotics for the next three to five days to minimize any risk of mediastinitis.[18] EUS-guided True-Cut needle biopsies should be avoided in suspected posterior mediastinal cysts because of the risk of mediastinitis.

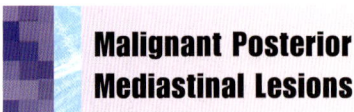

Malignant Posterior Mediastinal Lesions

EUS Appearance of Malignant Posterior Mediastinal Lymph Nodes

EUS findings associated with malignancy include round shape, short-axis diameter greater than 5–10 mm, hypoechoic echotexture, and well-demarcated borders.[24,25] If all 4 features are present in a lymph node, the chance of malignancy is 80-100%.[25,26] Because all four features are only seen in 25% of malignant lymph nodes, tissue sampling is important to obtain diagnostic material.[26]

The rate of a malignant diagnosis in EUS/FNA of posterior mediastinal nodes in patients without a known diagnosis of cancer varies depending on prior bronchoscopic evaluation and local referral patterns, but is approximately 50%.[8,27] The EUS distinction between a posterior mediastinal mass and lymph node can be difficult, because some lymph nodes are very large, while some masses are very small. Additionally, numerous lymph nodes matted together can form a "mass." Usually a mass is larger than an enlarged lymph node (i.e. several centimeters diameter), but there is no standardized terminology. The overall sensitivity, specificity, and accuracy for diagnosing malignancy in posterior mediastinal lesions with EUS/FNA is greater than 90%. (Table 11–2)

Lung Cancer Masses

Large lung cancer masses can abut the posterior mediastinum and be within reach of trans-esophageal EUS FNA. Often these tumors can also be diagnosed during bronchoscopy because of endobronchial tumor growth. Usually these are non-small-cell lung cancers. These are generally safe and easy to biopsy using trans-esophageal FNA technique. (Figures 11–6 A-D)

Metastatic Disease to the Posterior Mediastinum

A variety of tumors metastasize to the posterior mediastinum, appearing as either a lymph node or mass. The most common metastatic lesion is primary lung cancer, of which 80% is non-small-cell lung cancer (NSCLC), and the remaining 20% is small-cell carcinoma. Diagnosis and staging of non-small-cell lung

Table 11-2 Operating Characteristics of EUS FNA for Diagnosing Malignant Mediastinal Lesions

Reference	Year	n	Sensitivity (%)	Specificity (%)	Accuracy (%)	Positive Predictive Value	Negative Predictive Value
Wiersema[38]	2001	82	96	100	98	94	100
Larsen[39]	2002	79	92	100	94	100	80
Savides[27]	2004	59	96	100	98	100	97
Eloubeidi[40]	2005	104	93	100	97	100	97
OVERALL			92-96%	100%	94-97%	94-100%	80-100%

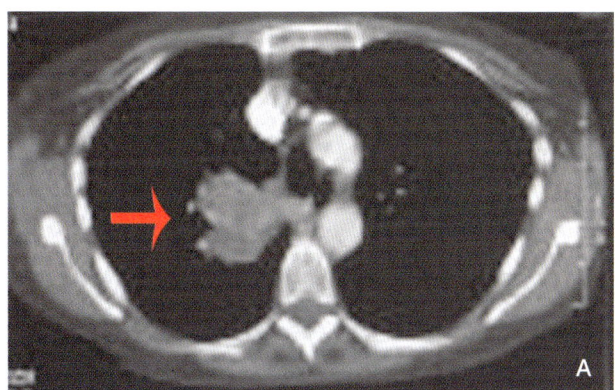
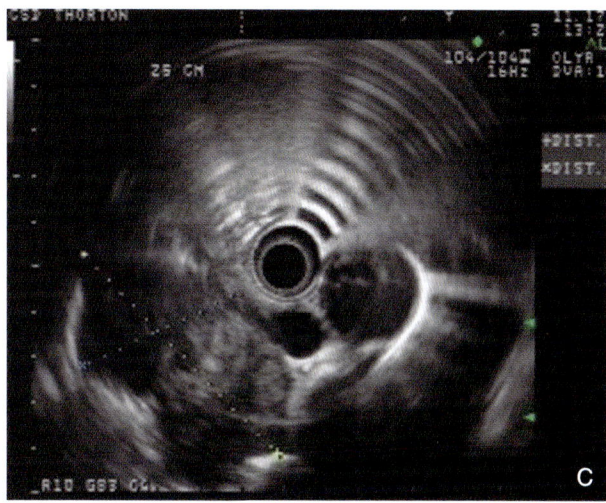
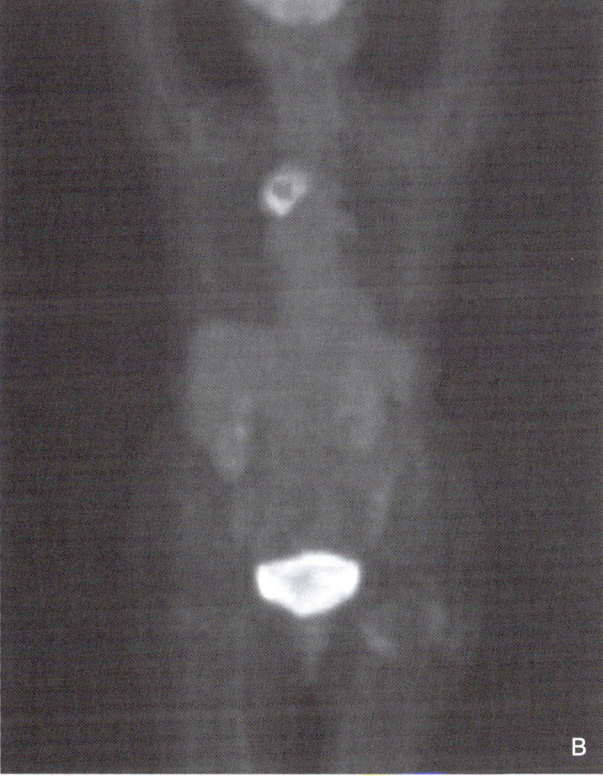
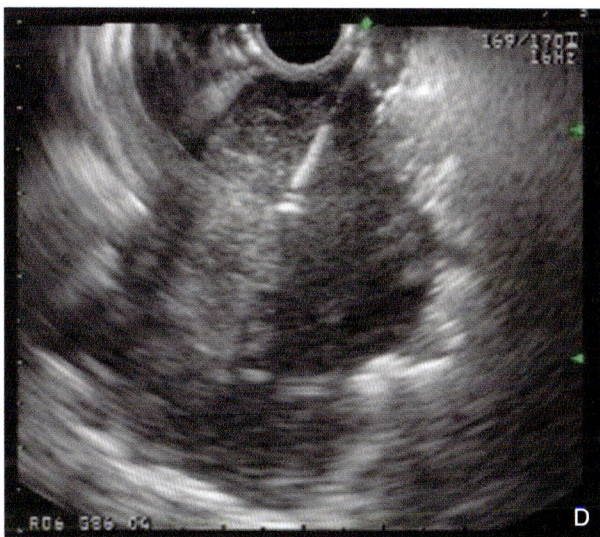

FIGURE 11-6. *A to D* (A) CT scan showing right upper lobe lung, non-small-cell lung cancer. (B) PET scan showing increased activity in the region of the right upper lobe mass. (C) Radial EUS of right upper lobe lung mass abutting the esophagus. (D) Transesophageal EUS FNA of right upper lobe mass, which revealed cells consistent with non-small-cell lung cancer.

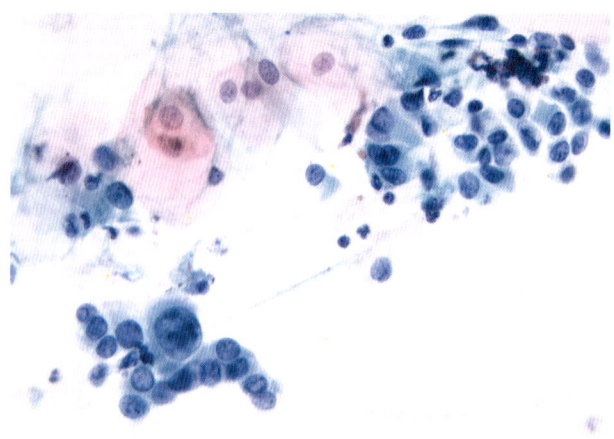

FIGURE 11-6. E (Continued) E Cytology showing non-small-cell carcinoma (Courstesy of Cynthia Behling, M.D., Ph.D.).

cancer is one of the most common indications for transesophageal EUS FNA. Usually there will be suspected lung cancer due to a peripheral lung mass with posterior mediastinal lymph nodes. The most common sites for EUS FNA of metastatic NSCLC are the subcarina (Figures 11–7 A-C) and posterior aortopulmonic window (Figures 11–8 A-C), although nodes can also be biopsied from the paratracheal and para-esophageal areas. Metastases from breast, colon, kidney, testis, larynx, pancreas, liver, and esophagus have been diagnosed by transesophageal EUS/FNA.[28][29-32]

Lymphoma

Mediastinal lymphoma will generally appear as multiple enlarged posterior mediastinal lymph nodes without peripheral lung mass (Figures 11–9 A, B). Histology can be either low grade or high grade (Figures 11–9 CD). Material from EUS/FNA

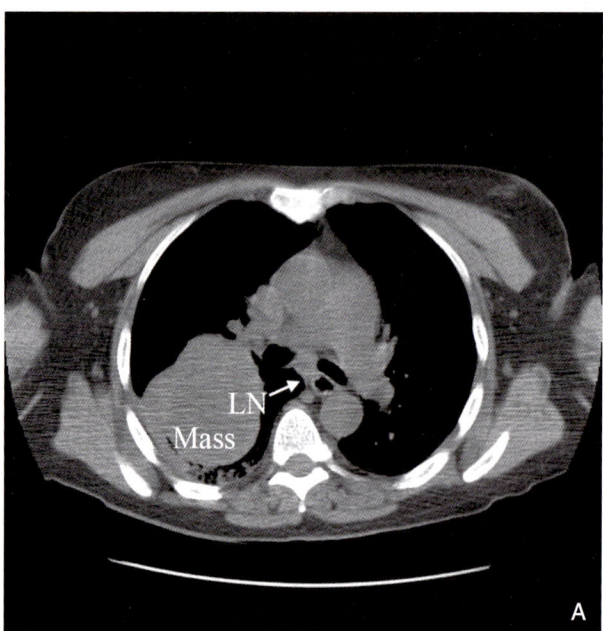

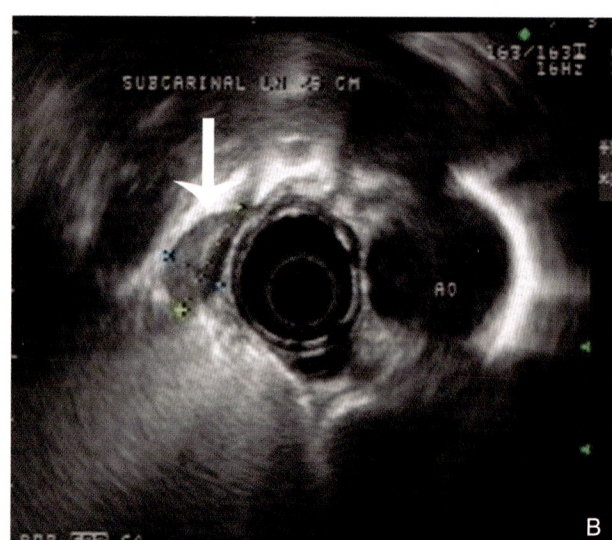

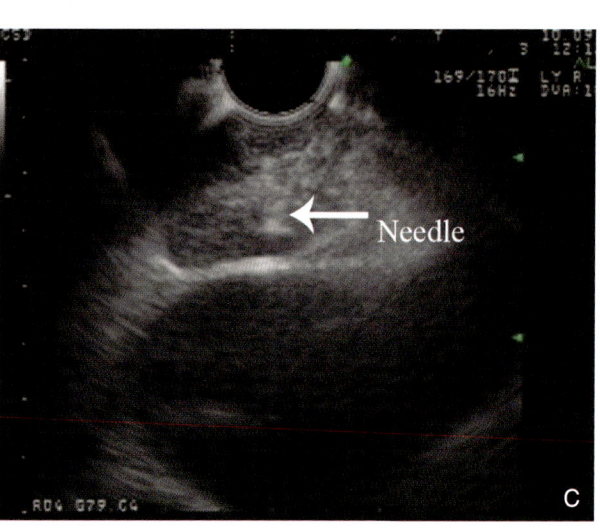

FIGURE 11-7. *A to C* (A) CT scan showing right lower lobe, non-small-cell lung cancer and subcarinal lymph node (arrow). (B) Radial EUS of subcarinal lymph node (18 mm × 9 mm) in NSCLC patient. (C) EUS FNA into the subcarinal lymph node.

EUS for Mediastinal Lymph Nodes and Masses

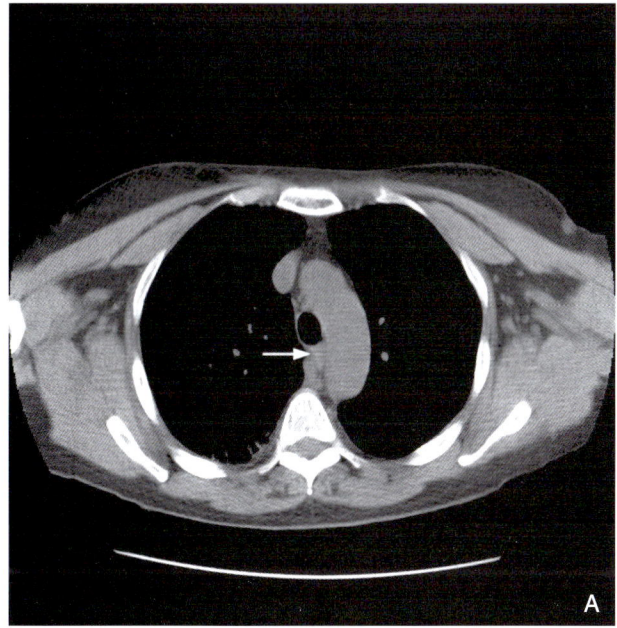
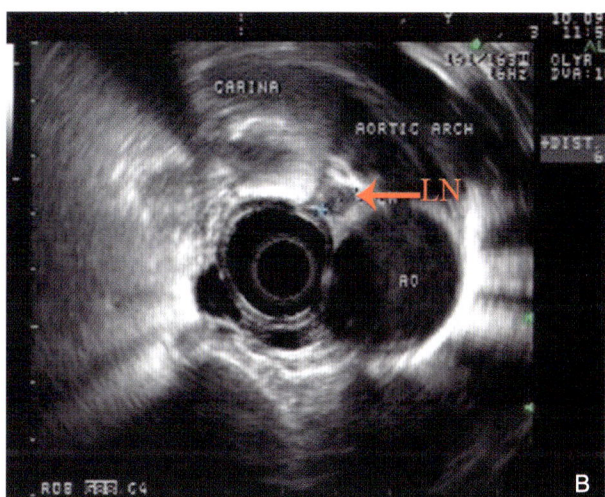
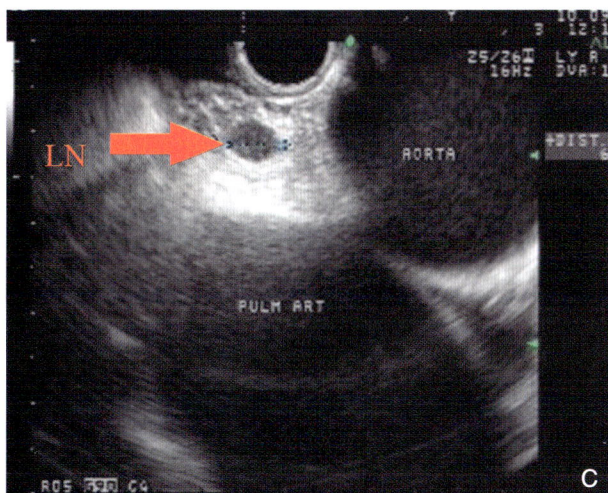

FIGURE 11–8. *A to C* (A) CT scan of a patient with right lower lobe NSCLC and posterior aortopulmonic window lymph node. (B) Radial EUS of aortopulmonic window lymph node (LN). Ao=aorta. (C) Linear EUS of aortopulmonic window lymph node (LN).

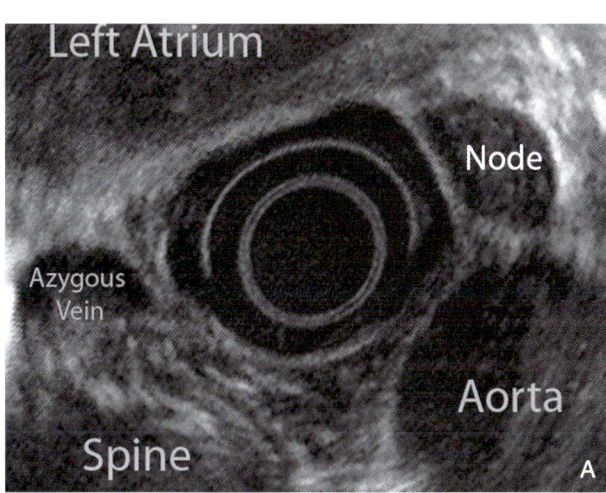
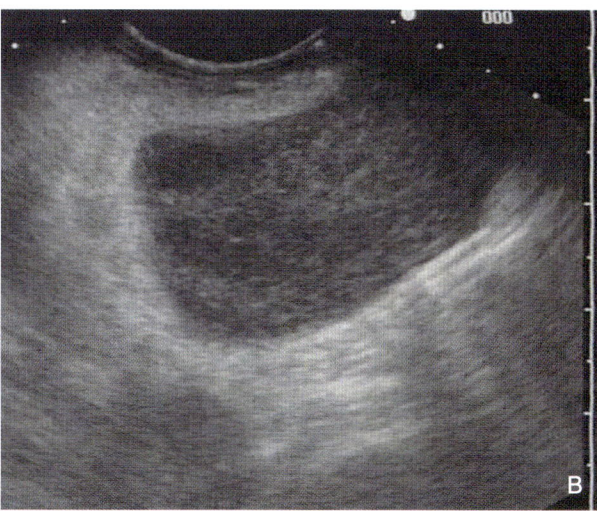

FIGURE 11–9. *A and B* (A) Radial array EUS of mediastinal low-grade lymphoma. This lymph node was aspirated during a staging procedure for early gastric cancer. (B) Linear array EUS of mediastinal large-cell lymphoma. (Courtesy Dr John Deutsch)

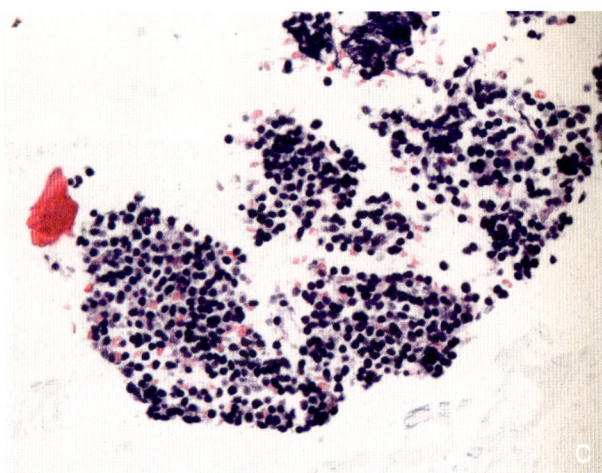 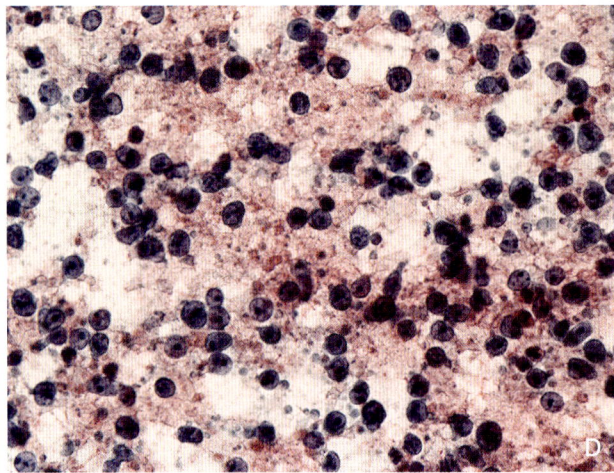

FIGURE 11–9. *C and D* (Continued) (C) Cytology from the node shown in Figure 8-9 A. Diagnosis of low-grade lymphoma was made by flow cytometry, which showed a lambda monoclonal B-cell lymphoproliferative disorder characterized by positivity for CD20 (moderate), CD19, CD5, CD22, CD11c (dim-variable), and CD23. Of note, CD38 is negative. The background T-cells expressed CD3 and CD5 normally. (Courtesy of Dr David Carter) (D) Papanicoaou stain from node shown in Figure 11-9 B showing prominent nucleoli in this large cell lymphoma (Courtesy of Dr David Carter)

can be evaluated by cytology, immunohistochemistry, and flow cytometry, allowing diagnosis and workup of lymphoma in posterior mediastinal lymph nodes.(Figure [33-36]) The sensitivity of diagnosing low-grade lymphoma can be increased (from 44% to 86%) by adding flow cytometry and immunocytochemistry.[33] For some lymphomas, such as low-grade follicular lesions, Tru-Cut biopsies may provide helpful architectural details.[1] A few series have found that lymphoma was able to de diagnosed with Tru-Cut biopsies when cytology was nondiagnostic, although it is not clear whether immediate cytologic evaluation, flow cytometry, and/or immunostains were done in these cases.[33,37]

Risks of Mediastinal EUS FNA

EUS FNA is an extremely safe procedure for sampling lymph nodes. The theoretical risks include perforation, bleeding, pneumothorax, and infection. Only mediastinitis has been repeatedly reported in the literature (Table 11–3). Most cases have involved FNA of cysts and/or use of Tru-Cut needle. Recently there have been reports of mediastinitis after EUS FNA of solid posterior mediastinal lesions. It is important to remember that any patient with chest pain or fever after mediastinal EUS FNA should be promptly evaluated for possible mediastinitis.

Overall Impact of EUS FNA for Mediastinal Lesions

A study of 59 patients referred to a surgeon for mediastinscopy in order to biopsy lymph nodes, but who instead first underwent EUS FNA, found that only 22% ultimately required surgery (mediastinoscopy or thoracotomy).[27] If there was a positive cytology for malignancy, only 4% of patients ultimately had surgery. If cytology was negative, only 33% ultimately had surgery. This data, obtained from a community-based integrated healthcare system, highlights that EUS FNA of these lesions is not only accurate but also significantly reduces the number of patients having surgery for diagnostic mediastinoscopy.

Table 11-3 Reported Cases of Transesophageal EUS-Guided FNA Causing Mediastinitis

Author (year)	Lesion Biopsied	FNA or Tru-Cut	Antibiotics	Complication	Management
Ryan[20] (2002)	Cyst	FNA	Yes	Incidental candida found at resection	Thoracotomy
Wildi[16] (2003)	Cyst (solid appearing)	FNA and Tru-Cut	No	Mediastinitis and sepsis	Thoracotomy
Annema[22] (2003)	Cyst	FNA	No	Mediastinitis (Strep pneumoniae)	Thoracotomy
Westerterp[17] (2004)	Cyst (solid) appearing	FNA	No	Mediastinitis	Endoscopic fenestration
Varadarajulu[23] (2004)	Cyst	Tru-Cut	No	Mediastinitis	Thoracotomy
Pai[41] (2005)	Mass (teratoma)	FNA	No	Mediastinitis	Thoracotomy
Will[32] (2005)	Lymph Node (malignant)	FNA	No	Mediastinitis and esophago-mediastinal fistula	Endoscopic treatment and antibiotics
Savides (2007)	Lymph node (benign)	FNA	No	Mediastinitis and osteomyelitis (Gemella morbillorum)	Antibiotics

Conclusion

Transesophageal EUS FNA is an extremely effective and safe method of biopsying posterior mediastinal lymph nodes and masses. It is playing an increasingly important role in diagnosing and staging lung cancer, as well as the evaluation of benign nodal disease. EUS FNA should be avoided in cystic lesions of the mediastinum, and recognition that mediastinitis can occur is important.

References

1. Levy, M. J., Jondal. M. L., Clain, J., Wiersema, M. J.: Preliminary experience with an EUS-guided Tru-Cut biopsy needle compared with EUS-guided FNA. Gastrointest Endosc 2003;57:101–106.
2. Mishra, G., Sahai, A. V., Penman, I. D., Williams, D. B., Judson, M. A., Lewin, D. N., Hawes, R. H., Hoffman, B. J.: Endoscopic ultrasonography with fine-needle aspiration: an accurate and simple diagnostic modality for sarcoidosis. Endoscopy 1999;31:377–382.
3. Fritscher-Ravens, A., Sriram, P. V., Topalidis, T., Hauber, H. P., Meyer, A., Soehendra, N., Pforte, A.: Diagnosing sarcoidosis using endosonography-guided fine-needle aspiration. Chest 2000;118:928–935.
4. Annema, J., Veselic, M., Rabe, K.: Endoscopic ultrasound guided fine needle aspiration for the diagnosis of sarcoidosis. 25 ed. 2005:1–5.
5. Wildi, S. M., Judson, M. A., Fraig, M., Fickling, W. E., Schmulewitz, N., Varadarajulu, S., Roberts, S. S., Prasad, P., Hawes, R. H., Wallace, M. B., Hoffman, B. J.: Is endosonography guided fine needle aspiration (EUS-FNA) for sarcoidosis as good as we think? Thorax 2004;59:794–799.
6. Wiersema, M. J., Chak, A., Wiersema, L. M.: Mediastinal histoplasmosis: evaluation with endosonography and endoscopic fine-needle aspiration biopsy. Gastrointest Endosc 1994;40:78–81.
7. Savides, T. J., Gress, F. G., Wheat, L. J., Ikenberry, S., Hawes, R. H.: Dysphagia due to mediastinal granulomas: diagnosis with endoscopic ultrasonography. Gastroenterology 1995;109:366–373.
8. Fritscher-Ravens, A., Sriram, P. V., Bobrowski, C., Pforte, A., Topalidis, T., Krause, C., Jaeckle, S., Thonke, F., Soehendra, N.: Mediastinal lymphadenopathy in patients with or without previous malignancy: EUS-FNA-based differential cytodiagnosis in 153 patients. Am J Gastroenterol 2000;95:2278–2284.
9. Hainaut, P, Monthe, A., Lesage, V., Weynand, B.: Tuberculous mediastinal lymphadenopathy. Acta Clin Belg 1998;53:114–116.
10. Kramer, H, Nieuwenhuis, J. A., Groen, H. J., Wempe, J. B.: Pulmonary tuberculosis diagnosed by esophageal endoscopic ultrasound with fine-needle aspiration. Int J Tuberc Lung Dis 2004;8:272–273.
11. Fritscher-Ravens, A., Schirrow, L., Pothmann, W., Knofel, W. T, Swain, P., Soehendra, N.: Critical care

transesophageal endosonography and guided fine-needle aspiration for diagnosis and management of posterior mediastinitis. Crit Care Med 2003;31:126–132.
12. Van, D. J., Rice, T. W., Sivak, M. V., Jr.: Endoscopic ultrasonography and endoscopically guided needle aspiration for the diagnosis of upper gastrointestinal tract foregut cysts. Am J Gastroenterol 1992;87:762–765.
13. Geller, A., Wang, K. K., DiMagno, E. P.: Diagnosis of foregut duplication cysts by endoscopic ultrasonography. Gastroenterology 1995;109:838–842.
14. Bhutani, M. S., Hoffman, B. J., Reed, C.: Endosonographic diagnosis of an esophageal duplication cyst. Endoscopy 1996;28:396–397.
15. Faigel, D. O., Burke, A., Ginsberg, G. G., Stotland, B. R., Kadish, S. L., Kochman, M. L.: The role of endoscopic ultrasound in the evaluation and management of foregut duplications. Gastrointest Endosc 1997;45:99–103.
16. Wildi, S. M., Hoda, R. S., Fickling, W., Schmulewitz, N., Varadarajulu, S., Roberts, S. S., Ferguson, B., Hoffman, B. J., Hawes, R. H., Wallace, M. B.: Diagnosis of benign cysts of the mediastinum: the role and risks of EUS and FNA. Gastrointest Endosc 2003;58:362–368.
17. Westerterp, M., van den Berg, J. G., van Lanschot, J. J., Fockens, P.: Intramural bronchogenic cysts mimicking solid tumors. Endoscopy 2004;36:1119–1122.
18. Fazel, A., Moezardalan, K., Varadarajulu, S., Draganov, P., Eloubeidi, M. A.: The utility and the safety of EUS-guided FNA in the evaluation of duplication cysts. Gastrointest Endosc 2005;62:575–580.
19. Eloubeidi, M. A., Cohn, M., Cerfolio, R. J., Chhieng, D. C., Jhala, N., Jhala, D., Eltoum, I. A.: Endoscopic ultrasound-guided fine-needle aspiration in the diagnosis of foregut duplication cysts: the value of demonstrating detached ciliary tufts in cyst fluid. Cancer 2004;102:253–258.
20. Ryan, A. G., Zamvar, V., Roberts, S. A.: Iatrogenic candidal infection of a mediastinal foregut cyst following endoscopic ultrasound-guided fine-needle aspiration. Endoscopy 2002;34:838–839.
21. Wiersema, M. J., Vilmann, P., Giovannini, M., Chang, K. J., Wiersema, L. M.: Endosonography-guided fine-needle aspiration biopsy: diagnostic accuracy and complication assessment. Gastroenterology 1997;112:1087–1095.
22. Annema, J. T., Veselic, M., Versteegh, M. I., Rabe, K. F.: Mediastinitis caused by EUS-FNA of a bronchogenic cyst. Endoscopy 2003;35:791–793.
23. Varadarajulu, S., Fraig, M., Schmulewitz, N., Roberts, S., Wildi, S., Hawes, R. H., Hoffman, B. J., Wallace, M. B.: Comparison of EUS-guided 19-gauge Tru-Cut needle biopsy with EUS-guided fine-needle aspiration. Endoscopy 2004;36:397–401.
24. Wiersema, M. J., Hassig, W. M., Hawes, R. H., Wonn, M. J.: Mediastinal lymph node detection with endosonography. Gastrointest Endosc 1993;39:788–793.
25. Catalano, M. F., Sivak, M. V., Jr., Rice, T., Gragg, L. A., Van Dam, J.: Endosonographic features predictive of lymph node metastasis. Gastrointest Endosc 1994;40:442–446.
26. Bhutani, M. S., Hawes, R. H., Hoffman, B. J.: A comparison of the accuracy of echo features during endoscopic ultrasound (EUS) and EUS-guided fine-needle aspiration for diagnosis of malignant lymph node invasion. Gastrointest Endosc 1997;45:474–479.
27. Savides, T. J., Perricone, A.: Impact of EUS-guided FNA of enlarged mediastinal lymph nodes on subsequent thoracic surgery rates. Gastrointest Endosc 2004;60:340–346.
28. Devereaux, B. M., LeBlanc, J. K., Yousif, E., Kesler, K., Brooks, J., Mathur, P., Sandler, A., Chappo, J., Lehman, G. A., Sherman, S., Gress, F., Ciaccia, D.: Clinical utility of EUS-guided fine-needle aspiration of mediastinal masses in the absence of known pulmonary malignancy. Gastrointest Endosc 2002;56:397–401.
29. DeWitt, J., Ghorai, S., Kahi, C., LeBlanc, J., McHenry, L., Chappo, J., Cramer, H., McGreevy, K., Chriswell, M., Sherman, S.: EUS-FNA of recurrent postoperative extraluminal and metastatic malignancy. Gastrointest Endosc 2003;58:542–548.
30. Kramer, H., Koeter, G. H., Sleijfer, D. T., van Putten, J. W., Groen, H. J.: Endoscopic ultrasound-guided fine-needle aspiration in patients with mediastinal abnormalities and previous extrathoracic malignancy. Eur J Cancer 2004;40:559–562.
31. Hahn, M., Faigel, D. O.: Frequency of mediastinal lymph node metastases in patients undergoing EUS evaluation of pancreaticobiliary masses. Gastrointest Endosc 2001;54:331–335.
32. Will, U., Meyer, F., Bosseckert, H.: Successful endoscopic management of iatrogenic mediastinal infection and subsequent esophagomediastinal fistula, following endosonographically guided fine-needle aspiration biopsy. Endoscopy 2005;37:88–90.
33. Ribeiro, A., Vazquez-Sequeiros, E., Wiersema, L. M., Wang, K. K., Clain, J. E., Wiersema, M. J.: EUS-guided fine-needle aspiration combined with flow cytometry and immunocytochemistry in the diagnosis of lymphoma. Gastrointest Endosc 2001;53:485–491.
34. Hoda, R. S., Picklesimer, L., Green, K. M., Self, S.: Fine-needle aspiration of a primary mediastinal large B-cell lymphoma: a case report with cytologic, histologic, and flow cytometric considerations. Diagn Cytopathol 2005;32:370–373.
35. Mehra, M., Tamhane, A., Eloubeidi, M. A.: EUS-guided FNA combined with flow cytometry in the diagnoses of suspected or recurrent intrathoracic or retroperitoneal lymphoma. Gastrointest Endosc 2005;62:508–513.
36. Noh, K. W., Wallace, M. B.: Can EUS-guided FNA with flow cytometry be used to diagnose lymphoma? Gastrointest Endosc 2005;62:514–516.
37. Storch, I., Jorda, M., Ribeiro, A.: EUS-guided biopsy in the diagnosis of pulmonary lymphoma in a patient with an esophagopulmonary fistula. Gastrointest Endosc 2005;61:904–906.
38. Wiersema, M. J., Vazquez-Sequeiros, E., Wiersema, L. M.: Evaluation of mediastinal lymphadenopathy with endoscopic US-guided fine-needle aspiration biopsy. Radiology 2001;219:252–257.
39. Larsen, S. S., Krasnik, M., Vilmann, P., Jacobsen, G. K., Pedersen, J. H., Faurschou, P., Folke, K.: Endoscopic ultrasound guided biopsy of mediastinal lesions has a major impact on patient management. Thorax 2002;57:98–103.
40. Eloubeidi, M. A., Cerfolio, R. J., Chen, V. K., Desmond, R., Syed, S., Ojha, B.: Endoscopic ultrasound-guided fine needle aspiration of mediastinal lymph node in patients with suspected lung cancer after positron emission tomography and computed tomography scans. Ann Thorac Surg 2005;79:263–268.
41. Pai, K. R., Page, R. D.: Mediastinitis after EUS-guided FNA biopsy of a posterior mediastinal metastatic teratoma. Gastrointest Endosc 2005;62:980–981.

CHAPTER 12

EUS Imaging and FNA of Primary Lung Tumors

Dr. J. T. Annema
Dr. L. Welker
Dr. M. Veseliç
Dr. K. F. Rabe

Introduction

Transesophageal ultrasound-guided fine needle aspiration (EUS-FNA) has been proven to be accurate for the analysis of mediastinal lymph nodes for patients with lung cancer.[1] In addition to mediastinal staging, primary intrapulmonary tumors that are located adjacent to the esophagus can be detected and aspirated by EUS-FNA as well. Besides establishing a tissue diagnosis, EUS can be of additional value in assessing the presence or absence of tumor invasion in the surrounding mediastinal tissue. In this chapter, the role of EUS-FNA will be evaluated for diagnosis and staging of primary lung tumors. Specific emphasis will be applied to the tissue handling and cytopathological evaluation of the fine needle aspirates.

Diagnosis of Primary Lung Tumors by EUS-FNA

In patients with suspected lung cancer, a tissue diagnosis is mandatory for treatment planning. Patients with non-small cell lung cancer (NSCLC) and small cell lung cancer (SCLC) have a different prognosis and vary in their therapeutic approach. Intrapulmonary lesions may also be caused by noncancerous lesions, such as tuberculosis, sarcoidosis, or hamartomas, in addition to lung cancer. In the diagnostic workup of patients with suspected lung cancer, bronchoscopy is the diagnostic method of choice. However, endoscopy fails to establish a diagnosis in up to 30% of cases, often because the intrapulmonary lesion is out of reach of the bronchoscope.[2] As the worldwide incidence of lung cancer is enormous—1.2 million[3] - the need for alternative tissue sampling methods is evident. In the subset of patients in whom the primary lung tumor is located adjacent to the esophagus (Figure 12–1), EUS-FNA might be considered the diagnostic procedure of choice after a nondiagnostic bronchoscopy. Intrapulmonary tumors typically present as a round hypoechoic mass with irregular borders (Figures 12–2, 12–6, 12–11) at ultrasound investigations performed via the esophagus. The irregular shape of the lung mass—caused by compromised lung tissue—is strikingly different from the shape of malignant mediastinal nodes that are commonly round and exhibit well-defined borders (Figure 12–10). Once an intrapulmonary lesion is identified, cells can be aspirated in a similar fashion to that of mediastinal nodes (Figures 12–2, 12–3, 12–4). Because larger masses tend to form central necrosis, clinicians prefer to sample the periphery of the lesion in order to avoid necrotic tissue.

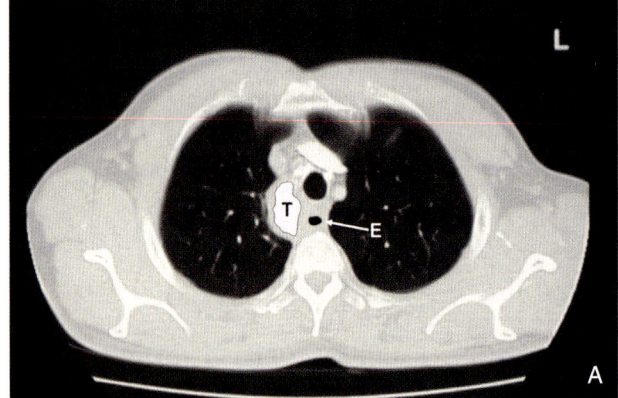
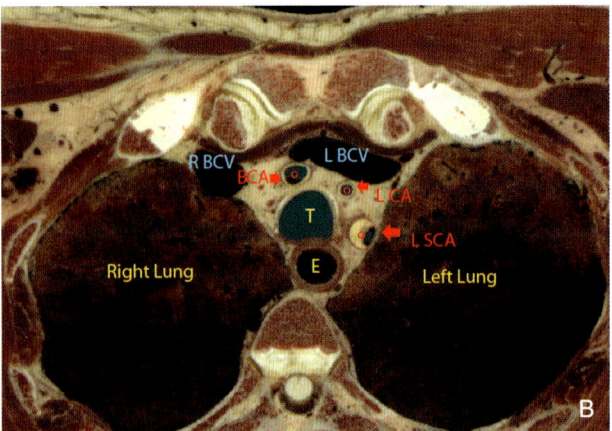

FIGURE 12–1. A and B A 47-year-old smoker presented with cough and fatigue. He had a primary lung tumor in the right lung, and there was no diagnosis after bronchoscopy. (A) Computed tomogram of the chest demonstrating a tumor in the right upper lobe (T) located immediately adjacent to the esophagus (E). (B) Corresponding visible human anatomy. BCA=brachiocephalic artery, L BCV= left brachiocephalic vein, RBCV=right brachiocephalic vein, L CA=left carotid artery, L SCA=Left subclavian artery, E=esophagus, T=trachea

Several studies have addressed the feasibility and yield of EUS-FNA for the analysis of primary intrapulmonary tumors. In a retrospective study of 18 patients with suspected lung cancer and a primary lung tumor located adjacent to the esophagus, all lesions were detected and sampled by EUS-FNA. The following diagnoses were established due to EUS-FNA findings: non-small cell lung cancer (NSCLC) [N=15], small cell lung cancer [n=1], lung metastases from other tumors [N=2].[4] In another study in which EUS-FNA was used for the diagnosis of intrapulmonary tumors following a nondiagnostic bronchoscopy, 32 consecutive patients with an intrapulmonary tumor without enlarged mediastinal nodes were investigated by EUS-FNA. The lung tumors were detected in all

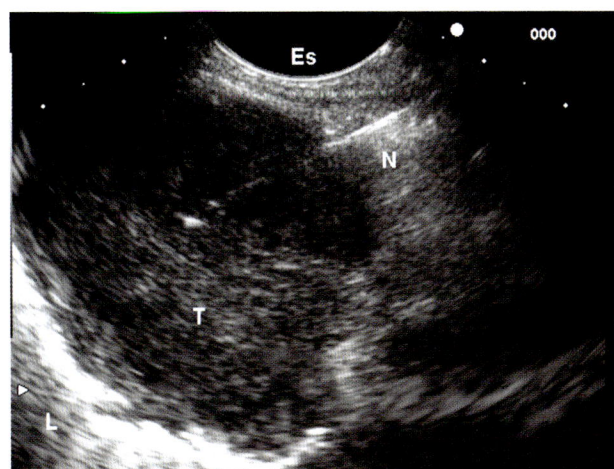

FIGURE 12–2. Corresponding EUS-FNA image demonstrating an irregularly shaped intrapulmonary mass (T) located adjacent to the esophagus. (L = compromised lung tissue, N = needle, Es = position of the linear ultrasound transducer in the esophagus)

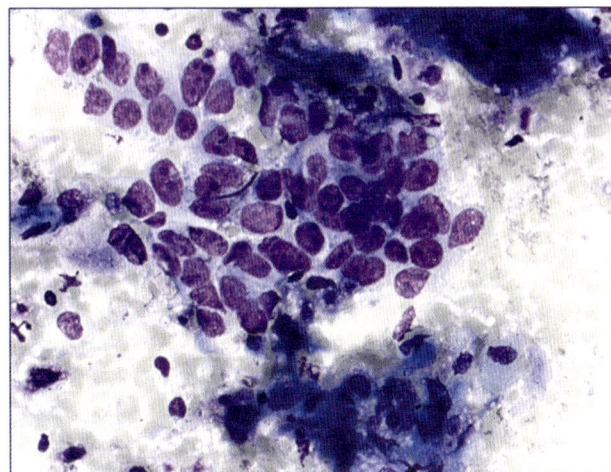

FIGURE 12–3. EUS guided fine needle aspirate of the primary lung tumor showing sheets of squamous cells with nuclear pleomorphism and macro nuclei with dense cytoplasm compatible with the diagnosis squamous cell carcinoma (HE, x 40).

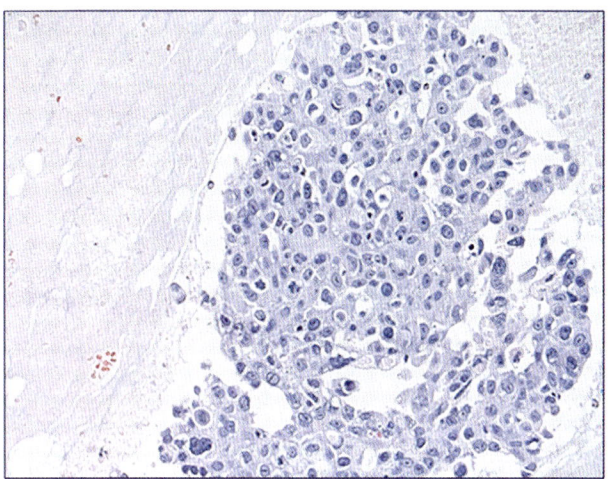

FIGURE 12–4. Corresponding cell block of the fine needle aspirate demonstrating squamous cell carcinoma with distinct intercellular bridges.

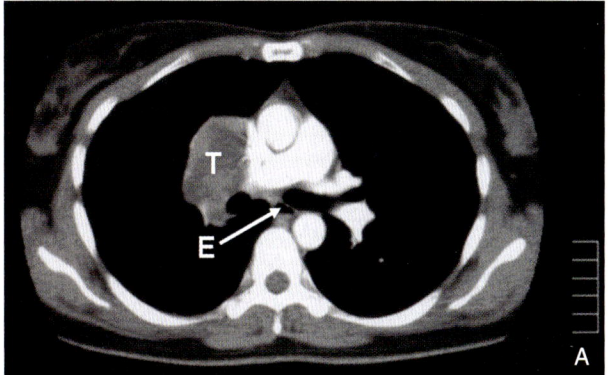

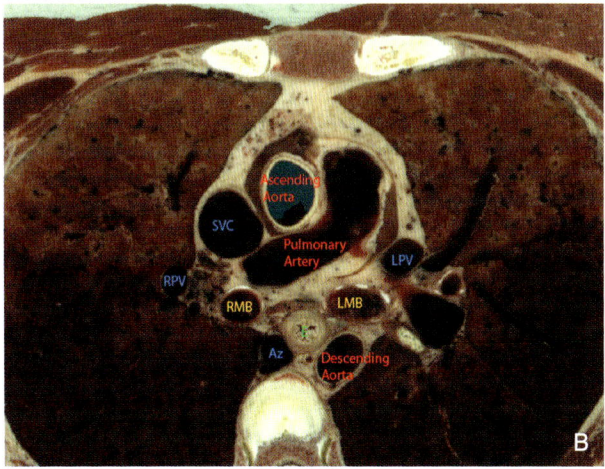

FIGURE 12–5. *A and B* A 40 year old woman with weight loss and a centrally located mass in the right lung. (A) Computed tomography of the chest (CT) demonstrating a centrally located intrapulmonary tumor (T). (E= esophagus). (B) corresponding Visible Human anatomy Az=azygous vein, E=esophagus, LMB =left mainstem bronchus, RMB=right mainstem bronchus, RPV=ascending right pulmonary vein, LPV=ascending left pulmonary vein, SVC=superior vena cava.

patients and the diagnosis NSCLC was established in 31 (97%).[5] In the 11 patients that were eligible for surgical resection of the tumor, EUS-FNA findings were confirmed by surgical-pathological staging in all cases. For one patient, in whom the aspirates were judged not to be representative for the target lesion, pneumonectomy demonstrated an intrapulmonary lymphoma. The aspiration of intrapulmonary tumors directly from the esophagus can theoretically lead to pneumothoraces, haemoptysis, and infection. So far, however, no complications have been recorded.[4,5]

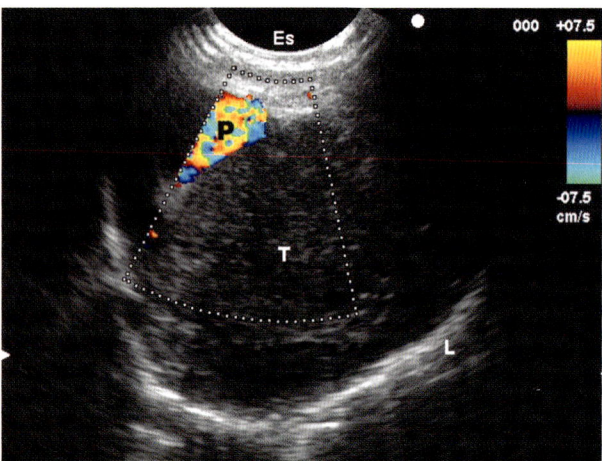

FIGURE 12–6. Corresponding EUS images demonstrating a large intrapulmonary tumor (T). Based on EUS imaging, there was suspicion of tumor invasion (T4) in the pulmonary artery (P). (L= compromised lung tissue, Es = position of the linear ultrasound transducer in the esophagus)

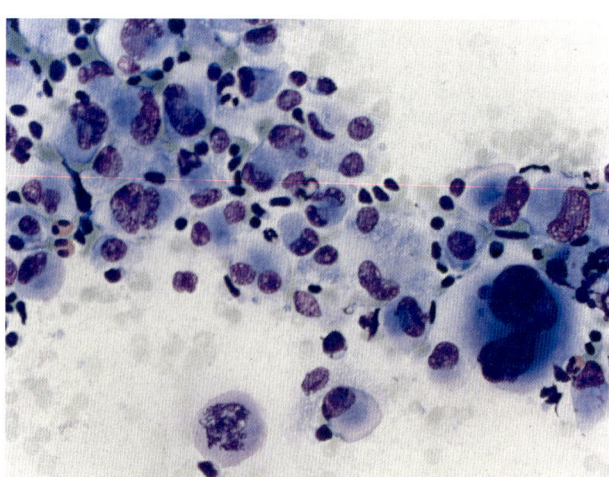

FIGURE 12–7. Corresponding fine needle aspirate showing syncytial groups and single malignant cells with pleomorphic giant cells compatible with the diagnosis giant cell carcinoma (HE, x 40)

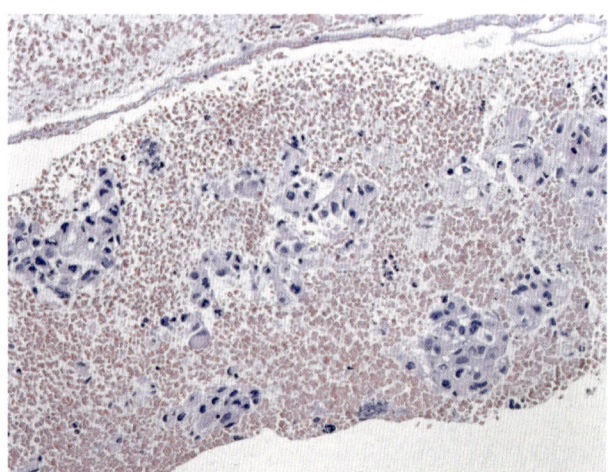

FIGURE 12–8. Corresponding cell block—resembling histology—demonstrating many small tumor fragments (HE, x 20).

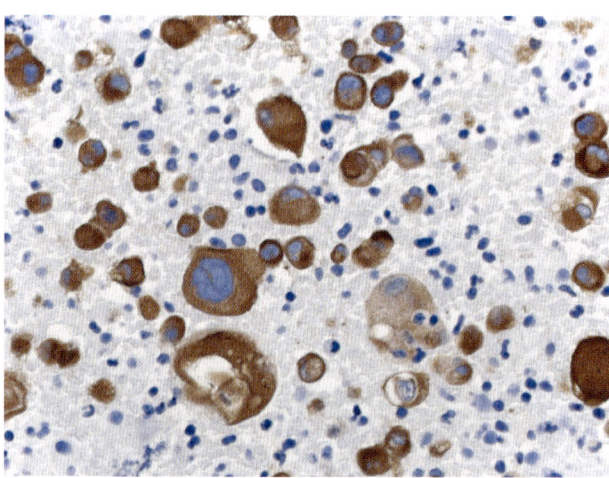

FIGURE 12–9. Keratin staining of the cell block, demonstrating the epithelial nature of the tumor cells.

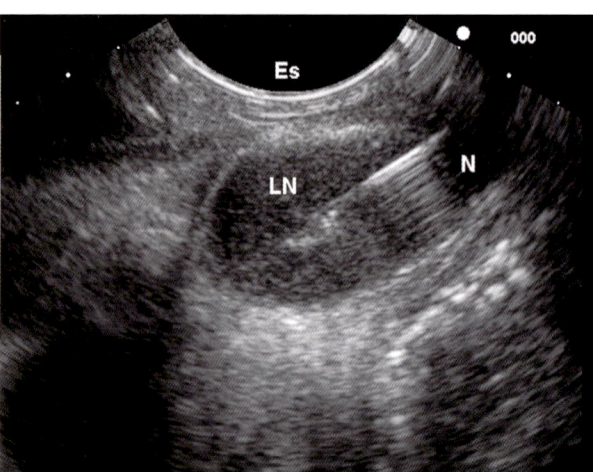

FIGURE 12–10. EUS-FNA of a subcarinal lymph node (LN). (N= Needle, Es = position of the linear ultrasound transducer in the esophagus)

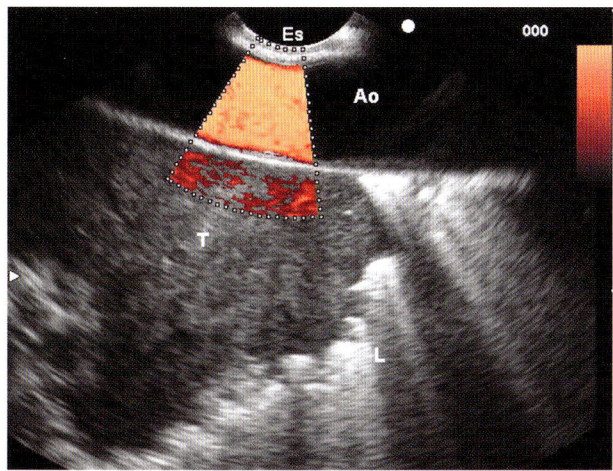

FIGURE 12–11. Tumor (T) in the left upper lobe located adjacent to the aorta (Ao). At EUS, there we no signs of invasion of the tumor (T4) in the lumen of the aorta (no T4). (Es = position of the linear ultrasound transducer in the esophagus)

 Cytopathology of Lung Tumors

Cytopathology is a very useful diagnostic method that enables accurate assessment of lymph nodes and respiratory tract tumors. The main objective of EUS-FNA is to determine the presence of a tumor and classify tumors according to the predominant "histological" type. Of primary importance is the identification of small-cell carcinomas versus no-small-cell neoplasms, as they are treated differently. In experienced hands, the accuracy of cytological diagnosis equals that of histological assessment [Koss L. G., Diagnostic Cytology and histopathologic bases, Philadelphia: Lippincott Williams & Wilkins, 5th edition, 2006, volume 1, chapter 20, p 645].

Tissue Handling

Diagnostic cytological criteria are based on morphologic cell criteria. Optimal smear preparation allows the distribution of well-preserved cells and small tissue fragments on the slide. It is important to prepare a thin and uniform smear. First of all, spraying and squeezing artefacts should be avoided. Another common problem is blood clotting. It distorts the architecture of cell clusters and may obscure microscopic details. Preferably, the endoscopist should examine the aspirated material macroscopically on site before sending it to the cytologist. Part of the aspirate, especially larger fragments and clotted blood particles, should be put into a tissue fixative for cell block preparation. Fixation techniques and smear preparations vary from laboratory to laboratory, but all have in common the reduction of artificial cell changes and producing an optimal cell sample. In many instances, both fixed and unfixed cell samples are required for optimal cytological evaluation. Air-dried samples are stained with haematological stains (May-Grünwald–Giemsa, Diff – Quick), whereas fixed material is commonly stained using the Papaniculaou method.

Cytological Analysis

A cytological preparation obtained by fine needle aspiration may be compared with a puzzle in which the components must be fitted together by the observer to form a familiar picture. While a histological section has essentially a flat, two-dimensional quality, the cytological preparation is often three-dimensional, as it may contain structured fragments of tissues removed entirely from their setting.

One of the most important aspects of cytological interpretation is the comprehensive knowledge of the normal environment of the tissue to be examined. A cytopathologist should be aware of the criteria that differentiate between noncancerous lesions and malignant neoplasms. Special attention should be given to intercellular relationships, such as cell cohesion, cell formation, and cell moulding. Cytological details, such as nuclear size and shape, chromatin, and amount of cytoplasm need to be assessed.

Typical features of specimens collected by direct ultrasound controlled FNA are large numbers of cancer cells and small tissue fragments. Single detached cells usually accompany the tissue fragments. The mere quantitative relationship between the tissue fragments or clusters and single detached cells is in itself a source of important information. A common property of cancer cells is their poor adhesiveness. Consequently, aspirates of malignant tumors often contain large populations of cancer cells selectively removed from the lesion. Thus, rich cellularity of smears and cell dispersion are landmarks of cancer. Aspirates of benign lesions are usually less cellular and contain fewer single cells.

Inadequate needle aspirates, containing large amounts of fibrous material or scanty tissue cellularity, and improper smear preparation may result in false negative EUS-FNA findings. The presence of onsite cytologic evaluation has been advocated to prevent delivery of inadequate material.[6] In contrast, a false-positive diagnosis is generally related to the interpretation of the aspirates. In such cases, a cytologist usually attempts to interpret scant material that contains only few abnormal cells.

Tumor Types

The WHO classification of respiratory tract tumors is used as the reference in describing the various tumor types [Sobin L. H. Histological typing of Lung and pleural tumors, 1999]. Because epithelial malignancies account for the vast majority of malignant lung tumors, they will be discussed in more detail. The main cytological features for smear preparations for the different types of lung cancer are:

Squamous Cell Carcinoma

- Pleomorphic single cells and syncytial sheets of cells with sharp cytoplasmic outlines and irregular cytoplasmic thinning manifested as caudate and spindle cells.
- Nuclei are irregular shaped and centrally located.
- Chromatin is coarsely granular.
- Keratinized squamous ghosts in a background of debris and blood.

Adenocarcinoma

- Large, three-dimensional cell groups, spherical or oval clusters, and acini with single cells.
- Individual cubical or columnar configured tumor cells, with basophilic or vacuolated cytoplasm.
- One or more prominent nuclei are present.
- Nuclei are eccentrically placed.
- Chromatin is finely granular to dusty.

Large-Cell Carcinoma

- Mixture of large, single cells and syncytial groups.
- Large, and round to oval-shaped nuclei
- Chromatin intermediate between squamous carcinoma and adenocarcinoma

Small-Cell Carcinoma

- Cells present in small clusters, clumps, and single cells with intercellular moulding.
- Apoptotic cells and mitotic figures.
- Nuclear moulding and single-file pattern.
- Nuclei vary from round to very irregular with salt-and-pepper chromatin (PAP) staining.
- Background with individual cell necrosis seen as small, dark, pyknotic nuclei.

There are also cytological criteria established for other neuroendocrine tumors (carcinoid tumors and large-cell neuroendocrine carcinoma).

The yield of cytology can be further enhanced by collecting material for cell block analysis. Cell block sections provide the advantage of a micro biopsy (Figures 12–4, 12–8, 12–9) and are highly recommended for examination of any specimen in which tiny tissue fragments are present or if there is residual material available after smears have been prepared [Koss, L. G.: Diagnostic Cytology and histopahologic bases, Philadelphia, Lippincott Williams & Wilkins: Auglage: 5th ed., 2005.]. Cell blocks, however, are not recommended as a substitute for conventional cytological evaluation. Adding cell block to conventional cytological evaluation provides clear advantages because it can disclose complex tissue patterns that may not be evident on smears. Additionally it enables immunohistochemistry evaluation as well as techniques like FISH[7] that can be helpful in differentiation between various tumor types (Figure 12–9) and therefore may prevent further diagnostic procedures.

Detection of Tumor Invasion by EUS

Once a primary lung tumor is detected by EUS, the relation between the tumor and the surrounding mediastinal tissues can be assessed. For staging purposes, it is important to asses whether the primary tumor invades mediastinal organs—such as the heart, large vessels and mediastinum—because those tumors are staged T4[8] and generally not treated by surgical resection.[9] Of the current imaging modalities, computed tomography (CT) has limited value[10] and positron emission tomography (PET) has no value[11] for the assessment of tumor invasion.

In those cases in which the primary tumor is situated immediately adjacent to vascular structures—such as the aorta (Figure 12–11), pulmonary artery (Figures 12–5, 12–6), azygos vene, and left atrium–the differences between the anechoic (blood) vessels and hypoechoic tumor are often great. Due to these ultrasound contrasts, an assessment can often be made regarding the presence (Figure 12–6) or absence (Figure 12–11) of tumor invasion. In a large staging study in 97 patients with a lung tumor located immediately adjacent to the aorta, EUS had an accuracy of 92% in assessing aortic tumor invasion. Importantly, surgical-pathological verification was available in all patients.[12] Assessing tumor invasion in the mediastinum is often difficult, due to the lack of ultrasound contrast between tumor and mediastinum (Figure 12–6). One study reported that EUS had a sensitivity of 88%, specificity of 98%, and positive predictive value of 70% for detecting tumor invasion.[13] The 30% false positive cases are worrying, because in these patients a potentially curative surgical resection of the tumor would be denied. In a prospective lung cancer staging study, the sensitivity, specificity, positive predictive value, negative predictive value, and accuracy of EUS and CT for tumor invasion were 44%, 100%, 100%, 88%, 89% and 38%,

88%, 38%, 88% and 79% respectively.[14] Due to the limited and conflicting data available, the definitive value of EUS in T4 staging requires further investigation. Whether EUS has a role in the assessment of mediastinal tumor invasion after induction chemotherapy also needs further exploration.

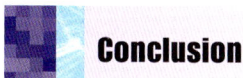

Conclusion

In patients with suspected lung cancer in which the lung mass is located adjacent the esophagus, EUS-FNA should be considered as a safe and minimally invasive method to establish a diagnosis. In addition to tissue sampling, an assessment regarding the presence or absence of tumor invasion in mediastinal structures (stage T4) can be made in selected cases. Adequate communication between respiratory physician, endosonographist, and cytopathologist regarding clinical information and tissue handling is a prerequisite for obtaining optimal results.

References

1. Annema, J. T., Rabe, K. F.: State of the art lecture: EUS and EBUS in pulmonary medicine. Endoscopy 2006; 38 Suppl 1:S118–S122.
2. Mazzone P., Jain, P., Arroliga, A.C., Matthay, R.A.: Bronchoscopy and needle biopsy techniques for diagnosis and staging of lung cancer. Clin Chest Med 2002; 23(1):137-58, ix.
3. Parkin, D.M.: Global cancer statistics in the year 2000. Lancet Oncol 2001;2(9):533–543.
4. Varadarajulu, S., Hoffman, B. J., Hawes, R.H., Eloubeidi, M. A.: EUS-guided FNA of lung masses adjacent to or abutting the esophagus after unrevealing CT-guided biopsy or bronchoscopy. Gastrointest Endosc 2004; 60(2):293–297.
5. Annema, J. T., Veselic, M., Rabe, K.F.: EUS-guided FNA of centrally located lung tumors following a nondiagnostic bronchoscopy. Lung Cancer 2005;48(3): 357–361.
6. Tourno,y K.G., Praet, M.M., Van Maele, G., van Meerbeeck, J.P.: Esophageal endoscopic ultrasound with fine-needle aspiration with an on-site cytopathologist: high accuracy for the diagnosis of mediastinal lymphadenopathy. Chest 2005; 128(4):3004–3009.
7. Karnauchow, P. N., Bonin, R. E:. "Cell-block" technique for fine needle aspiration biopsy. J Clin Pathol 1982; 35(6):688.
8. Mountain, C. F., Dresler, C. M.: Regional lymph node classification for lung cancer staging. Chest 1997; 111(6):1718–1723.
9. Martini, N., Yellin, A., Ginsberg, R. J., Bains, M. S., Burt, M. E., McCormack, P.M., et al.: Management of non-small cell lung cancer with direct mediastinal involvement. Ann Thorac Surg 1994;58(5):1447–1451.
10. Gdeedo, A., Van Schil, P., Corthouts, B., Van Mieghem, F., Van Meerbeeck, J., Van Marck, E.: Comparison of imaging TNM [(i)TNM] and pathological TNM [pTNM] in staging of bronchogenic carcinoma. Eur J Cardiothorac Surg 1997;12(2):224–227.
11. Pieterman, R. M., van Putten, J.W., Meuzelaar ,J. J., Mooyaart, E. L., Vaalburg, W., Koeter, G. H. et al.: Preoperative staging of non-small-cell lung cancer with positron-emission tomography. N Engl J Med 2000 Jul 27;343 (4):254 -61 2000; 343:254–261.
12. Schrode,r C., Schonhofer, .B, Vogel, B.: Transesophageal echographic determination of aortic invasion by lung cancer. Chest 2005;127(2):438–442.
13. Varadarajulu, S., Schmulewitz, N., Wildi, S. F., Roberts, S., Ravenel. J., Reed. C. E. et al.: Accuracy of EUS in staging of T4 lung cancer. Gastrointest Endosc 2004; 59(3):345–348.
14. Annema, J. T., Versteegh, M. I., Veselic, M., Welker, L., Mauad, T., Sont, J. K. et al.: Endoscopic ultrasound added to mediastinoscopy for preoperative staging of patients with lung cancer. JAMA 2005;294(8):931–936.

CHAPTER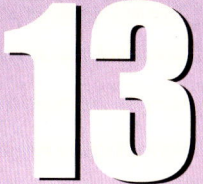

Transbronchial Ultrasound

Dr. Shivakumar Vignesh
Dr. Brad Vincent
Dr. Gerard A. Silvestri
Dr. Brenda Hoffman

Background

The treatment of non-small-cell lung cancer (NSCLC) is dictated by the presence or absence of metastatic disease at the time of diagnosis. For stages I and II of the disease, surgical resection may be curative with five-year survival rates at approximately 70–80%.[63] The survival rate decreases considerably once metastases to regional (hilar and mediastinal) lymph nodes are present. Mediastinal lymph node metastases are discovered in 26–44% of newly diagnosed NSCLC, and patients with multiple-level mediastinal nodal involvement have a very poor prognosis with five-year survival rates of 5–17%.[2,3,4,6,9–15] Currently the mainstay of therapy for patients with ipsilateral and/or contralateral mediastinal nodal metastases is platinum-based chemotherapy with or without thoracic irradiation. Patients in stage IIIA of the disease may be treated surgically following neoadjuvant chemotherapy, but this approach has not yet been proven to be of benefit and is currently being investigated.[7,8,16–19] Nevertheless, mediastinal lymph node staging* remains a vital step in the comprehensive evaluation of NSCLC. Current methods of mediastinal lymph node staging include noninvasive radiologic methods and invasive sampling of nodal tissue.

Noninvasive Staging Modalities

Noninvasive assessment of the mediastinal lymph nodes usually begins with computed tomography (CT). CT can localize enlarged lymph nodes, but it is an unreliable predictor of metastatic nodal involvement, with an unacceptably high false-negative rate of 17–20%, false-positive rate of 32–44%,[10,45] probability toward interobserver variability.[10] CT has a sensitivity, specificity, and overall accuracy of 57–79%, 78–82%, and 58–80%, respectively.[10,25] 18-Fluoro-Deoxyglucose positron emission tomography (FDG-PET) measures the metabolic activity of tissue. A standard uptake value (SUV) is assigned to the corresponding digital image, based on the intensity of metabolic activity. FDG-PET has become a valuable tool in the staging of NSCLC, especially in the detection of extrathoracic metastases.[10,25-28,36,38,39,40-44] Benign disease processes, such as infection or inflammation, however, may also show increased metabolic uptake. The false-positive rate of FDG-PET ranges from 11 to 21% when compared to pathologically obtained tissue[10,25-28,36,38,39,40-44] though simultaneous-acquisition FDG-PET/CT imaging has been shown to be superior to either modality alone.[99] Ultimately, FDG-PET has not been shown to reduce the need for pathologic lymph node examination.[45]

Inaccurate staging may lead to inappropriate therapy resulting in increased mortality, morbidity, and cost of care.[40] Proper staging requires tissue sampling of radiologically abnormal and, perhaps even radiologically normal mediastinal nodes.[75] Current guidelines[45,46] recommend that patients with abnormal mediastinal nodes, with suspected or proven NSCLC, should undergo tissue sampling before undergoing surgical interventions.

Invasive Staging Modalities

Invasive staging of mediastinal lymph nodes should be performed on any patient with NSCLC and a radiologically abnormal mediastinum and, perhaps even on patients with a radiologically normal mediastinum.[9,22,29,30,46,48] Invasive lymph node sampling can be performed in a number of ways.

Mediastinoscopy is considered the gold standard and has a high sensitivity and specificity with a low complication rate.[5,9,21-23,29,30] Access to the posterior and inferior mediastinum requires either extended cervical mediastinoscopy or thoracoscopy, neither of which is commonly performed. Practice patterns are highly variable with only 40% of mediastinoscopies conforming to "gold standard" techniques in one large study [98]. In another large study in the United States, mediastinoscopy was performed in only in about 25% of surgical candidates with diagnostic lymphoid tissue being obtained in only one-third of those patients.[70] Mediastinoscopy requires general anesthesia, but is generally safe with associated morbidity of 1-2% and mortality of 0.3%.[48]

CT-guided transthoracic needle aspiration (TTNA) of hilar and mediastinal lymph nodes has been described[1] but requires specialized training and is not widely used. It can result in pneumothorax, bleeding, recurrent laryngeal nerve injury, and arrhythmias.[30]

Blind transbronchial needle aspiration (TBNA) is an underutilized bronchoscopic modality in which a 19- or 21-gauge needle is used to biopsy accessible lymph nodes.[24,38] Because the target cannot be visualized in real-time with blind TBNA, aspiration is directed by knowledge of thoracic anatomy and prior imaging, usually CT. The overall sensitivity of TBNA ranges from 72% to 79%, and the specificity ranges from 91% to 100%, with a false-negative rate of up to 30%, and NPV ranges from 36 to 100%.[9,30] The

---

*In this chapter mediastinal staging refers only to non-small-cell lung cancer (NSCLC)

diagnostic yield ranges from 15% to more than 85%,[30,64] but yield increases at the right paratracheal and subcarinal lymph node stations.[9,50-54] In general the diagnostic yield of TBNA varies depending on lymph node size, location, and the operator's experience[30] but is still poor when compared to mediastinoscopy.[9] TBNA is underutilized for a number of reasons, including lack of proper training, fear of damage to mediastinal structures, and poor yield being commonly cited.[30,50-54] CT fluoroscopy guidance has been added to blind TBNA with little-to-no improvement in diagnostic yield.[21,55,56]

Endoscopes equipped with curved linear array ultrasound probes allow localization of the lymph node and visualization of needle aspiration on a real-time basis, thus providing safe and accurate transesophageal mediastinal nodal sampling. Figure 13–1 shows some of the anatomy of this region, and the relation of the esophagus to the trachea, the bronchopulmonary nodes, and the aorta. Endoscopic ultrasound guided with fine needle aspiration (EUS-FNA) is able to access the posterior mediastinum, including the left paratracheal nodes (2L, 4L) and stations 7, 8 and 9, but right paratracheal nodes (2R, 4R) and the pretracheal space are generally not accessible with this modality. (Figure 13–2);[22,23,31-34,47] [Chapter 11]. Not all aortopulmonary window or paraaortic lymph nodes can by safely sampled with EUS-FNA because of the interposition of the pulmonary artery and aorta. The utility, safety, and accuracy of EUS-FNA for mediastinal staging is well established[10,30-34,80,82-94] and it may obviate the need for mediastinoscopy or thoracotomy.[92,93,97]

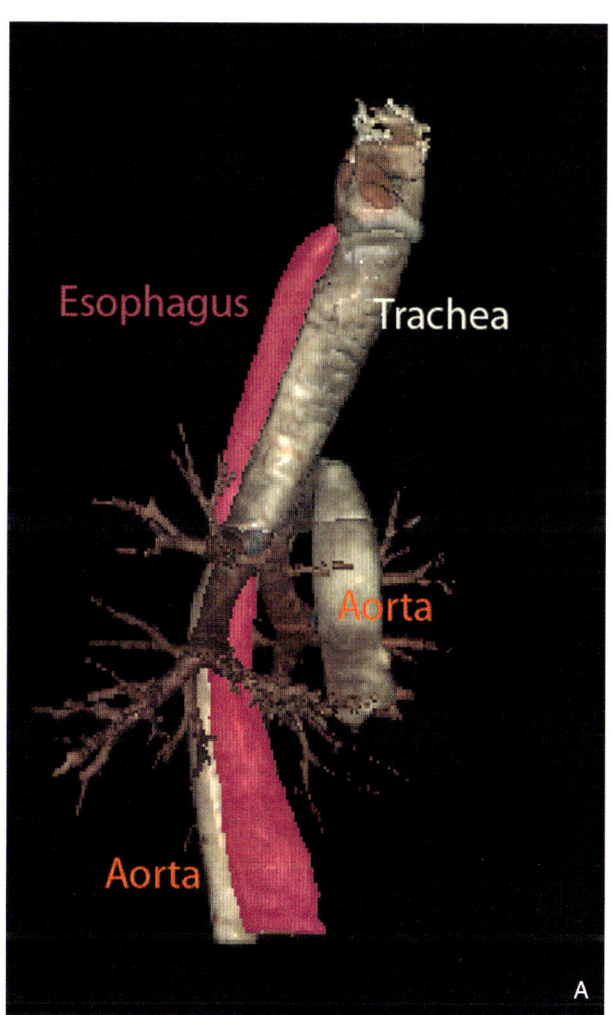 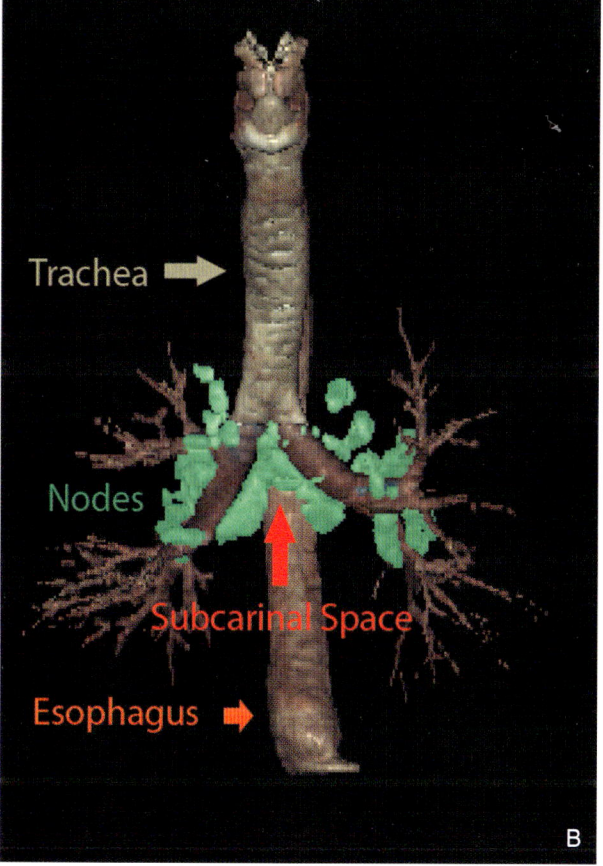

FIGURE 13–1. *A and B* Visible Human Anatomy from the TolTech dissector showing the relation of various mediastinal structures. (A) Esophagus, bronchial tree, and the aorta. (B) Anterior view showing trachea, esophagus, nodes, and subcarinal space.

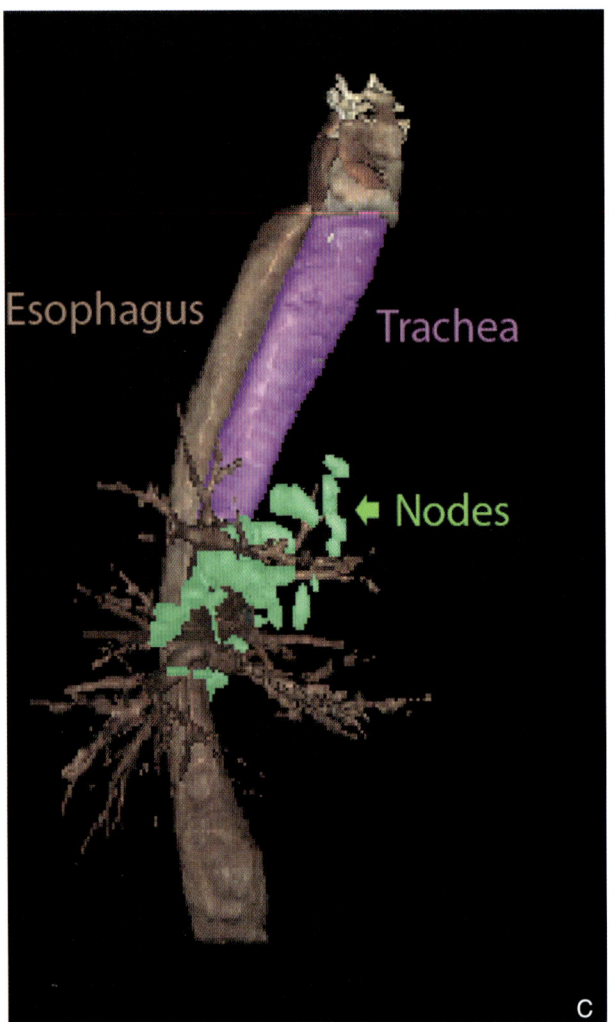
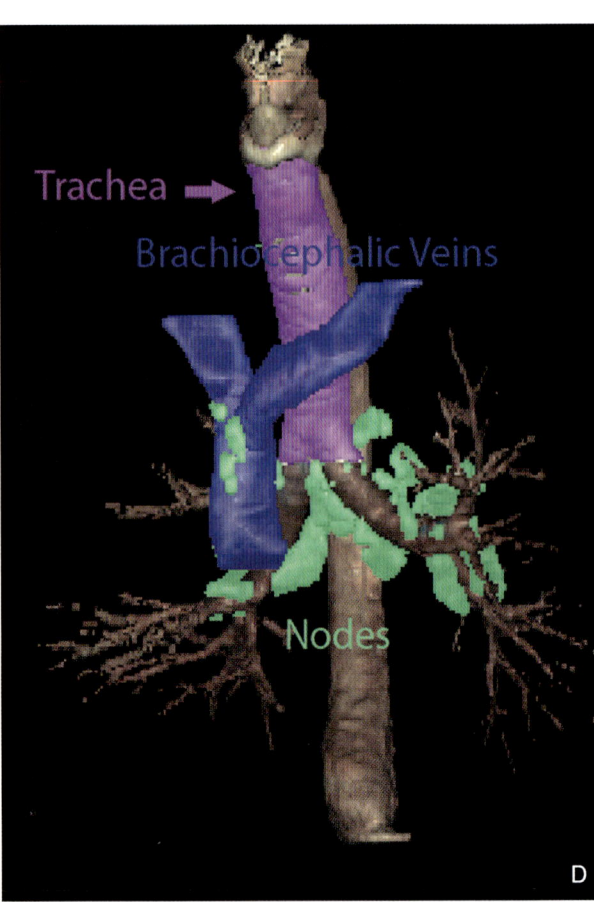

FIGURE 13–1. *C and D* (C) Lateral view showing trachea, nodes, and esophagus (D) Includes brachiocephalic vein and superior vena cava.

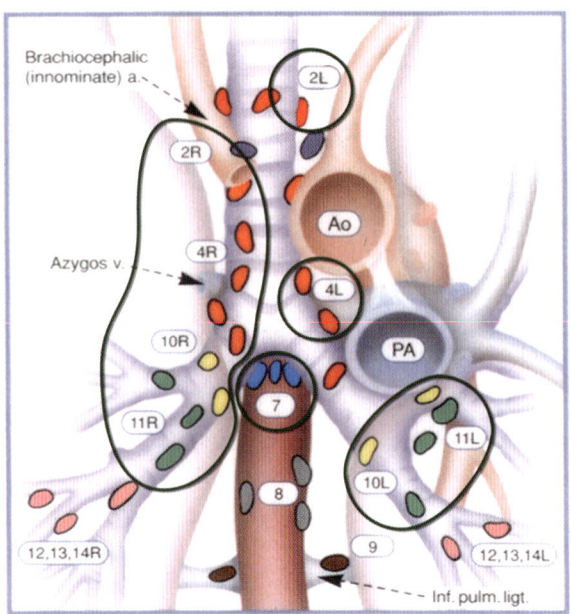

FIGURE 13–2. Mediastinal lymph node stations and access of endobronchial ultrasound (EBUS)

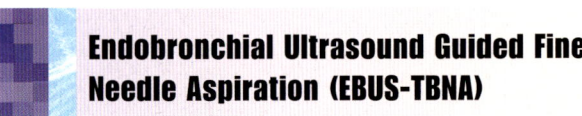

Endobronchial Ultrasound Guided Fine Needle Aspiration (EBUS-TBNA)

Borrowing upon the technology used in EUS-FNA, recently curvilinear array ultrasound has also been added to the videobronchoscope. The instrument has an outer diameter of 6.9 mm, a 2.0-mm instrument channel, and 30° oblique forward-viewing optics. An electronic convex array ultrasound transducer is mounted at the distal tip and is covered by a water-inflatable balloon sheath. Scanning is performed at a frequency of 7.5 MHz, and the angle of view is 90°,[64,65] [Figure 13–3]. The needle exits the outer covering of the insertion tube at 20° and has a stylet, which is withdrawn after passing the bronchial wall, avoiding contamination during TBNA.[65]; [Figure 13–4]. The transbronchial passage of the needle is visualized in real-time. Color-power Doppler ultrasound is available to evaluate vascular structures.

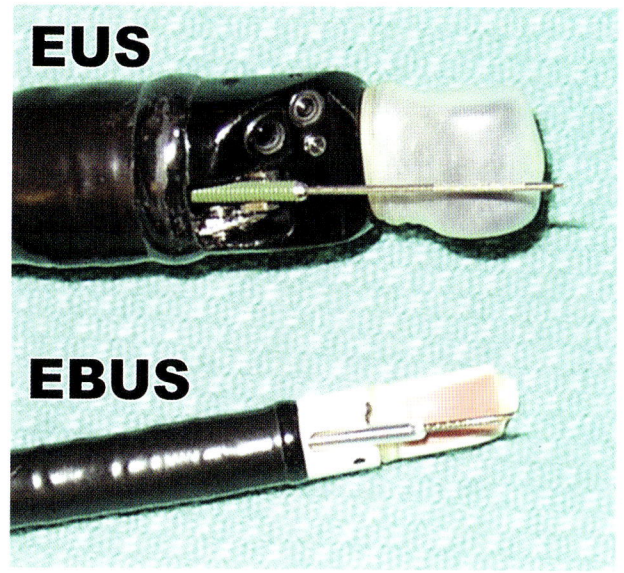

FIGURE 13-3. Endobronchial Ultrasound (EBUS) and Endoscopic ultrasound (EUS) echoendoscopes

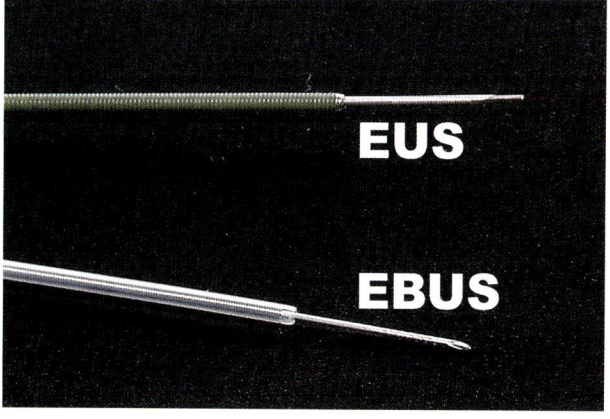

FIGURE 13-4. Aspiration needles used for EUS and EBUS

Mediastinal nodal staging in known or suspected NSCLC, undiagnosed intrathoracic lymphadenopathy, and diagnosis of intrapulmonary tumors located adjacent to the main bronchi are the indications for EBUS-TBNA.[35,59-62] As shown in the digital human anatomy in Figure 13–1, the trachea and bronchi are surrounded by the bronchopulmonary lymph nodes making access via the trachea a relatively straight forward process. In a large, randomized trial, EBUS-TBNA significantly increased the diagnostic yield at all nodal stations except the subcarinal (84% versus 58%) when compared with conventional TBNA.[66] EBUS-TBNA is a highly accurate and safe method for sampling mediastinal lymph nodes[22,35-37,57,58,66,75] and can access stations 1,2R, 2L, 3, 4R, 4L, 7, 10R, 10L, 11R, 11L and 12 (Figures 13–2 and 13–5–13–11). In addition to being able to access all mediastinal nodal stations within reach of standard mediastinoscopy, EBUS-TBNA has the advantage of also being able to routinely access posterior mediastinal (Station 7; Figure 13–11) and hilar lymph nodes (levels 10 and 11; Figures 13–8, 13–9, 13–10).[58,66] EBUS-TBNA can be done as an outpatient procedure with conscious sedation and may be a minimally invasive alternative to mediastinoscopy.

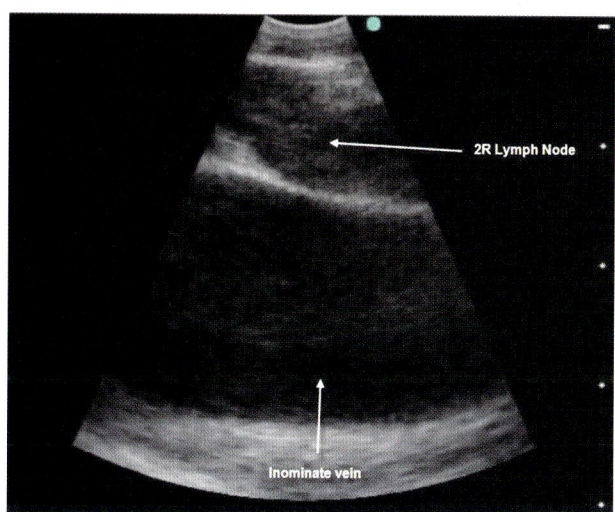

FIGURE 13-5. Right upper paratracheal nodes (2R) located between intersection of caudal margin of innominate vein with trachea and the apex of the lung (supra-innominate nodes)

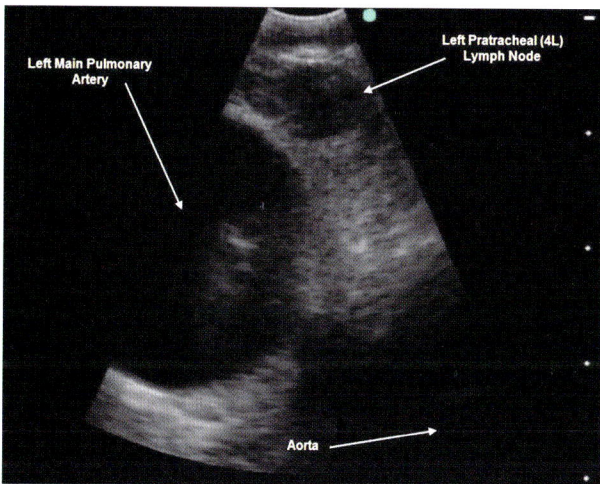

FIGURE 13-6. Left lower paratracheal nodes (4L) located between top of aortic arch and carina (medial to ligamentum arteriosum)

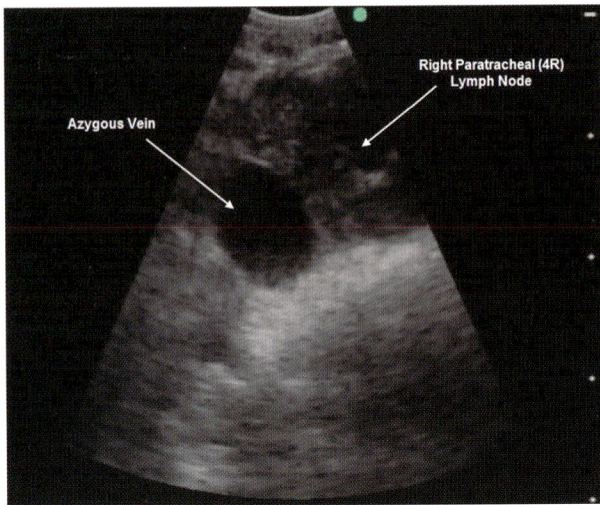

FIGURE 13–7. Right lower paratracheal nodes (4R) located between insertion of caudal margin of innomniate vein with trachea and cephalic border of azygos vein

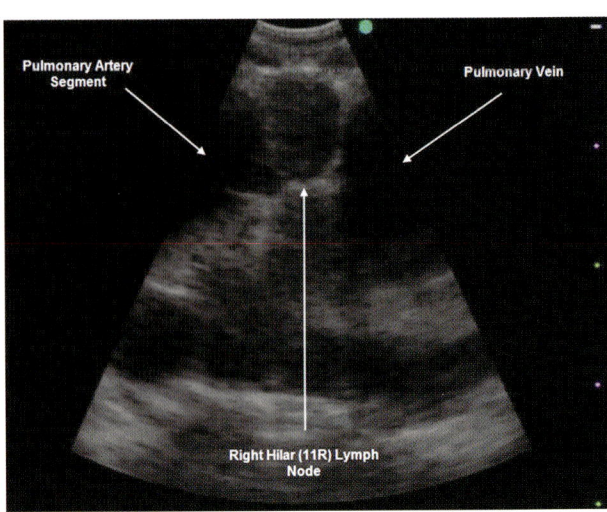

FIGURE 13–10. Right Interlobar (11R)

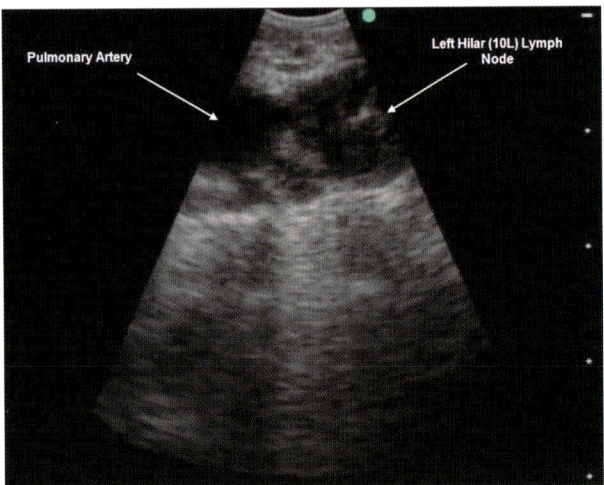

FIGURE 13–8. Left tracheobronchial angle nodes or Left Hilar (10L)

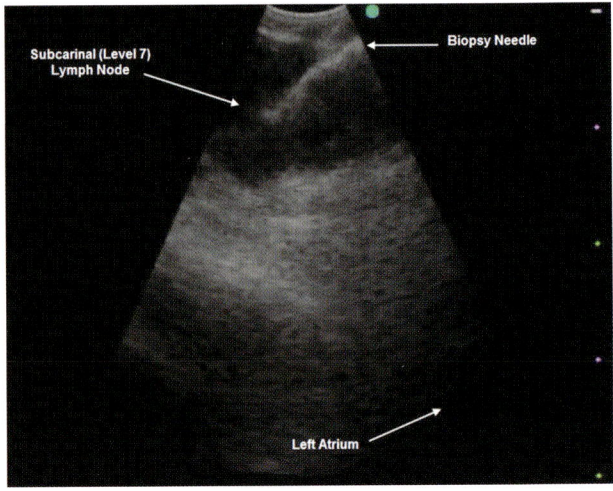

FIGURE 13–11. Subcarinal (7) located caudal to the carina of the trachea

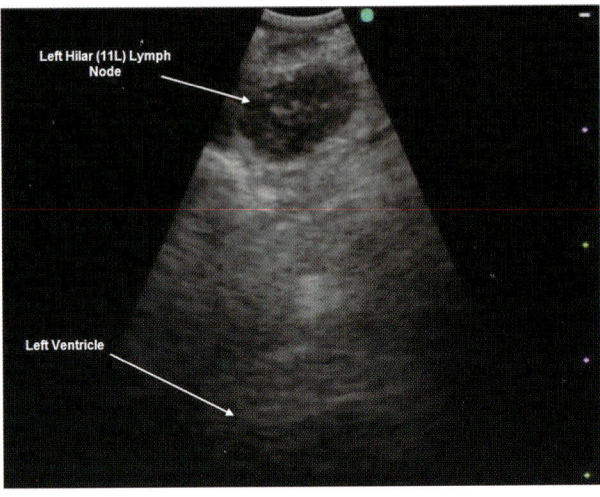

FIGURE 13–9. Left interlobar (11L)

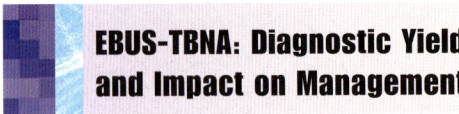

EBUS-TBNA: Diagnostic Yield and Impact on Management

The sensitivity, specificity, and accuracy of EBUS-TBNA for mediastinal staging in patients with NSCLC are 94%, 100%, and 95% respectively.[72-75] Rapid onsite cytopathology (ROSE) in conjunction with EBUS-TBNA can increase diagnostic yield[86]; [Figure 13–12] and shorten procedure times.[86] In several studies, EBUS-TBNA has been shown to decrease surgical interventions including mediastinoscopies, and thoracotomies.[73,74] In the largest published series of EBUS-TBNA (n=502), the range of lymph nodes

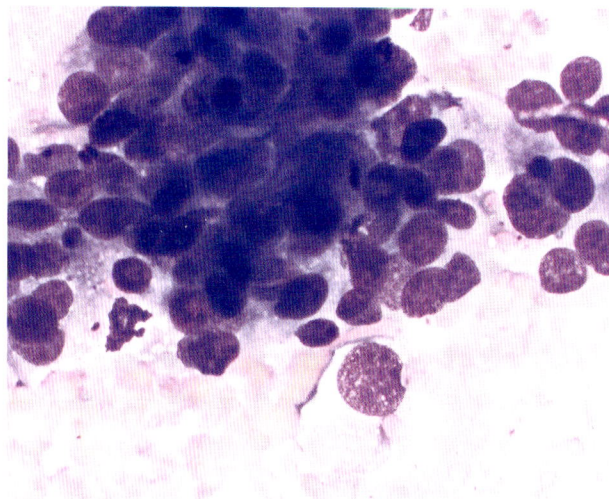

FIGURE 13–12. Cytology from EBUS-TBNA showing metastatic adenocarcinoma in left hilar node (10L)

accessed included levels 2R, 2L, 3, 4R, 4L, 7, 10R, 10L, 11R and 11L. Adequate specimen (lymphocytes present) was obtained in 94.5% of cases, and the diagnosis was established in 93.5% of cases.[74] Some of these lymph node stations (10L, 10L, 11R, 11L) are inaccessible by any other modality. One criticism of minimally invasive techniques (blind TBNA, EUS-FNA or EBUS-TBNA) is that the patients who undergo these procedures have bulky disease, while those who undergo mediastinoscopy have either single-station nodal disease or no obvious disease radiographically. However, in 100 patients scheduled for surgery with a normal mediastinum on CT, EBUS-TBNA had a sensitivity of 92%, a specificity of 100%, and a negative predictive value of 96.3%—with surgical confirmation in 119 sampled lymph nodes. Cancer was found in lymph nodes of 1 of every 6 patients.[75] These findings compare favorably to mediastinoscopy.

Mortality related to EBUS-TBNA has not been reported. Pneumothorax, pneumomediastinum, hemomediastinum, bacteremia, and pericarditis are known but rare complications of blind TBNA.[21,24,30,50–54]

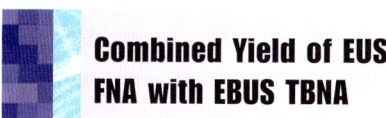

Combined Yield of EUS FNA with EBUS TBNA

EBUS-TBNA may be combined with EUS-FNA in the same procedural setting with synergistic effects.[22,37] The combination of EBUS-TBNA with EUS-FNA makes it possible to examine the upper mediastinal, hilar, and posterior-inferior lymph node stations. The only mediastinal nodal groups that are not routinely accessible to either approach are station 5 (aortopulmonary window lateral to the ligamentum arteriosum) and station 6 (para-aortic). The yield of EBUS-TBNA seems comparable to EUS-FNA.[80,82,95] In one study, EUS-FNA and EBUS-TBNA were compared in 33 patients (119 lesions sampled by either EUS-FNA or EBUS-TBNA), for mediastinal staging in patients with known or suspected NSCLC. Eleven additional cancer diagnoses and three samples with cells suspicious for carcinoma were obtained by EBUS-TBNA that had not been obtained by EUS-FNA. Conversely, EUS-FNA established twelve additional cancer diagnoses, one instance of suspicion for carcinoma, and one case of sarcoidosis compared to patients who had undergone EBUS-TBNA. The combined accuracy of EUS-FNA and EBUS-TBNA for mediastinal nodal involvement was 100%.[79]

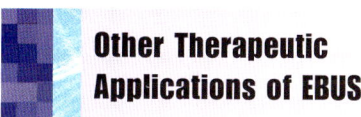

Other Therapeutic Applications of EBUS

EBUS may also have therapeutic airway applications. In one study, including tumor debridement with Neodymium: yttrium aluminum garnet (Nd: YAG), laser and argon plasma coagulation, brachytherapy, foreign body removal, and airway stent placement, EBUS was also used successfully in endoscopic drainage of abscesses and had a low overall complication rate. [96]

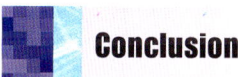

Conclusion

EBUS-TBNA is a safe, accurate, and minimally invasive method for mediastinal staging and diagnosis of mediastinal lesions. EBUS-TBNA and EUS-FNA can also complement each other in terms of diagnostic reach. The combination of these two similar techniques complement and may potentially replace more invasive and costly procedures, including mediastinoscopy. These techniques have certain advantages over mediastinoscopy, not the least of which is the breadth and scope of accessible lymph nodes.

The staging algorithm of the future could include radiologic evaluation, such as FDG-PET and CT, as well as routinely performed EBUS TBNA with or without EUS FNA. Mediastinoscopy might only be necessary in situations where other staging studies are either unsuccessful or when additional tissue is needed for histological or molecular confirmation.

References

1. Zwischenberger, J. B., Savage, C., Alpard, S. K., Anderson, C. M., Marroquin, S., Goodacre, B. W.: Mediastinal Transthoracic Needle and Core Lymph Node Biopsy: Should it Replace Mediastinoscopy? Chest 2002;121:1165-1170
2. Dillemans, B., Deneffe, G., Verschakelen, J., Decramer, M.: Value of computed tomography and mediastinoscopy in preoperative evaluation of mediastinal nodes in non-small cell lung cancer. A study of 569 patients. E J Cardiothoracic Surg 1994;8:37–42.
3. Gross, B. H., Glazer, G. M., Orringer, M. B., Spizarny, D. L., Flint, A.: Bronchogenic carcinoma metastatic to normal-sized lymph nodes: frequency and significance. Radiology 1988;166:71–74.
4. McLoud, T. C., Bourgouin, P. M., Greenberg, R. W., et al.: Bronchogenic carcinoma: analysis of staging in the mediastinum with CT by correlative lymph node mapping and sampling. Radiology 1992;182:319–323.
5. Sihoe, A. D., Yim, A. P.: Lung cancer staging. J Surg Res 2004;117:92–106.
6. Spira, A., Ettinger, D. S.: Multidisciplinary management of lung cancer. N Engl J Med 2004;350:379–92.
7. Albain, K. S.:.Induction chemotherapy or chemoradiotherapy before surgery for non-small-cell lung cancer. Curr Oncol Rep. 2000 Jan;2(1):54–63.
8. Albain K. S.: Induction chemotherapy with/without radiation followed by surgery in stage III non-small-cell lung cancer. Oncology (Williston Park). 1997 Sep;11(9 Suppl 9):51-7.
9. Toloza, E. M., Harpole, L., Detterbeck, F., McCrory, D. C.: Invasive staging of non-small-cell lung cancer: a review of the current evidence. Chest 2003; 123: Suppl. 1, 157S–166S
10. Toloza, E. M., Harpole, L., McCrory, D. C.: Noninvasive staging of non-small-cell lung cancer: a review of the current evidence. Chest 2003;123: Suppl. 1, 137S–146S.
11. Watanabe, Y., Hayashi, Y., Shimizu, J., Oda, M., and Iwa, T.: Mediastinal nodal involvement and the prognosis of non-small cell lung cancer Chest, Vol 100, 422-428
12. Peter Goldstraw, FRCS, Gopi C. Mannam, FRCSEd, FRCS(Glas), David K. Kaplan, FRCS, CT, Panos Michail, MDSurgical management of non-small-cell lung cancer with ipsilateral mediastinal node metastasis (N2 disease) Thorac Cardiovasc Surg 1994;107:19-28.
13. Naruke, T., Suemasu, K., and Ishikawa, S.: Lymph node mapping and curability at various levels of metastasis in resected lung cancer The Journal of Thoracic and Cardiovascular Surgery, Vol 76, 832–839.
14. Vansteenkiste, J. F., De Leyn, P. R., Deneffe, G. J., et al.: Survival and Prognostic Factors in Resected N2 Non–Small Cell Lung Cancer: A Study of 140 Cases Ann Thorac Surg 1997;63:1441–1450.
15. Andre, F., Grunenwald, D., Pignon, J. P., Dujon, A., Pujol, J. L., et al: Survival of patients with resected N2 non-small-cell lung cancer: evidence for a subclassification and implications. J Clin Oncol. 2000 Aug;18(16):2981–9.
16. Depierre, A., Milleron, B., Moro-Sibilot, D., et al. : Preoperative chemotherapy followed by surgery compared with primary surgery in resectable stage I, II, and IIIa non-small-cell lung cancer. J Clin Oncol 2002;20:247–53
17. Fossella, F. V., Rivera, E., Roth, J. A.: Preoperative chemotherapy for stage IIIa non-small-cell lung cancer. Curr Opin Oncol 1996;8:106 –11.
18. Zatopek, N. K., Holoye, P. Y., Ellerbroek, N. A., et al.: Resectability of small-cell lung cancer following induction chemotherapy in patients with limited disease (stage II-IIIb). Am J Clin Oncol 1991;14:427–32.
19. Mountain, C. F.: Revisions in the international system for staging lung cancer. Chest 1997;111:1710–7.
20. Mountain, C. F., Dresler, C. M.: Regional lymph node classification for lung cancer staging. Chest 1997;111:1718–23
21. Garpestad, E., Goldberg, S., Herth, F., et al.: CT fluoroscopy guidance for transbronchial needle aspiration: an experience in 35 patients. Chest 2001;119:329–32.
22. Silvestri, G. A., Hoffman, B., Reed, C. E.: One From Column A: Choosing Between CT, Positron Emission Tomography, Endoscopic Ultrasound with Fine-Needle Aspiration, Transbronchial Needle Aspiration, Thoracoscopy, Mediastinoscopy and Mediastinotomy for Staging Lung Cancer. Chest 2003; 123: 333–335
23. Jacobson, B. C., Hirota, W. K., Goldstein, J. L., et al.: The role of EUS for evaluation of mediastinal adenopathy. Gastrointest Endoscopy 2003;58:819–821.
24. Harrow, E. M., Abi-Saleh, W., Blum, J., et al.: The Utility of Transbronchial Needle Aspiration in the staging of Bronchogenic Carcinoma. Am J Respir Crit Care Med 2000;161: 601–607.
25. Gould, M. K., Kuschner, W. G., Rydzak, C. E., et al.: Test performance of positron emission tomography and computed tomography for mediastinal staging in patients with non-small-cell lung cancer: a meta-analysis. Ann Intern Med 2003;139:879–892
26. Gonzales-Stawinski, G. V., Lemaire, A., Merchant, F., et al. : A comparative analysis of positron emission tomography and mediastinoscopy in staging non-small cell lung cancer. J Thorac Cardiovasc Surg 2003;126: 1900–1905
27. Kernstine, K. H., McLaughlin, K. A., Menda, Y., et al.: Can FDG-PET reduce the need for mediastinoscopy in potentially surgically resectable nonsmall cell lung cancer? Ann Thorac Surg 2002;73:394-402.
28. Brim, O., Kappetein, A. P., Stijnen, T., Bogers, A. J.: Meta-analysis of positron emission tomographic and computed tomographic imaging in detecting mediastinal lymph node metastases in nonsmall cell lung cancer. Ann Thorac Surg 2005;79:375–382.
29. Hoffmann, H. Invasive staging of lung cancer by mediastinoscopy and video-assisted thoracoscopy. Lung Cancer 2001;34:3–5.
30. Detterbeck, F. C., DeCamp, M. M., Jr., Kohman, L. J., Silvestri, G. A; American College of Chest Physicians. Lung cancer. Invasive staging: the guidelines. Chest. 2003 Jan;123(1 Suppl):167S-175S.
31. Wallace, M. B., Woodward, T. A., Raimondo, M.: Endoscopic ultrasound and staging of non-small-cell lung cancer. Gastrointest Endosc Clin N Am 2005;5: 157–167.
32. Annema, J. T., Versteegh, M. I., Veselic, M., Voigt, P., Rabe, K. F.: Endoscopic ultrasound-guided fine-needle aspiration in the diagnosis and staging of lung cancer and its impact on surgical staging. J Clin Oncol 2005;23:8357–8361.
33. Annema, J. T., Versteegh, M. I., Veselic, M., et al.: Endoscopic ultrasound added to mediastinoscopy for preoperative staging of patients with lung cancer. JAMA 2005;294:931–936.
34. Fritscher-Ravens, A., Bohuslavizki, K. H., Brandt, L., et al.: Mediastinal lymph node involvement in potentially respectable lung cancer: comparison of CT, positron emission tomography, and endoscopic ultrasonography

with and without fine-needle aspiration. Chest 2003; 123:442–51.
35. Krasnik, M., Vilmann, P., Larsen, S. S., Jacobsen, G. K.: Preliminary experience with a new method of endoscopic transbronchial real time ultrasound guided biopsy for diagnosis of mediastinal and hilar lesions. *Thorax* 2003;58:1083–1088.
36. Yasufuku, K., Nakajima, T., Motoori, K., et al.: Comparison of Endobronchial Ultrasound, Positron Emission Tomography and CT for Lymph Node Staging of Lung Cancer. Chest 2006;130:710–718.
37. Rintoul, R. C., Skwarski, K. M., Murchison, J. T., Hill, A., Walker, W. S., Penman, I. D.: Endoscopic and Endobronchial Ultrasound Real-time Fine-Needle Aspiration for Staging of the Mediastinum in Lung Cancer. Chest 2004; 126: 2020–2022.
38. Mazzone, P., Jain, P., Arroliga, A. C., Matthay, R. A.: Bronchoscopy and Needle biopsy techniques for diagnosis and staging of lung cancer. Clin Chest Med 2002; 23:137–158.
39. Cerfolio, R. J., Ojha, B., Bryant, A., Bass, C. S., Bartalucci, A. A., Mountz, J. M..: The role of FDG-PET scan in staging patients with non-small cell lung cancer. Ann Thorac Surg 2003;76:861–866.
40. Kernstine, K. H., Stanford. W., Mullan, B. F., et al.: PET, CT, and MRI with Combidex for mediastinal staging in non-small-cell lung carcinoma. *Ann Thorac Surg.* 1999; 68:1022–1028.
41. Downey, R. J., Akhurst, T., Gonen, M., et al.: Preoperative F-18 fluorodeoxyglucose-positron emission tomography maximal standardized uptake value predicts survival after lung cancer resection. J Clin Oncol 22:3255–3260, 2004.
42. Weder, W., Schmid, R. A., Bruchhaus, H., et al.: Detection of extrathoracic metastases by positron emission tomography in lung cancer. Ann Thorac Surg 66:886–893, 1998.
43. Viney, R. C., Boyer, M. J., King, M. T., et al.: Randomized controlled trial of the role of positron emission tomography in the management of stage I and II non-small-cell lung cancer. J Clin Oncol 22:2357–2362, 2004.
44. Pozo-Rodriguez, F., Martin de Nicolás, J. L., Sánchez-Nistal, M. A., et al: Accuracy of helical CT and FDG-PET for identifying lymph node mediastinal metastases in potentially resectable non–small-cell lung cancer. J Clin Oncol 23:8348–8356, 2005
45. Silvestri, G. A., Tanoue, L. T., Margolis, M. L., Barker, J., Detterbeck, F.: American College of Chest Physicians. The noninvasivestaging of non-small cell lung cancer: the guidelines. Chest2003;123(1 Suppl):147S–156S.
46. Detterbeck, F. C., DeCamp, M. M. Jr, Kohman, L. J., Silvestri, G. A.: American College of Chest Physicians. Lung cancer. Invasivestaging: the guidelines. Chest 2003;123(1 Suppl):167S–175S.
47. Chang, K. J., Erickson, R. A., Nguyen, P.: Endoscopic ultrasound (EUS) and EUS-guided fine-needle aspiration of the left adrenal gland. Gastrointest Endosc 1996;44:568–72.
48. Abolhoda, A., Keller, S.: Mediastinal staging of lung cancer. In: Pass, H. I., Michell, J. B., Johnson, D. H., Turrisi, A. T., Minna, J. D., eds.: Lung Cancer: Principles and Practice. Philadephia: Lippincott, Williams, and Wilkins, 2000.
49. Ginsberg, R. J., Rice, T.W., Goldberg, M., Waters, P. F., Schmocker, B. J.: Extended cervical mediastinoscopy. A single staging procedure for bronchogenic carcinoma of the left upper lobeThe Journal of Thoracic and Cardiovascular Surgery, Vol 94, 673–678.
50. N. J. Pastis, P. J. Nietert, G. A. Silvestri, and for the American College of Chest Physicians Inter Variation in Training for Interventional Pulmonary Procedures Among US Pulmonary/Critical Care Fellowships: A Survey of Fellowship Directors
Chest, May 1, 2005; 127(5): 1614–1621.
51. Amir Sharafkhaneh, Walid Baaklini, Arnold B. Gorin, and Linda Green Yield of Transbronchial Needle Aspiration in Diagnosis of Mediastinal Lesions *Chest* 2003;124;2131–2135.
52. Frank, H. W. Hermensa, Ton, C. A., Van Engelenburgb, Frank J. Vissera: Diagnostic Yield of Transbronchial Histology Needle Aspiration in Patients with Mediastinal Lymph Node Enlargement. Respiration 2003;70:631–635.
53. Dasgupta, A., Jain, P., Minai, O. A. et al: Utility of transbronchial needle aspiration in the diagnosis of endobronchial lesions. Chest 1999;115,1237–1241.
54. Haponik, E. F., Russell, G. B., Beamis, J. F. J., et al.: Bronchoscopytraining: current fellows' experiences and some concerns for the future. Chest 2000;118:625–630.
55. White, C. S., Weiner, E. A., Patel, P., et al.: Transbronchial needle aspiration: guidance with CT fluoroscopy. Chest 2000;118,1630–1638.
56. Goldberg, S. N., Raptopoulos, V., Boiselle, P. M., et al.: Mediastinal lymphadenopathy: diagnostic yield of transbronchial mediastinal lymph node biopsy with CT fluoroscopic guidance-initial experience. Radiology 2000; 216,764–767.
57. Shannon, J. J., Bude, R.O., Orens, J.B., et al.: Endobronchial ultrasound-guided needle aspiration of mediastinal adenopathy. Am J Respir Crit Care Med 1996;153,1424–1430.
58. Herth, F. J., Becker, H. D., Ernst, A.: Ultrasound-guided transbronchial needle aspiration: an experience in 242 patients. Chest 2003;123,604–607.
59. Becker, H. D., Herth, F.: Endobronchial ultrasound of the airways and mediastinum. Bolliger, CT Mathur, PN eds. Interventional bronchoscopy (vol 30) 2000,80–93 Karger. Basel, Switzerland.
60. Goldberg, B. B., Steiner, R. M., Liu, J. B., et al.: US-assisted bronchoscopy with use of miniature transducer-containing catheters. Radiology 1994;190,233–237.
61. Kurimoto, N., Murayama, M., Yoshioka, S., et al.: Assessment of usefulness of endobronchial ultrasonography in determination of depth of tracheobronchial tumor invasion. Chest 1999;115,1500–1506.
62. Miyazu, Y., Miyazawa, T., Kurimoto, N., et al.: Endobronchial ultrasonography in the assessment of centrally located early-stage lung cancer before photodynamic therapy. Am J Respir Crit Care Med 2002;165, 832–837.
63. Henschke, C. I., Yankelevitz, D. F., Libby, D. M., Pasmantier, M. W., Smith, J. P., Miettinen, O. S.: Survival of Patients with Stage I Lung Cancer Detected on CT Screening, The International Early Lung Cancer Action Program Investigators N Engl J Med. 2006 Oct 26;355 (17):1763–71.
64. F. J. F. Herth, K. F. Rabe, S. Gasparini, and J. T. Annema: Transbronchial and transoesophageal (ultrasound-guided) needle aspirations for the analysis of mediastinal lesions Eur Respir J 2006; 28:1264–1275.
65. Falcone, F., Fois, F., Grosso, D.: Endobronchial ultrasound. Respiration 2003;70,179–194.
66. Herth, F. J., Becker, H. D., Ernst, A.: Conventional vs endobronchial ultrasound-guided transbronchial needle aspiration: a randomized trial. Chest 2004;125, 322-325.

69. Pitz, C., Mass, K., Swieten, H., et al.: Surgery as part of combined modality treatment in stage IIIB non-small cell lung cancer. Ann Thorac Surg 2002; 74: 164–169.
70. Little, A. G., Rusch, V. W., Bonner, J. A., et al.: Patterns of Surgical Care of Lung Cancer Patients. Ann Thorac Surg 2005;80:2051–56.
71. Okamoto, H., Watanabe, K., Nagatomo, A., et al.: Endobronchial ultrasonography for mediastinal and hilar lymph node metastases of lung cancer. *Chest* 2002;121:1498–1506.
72. Yasufuku, K., Chiyo, M., Sekine, Y., et al.: Real-time endobronchial ultrasound-guided transbronchial needle aspiration of mediastinal and hilar lymph nodes. *Chest* 2004;126:122–128.
73. Yasufuku, K., Chiyo, M., Koh, E., et al.: Endobronchial ultrasound guided transbronchial needle aspiration for staging of lung cancer. *Lung Cancer* 2005;50: 347–354.
74. Herth, F. J., Eberhardt, R., Vilmann, P., Krasnik, M., Ernst, A.: Real-time, endobronchial ultrasound-guided, transbronchial needle aspiration: a new method for sampling mediastinal lymph nodes. *Thorax* 2006;61: 795–798.
75. Herth, F. J., Ernst, A., Eberhardt, R., Vilmann, P., Dienemann, H., Krasnik, M.: Endobronchial ultrasound-guided transbronchial needle aspiration of lymph nodes in the radiologically normal mediastinum. *Eur Respir J* 2006;28:910–914.
76. Hoffmann, H.: Invasive staging of lung cancer by mediastinoscopy and video-assisted thoracoscopy. *Lung Cancer* 2001;34:3–5.
77. Luke, W. P., Pearson, F. G., Todd, T. R., Patterson, G. A., Cooper, J. D.: Prospective evaluation of mediastinoscopy for assessment of carcinoma of the lung. *J Thorac Cardiovasc Surg* 1986;91:53–56.
78. Coughlin, M., Deslauriers, J., Beaulieu, M., et al. : Role of mediastinoscopy in pretreatment staging of patients with primary lung cancer. *Ann Thorac Surg* 1985;40: 556–560.
79. P. Vilmann, M. Krasnik, S. S. Larsen, G. K. Jacobsen, P. Clementsen: Transesophageal Endoscopic Ultrasound-Guided Fine-Needle Aspiration (EUS-FNA) and Endobronchial Ultrasound-Guided Transbronchial Needle Aspiration (EBUS-TBNA) Biopsy: A Combined Approach in the Evaluation of Mediastinal Lesions. Endoscopy 2005;37:833–839.
80. Rintoul, R. C., Skwarski, K. M., Murchison, J. T., Wallace, W. A., Walker, W. S., Penman, I. D.: Endobronchial and endoscopic ultrasound-guided real-time fine-needle aspiration for mediastinal staging. *Eur Respir J* 2005;25: 416–421.
81. Sterling, B. E.: Complication with a transbronchial histology needle. *Chest* 1990;98:783–784.
82. Wallace, M. B., Ravenel, J., Block, M. I., et al.: Endoscopic ultrasound in lung cancer patients with a normal mediastinum on computed tomography. Ann Thorac Surg 77:1763–1768, 2004.
83. Wallace, M. B., Silvestri, G. A., Sahai, A. V., et al.: Endoscopic ultrasound-guided fine needle aspiration for staging patients with carcinoma of the lung. Ann Thorac Surg 72:1861–1867, 2001.
84. Fritscher-Ravens, A., Davidson, B. L., Hauber, H. P., et al.: Endoscopic ultrasound, positron emission tomography, and computerized tomography for lung cancer. Am J Respir Crit Care Med 168:1293–1297, 2003.
85. Wiersema, M. J., Vazquez-Sequeiros, E., Wiersema, L. M.: Evaluation of mediastinal lymphadenopathy with endoscopic US-guided fine-needle aspiration biopsy. Radiology 219:252–257, 2001.
86. Baram, D., Garcia, R. B., Richman, P. S.: Impact of Rapid On-Site Cytologic Evaluation During Transbronchial Needle Aspiration. Chest 2005; 128: 869–875.
87. Aabakken, L., Silvestri, G. A., Hawes, R., Reed, C. E., Marsi, V., Hoffman, B.: Cost-efficacy of endoscopic ultrasonography with fine-needle aspiration vs. mediastinotomy in patients with lung cancer and suspected mediastinal adenopathy. Endoscopy 1999;31:707–711.
88. Silvestri, G. A., Hoffman, B. J., Bhutani, M. S., Hawes, R. H., Coppage, L., Sanders-Cliette, A., et al.: Endoscopic ultrasound with fine-needle aspiration in the diagnosis and staging of lung cancer. Ann Thorac Surg 1996;61:1441–1446.
89. Gress, F. G., Savides, T. J., Sandler, A., Kesler, K., Conces, D., Cummings. O., et al.: Endoscopic ultrasonography, fine-needle aspiration biopsy guided by endoscopic ultrasonography, and computed tomography in the preoperative staging of non-small-cell lung cancer: a comparison study. Ann Intern Med 1997;127:604–612.
90. Kramer, H., van Putten, J. W., Post, W. J., et al.: Oesophageal endoscopic ultrasound with fine needle aspiration improves and simplifies the staging of lung cancer. Thorax. 2004 Jul;59(7):596–601.
91. Annema, J. T., Hoekstra, O. S., Smit, E. F., et al.: Towards a minimally invasive staging strategy in NSCLC: analysis of PET positive mediastinal lesions by EUS-FNA. Lung Cancer. 2004 Apr;44(1):53–60.
92. Larsen, S. S., Krasnik, M., Vilmann, P., Jacobsen, G. K., Pederson, J. H., Faurschou, P., et al.: Endoscopic ultrasound guided biopsy of mediastinal lesions has a major impact on patient management. Thorax 2002;57: 98–103.
93. Savides, T. J., Perricone, A.: Impact of EUS-guided FNA of enlarged mediastinal lymph nodes on subsequent thoracic surgery rates. Gastrointest Endosc 2004;60: 340–350.
94. Fritscher-Ravens, A., Sririam, P. V. J., Bobrowski, C., Pforte, A., Topalidis, T., Krause, C., et al.: Mediastinal lymphadenopathy in patients with or without previous malignancy: EUS FNA-based differential cytodiagnosis in 153 patients. Am J Gastroenterol 2000;95:2278–2284.
95. LeBlanc, J. K., Devereaux, B. M., Imperiale, T. F., et al.: Endoscopic ultrasound in non-small cell lung cancer and negative mediastinum on computed tomography. *Am J Respir Crit Care Med* 2005;171:177–182.
96. F. Herth[1], H.D. Becker[1], J. LoCicero, III[2] and A. Ernst[3] Endobronchial ultrasound in therapeutic bronchoscopy Eur Respir J 2002; 20:118–121.
97. Larsen, S. S., Vilman, P., Krasnik, M.: Endoscopic Ultrasound-Guided Biopsy Performed Routinely in Lung Cancer Staging Spares Futile Thoracotomies: Preliminary Results from a Randomised Clinical Trial. Lung Cancer 2005; 49: 377–385.
98. Smulder, S. A., Smeenk, F. W. J. M., Janssen-Heijnen, M. L. G., de Munck, D. R. A. J. , Postmus, P. E.: Surgical Mediastinal Staging in Everyday practice. Lung Cancer 2005; 47: 243–51.
99. Gerald Antoch, M. D., Jörg Stattaus, M. D., Andre T. Nemat, M. D., Non–Small-Cell Lung Cancer: Dual-Modality PET/CT in Preoperative Staging Radiology 2003; 229:526–533.

SECTION II

Hepatopancreatobiliary/ Abdomen

CHAPTER 14

Pancreatic Carcinoma: Detection and Staging

Dr. Jeffrey H. Lee
Dr. Eric P. Tamm

Background

Pancreatic adenocarcinoma is the fourth-leading cause for cancer-related death in the United States. Pancreatic cancers can arise from both the exocrine and endocrine portions of the pancreas. Of pancreatic tumors, 95% develop from the exocrine portion of the pancreas, including the ductal epithelium, acinar cells, connective tissue, and lymphatic tissue. Given a five-year survival rate of 4% of pancreatic adenocarcinoma, the emphasis has been on early detection and prompt management.[1]

For most facilities, computed tomography (CT) is the preferred modality for the initial cross-sectional imaging workup of pancreatic cancer. CT has the advantage of being rapid, operator independent, and capable of handling a wide variety of patients, typically avoiding the need for sedation. The rapid evolution of the newest multidetector row CT scanners (MDCT), now allows for submillimeter sections of the entire abdomen within a five second breathhold.

As with CT, MRI can provide information for all aspects of staging, including vascular involvement, nodal disease, and liver metastases. Multiple developments, including multichannel coils, parallel imaging, and higher field strength clinical imaging platforms, have resulted in significant improvements in the image quality of MRI. MRI offers inherently better soft tissue contrast than CT, even without the use of intravenous contrast agents, but has lower spatial resolution than CT. Currently images must be obtained at a greater slice thickness than MDCT for coverage of the entire abdomen.

Although CT has been considered the first test for preoperative staging of suspected pancreatic cancer, the role of endoscopic ultrasound (EUS) as an adjunct to diagnosing and staging for locoregional involvement has gradually increased during the past fifteen years. While EUS alone cannot provide complete staging of pancreatic malignancy due to its limited depth of penetration, complete staging can be established in conjunction with CT or MRI. In this chapter, we will discuss some of the strengths of CT, MRI, and EUS and how they complement each other in accurately staging pancreatic malignancy.

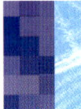

Description of Equipment and Techniques of CT, MRI, and EUS

CT

Key to optimizing image quality is the use of a large bolus of contrast (typically 120–150 cc of iodinated contrast) injected rapidly (4–5cc/sec) through peripheral veins to improve tumor conspicuity and to best delineate the tumor from adjacent vasculature.[2-4] Two passes are commonly made through the abdomen following the start of contrast injection. The first pass is obtained during the phase of peak pancreatic enhancement, typically 35–50 seconds after the start of contrast injection, to maximize the conspicuity of pancreatic adenocarcinoma. The second phase is obtained during the phase of peak liver enhancement, typically 50-70 seconds after the start of the injection, to maximize detection of liver metastases and during which the superior mesenteric, portal, and splenic veins are well opacified.[5] If iodinated intravenous contrast cannot be administered, for reasons such as dye allergy or renal failure, an alternative modality (MRI, CT/PET) can be obtained to provide cross-sectional information and staging information.

MRI

A typical MRI protocol for imaging the pancreas includes pre-enhanced T1 and fat-suppressed T2 weighted images, and enhanced, dynamically obtained, 3D gradient recalled echo (GRE) sequence with T1 weighting and fat suppression. These images can be obtained in a single breath-hold as thin section, overlapping images than can provide improved detail in imaging the pancreas. The additional use of magnetic resonance cholangiopancreatogoraphy can be useful in visualizing ductal anatomy and in imaging the internal characteristics of cystic lesions.

EUS

There are two modes in EUS, radial and curvilinear array. The radial array provides a 270–360 degree panoramic view as in CT scan. The curvilinear array provides a 120-degree long-axis view with capacity for fine needle aspiration (FNA). Equipped with Doppler imaging, it allows tissue sampling by FNA, while avoiding the major vessels. The available needles for FNA are 19, 22, and 25 gauges.

Once the specimens are obtained, approximately half of the smears are air-dried and stained with Diff-Quik (Mercedes Medical, Sarasota, FL), while the remaining smears are fixed in 95% alcohol for Papanicolaou's staining. Any additional material is collected in saline solution or formalin for cell block, which is stained with Hematoxylin and Eosin and in immunohistochemical stains, if necessary. The immediate staining and review by an experienced cytologist would confirm tissue diagnosis before the EUS session is terminated. During the session of EUS FNA, endoscopic retrograde cholangiopancreatography (ERCP) can also be performed to alleviate the symptoms of obstructive jaundice.

Diagnosis and Staging by CT, MRI, and EUS

The anatomy of the regions to be discussed is illustrated with a series of transaxial cross-sections taken from the visible Human Anatomy Data Set (Figure 14–1 A to C)

CT

Pancreatic cancer most commonly manifests as a hypodense mass with ill-defined margins. Most tumors (approximately 60%) are identified in the pancreatic head, involving then the body and tail in order of decreasing frequency.[6] Thin section imaging (0.625-2.5 mm) avoids the problem of obscuration of small tumors secondary to volume averaging of tumors with normal pancreatic parenchyma within the same slice thickness. It also provides for better visualization of the interface of tumor and vessel, especially those vessels (common hepatic, celiac, and superior mesenteric arteries) that have subcentimeter diameters.

Dual-phase imaging is crucial; up to 40% of tumors will have the same density as adjacent normal pancreatic parenchyma on the portal venous phase of imaging.[7] (Figure 14–2)

It is also necessary to pay close attention to the secondary effects of the tumor. These include pancreatic duct and/or common bile duct dilatation and/or cutoff of ducts (Figure 14–3), distortion of the pancreatic contour, replacement of the normal pattern of the pancreatic parenchyma, focal enlargement of the pancreas, upstream atrophy of the pancreas, soft tissue density infiltration toward adjacent vessels, and regional adenopathy. A retrospective study identified duct dilatation and cutoff as being visible in 50% of cases 2–18 months prior to definitively determining a diagnosis of pancreatic cancer.[8]

The differential diagnosis for pancreatic adenocarcinoma includes chronic pancreatitis,[9] (Figure 14–4) primary or secondary involvement by lymphoma (Figure 14–5), and metastatic disease from tumors originating in such organs as the intrapancreatic common bile duct, breast, lung, stomach, duodenum and colon. Sarcomas can also metastasize to the pancreas (Figure 14–6). Islet cell tumors are

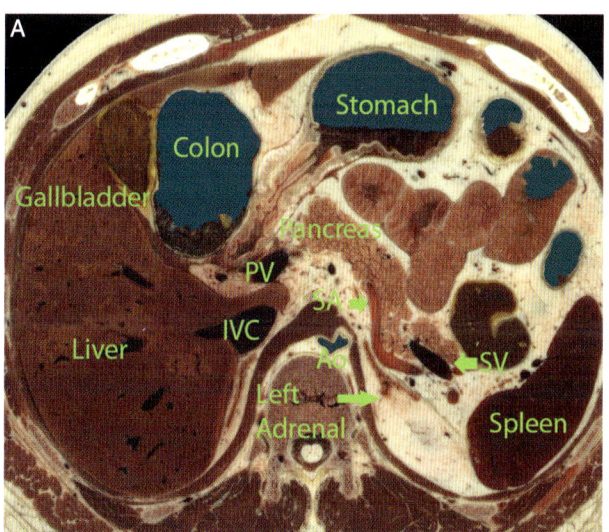

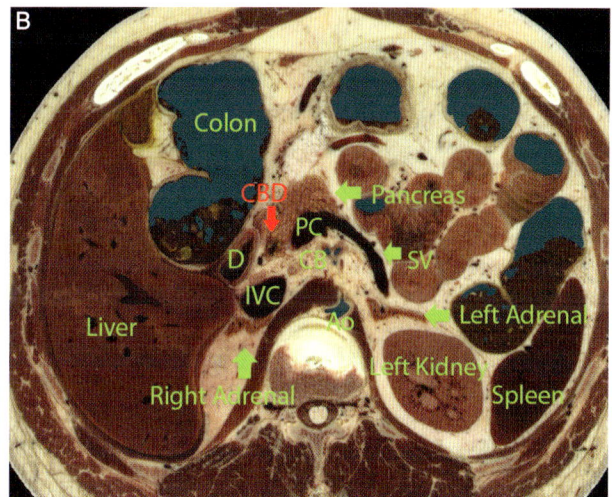

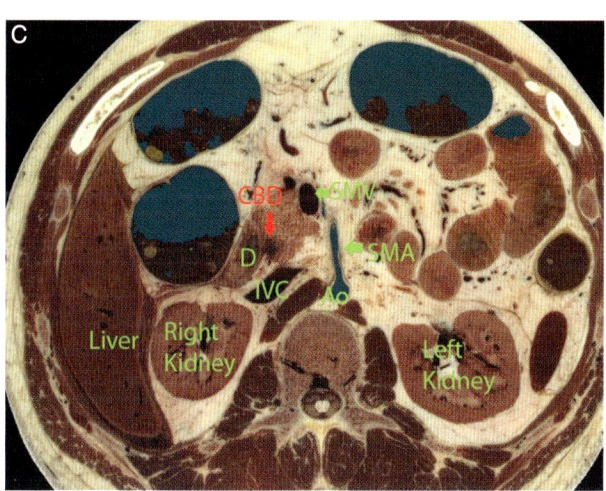

FIGURE 14–1. *A to C* Visible Human transaxial cross-sections at the level of the pancreatic body (A) celiac artery bifurcation (B) and superior mesenteric artery insertion into the aorta. (C) Ao=aorta, IVC=inferior vena cava, SA=splenic artery, SV=splenic vein, PV=portal vein, CB=celiac bifurcation, CBD(red)=common bile duct, D=duodenum, SMA=superior mesenteric artery, SMV=superior mesenteric vein

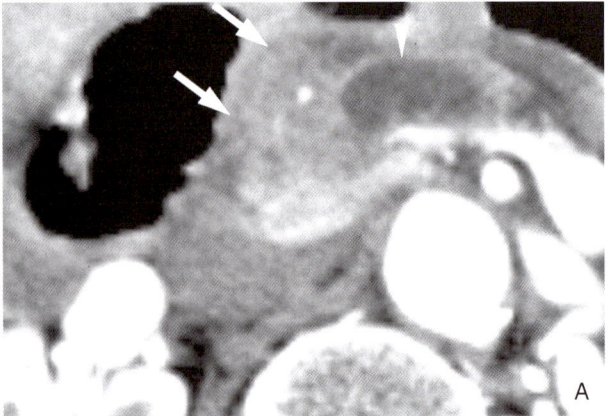
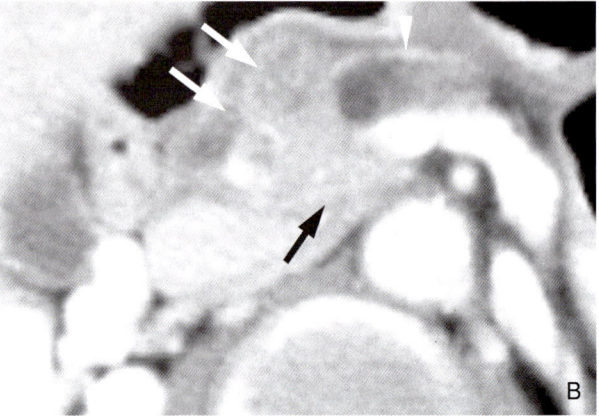

FIGURE 14–2. *A and B* A 72-year-old female with a history of pancreatic cancer. Mass (white arrows) in the superior pancreatic head, associated with pancreatic duct obstruction (white arrowheads) is better seen on the pancreatic parenchymal phase (A) than on the portal venous phase (B). Note the similarity of enhancement of the tumor to the uncinate (black arrow) in (B).

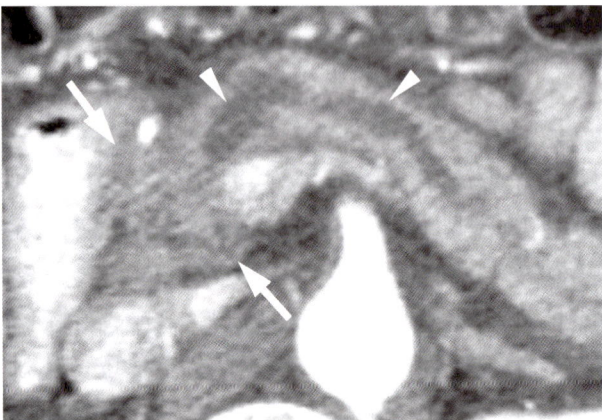

FIGURE 14–3. A 55-year-old male with diagnosis of pancreatic cancer. Pancreatic duct dilatation (arrowheads) is seen secondary to an obstructing pancreatic cancer (white arrows).

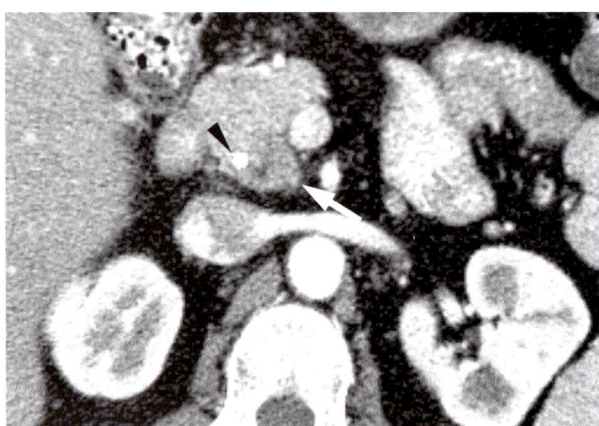

FIGURE 14–4. A 54-year-old female with common bile duct stricture and mass seen on CT. Images from the pancreatic parenchymal phase of a contrast enhanced CT show a mass (white arrow) associated with obstruction of the common bile duct. A stent is present (black arrowhead). Surgical pathology showed chronic pancreatitis.

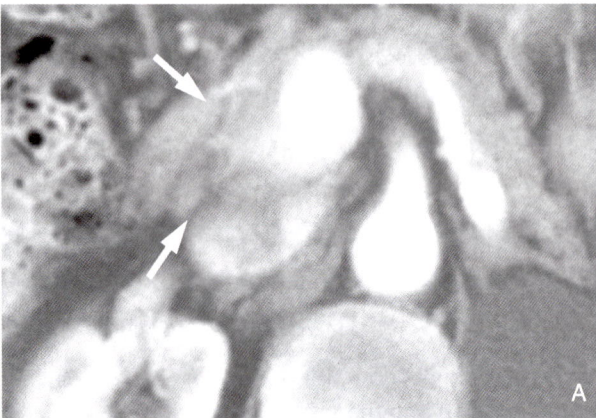
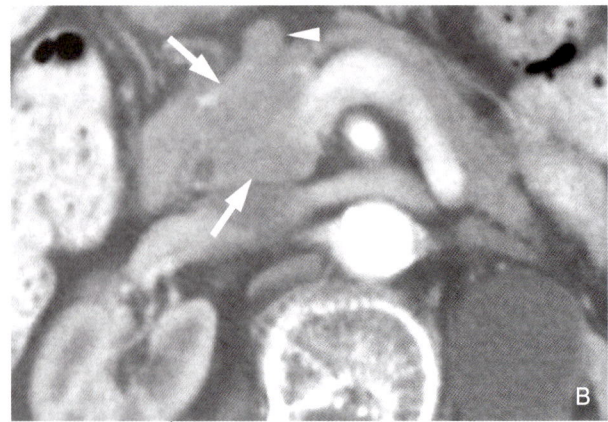

FIGURE 14–5. *A and B* A 75-year-old female with a history of lymphoma. A baseline study showed no evidence of pancreatic involvement. Pancreatic head and neck (A) appeared normal or slightly atrophic (white arrows). Follow-up imaging (B) showed gradual diffuse enlargement of the pancreatic head and neck consistent with lymphomatous infiltration (white arrows). Lobular mass (white arrowhead) represents volume averaging artifact of the pancreas.

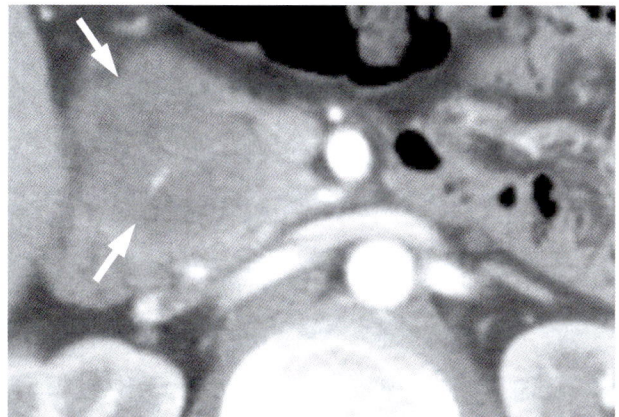

FIGURE 14–6. A 23-year-old male with a history of Ewing sarcoma with metastasis (white arrows) to the pancreatic head.

commonly hypervascular, but can rarely mimic pancreatic cancer.

Overall, the sensitivity of MDCT for pancreatic adenocarcinoma is 86–97%, with sensitivity decreasing for smaller lesions (approximately 77% for tumors less than 2 cm).[5,10-12] It is important to obtain cross-sectional imaging prior to any intervention. Inflammatory changes following biopsy, stent placement, and ERCP (with or without brushings) can obscure tumors and overestimate the extent of disease because of peripancreatic inflammation. Indeed, once a biliary stent has been placed, the point of obstruction can no longer be visualized, limiting the ability to localize the tumor.

Pancreatic cancer staging means identification of vascular involvement, nodal disease, and the presence of distant metastases (liver, lung, peritoneum). Involvement of the superior mesenteric, celiac, or common hepatic arteries typically means unresectable disease.[13] The recent development of venous interposition grafts means that, in several institutions, but not all, venous involvement without arterial involvement, short of venous obstruction, is still resectable disease. It is therefore important to be knowledgeable of what represents resectable disease at the institution at which one is practicing. Patients may also seek second opinions at institutions that may utilize such grafts; for this reason, reports should include a complete description of the extent of disease to allow a variety of practitioners to decide whether disease is resectable according to their institution's criteria.

Probably the most commonly utilized criteria for identifying resectable disease is that of the circumferential degrees of involvement of a given vessel by the tumor. Lu et al showed that using a threshold of 180 degrees of vascular involvement (greater than 180 degrees being unresectable disease) yielded a sensitivity of 84%, with specificity of 98% for unresectable disease.[14] (Figures 14–7, 14–8)

The commonly used CT criteria for nodal involvement by tumor is that of nodal enlargement to greater than 1 cm in short axis (Figure 14–9). Unfortunately, sensitivity for nodal disease is very limited as micrometastases can be present in nodes much smaller than 1cm, and hyperplastic nodes, without any evidence of tumor, can be larger than 1 cm. In a study by Valls et al, CT identified only 16.7% (3/18) of patients with adenopathy at surgery; however, only 5.9% (2/34) were actually unresectable because of adenopathy.[15] Therefore, while CT has limited sensitivity, the apparent impact of this limitation is less than expected. Of greater importance is the identification of suspicious nodes outside of the typical surgical field. This would include para-aortic adenopathy, adenopathy to the left of the superior mesenteric vessels, and adenopathy in the jejunal, or less commonly, ileocolic mesentery. Distant adenopathy can also be identified uncommonly in the pelvis.

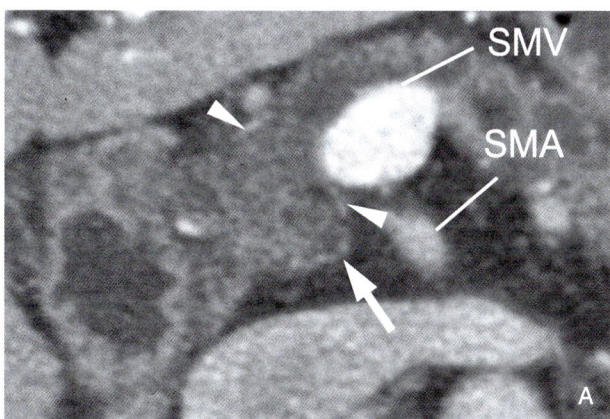 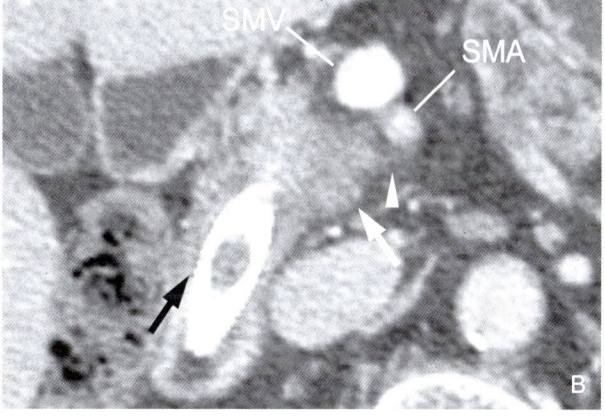

FIGURE 14–7. A and B   A 73-year-old female with a history of pancreatic cancer. Baseline CT during the (A) pancreatic parenchymal phase and (B) portal venous phase show a pancreatic head mass (white arrows) contacting the SMV in (A) and the SMA in (B) over less than 180 degrees of their circumference (arrowheads). A metallic stent is present (black arrow) in the common bile duct. SMV—superior mesenteric vein, SMA—superior mesenteric artery.

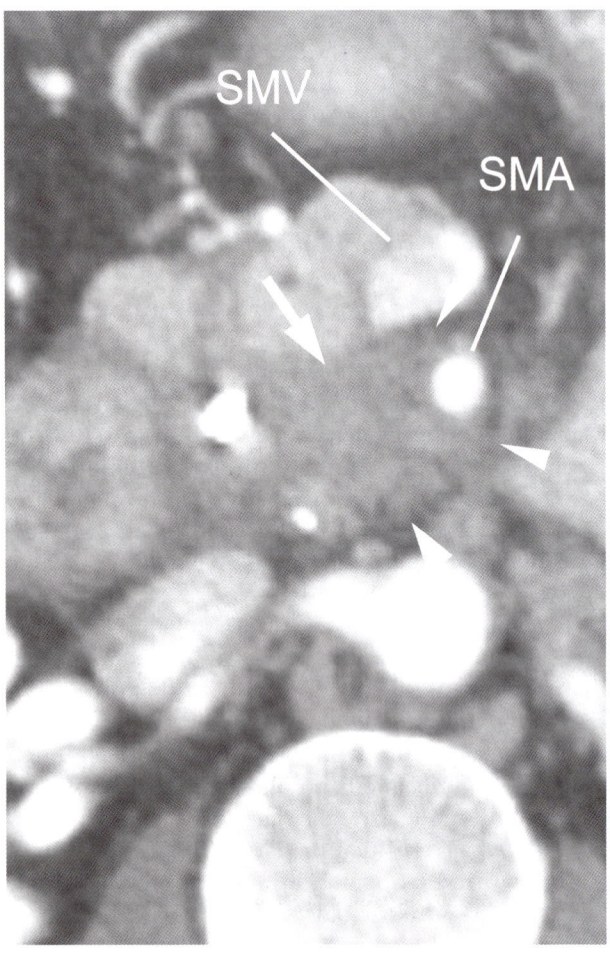

FIGURE 14–8. A 53-year-old female with pancreatic cancer. CT image obtained during the pancreatic parenchymal phase of enhancement shows tumor (white arows) contacting greater than 180 degrees of the circumference (white arrowheads) of the superior mesenteric artery (SMA). (SMV) Superior mesenteric vein

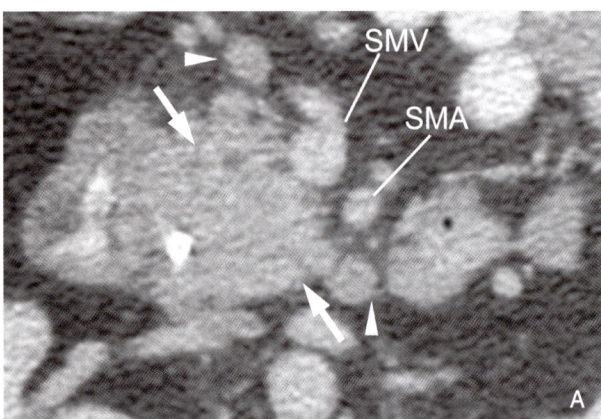
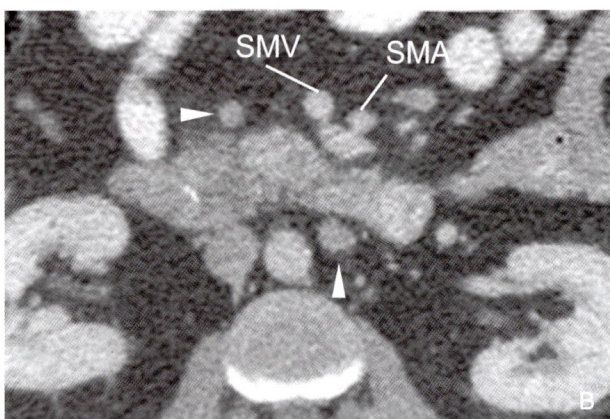

FIGURE 14–9. *A and B* A 57-year-old male with pancreatic cancer. On the portal venous phase of enhancement (A) a pancreatic mass (white arrows) isodense to normal pancreas is associated with multiple sites of adenopathy (white arrowheads) near the superior mesenteric vein (SMV), posterior and medial to the superior mesenteric artery (SMA). At a more inferior level (B) adenopathy is seen in the left para-aortic region.

On CT, liver metastases typically have a hypodense appearance with ill-defined borders during the portal venous phase of imaging (Figure 14–10). They may show a slightly hypervascular rim on the pancreatic parenchymal phase of imaging. The size of liver metastases is variable, ranging from low volume (1-2 cm) to significantly larger. In the study by Valls, 9 out of 34 cases called resectable at CT were unresectable at surgery due to small liver metastases with an average size of 8 mm.[15] Lesions less than 1 cm typically cannot be adequately characterized on CT. For those patients who will undergo preoperative therapy (chemotherapy and/or radiation therapy), follow-up CT after therapy may provide better characterization as metastatic disease would be expected to progress.

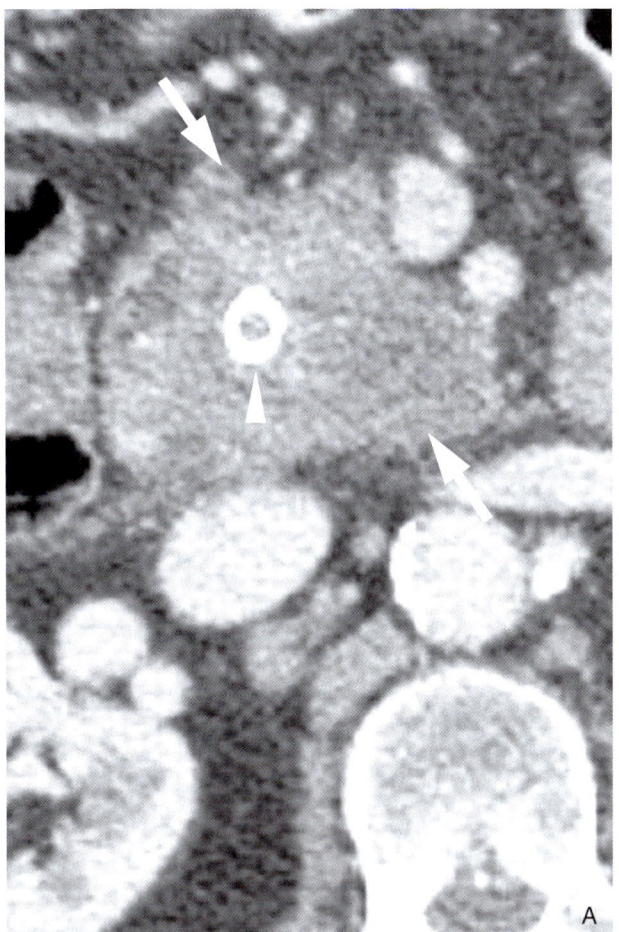
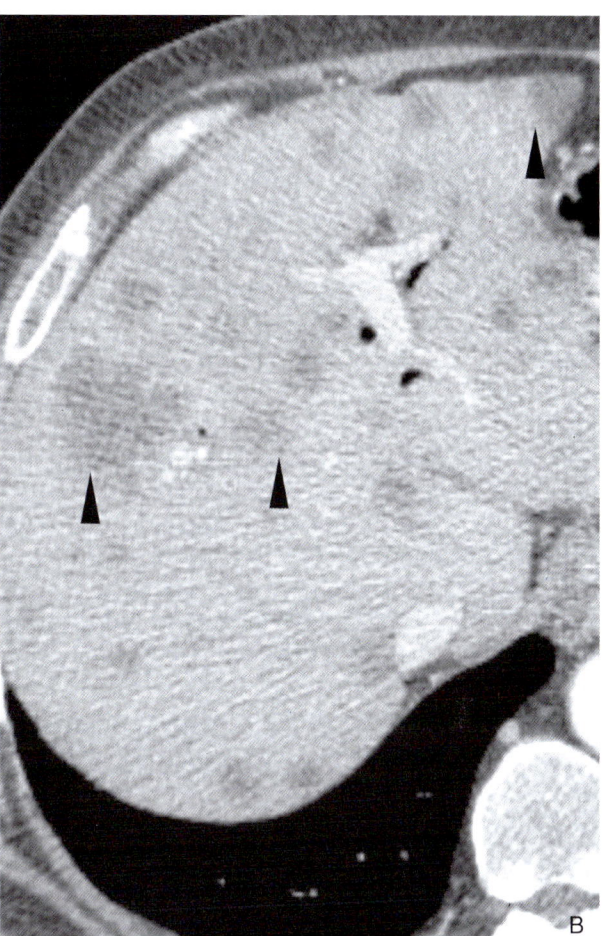

FIGURE 14–10. *A and B* A 68-year-old male with a history of pancreatic cancer. Portal venous phase axial images show (A) a large mass in the pancreatic head (white arrows) encompassing a metallic stent (white arrowhead), and (B) multiple liver metastases (black arrowheads indicate the three largest).

Metastatic disease to the peritoneum is most commonly very small in size, having the appearance of small, subcentimeter nodules. But it can be variable and significantly larger in advanced peritoneal disease (Figure 14–11). While detectable at surgery, it can be very difficult to identify at CT. It is most commonly identified along the peritoneal ligaments nearest the site of primary tumor, such as the transverse mesocolon, spreading outward to involve the omentum, and the paracolic gutters. While much less specific than the finding of peritoneal nodules, ascites can be considered a sign of peritoneal disease, but can also be

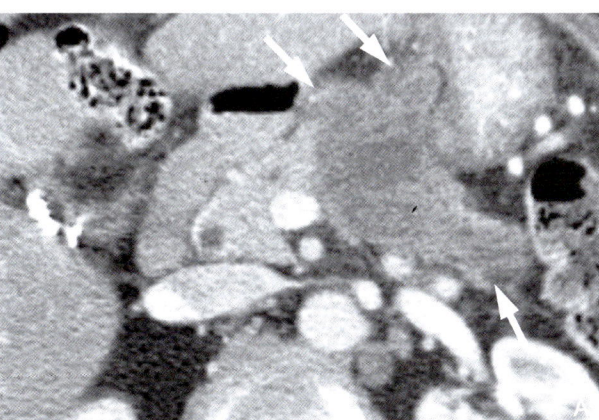
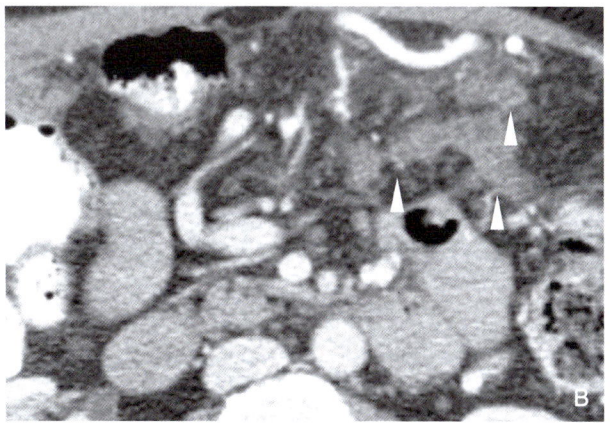

FIGURE 14–11. *A and B* A 63-year-old female with pancreatic cancer. Axial image at the level of the pancreas (A) shows a large pancreatic tail mass (white arrows). More inferiorly located axial image (B) shows peritoneal disease (white arrowheads) extending from the mesentery to the left anterior abdominal wall.

secondary to portal/mesenteric venous compromise, cirrhosis, or hypoproteinemia. While laparoscopic examination has been suggested as a preoperative adjunct to identify peritoneal disease, a recent review of the literature shows that, when accounting for already present locally advanced disease, or liver metastases, identified on cross-sectional imaging, laparoscopy would have changed management in 4–13% of patients.[16]

MRI

As on CT, pancreatic ductal adenocarcinomas are typically hypointense to normal pancreatic parenchyma both before, and after, contrast enhancement (Figure 14–12), but often becomes isointense to normal pancreatic parenchyma on portal venous phase (or later) images.[17,18] Unfortunately, atrophic pancreatic parenchyma proximal to the site of the tumor, secondary to longstanding duct obstruction, will also appear hypointense and can sometimes be difficult to differentiate from the tumor.[19] As seen on CT, pancreatic cancer is often associated with pancreatic or common bile duct obstruction. Indeed, the use of MRCP alone has been reported to have a sensitivity of 84% and a specificity of 97% for a tumor.[20] Obstruction of both the common bile duct and pancreatic duct is very concerning for the presence of a tumor.[18] However, MRCP alone is unable to provide a full-assessment of the pancreas necessary for adequate staging.

The differential for pancreatic cancer on MRI is the same as that for CT, namely, chronic pancreatitis, lymphoma, and metastatic disease.

As with CT, MRI can provide information for all aspects of staging, including vascular involvement, nodal disease, and liver metastases. T1-weighted images without fat suppression provide good contrast between extra-pancreatic extension of a tumor and adjacent vasculature. Enhancing the tumor can also help to differentiate it from vessels on post-contrast 3D GRE images, but the tumor often enhances poorly on the early phases of dynamic imaging and may be difficult to delineate from suppressed fat; therefore, close attention to delayed phases is often useful. As with CT, tumor involvement of vasculature can be measured by the degrees of involvement of a vessel's circumference. In a study by Arslan et al. that compared MR and MR angiography with CT and CT angiography, where greater than 180 of tumor contact or distortion of vascular contour were the criteria for unresectable disease, no statistical significance in staging accuracy was seen between the two modalities.[21]

MRI shares the limited accuracy of CT for nodal disease. As with CT, a size of greater than 1cm in short axis is the criterion commonly used for identifying nodal involvement by a tumor. Lymph nodes are best appreciated on fat-suppressed T2- weighted images, appearing bright against the suppressed fat (Figure 14–12).

MRI is frequently used as a problem solving tool in the workup of questionable liver metastases. Liver metastases are typically hypointense on T1 and post-contrast fat-suppressed T1-W images, while slightly hyperintense on T2- weighted images.(Figure 14–13) Liver specific agents that are taken up either by hepatocytes, or, in the case of ferumoxides, by reticuloendothelial cells, can improve the sensitivity and specificity of MRI for liver metastases. Ferumoxides cause the normal liver to drop in signal, causing metastases, which lack reticuloendothelial cells, to stand out more prominently on fat-suppressed, T2-weighted images.[22]

Unfortunately the small size of typical pancreatic peritoneal metastases makes them very difficult to visualize on MRI. Therefore, MRI currently has only a limited role in this area.

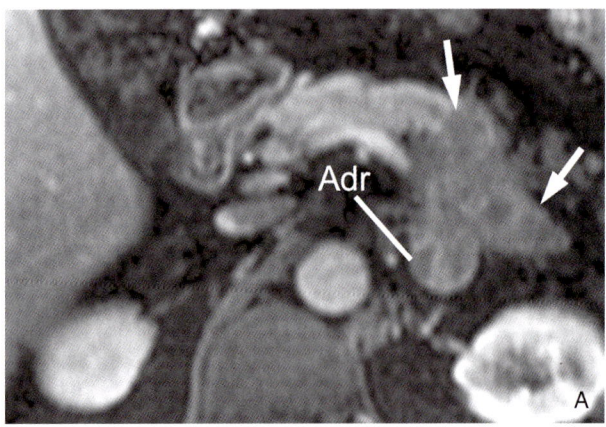

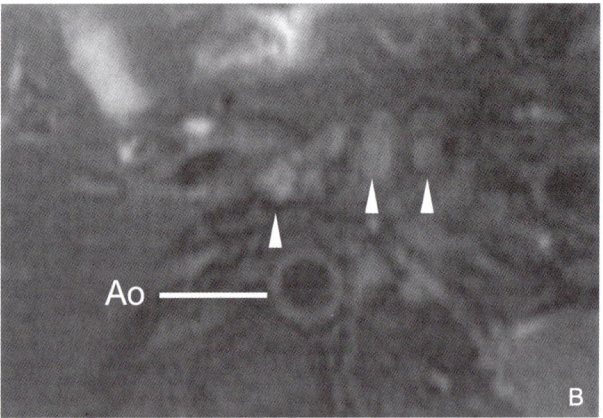

FIGURE 14–12. *A and B* A 72-year-old male with history of pancreatic cancer. (A) Gadolinium-enhanced, fat-suppressed, T1-weighted MRI image shows a pancreatic tail mass (white arrows) that has extended posteriorly to involve the left adrenal gland (Adr). (B) Fat-suppressed, T2-weighted MRI image shows adenopathy (white arrowheads) superior the celiac axis (not shown) anterior to the aorta (Ao).

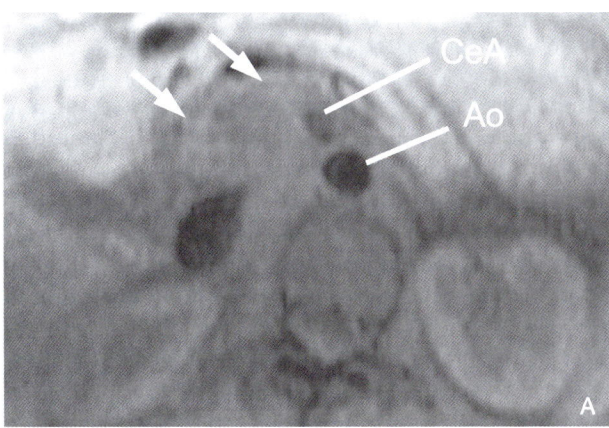
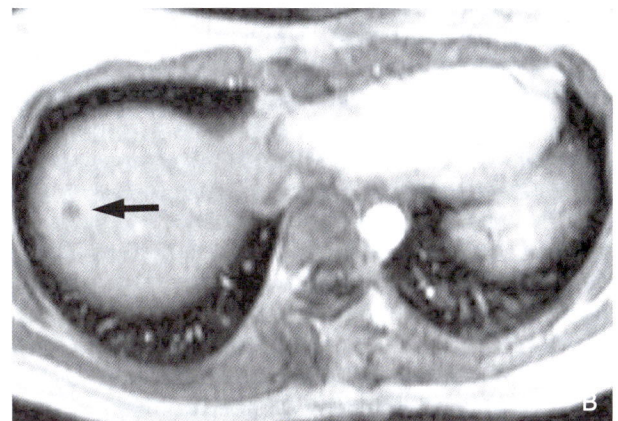

FIGURE 14–13. *A and B* A 30-year-old female with a history of pancreatic cancer shown on biopsy to be adenocarcinoma. (A) Axial fat suppressed T1 weighted image shows large pancreatic tumor (white arrows) surrounding the celiac artery trunk (CeA). (B) T1-weighted, post-contrast image shows ring-enhancing lesion (black arrow) at dome of liver, consistent with a metastasis. Ao-Aorta

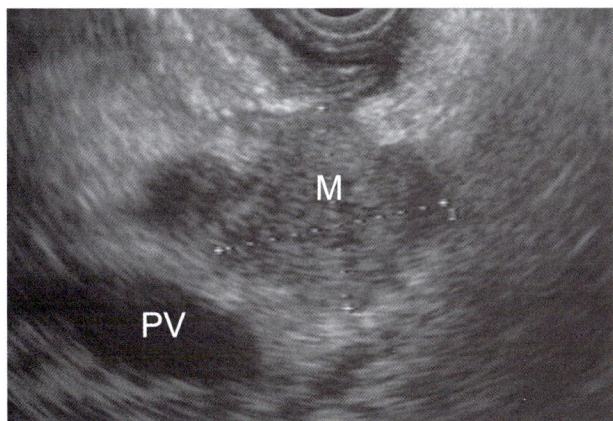

FIGURE 14–14. The linear EUS exam shows a hypoechoic mass with an irregular border in the head of the pancreas. There is a clear echoplane between the mass and the portal vein. FNA confirmed adenocarcinoma: M: mass, PV: portal vein.

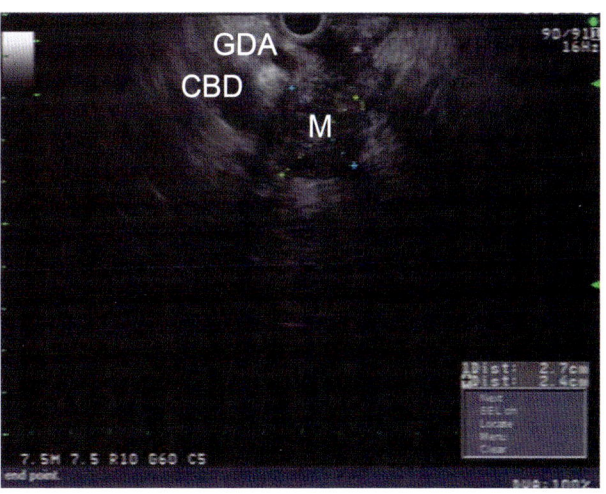

FIGURE 14–15. The linear EUS shows a 2.7 × 2.4 cm hypoechoir round mass with a regular border compressing on the distal bile duct, causing obstructive jaundice. The gastroduodenal artery is running closely and superiorly to the mass. FNA confirmed adenocarcinoma: CBD: common bile duct, GDA: gastroduodenal artery, M: mass.

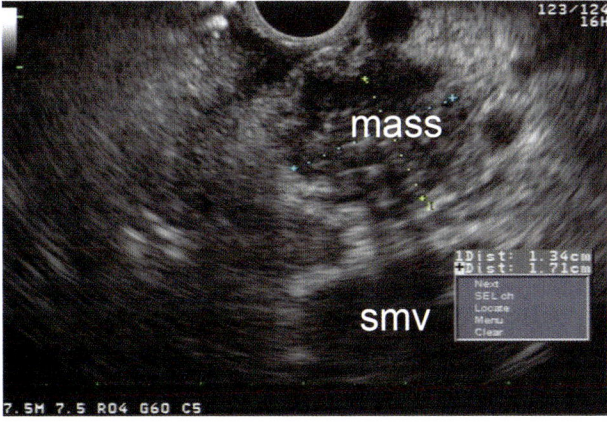

FIGURE 14–16. The linear EUS exam shows a 1.34 × 1.71 cm hypoechoic mass with hyperechoic strands, with an irregular border in the head of the pancreas. A clear echoplane between the mass and superior mesenteric vein (SMV) is seen. FNA confirmed adenocarcinoma.

Table 14–1. EUS Staging of Pancreatic Adenocarcinoma

Primary Tumor (T)

T0	No evidence of primary
Tis	In situ
T1	Tumor limited to pancreas, ≤ 2cm
T2	Tumor limited to pancreas, > 2cm
T3	Tumor extends beyond pancreas, no involvement of CA or SMA
T4	Tumor involves CA or SMA

Regional Lymph Nodes (N)

N0	No nodal metastasis
N1	Regional lymph node meastasis

Distant Metastasis (M)

M0	No distant metastasis
M1	Distant metastasis

Stage Groupings

Stage 0	Tis N0 M0
Stage I	IA T1 N0 M0
	IB T2 N0 M0
Stage II	IIA T3 N0 M0
	IIB T1-3 N1 M0
Stage III	T4 N0-1 M0
Stage IV	T1-4 N0-1 M1

Abbreviations: CA, celiac axis; SMA, superior mesenteric artery
American Joint Committee on Cancer, 6th Edition[46]

EUS

When a pancreatic mass is found on CT scan, the next step should be, if indicated, performing EUS and fine needle aspiration (FNA) to obtain local tumor staging and tissue diagnosis.(Table 14–1) EUS is able to distinguish solid lesions from cystic lesions.

EUS can also define the tumor size, location, and possible vascular or lymph node involvement. (Figure 14–14, 14–15, 14–16, 14–17) Because ERCP with cytologic brushing has a low sensitivity (30–56%), the cytological specimen obtained by EUS-guided FNA not only helps differentiate between benign and malignant lesions seen on EUS alone, but also what type of the tumor it is. (Figures 14–18, 14–19, 14–20)

The diagnostic accuracy of EUS FNA for pancreatic cancer has been well established. A report from Mayo clinic showed the accuracy of EUS FNA to be 88%, sensitivity to be 86%, specificity to be 94%, a positive predictive value of 100%, and a negative predictive value of 86%.[23] In other reports, T-stage accuracy ranges from 78% to 94%, and N-stage varies from 64% to 82%.[24-29] Although earlier studies suggested that EUS was superior to CT, recent reports found that helical CT is more accurate for T-staging and equivalent for N-staging.[11] As described earlier, use of dual-phase post-injection image acquisition clearly improved staging accuracy for CT. Use of MDCT might have improved detection of smaller tumors. This advancement in CT imaging appears to have narrowed the difference. In a prospective blind study, using the surgical results as the gold standard, helical CT was superior to EUS and MRI in assessing locore-

FIGURE 14-17. The linear EUS exam shows a 4.02 × 3.50 cm hypoechoic mass with a mildly irregular border in the head of the pancreas. The portal vein is running into the mass. FNA confirmed adenocarcinoma: M: mass, PV: portal vein.

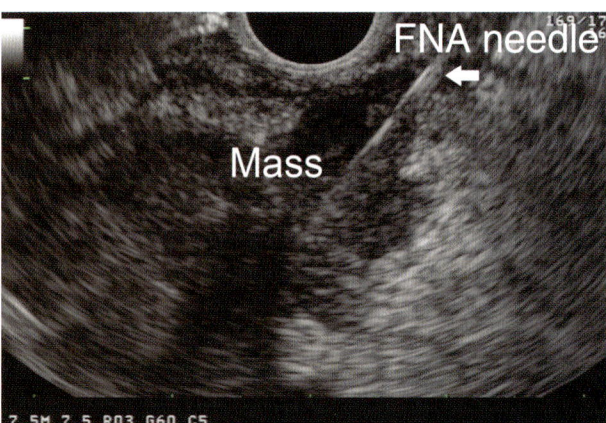

FIGURE 14–18. The linear EUS exam shows a large hypoechoic mass with an irregular border, with some hyperechoic strands in the head and neck of the pancreas. Without any signs of vascular or duodenal involvement, FNA confirmed pancreas lymphoma.

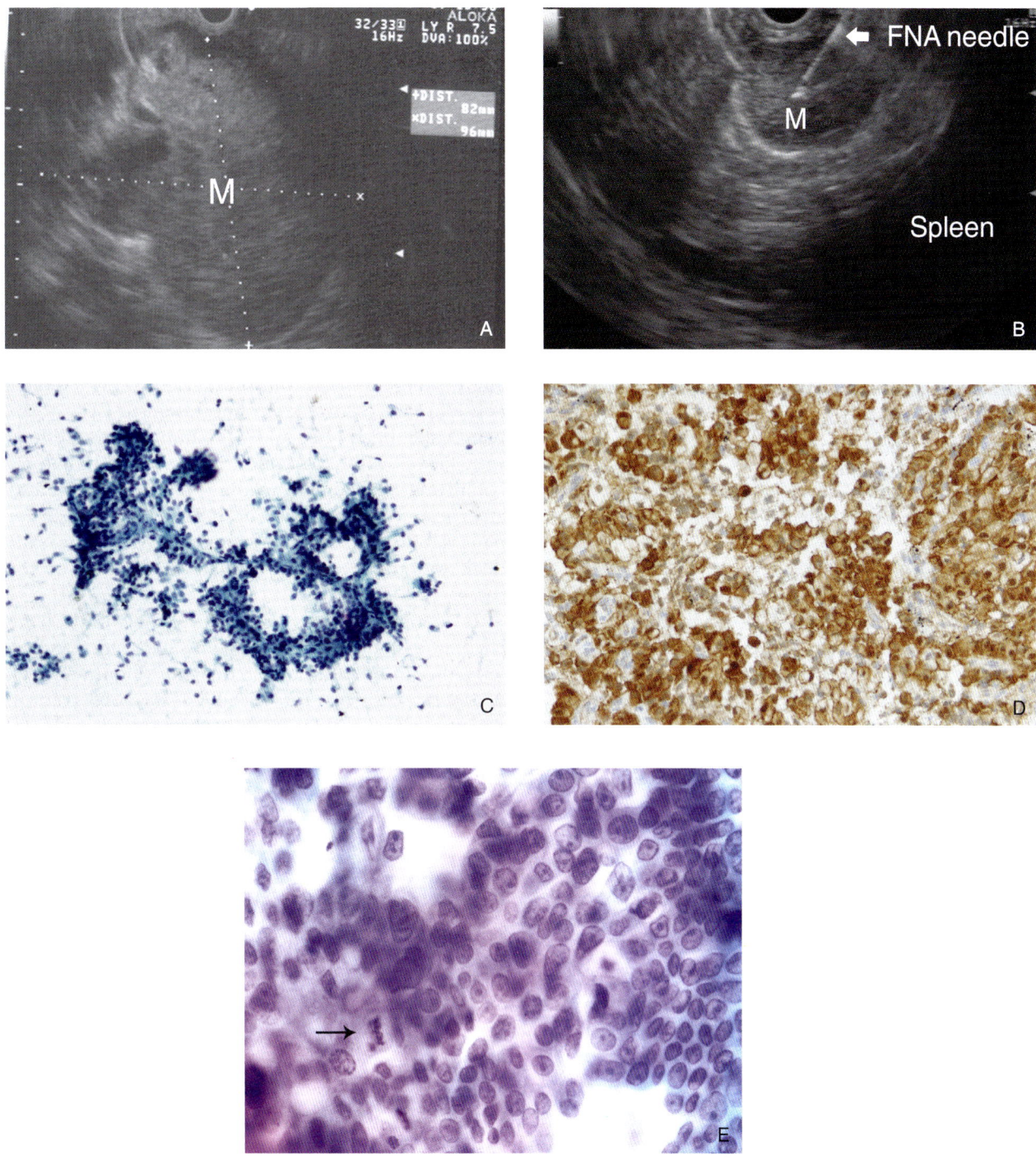

FIGURE 14–19. *A to E* (A) The linear EUS exam shows a large 8.2 × 9.6 cm hypoechoic mass with some hyperechoic and anechoic components and a regular border in the body of the pancreas. FNA confirmed pseudopapillary tumor of the pancreas: M: mass. (B) The linear EUS exam shows a hypoechoic mass with some hyperechoic component with a regular boder in the tail of the pancreas near the spleen. FNA confirmed pseudopapillary tumor of the pancreas. M: mass. (C) Solid-pseudopapillary tumor of the pancreas (Papanicoloau stain, 100x): Tumor cells are seen radiating from a central fibrovascular core creating a papillary-like appearance; cells farthest from the vessels lose cohesion and become the single cells seen in the background. (D) Solid-pseudopapillary tumor (histologic preparation, beta-catenin immunoperoxidase stain, 200×). Tumor cells demonstrate positive staining for beta-catenin. (E) Pancreatic Adenocarcinoma (Papanicolaou stained slide preparation, 300×): In contrast to the previous cytology slides (Figures 14–18 C and 14–18 D), this slide shows malignant ductal epithelium demonstrating significant nuclear overlap and crowding, variation in nuclear size volumes (exceeding a 4:1 ratio), nuclear contour irregularity and mitotic activity (arrow).

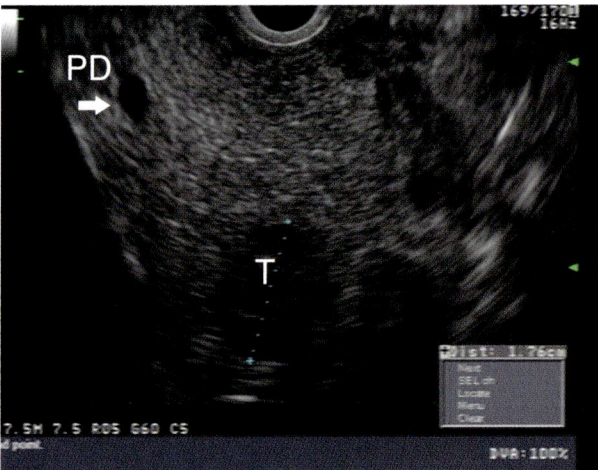

FIGURE 14–20. The linear EUS exam shows a 1.76 cm round hypoechoic mass with a regular border in the body of the pancreas without any major vascular involvement. FNA confirmed a pancreatic endocrine neoplasm: T: tumor, PD: pancreatic duct.

gional extension of the tumor (T-staging). Accuracy of EUS was at 62%; CT at 74%; MRI at 68%. For lymph node involvement (N-staging), the accuracy was reported as EUS at 65%, CT at 62%, and MRI at 61%. For vascular invasion, the accuracy was reported as EUS at 76%, CT at 83%, MRI at 74%, and angiography at 67%.[30] The T- and N-staging accuracy of EUS may be affected by peritumoral inflammation and large tumor size. However, EUS was reported to be still more sensitive than CT for detection of pancreatic masses smaller than 3 cm in diameter.[31] Mertz et al reported PET scanning having a sensitivity similar to that of EUS for the diagnosis of local pancreatic disease.[32] In this study, PET helped to clarify ambiguous CT findings and identified unsuspected metastases leading to avoidance of operation in five cases.

When assessing resectability, major vessels need to be carefully inspected. Again, the absolute contraindication for surgical resection at our institution is involvement of SMA or the celiac artery. EUS can easily assess the portal vein, SMV, splenic artery, splenic vein, celiac artery, and common hepatic artery. The SMA is, at times, difficult to completely assess by EUS.

Sensitivity for detecting vascular invasion and predicting surgical resectability has been greater than 90% in some studies.[24,25,33] However, the limitations of EUS in assessing vascular involvement were well described by Aslanian et al., where EUS had a sensitivity of 63%, specificity of 64%, positive predictive value (PPV) of 43%, and negative predictive value (NVP) of 80% for vascular adherence. The rates were 50%, 58%, 28%, and 82%, respectively for vascular invasion.[34] In this study, the authors found loss of echoplane to be a poor predictor of vascular involvement. Only 29% of cases with loss of echoplane alone had vascular adherence, and none had vascular invasion histologically.

FNA can be performed under CT or EUS guidance. EUS-guided FNA is more convenient for patients because it can be done along with EUS examination on the same day, as opposed to a two-step approach, with CT one day and CT-guided FNA on another day. EUS FNA is not without limitation; Volmar et al reported a false-positive rate of 0.3% and a false-negative rate of 14.3% for FNA of pancreatic neoplasia.[31]

EUS is challenging in the setting of surgically altered anatomy. Prior Bilroth II gastrectomy was once considered a relative contraindication to EUS of the pancreatic head. Lee and Topazian reported that, with linear echoendoscope, the pancreatic anatomy could well be defined including the inferior pancreatic head, ampulla, periampullary ducts, superior pancreatic head, and porta hepatis. The pancreatic neck was, however, only visualized in 60% of the cases.[35]

It is important to emphasize that underlying chronic pancreatitis (CP) presents a significant challenge because it affects EUS imaging (Figure 14–21). A lower sensitivity for EUS-FNA was observed in patients with CP than in those without CP (73.9 vs.

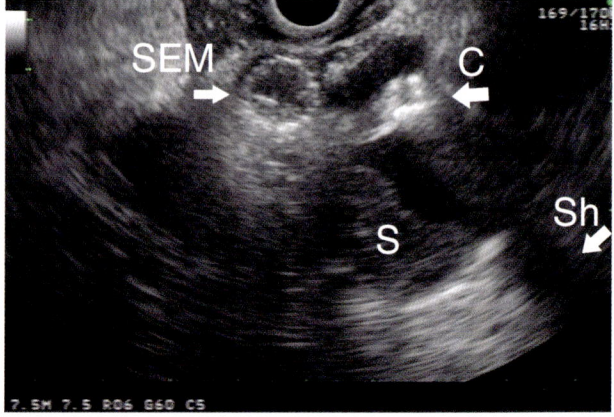

FIGURE 14–21. The linear EUS exam shows a hypoechoic mass with a cystic component in the head of the pancreas compressing on the distal bile duct causing obstructive jaundice. The patient had a metal biliary stent placement at an outside facility before coming to MD Anderson Cancer Center. A small calcification within the mass is casting a classic shadow: FNA showed marked inflammation without any malignant cells; the clinical history along with the imaging studies and cytology finding was consistent with chronic pancreatitis: SEM: self-expanding metal stent, C: calcification, S: solid componet in the mass, Sh: shadow from calcification.

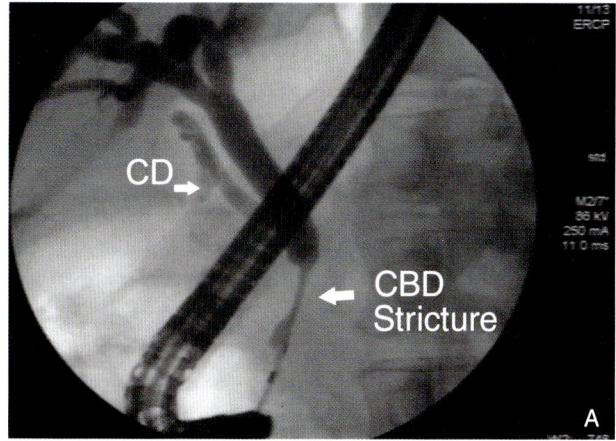 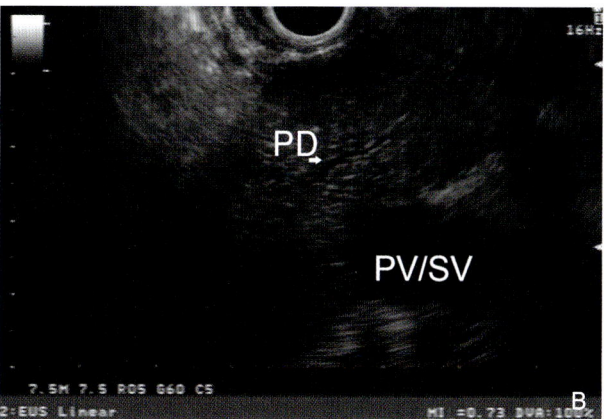

FIGURE 14–22. *A and B* (A) The cholangiogram shows a 1 cm stricture in the common bile duct of intrapancreatic segment with prestenotic mild dilation. CD: cystic duct, CBD: common bile duct. The biliary brushing was negative for malignant cells. (B) The linear EUS exam in the same patient as in Figure 14–21 A shows a diffusely hypoechoic, enlarged pancreas with thin, irregular, tortuous pancreatic duct. The immunoglobulin G subclass 4 (Ig G4) was markedly elevated. These findings and clinical course were consistent with autoimmune pancreatitis. PD: pancreatic duct, PV: portal vein, SV: splenic vein.

91.3%; p = 0.02). However, no significant difference was noted for specificity (100 vs. 93.8%), PPV (100 vs. 99.5%), and accuracy (91.5 vs. 91.4%).[36] In the study by Mertz et al, chronic pancreatitis impaired accuracy, leading to two false-negative results by EUS and PET.[32] Autoimmune pancreatitis can present with obstructive jaundice and questionable mass in CT or EUS (Figure 14–22). Restaging after neoadjuvant therapy is also limited because EUS cannot distinguish a tumor from post-treatment effects.

General Limitations and Complications of EUS

The potential complications of EUS include bleeding, perforation, pancreatitis, abdominal pain, infection, sedation related issues, etc... Nonetheless, in experienced hands, the complication rate in EUS-FNA of solid pancreatic masses was found to be similar to that of upper endoscopy.[37] The most clinically relevant adverse events occur within a week of the procedure.

In a prospective study of 355 patients, the overall complication rate was reported to be 2.54% with 0 mortality; the complications were acute pancreatitis, abdominal pain, fever, and oversedation.[37] The risk of pancreatitis after EUS-FNA of the pancreas was reported to be 0.29 (retrospective study), −0.85 % (prospective study), as opposed to 3% by percutaneous FNA of the pancreas.[38-40]

Other important potential limitations include operator-dependency, need for adequate sedation, length of the procedure (compared to CT scan), need for an experienced gastrointestinal cytologist, and the limited availability of EUS in the community.

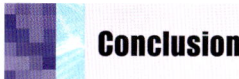

Conclusion

With ongoing development of new and improved tools and technology, there has been a giant leap in accuracy and efficiency in diagnosing and staging of pancreatic malignancy. This success was possible with CT or MRI, and EUS each playing a complimentary role in achieving the same goal, that is, prompt and accurate diagnosis and staging without having patients undergo surgical exploration. These imaging modalities will continue to advance and contribute to optimizing management of pancreatic cancer. While, EUS FNA has been utilized more as a diagnostic tool, the future of EUS-guided therapy of pancreatic cancer has promising potential. Chang et al has already reported delivering allogeneic mixed lymphocyte culture by EUS-guided fine needle injection (EUS-FNI) directly into advanced pancreatic cancer.[41] Sangro et al also reported injection of Ad.IL-12 (an adenovirus encoding interleukin-12), an adenoviral vector that expresses the human interleukin-12 in patients with advanced pancreatic cancer.[42] Hecht et al examined the feasibility, tolerability, and efficacy of ONYX-015 (an E1B-55kD gene-deleted replication-selective adenovirus) delivered by EUS FNI into the primary pancreatic tumor in conjunction with intravenous gemcitabine in patients with advanced pancreatic cancer; partial response was observed.[43] In a multicenter trial, TNFerade, a replication-deficient adenoviral vector containing the human tumor necrosis factor-alpha gene, was delivered by EUS FNI (or percutaneously) into locally advanced pancreatic cancer with concurrent chemoradiation.[44] Lastly, Matthes et al., investigated EUS FNI of OncoGel (ReGel/paclitaxel, a new formulation for intralesional injection of paclitaxel); EUS-FNI of OncoGel into the pancreas of Yorkshire pigs provided high and sustained localized concentrations of paclitaxel.[45] EUS FNI of chemotherapeutic agents into advanced pancreatic cancer facilitates achievement of therapeutic tissue levels of the agents with only minimal systemic toxicity. As failure in the treatment of pancreatic cancer often stems from the systemic nature of the disease, intralesional injection of an anti-tumor agent, when used alone, is not likely to bring a significant benefit. However, as it has occurred in the history of endoscopic retrograde cholangiopancreatography, the utility of UES will continue to move from the realm of diagnostic modality to therapeutic application. We look forward to seeing new advances and applications for EUS in the near future.

References

1. Jemal, A., Siegel, R., Ward, E., et al.: Cancer Statistics, 2008. CA Cancer J Clin., 2008; 58:71.
2. Kim, T., Murakami, T., Takahashi, S., et al.: Pancreatic CT imaging: effects of different injection rates and doses of contrast material. Radiology 1999;212(1): 219–225.
3. Schueller, G., Schima, W., Schueller-Weidekamm, C., et al.: Multidetector CT of pancreas: effects of contrast material flow rate and individualized scan delay on enhancement of pancreas and tumor contrast. Radiology 2006;241(2):441–448.
4. Tublin, M. E., Tessler, F. N., Cheng, S. L., et al.: Effect of injection rate of contrast medium on pancreatic and hepatic helical CT. Radiology 1999;210(1):97–101.
5. Fletcher, J. G., Wiersema, M. J., Farrell, M. A., et al.: Pancreatic malignancy: value of arterial, pancreatic, and hepatic phase imaging with multi-detector row CT. Radiology 2003;229(1):81–90.
6. Clark, L. R., Jaffe, M. H., Choyke, P. L., et al.: Pancreatic imaging. Radiol Clin North Am 1985;23(3):489–501.
7. Lu, D. S., Vedantham, S., Krasny, R. M., et al.: Two-phase helical CT for pancreatic tumors pancreatic versus hepatic phase enhancement for tumor, pancreas and vascular structures. Radiology 1996;199(3):697–701.
8. Gangi, S., Fletcher, J. G., Nathan, M. A., et al.: Time interval between abnormalities seen on CT and the clinical diagnosis of pancreatic cancer: retrospective review of CT scans obtained before diagnosis. Am J Roentgenol 2004;182(4):897–903.
9. Kim, T., Murakami, T., Takamura, M., et al.: Pancreatic mass due to chronic pancreatitis: correlation of CT and MR imaging features with pathologic findings. Am J Roentgenol 2001;177(2):367–71.
10. Agarwal, B., Abu-Hamda, E., Molke, K. L., et al.: Endoscopic ultrasound-guided fine needle aspiration and multidetector spiral CT in the diagnosis of pancreatic cancer. Am J Gastroenterol 2004;99(5):844–850.
11. DeWitt, J., Devereaux, B., Chriswell, M., et al.: Comparison of endoscopic ultrasound and multidetector computed tomography for the detection and staging of pancreatic cancer. Ann Intern Med 2004;141: 753–763.
12. Bronstein, Y. L., Loyer, E. M., Kaur, H., et al.: Detection of small pancreatic tumors with multiphasic helical CT. Am J Roentgenol 2004;182(3):619–623.
13. Pancreas. In Sobin, L., Wittekind, C., eds.: TNM classification of malignant tumors. Baltimore: Wiley-Liss, 2002:93–96.
14. Lu, D. S., Reber, H. A., Krasny, R. M., et al.: Local staging of pancreatic cancer: criteria for unresectability of major vessels as revealed by pancreatic-phase, thin-section helical CT. Am J Roentgenol 1997;168(6): 1439–1443.
15. Valls, C., Andia, E., Sanchez, A., et al.: Dual-phase helical CT of pancreatic adenocarcinoma: assessment of resectability before surgery. Am J Roentgenol 2002; 178(4):821–826.
16. Pisters, P. W., Lee, J. E., Vauthey, J. N., et al.: Laparoscopy in the staging of pancreatic cancer. Br J Surg 2001; 88(3):325–337.
17. Ly, J. N., Miller, F. H.: MR imaging of the pancreas: a practical approach. Radiol Clin North Am 2002; 40(6):1289–1306.
18. Fayad, L. M., Mitchell, D. G.: Magnetic resonance imaging of pancreatic adenocarcinoma. Int J Gastrointest Cancer 2001;30(1-2):19–25.
19. Pamuklar, E., Semelka, R. C.: MR imaging of the pancreas. Magnetic Resonance Imaging Clinics of North America 2005;13(2):313–330.
20. Adamek, H. E., Albert, J., Breer, H., et al.: Pancreatic cancer detection with magnetic resonance cholangiopancreatography and endoscopic retrograde cholangiopancreatography: a prospective controlled study. Lancet 2000;356(9225):190–193.
21. Arslan, A., Buanes, T., Geitung, J. T.: Pancreatic carcinoma: MR, MR angiography and dynamic helical CT in the evaluation of vascular invasion. Eur J Radiol 2001;38(2):151–159.
22. Gandhi, S. N., Brown, M. A., Wong, J. G., et al.: MR contrast agents for liver imaging: what, when, how. Radiographics 2006;26(6):1621–1636.
23. Wiersema, M. J., Vilmann, P., Giovannini, M., et al.: Endosonography-guided fine-needle aspiration biopsy: diagnostic accuracy and complication assessment. Gastroenterology 1997;112(4):1087–1095.
24. Gress, F., Hawes, R. H., Savides, T. J., et al.: Role of EUS in the preoperative staging of pancreatic cancer: a large single-center experience. Gastrointest Endosc 1999;50:786–791.
25. Palazzo, L., Roseau, G., Gayer, B., et al.: Endoscopio ultrasonography in the diagnosis and staging of pancreatic adencarcinoma. Endoscopy 1993;25:143–150.
26. Tio, T. L., Tytgat, G. N., Cikot, R. J., et al.: Ampullopancreatic carcinoma: preoperative TNM classification with endosonography. Radiology 1990;175:455–461.
27. Grimm, H., Maydeo, A., Soehendra, N.: Endoluminal ultrasound for the diagnosis and staging of pancreatic cancer. Baillieres Clin Gastgroenterol 1990;4:869–887.
28. Muller, M. F., Meyenberger, C., Bertschinger, P., et al.: Pancreatic tumors: evaluation with endoscopic US, CT, and MR imaging. Radiology 1994;190:745–751.
29. Yasuda, K., Mukai, H., Nakajima, M., et al.: Staging of pancreatic carcinoma by endoscopic ultrasonography. Endoscopy. 1993;25:151–155.
30. Soriano, A., Castells, A., Ayuso, C., et al.: Preoperative staging and tumor resectability assessment of pancreatic cancer: prospective study comparing endoscopic ultra-

sonography, helical computed tomography, magnetic resonante imaging, and angiography. Am J Gastroenterol 2004;99:492–501.
31. Volmar, K., Vollmer, R., Jowell, P., et al.: Pancreatic FNA in 1000 cases: a comparison of imaging modalities. Gastrointest Endosc 2005;61(7):854–861.
32. Mertz, H., Sechopoulos, P., Delbeke, D., et al.: EUS, PET, and CT scanning for evaluation of pancreatic adenocarcinoma. Gastrointest Endosc 2000;52:367–371
33. Rosch, T., Braig, C., Gain, T., et al.: Staging of pancreatic and ampullary carcinoma by endoscopic ultrasonography. Gastroenterology 1992;102:188–199.
34. Aslanian, H., Salem, R., Lee, J. H,. et al.: EUS diagnosis of vascular invasion in pancreatic cancer: Surgical and histologic correlates. Am J Gastroenterol. 2005;100: 1381–1385.
35. Lee, J. H., Topazian, M.: Pancreatic Endosonography after Billroth II Gastrectomy. Endoscopy. 2004;36(11): 972–975.
36. Varadarajulu, S., Tamhane, A., Eloubeidi, M.: Yield of EUS-guided FNA of pancreatic masses in the presence or the absence of chronic pancreatitis. Gastrointest Endosc 2005;62(5):728–736.
37. Eloubeidi, M. A., Chen, V. K., Eltoum, I. A., et al.: Endoscopic ultrasound-guided fine needle aspiration biopsy of patients with suspected pancreatic cancer: diagnostic accuracy and acute and 30-day complications. Am J Gastroenterol 2003;98:37. 2663–2668.
38. Eloubeidi, M. A., Tamhane, A., Varadarajulu, S., et al.: Frequency of major complications after EUS-guided FNA of solid pancreatic masses: a prospective evaluation. Gastrointest Endosc 2006;63(4):622–629.
39. Eloubeidi, M. A., Gress, F. G., Savides, T. J., et al.: Acute pancreatitis after EUS-guided FNA of solid pancreatic masses: a pooled analysis from EUS centers in the United States. Gastrointest Endosc 1998;48:18–25.
40. Mueller, P. R., Miketic, L. M., Simeone, J. F., et al.: Severe acute pancreatitis after percutaneous biopsy of the pancreas. Am J Roentgenol 1988;15:493–494.
41. Chang, K. J., Nguyen, P. T., Thompson, J. A., et al.: Phase I Clinical Trial of Allogeneic Mixed Lymphocyte Culture (Cytoimplant) Delivered by Endoscopic Ultrasound-Guided Fine-Needle Injection in Patients with Advanced Pancreatic Carcinoma. Cancer 2000; 88(6):1325–1335.
42. Sangro, B., Mazzolini, G., Ruiz, J., et al.: Phase I Trial of Intratumoral Injection of an Adenovirus Encoding Interleukin-12 for Advanced Digestive Tumors. Journal Clin Oncology 2004;22(8):1389–1397.
43. Hecht, J. R., Bedford, R., Abbruzzese, J. L., et al.: A phase I/II trial of intratumoral endoscopic ultrasound injection of ONYX-015 with intravenous gemcitabine in unresectable pancreatic carcinoma. Clin Cancer Res 2003;9(2):555–561.
44. Farrell, J. J., Senzer, N., Hecht, J. R., et al.: Long-Term Data for Endoscopic Ultrasound (EUS) and Percutaneous (PTA) Guided Intratumoral TNFerade Gene Delivery Combined with Chemoradiation in the Treatment of Locally Advanced Pancreatic Cancer (LAPC) Gastrointest Endosc 2006;63(5):AB580
45. Matthes, K., Mino-Kenudson, M., Sahani, V., et al.: EUS-guided injection of paclitaxel (OncoGel) provides therapeutic drug concentrations in the porcine pancreas. Gastrointest Endosc 2007;65(3):448–453.
46. Exocrine pancreas. In American Joint Committee on Cancer: AJCC Cancer Staging Manual. New York: Springer, 2002, 6th ed., pp. 157-164.

CHAPTER 15

Pancreatic Neuroendocrine Tumors

Dr. John C. Deutsch

Neuroendocrine tumors are interesting neoplastic lesions that can be benign or malignant, hormonally active or inactive, symptomatic or asymptomatic. Although uncommon, when they occur, they often originate in the pancreas. EUS has been an important modality in the evaluation of pancreatic and peripancreatic neuroendocrine tumors for many years, particularly following the multicenter report by Rosch, et al in 1992[1] about the value of EUS in the evaluation of these lesions. In that report, EUS localized 32 of 39 neuroendocrine tumors not identified by previous imaging.

EUS FNA allows one to obtain tissue confirmation of the diagnosis. For example, Figure 15–1 shows diagnostic immunohistochemistry using synaptophysin on tissue obtained during EUS FNA from a cystic pancreatic tumor (EUS image shown in Figure 15–14).

In the past, neuroendocrine tumors of the pancreas were often first brought to medical attention due to syndromes related to the ectopic production of hormones, including insulin, gastrin, glucogon, and vasoactive intestinal peptide. Possibly due to better imaging and the availability of EUS, the incidence of nonfunctioning tumors seems to be increasing. For instance, a review of the University of Pittsburg experience by Jani et al reported only 4 of the 22 pancreatic neuroendocrine tumors evaluated in the two previous years were functional.[2]

In general, neuroendocrine tumors are found by EUS in three circumstances:

1) When a previous imaging study (generally a CT scan or ultrasound) has identified a mass lesion
2) With an incidental finding during EUS evaluation for some other reason
3) During evaluation of a suspected ectopic hormone syndrome (generally for insulinomas and gastrinomas)

Neuroendocrine tumors can occur in any part of the pancreas. As a rule, tumors seem to occur more frequently in the head of the pancreas[3] although some literature suggests certain subtypes (VIPoma, glucogonoma) are more frequent in the tail.[4,5] Gastrinomas seem to primarily occur in the pancreas or duodenum in an area known as the gastrinoma triangle[6] (Figure 15–2), which is an anatomic area defined by the junction of the cystic and common bile ducts superiorly, the junction of the second and third portions of the duodenum inferiorly, and the junction of the neck and body of the pancreas medially.

Therefore, when evaluating a patient for neuroendocrine tumors, it is important to perform a complete EUS evaluation of the pancreas from the tip of the tail near the splenic hilum (Figure 15–3) through the uncinate process at the point that the superior mesenteric artery crosses the duodenum (Figures 15–4, 15–5) as well as a close inspection of the intestinal lumen. Peripancreatic adenopathy and liver lesions should also be sought.

Neuroendocrine tumors are generally round and tend to be hypoechoic with well-defined margins (see images that follow). This chapter shows examples of neuroendocrine tumors using various EUS instruments, including the Olympus GFUM30 and GFUM130 rotating radial array and ALOKA GFUE 160 and GFUE-140p equipment, as well as the Pentax FG35UX and EG3630 series of solid-state radial and linear array echoendoscopes.

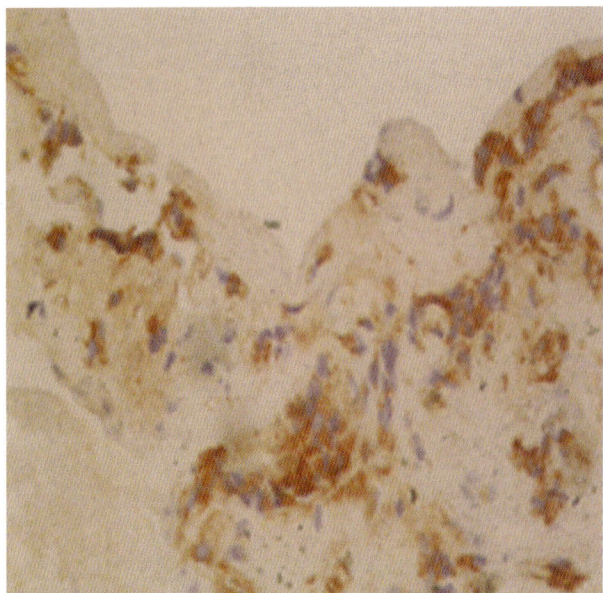

FIGURE 15–1. Synaptophysin staining of cells obtained from a cystic pancreatic lesion (See Figure 15–14)

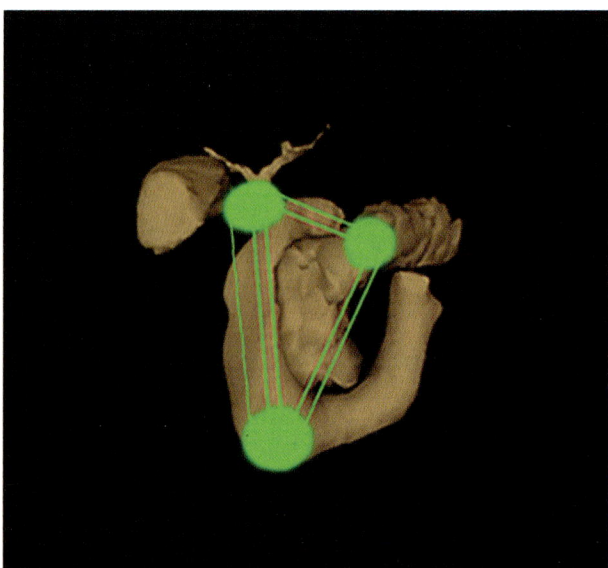

FIGURE 15–2. Visible Human Data Set model of duodenum, pancreas, and biliary tree. The green dots outline the "gastrinoma triangle."

Pancreatic Neuroendocrine Tumors   167

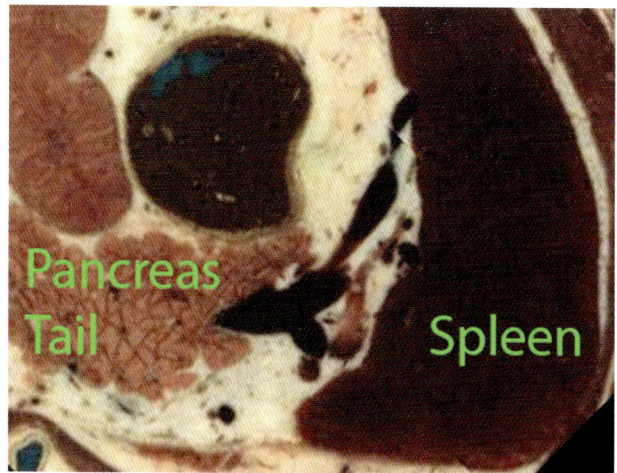

FIGURE 15–3. Visible Human Data Set image of pancreas tail and splenic hilum

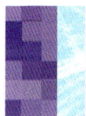 **LOCALIZED FUNCTIONAL PANCREATIC NEUROENDOCRINE TUMORS**

Figures 15–6 - 15–9 demonstrate two examples of insulinomas identified during evaluations for hypoglycemia. Neither were visualized by previous CT

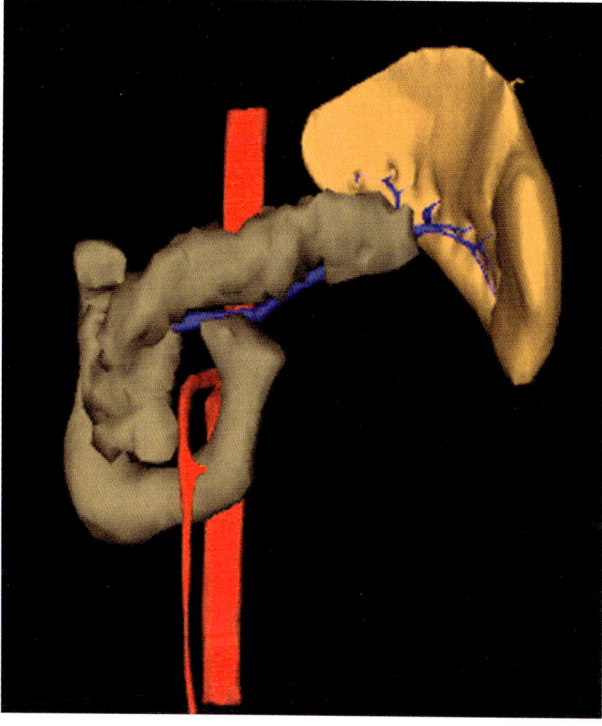

FIGURE 15–5. Visible Human Data Set model of pancreas, spleen, duodenum, aorta and superior mesenteric artery

scans. The first case (Figures 15–6, 15–7) is a 1 cm tumor found adjacent to the splenic artery found during an investigation for hypoglycemia, elevated insulin, and C-peptide levels, and low beta-hydroxybutyrate and sulfonourea levels. The second case (Figures 15–8, 15–9) shows a 2.2 cm tumor found in the tail of the pancreas during an evaluation of fasting hypoglycemia. This patient had elevated insulin levels in pancreatic venous drainage. As shown, these tumors are round and hypoechoic as expected for insulinomas. In both patients, removal of the tumors resolved the hypoglycemia.

Two examples of neuroendocrine tumors found in patients with elevated serum glucogon levels are shown in Figures 15–10 and 15–11. Each tumor was

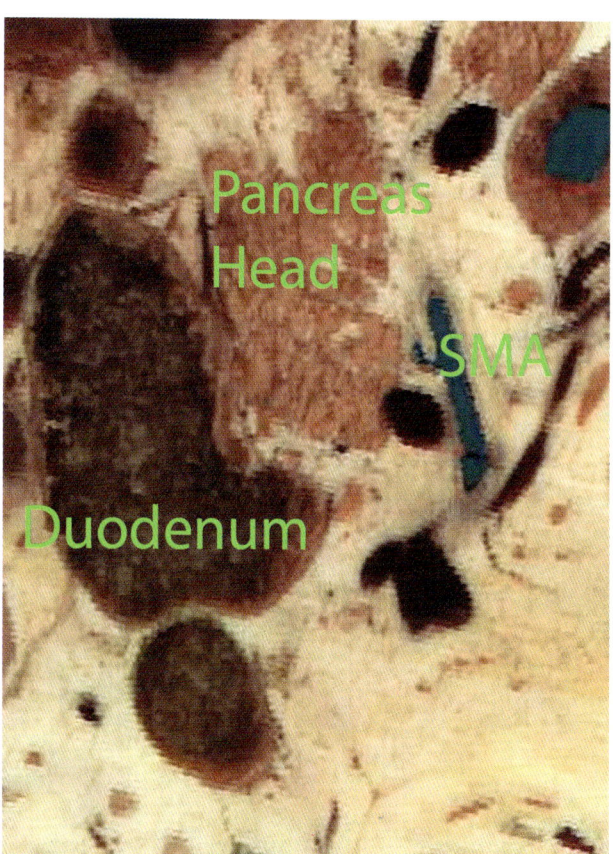

FIGURE 15–4. Visible Human Data Set image of pancreas head, superior mesenteric artery (SMA), and duodenum

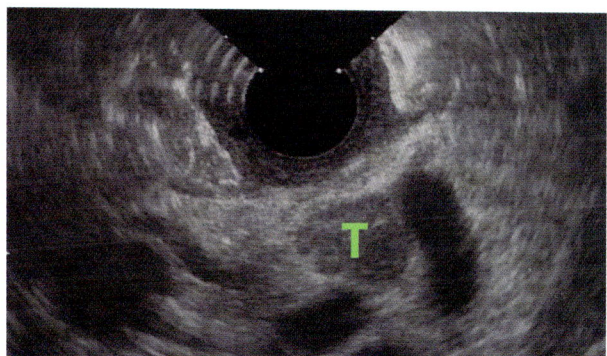

FIGURE 15–6. Radial EUS of an insulinoma (T) in the body of the pancreas against the splenic artery

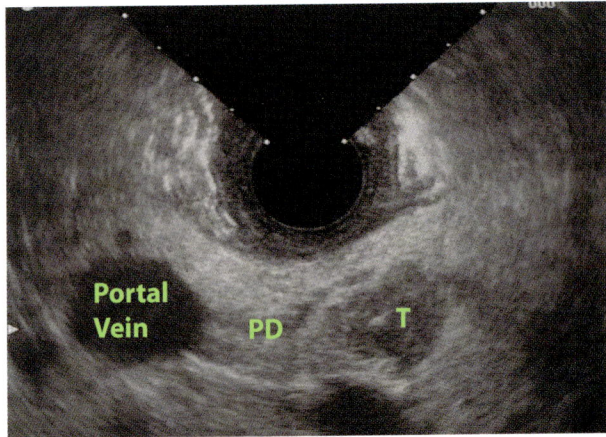

FIGURE 15–7. A radial EUS image of the same patient in Figure 15-6 showing the insulinoma (T) as it relates to the portal confluence and pancreatic duct (PD).

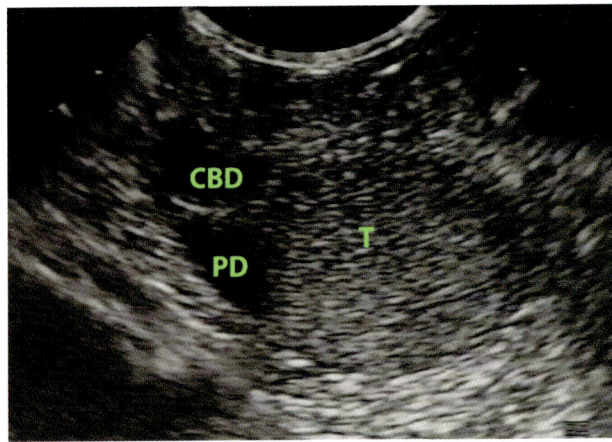

FIGURE 15–10. Linear EUS view of pancreatic head showing a glucagonoma (T) against the common bile duct (CBD) and pancreatic duct (PD). Image courtesy of Dr John Bosco, Brunswick Gastroenterology Associates, Brunswick, ME.

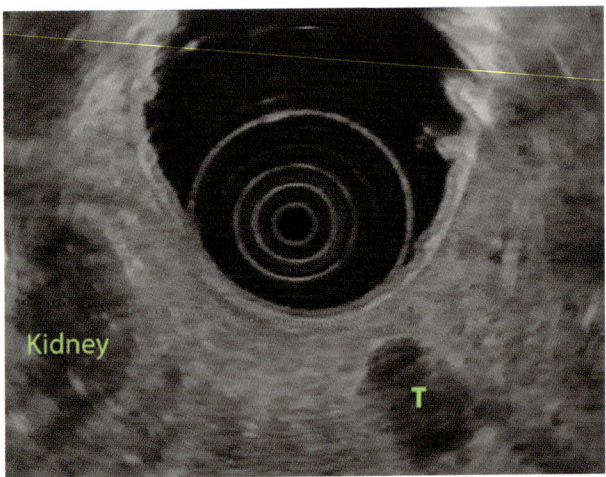

FIGURE 15–8. A radial EUS image of an insulinoma (T) in the tail of the pancreas

approximately 2 cm in size and they were found in the head and tail of the pancreas respectively. Both subjects were identified during CT evaluations for abdominal pain. Neither patient had necrolytic migratory erythema, (a crusty, blistering rash typical of glucogonoma,[7] although both patients had glucose intolerance.

LOCALIZED NONFUNCTIONAL PANCREATIC NEUROENDOCRINE TUMORS

As mentioned earlier, nonfunctioning tumors appear to be much more common than functioning tumors. A variety of presentations are shown below.

Figure 15–12 shows a 1 cm lesion in the head of the pancreas. This tumor came to attention during a

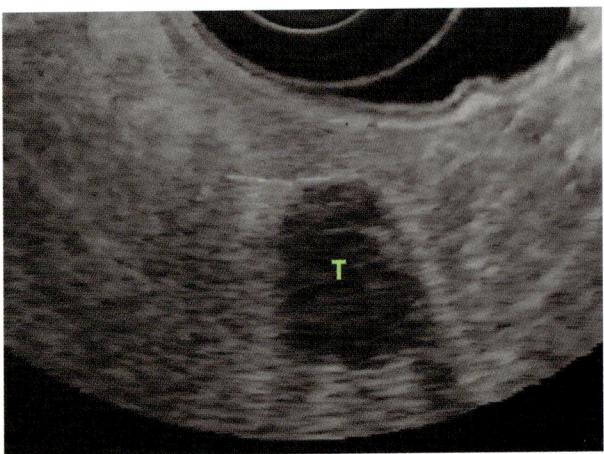

FIGURE 15–9. A close-up radial EUS view of the insulinoma (T) in Figure 15–8

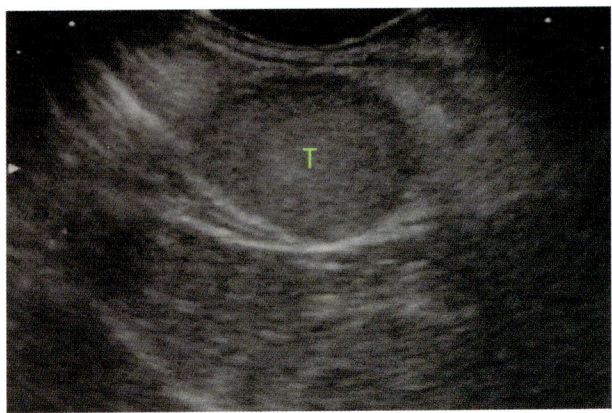

FIGURE 15–11. Linear array view of pancreas body showing a glucagonoma (T)

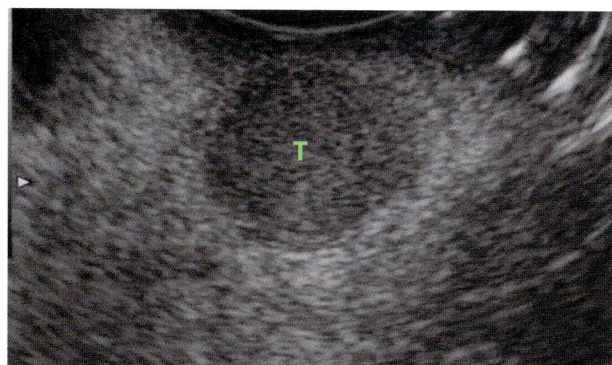

FIGURE 15–12. Linear EUS image of a 1 cm pancreatic head nonfunctioning neuroendocrine tumor (T).

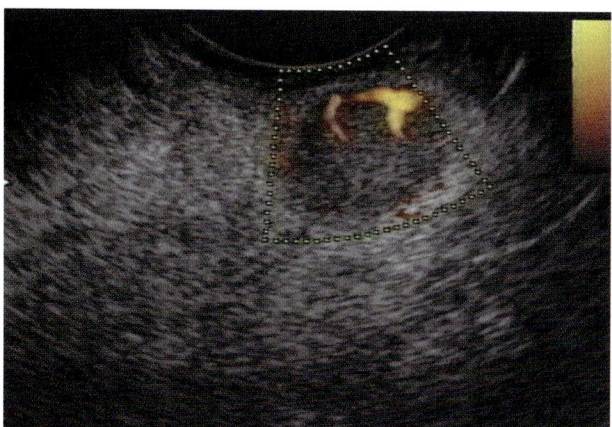

FIGURE 15–13. Color Doppler of the tumor in Figure 15–12 showing vascular flow

screening abdominal ultrasound performed by the patient's primary provider. The patient had requested the ultrasound because her friend had just been diagnosed with a liver tumor. The vascular nature of this neuroendocrine tumor can be appreciated by the color Doppler image (Figure 15–13).

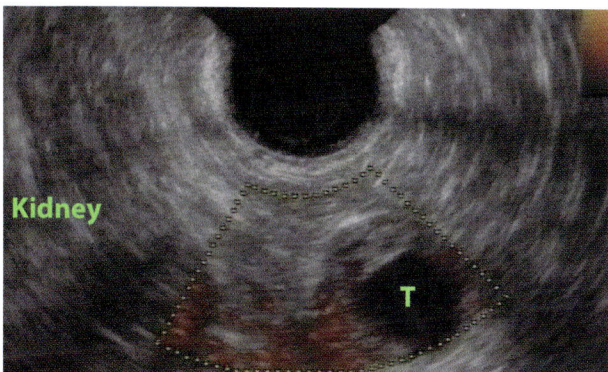

FIGURE 15–14. Radial EUS with color Doppler image of a 2 cm cystic nonfunctioning neuroendocrine tumor (T) of the pancreas tail. FNA from this lesion is shown in Figure 15–1.

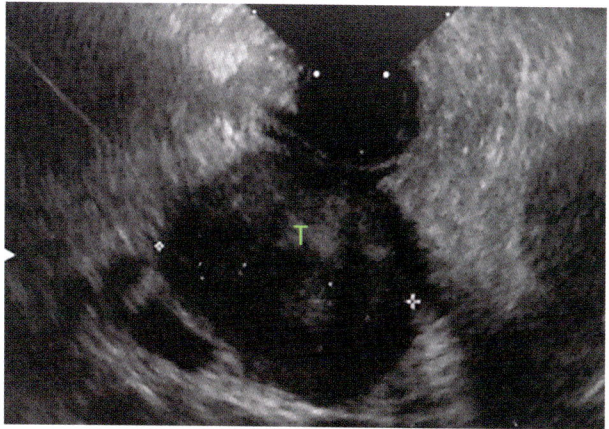

FIGURE 15–15. Radial EUS image of a 3 cm nonfunctioning neuroendocrine tumor (T). Lymph node metastasis were present at the time of surgery.

Neuroendocrine tumors can undergo cystic degeneration. Figure 15–14 shows an example of a 2 cm cystic/solid lesion in the pancreatic tail. Lack of persistant Doppler flow suggested this was not a vascular process. The lesion was aspirated by EUS (Video 15–1) and revealed a neoplastic process. The immunohistochemistry demonstrated synaptophysin reactivity, consistent with neuroendocrine origin (Figure 15–1).

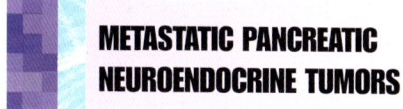

METASTATIC PANCREATIC NEUROENDOCRINE TUMORS

Prognosis worsens and frequency of metastasis seem to increase as tumors enlarge.[8] The following examples show tumors that were each approximately 3 cm in size with localregional or systemic metastasis. The patient with the tumor shown in Figure 15-15 was found during surgery to have nodal metastasis, which

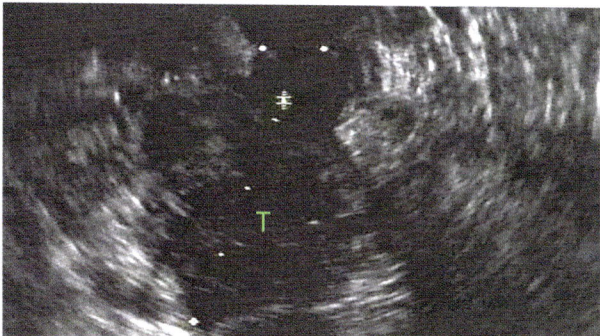

FIGURE 15–16. Radial EUS image of a 3 cm nonfunctioning neuroendocrine tumor (T). A 5 mm liver lesion was seen during EUS and biopsied, showing metastatic disease.

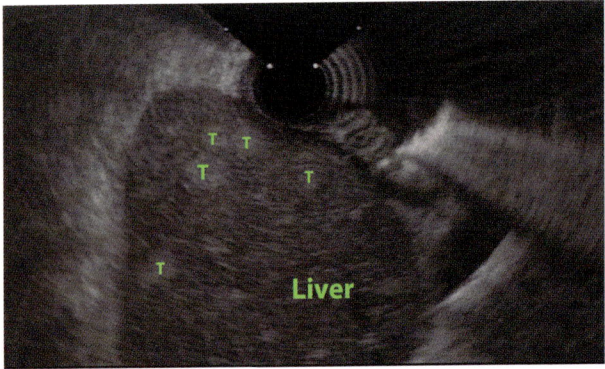

FIGURE 15–17. Radial EUS of the liver showing multiple metastasis of a neuroendocrine tumor (T). A primary site was not positively identified but the patient was found to have a 5 mm lesion in the pancreas Figure 15–18.

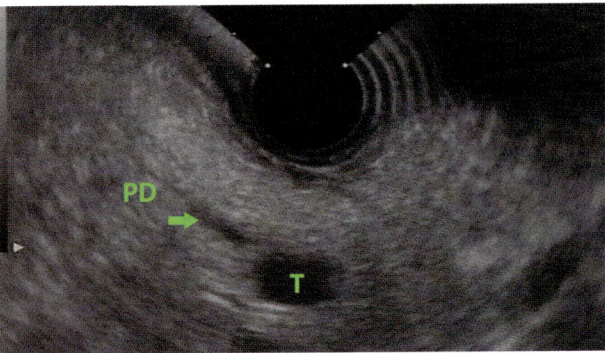

FIGURE 15–18. Radial EUS of the pancreas showing a 5 mm lesion (T) that was not biopsied adjacent to the pancreatic duct (PD). The patient presented with multiple liver lesions, shown in Figure 15–17.

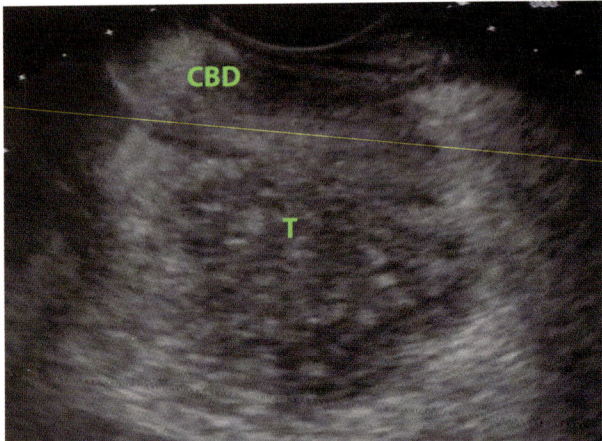

FIGURE 15–19. Linear EUS of the pancreatic head showing a mass (T), which was found to have small cell carcinoma and was obstructing the common bile duct (CBD).

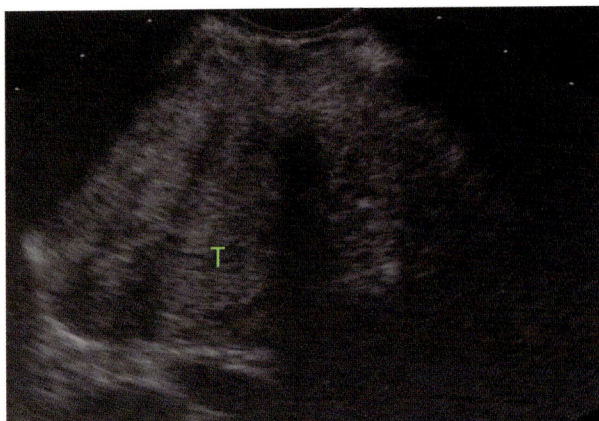

FIGURE 15–20. Linear EUS of an 8cm tumor (T) found in a young patient during imaging following a motor vehicle accident. Involved lymph nodes were found at the time of surgery.

were not apparent during the EUS evaluation. The irregularly shaped tumor shown in Figure 15–16 was found to have a 5 mm metastatic focus in the liver during the initial EUS, which was confirmed by FNA.

Figure 15–17 shows an example of another patient with extensive small liver metastasis from a neuroendocrine tumor. A primary site was never positively identified in this patient, although there was a 0.5 cm pancreatic body lesion discovered, as shown in Figure 15–18, which was not biopsied.

A very aggressive neuroendocrine tumor in the head of the pancreas is shown in Figure 15–19. This patient presented with biliary obstruction. Histology showed small-cell carcinoma. During the EUS examination, unsuspected enlarged subcarinal lymph nodes were found and biopsied. These also contained small-cell carcinoma. This suggested the disease was likely metastatic to the pancreas from an occult pulmonary primary. A primary pancreatic small-cell cancer is also possible, but much less common.

On occasion, the primary tumor is quite large and without evident symptoms. Figure 15–20 shows a tumor identified in a 37-year-old patient during evaluation for blunt abdominal trauma. The pancreatic head tumor is so large (8 cm) that if fills the entire field of view. Video 15–2 better shows the extent of this tumor adjacent to the common bile duct and gastroduodenal artery. The patient had endoscopic evidence of duodenal compression (Figure 15–21).

LUMINAL NEUROENDOCRINE TUMORS

Neuroendocrine tumors can present as masses adjacent to the pancreas. This can be due to nodal involvement. Figure 15–22 shows a tumor found next

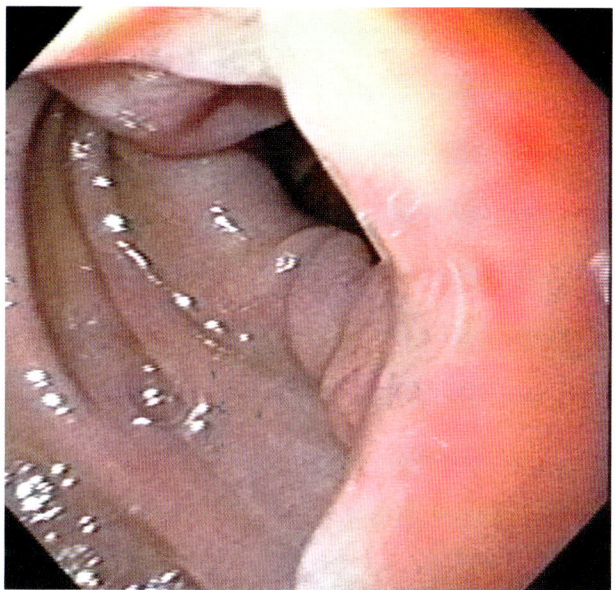

FIGURE 15–21. Endoscopy from the patient shown in Figure 15–20. The duodenum is compressed by this tumor.

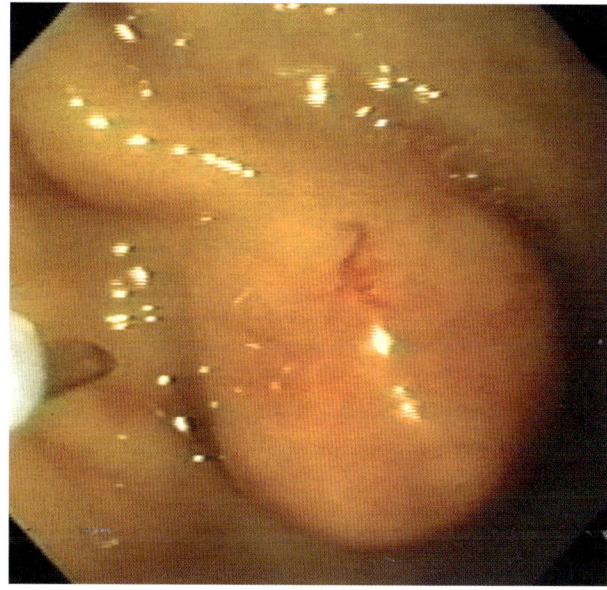

FIGURE 15–23. Endoscopic view of a 1 cm gastric carcinoid

to the third part of the duodenum. Neuroendocrine features were confirmed by FNA. This patient had undergone resection of an ileal carcinoid tumor 10 years earlier and this peripancreatic mass was felt to be a nodal metastasis.

Neuroendocrine tumors in the upper abdomen including carcinoids or gastrinomas, will on occasion be found in the gastrointestinal wall. Figure 15–23 shows a gastric nodule, which was biopsied and shown to be a carcinoid tumor. EUS revealed the lesion to be 1 cm in diameter and confined to the upper layer of the stomach (Figure 15–24). No metastasis were identified. Endoscopic removal was attempted, but the tumor did not lift away from the muscularis propria. Therefore laparoscopic resection was performed.

Figure 15–25 shows a small duodenal bulbar lesion. Biopsies revealed a carcinoid tumor. EUS showed this to be 3 mm in size, superficial and away from the gastroduodenal artery (Figure 15–26). Endoscopic removal was performed, and the patient is now 24 months from the resection with no evidence of reoccurance.

Figure 15–27 shows a duodenal neuroendocrine tumor that was found during evaluation for gastrinoma syndrome. EUS demonstrated an isolated duodenal mass and an unremarkable pancreas (Figure 15–28). The duodenal lesion was removed, and the symptoms of gastrinoma disappeared.

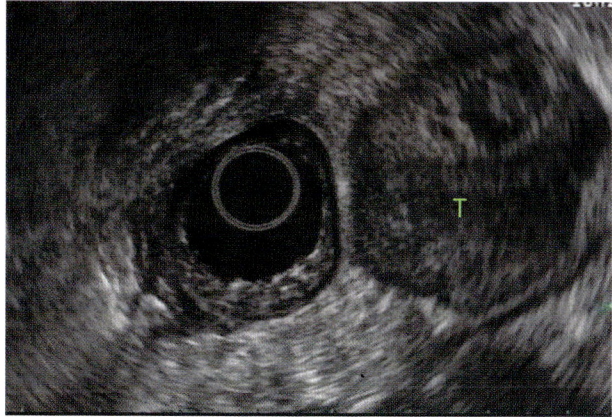

FIGURE 15–22. Radial EUS of a peripancreatic neuroendocrine tumor (T) near the third part of the duodenum. The patient had an ileal carcinoid removed 10 years earlier, and this was suspected to be a metastatic lymph node.

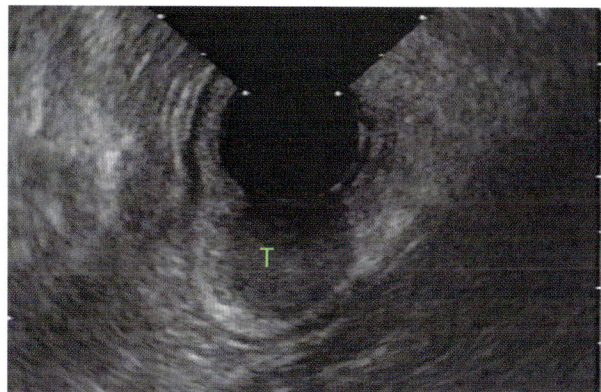

FIGURE 15–24. Radial EUS of the gastric carcinoid (T) shown in Figure 15–23

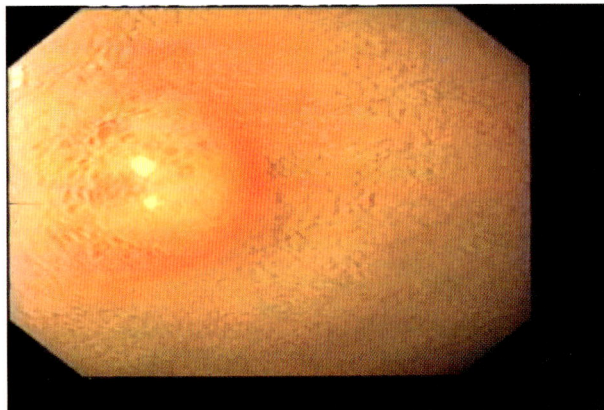

FIGURE 15–25. Endoscopic view of a 4 mm duodenal carcinoid (T)

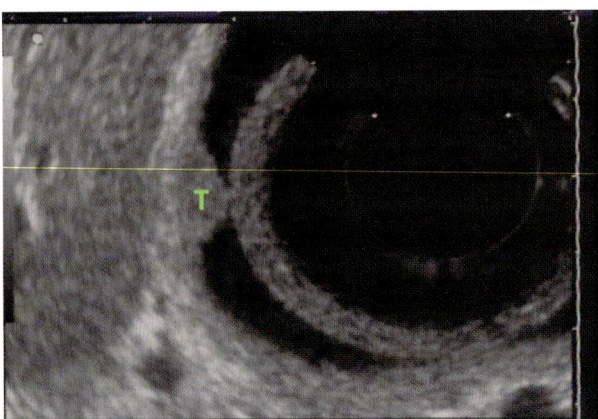

FIGURE 15–26. Radial EUS of a small duodenal carcinoid

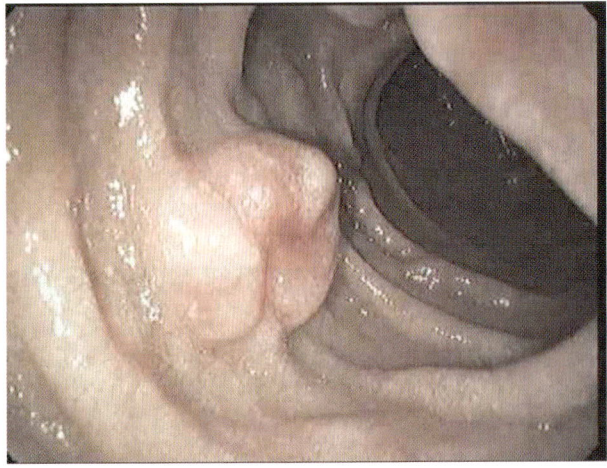

FIGURE 15–27. Endoscopic view of a duodenal gastrinoma (Courtesy of Dr. Kevin McGrath, University of Pittsburg)

Videos: Available at www.pmph-usa.com/bhutani
Video 15-1: Linear EUS of cystic neuroendocrine tumor, with color Doppler, FNA, and histology.

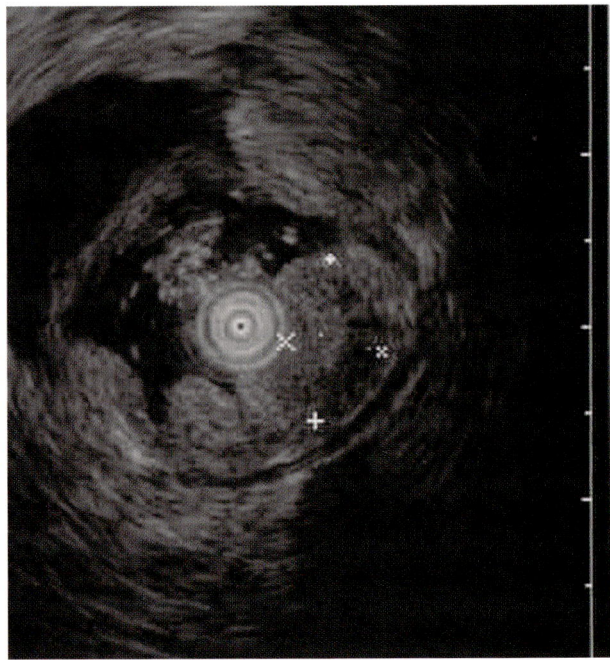

FIGURE 15–28. Radial EUS of the lesion shown in Figure 15-27 (Courtesy of Dr. Kevin McGrath, University of Pittsburg)

Video 15-2: Linear EUS of large neuroendocrine tumor showing partial biliary obstruction.

References

1. Rosch, T., Lightdale, C. J., Botet, J. F., Boyce, G. A., Sivak, M. V., Jr., Yasuda, K., Heyder, N., Palazzo, L., Dancygier, H., Schusdziarra, V., et al: Localization of pancreatic endocrine tumors by endoscopic ultrasonography. N Engl J Med. 1992 Jun 25;326(26):1721–1726.
2. Jani, N., Khalid, A., McGrath, K.: Pancreatic Endocrine Tumors, http://www.vhjoe.org/Volume3Issue3/3-3-2.htm, 2004.
3. Anderson, M. A., Carpenter, S., Thompson, N. W., Nostrant, T. T., Elta, G. H., Scheiman, J. M.: Endoscopic ultrasound is highly accurate and directs management in patients with neuroendocrine tumors of the pancreas. Am J Gastroenterol. 2000 Sep;95(9):2271–2277.
4. Stacpoole, P. W.: The glucagonoma syndrome: clinical features, diagnosis, and treatment. Endocr Rev. 1981 Summer;2(3):347–361. Review.
5. Smith, S. L., Branton, S. A., Avino, A. J., Martin, J. K., Klingler, P. J., Thompson, G. B., Grant, C. S., van Heerden, J. A: Vasoactive intestinal polypeptide secreting islet cell tumors: A 15-year experience and review of the literature. Surgery. 1998 Dec;124(6):1050—1055.
6. Stabile, B. E., Morrow, D. J., Passaro, E., Jr.: The gastrinoma triangle: operative implications. Am J Surg. 1984 Jan;147(1):25–31.
7. DermNetNZ, Necrolytic migratory erythema, http://dermnetnz.org/systemic/necrolytic-erythema.html
8. Gullo, L., Migliori, M., Falconi, M., Pederzoli, P., Bettini, R., Casadei, R., Delle Fave, G., Corleto, V. D., Ceccarelli, C., Santini, D., Tomassetti, P.: Nonfunctioning pancreatic endocrine tumors: a multicenter clinical study. Am J Gastroenterol. 2003 98(11):2435–2439.

CHAPTER 16

Pancreatic Metastases

Dr. John DeWitt

Introduction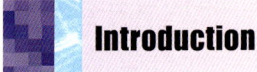

Most solid pancreatic masses represent primary pancreatic neoplasms or focal chronic pancreatitis. However, secondary involvement of the pancreas by systemic malignancy may rarely occur. Recent large surgical series have shown that pancreatic metastases represent 2–3% of all pancreatic resections.[1-3] Accurate identification of isolated pancreatic metastases is clinically important because aggressive surgical resection in selected patients may permit long-term survival.[4-6] In other patients, however, proper diagnosis may avoid unnecessary surgery and permit triage to more appropriate nonoperative therapy.

The most common primary malignancies that metastasize to the pancreas are lung cancer and renal cell carcinoma (RCC). In a recent review of 333 cases of pancreatic metastases up to the year 2003, Minni et al.[7] found that the most frequent site of metastasis originated from the kidney, which represented 150, or 45%, of the study population. These authors found other common sites of primary cancer included: lung, breast, colorectal, and skin (melanoma). Another feature highlighted by this review was the often long delay between the diagnosis of the primary malignancy and subsequent pancreatic metastasis. The mean time between diagnosis and recurrence in the pancreas for all patients in this series was 9.2 years. In another review of 699 cases of pancreatic metastases diagnosed by biopsy/FNA (n=236) or autopsy (n=463), Mesa et al.[8] found that primary lung cancer (19%) was more common than RCC (16%). The variations in diagnoses found by these two studies may reflect differences in how the diagnosis was established (biopsy vs. autopsy)

Secondary involvement of the pancreas by malignancy is usually seen in one of three settings: a) one site among widely metastatic cancer; b) single metastatic focus without other known site of tumor spread or; c) direct extension from an adjacent site.[6] Within the pancreas, there have similarly been three main patterns of tumor spread noted by computed tomography (CT) imaging: large solitary masses, multinodular lesions, and diffuse pancreatic enlargement without focal signs.[8-10] The appearance of pancreatic metastases by CT imaging is well described.[5,9-12] In a review of 66 metastatic lesions, Klein et al[12] found that these lesions may involve all parts of the pancreas and usually have discrete margins with smooth borders. Dual-phase CT imaging is recommended for suspected metastatic RCC (and most other suspected metastases), because these lesions enhance during the early phases of dual-phase helical CT imaging.[12]

Endoscopic ultrasound (EUS)-guided fine-needle aspiration (EUS-FNA) has been demonstrated to be a safe and accurate method for the diagnosis of primary pancreatic cancer with a reported sensitivity of about 85% and a specificity approaching 100%.[13-19] Large case series[8,20-24] and case reports[25-30] in a total of 94 patients (Table 16–1) have also documented the role

Table 16–1 Summary of Previously Published Articles on the Role of EUS and EUS-FNA of Pancreatic Metastases. The number of total metastatic lesions including those with renal cell carcinoma (RCC) or other tumors is included.

Author (year)	Reference	Type of Study	Pancreatic Metastases (n)	EUS-FNA Utilized	RCC (n)	Other Metastases (n)
Palazzo (1996)	20	Retrospective, single center	7	No	4	ovary (1), chrondosarcoma (1), gallbladder (1)
Fritscher-Ravens (2001)	21	Retrospective, single center	12	Yes	3	breast (2), esophageal (2), colon (2), lung (1), lymphoma (1), ovary (1)
Béchade (2003)	22	Retrospective, single center	11	Yes	11	None
Mesa (2004)	8	Retrospective, single center	11	Yes	1	lung (4), breast (2), colon (1), uterus (1), ovary (1), lymphoma (1)

(Continued on following page)

Table 16-1 (Continued)

Author (year)	Reference	Type of Study	Pancreatic Metastases (n)	EUS-FNA Utilized	RCC (n)	Other Metastases (n)
Moussa (2004)	23	Retrospective, multicenter.	22	Yes	10	colon (4), lung (4), breast (2), melanoma (1), ileal carcinoid (1)
DeWitt (2005)	24	Retrospective, multicenter*	24	Yes	10	melanoma (6), lung (4), colon (2), liver (1), stomach (1)
Sweeny (2002)	26	Case report	1	Yes	0	uterus (1)
Eloubeidi (2002)	25	Case report	1	Yes	1	None
DeWitt (2003)	27	Case series	2	Yes	0	melanoma (2)
Rengen (2006)	28	Case report	1	Yes	0	colon (1)
Siddiqui (2006)	29	Case report	1	Yes	0	thyroid (1)
Silva (2006)	30	Case report	1	Yes +	0	ovary (1)
TOTAL	-	-	94	-	40	lung (13), colon (10), melanoma (9), breast (6), ovary (4), esophageal (2), lymphoma (2), uterus (2), chrondrosarcoma (1), gallbladder (1), liver (1), stomach (1), carcinoid (1), thyroid (1)

* Includes 2 cases in reference 26
\+ EUS-Trucut biopsy also used

of EUS imaging and EUS-FNA for the diagnosis of metastatic lesions in the pancreas. Of these 94 patients, 43% have been from primary renal cancer. Interestingly, this frequency of metastatic RCC is similar to that (45%) reported by Minni et al.[7] in 333 patients.

Nearly all patients with pancreatic metastases evaluated by EUS or EUS-FNA have a pancreatic mass visualized by previous CT scan. These patients usually undergo CT for staging of a recently diagnosed cancer or surveillance of a suspected cancer in remission with or without symptoms such as weight loss or abdominal pain. EUS-FNA of pancreatic metastases have been reported in patients undergoing routine CT surveillance of a previously diagnosed cancer,[23,24] even after previously negative or equivocal CT scans.[24]

A trans axial digital anatomy image from the Visible Human Data Set is shown in Figure 16-1. This image shows some of the relevant structures associated with the pancreas head, and roughly corresponds to the CT images that follow.

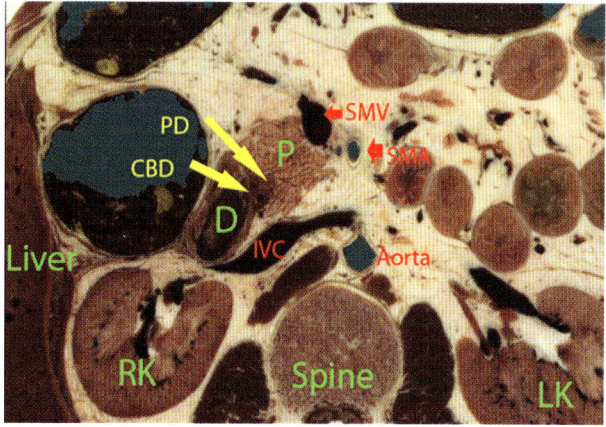

FIGURE 16–1. Transaxial Visible Human image at the level of the pancreatic head. P is pancreas, D is duodenum, PD is pancreatic duct, CBD is common bile duct, SMV is superior mesenteric vein, SMA is superior mesenteric artery, RK is right kidney, and LK is left kidney. The "spine" is shown at the level of the first lumbar vertebra.

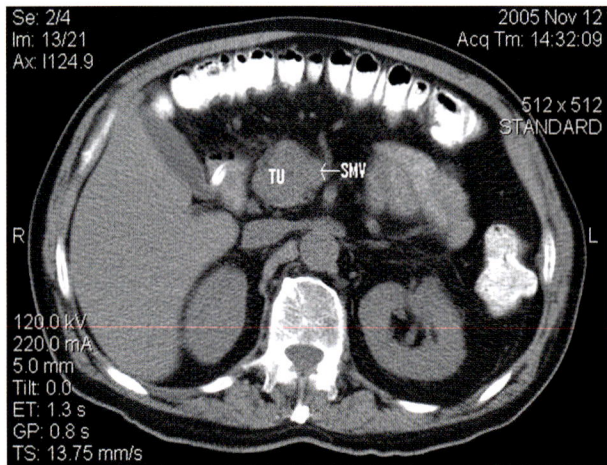

FIGURE 16–2. Abdominal CT scan in a 66-year-old male smoker with small-cell lung cancer (SCLC) diagnosed two months prior to the exam. A well-defined mass (TU) is present in the head of the pancreas adjacent to the superior mesenteric vein (SMV).

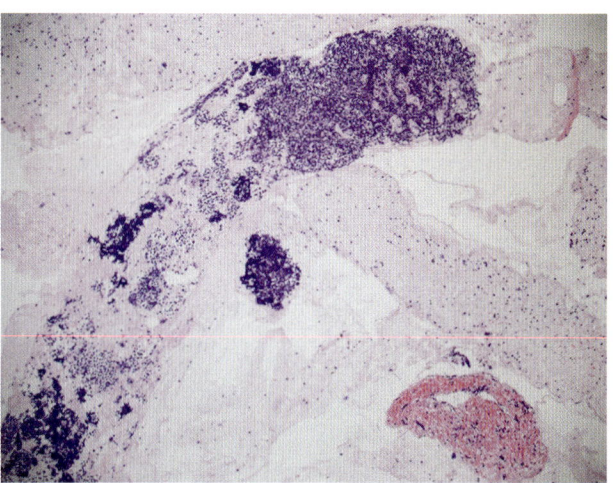

FIGURE 16–4. Photomicrograph of low power view from EUS-FNA showing a 'core-biopsy'-like group of blue-colored tumor cells (H&E; 100x).

Compared to EUS imaging of primary pancreatic cancer, pancreatic metastases are more likely to have well-defined peripheral margins (Figures 16–2 - 16–5).[24] Otherwise, EUS morphology alone cannot distinguish a primary cancer from a metastatic lesion.[21,24] Béchade et al[22] similarly reported that 10 of 11 patients with metastatic RCC to the pancreas had EUS evidence of well-defined tumor margins. Because RCC is a hypervascular tumor, EUS imaging

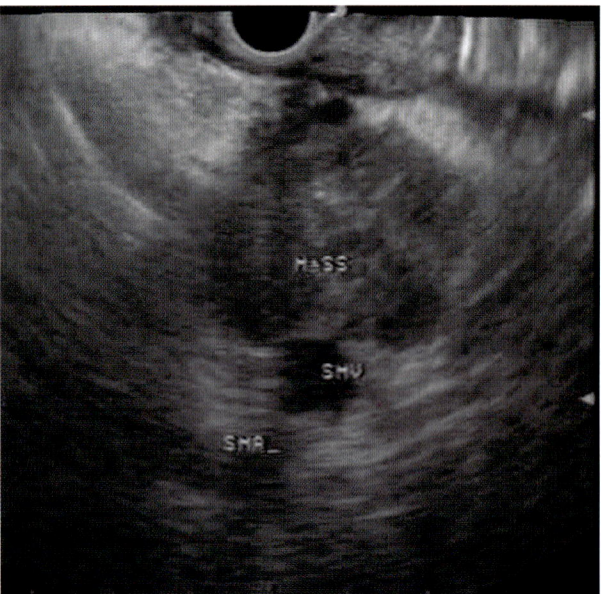

FIGURE 16–3. Linear EUS (6 MHz) view of the same mass in Figure 16–1 demonstrating a 3.5 cm hypoechoic, well-defined tumor adherent to the SMV. The superior mesenteric artery (SMA) is not involved by the mass.

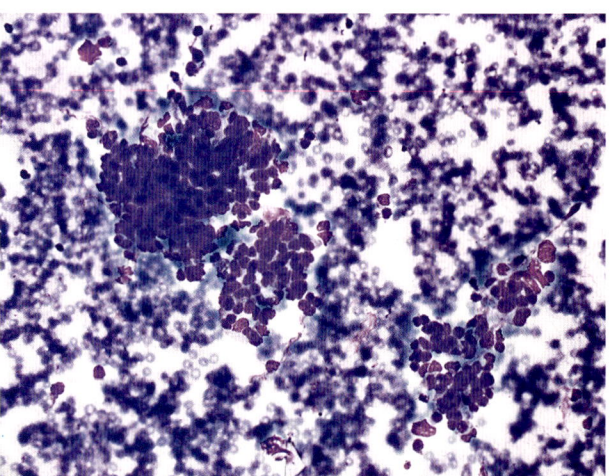

FIGURE 16–5. Higher power view of tumor cells demonstrating scant cytoplasm and nuclear molding (Diff-Quik; 400×). Tumor cells also stained positive for keratin cocktail and chromogranin, and weakly positive for synaptophysin. The cytomorphologic and immunostaining patterns are consistent with metastatic SCLC.

of metastases is usually associated with peripheral enhancement of the ultrasound beam (Figures 16–6 - 16–9).[20,22] Metastatic RCC is characteristically homogeneous and solid, but may have cystic spaces. Video 16–1 shows an example of FNA of a metastatic RCC in the pancreas. Pancreatic metastases collectively are usually solid, but EUS appearance may be cystic alone[27] or a mixed solid and cystic lesion.[24,27,30] These tumors are usually unilocular by EUS imaging, but may also present (particularly RCC) as multifocal lesions within the pancreas.[21,22,24,26] An endosonographer should consider the diagnosis of a pancreatic metastasis in a patient with a remote history or

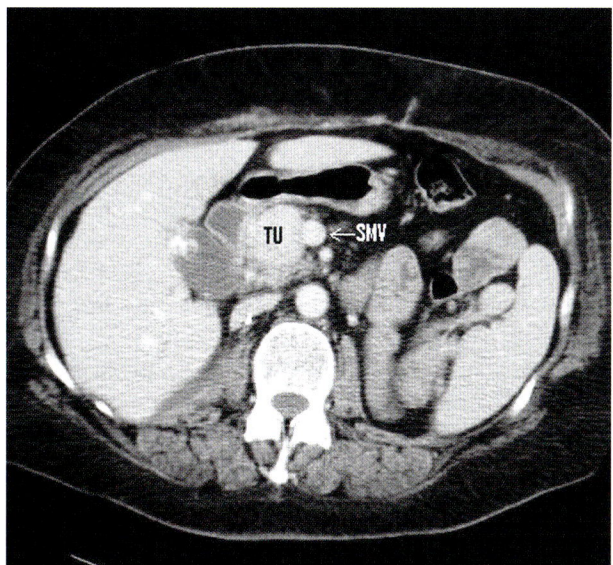

FIGURE 16–6. Abdominal CT scan in a 58-year-old female who underwent bilateral nephrectomies for renal cell carcinoma (RCC) 12 months prior to the exam. A high attenuation, well-defined 4 cm mass (TU) in the head of the pancreas. There is no evidence of invasion of the superior mesenteric vein (SMV).

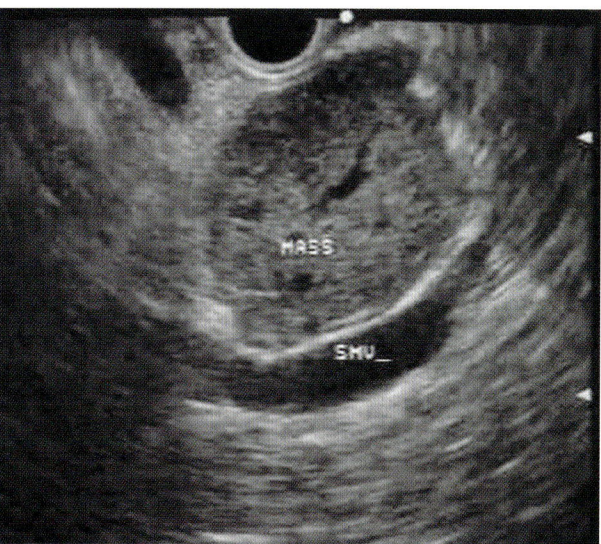

FIGURE 16–7. Linear EUS (7.5 MHz) view of the mass in the same patient in Figure 16–5. The tumor is well defined with cystic spaces internally. There is distal enhancement of the ultrasound beam consistent with a hypervascular mass. The echorich plane between the tumor and SMV is preserved indicating a lack of invasion.

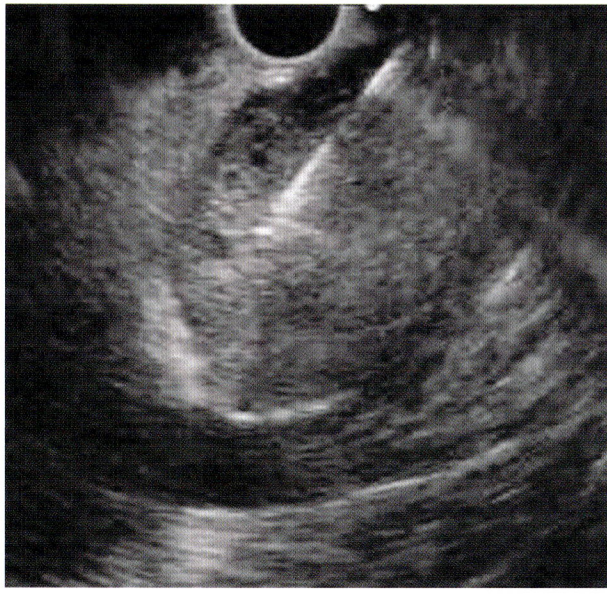

FIGURE 16–8. EUS-FNA of the pancreatic mass with the tip of the needle clearly seen within the lesion

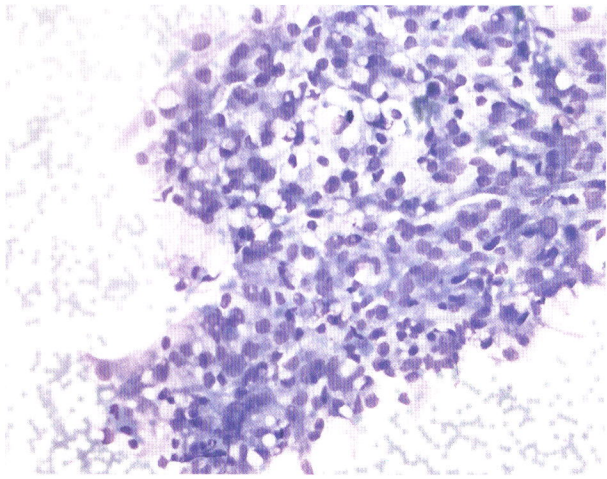

FIGURE 16–9. Photomicrograph of the specimen from the patient in Figures 16–5 to 16–8 demonstrating malignant cells with abundant vacuolated cytoplasm, large round nuclei, and prominent nucleoli consistent with metastatic renal cell carcinoma. (Diff-Quik; 200×)

recently diagnosed extrapancreatic cancer, and an abdominal imaging study that demonstrates one or more well-rounded solid or cystic pancreatic masses.

Because imaging alone cannot usually distinguish primary pancreatic cancer from metastatic lesions, EUS-FNA or EUS-guided Tru-cut biopsy (EUS-TCB) of these lesions may provide additional diagnostic information. To maximize yield and minimize nondiagnostic biopsies, EUS-FNA is best done with on-site, real-time cytology interpretation.[31] Two slide preparations from each fine-needle aspirate are recommended. One slide is stained (i.e. modified Giemsa stains) for on-site evaluation, while the other is ethanol-fixed and stained (i.e. Pap stain) later for future interpretation. If on-site cytology interpretation and/or patient history suggest a possible metastatic lesion in the pancreas, then additional FNA passes should be made for cell block examination. Furthermore, if on-site interpretation is not available, a cell block preparation should also be made. The cell block preparation is fixed in formalin and embedded in paraffin. Hematoxylin-eosin (H&E) stains and possible immunocytochemistry (ICC) on the cell block may aid in the diagnosis of the suspected metastatic lesion (Figures 16–10 - 16–14).[8,24] To aid the pathologist, the endosonographer should provide the date, method used, and anatomical site sampled to diagnosis any previous malignancy in these

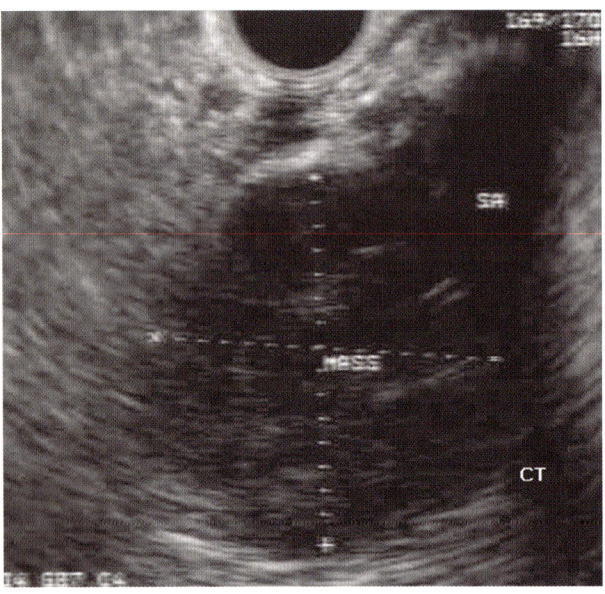

FIGURE 16–10. Linear EUS (6 MHz) image of a well-defined 3 cm mass in the body of the pancreas with invasion of the celiac trunk (CT) and proximal splenic artery (SA). The patient was a 58-year-old male with previous right nephrectomy for RCC, who presented with acute pancreatitis. Previous cholecystectomy had revealed melanoma within the gallbladder without a known primary tumor on the skin. CT scan eight weeks prior to EUS revealed peripancreatic inflammatory changes, but no pancreatic mass.

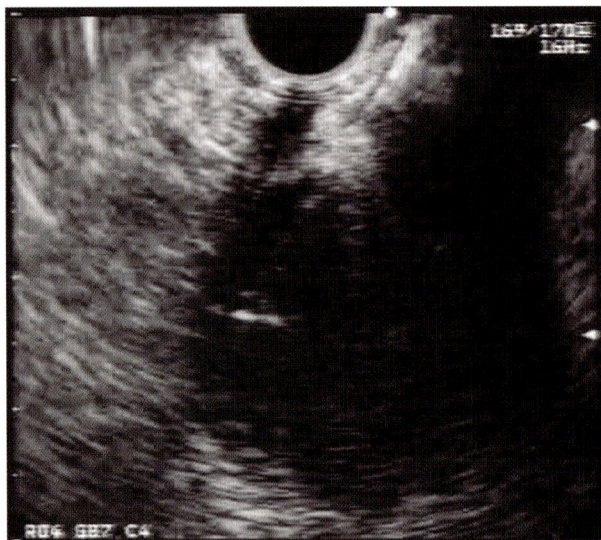

FIGURE 16–11. EUS-FNA of the mass within the body of the pancreas from the patient in Figure 16–10.

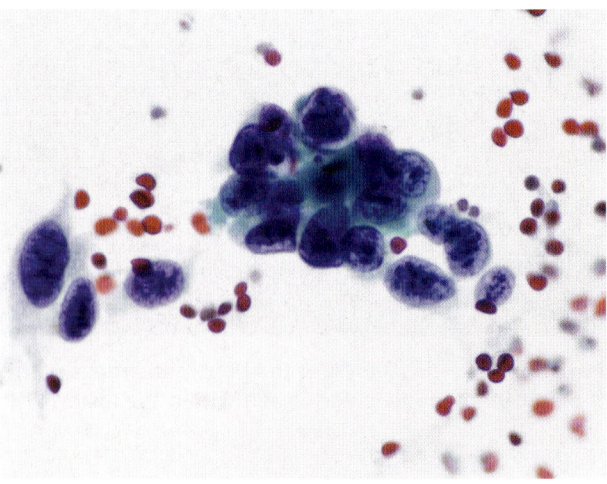

FIGURE 16–12. Photomicrograph of high power view of malignant plasmacytoid cells with large nuclei and sparse cytoplasm (Papanicolaou stain; 400×). The cytomorphologic appearance alone is diagnostic of melanoma although immunostains were performed for confirmation.

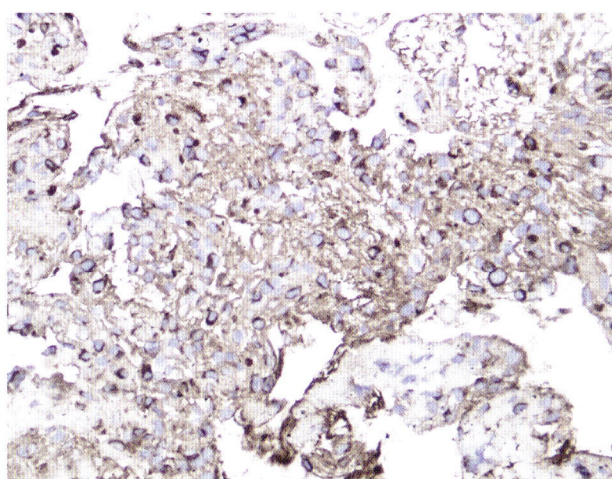

FIGURE 16–13. Photomicrograph of cell block specimen from Figure 16–11 (100×) after staining with HMB-45. The intracytoplasmic melanin with the melanocytes is strongly stained by HMB-45 consistent with melanoma.

patients. Comparison of tissue sampling from EUS with any other pathology specimen from the tumor may prove critical to confirm the suspected diagnosis of metastasis to the pancreas.

There are limited published data in a large series of patients that describe the criteria required for the cytologic diagnosis of pancreatic metastases. From a consensus among the pathologists from two institutions (Indiana University and Duke University),[24] it was agreed that cytomorphology alone (without the use of ICC) is sufficient to diagnose metastatic RCC, small-cell lung carcinoma (SCLC), hepatocellular carcinoma (HCC), and melanoma (although ICC is usually used for the latter). Furthermore, cytomorphology alone was often deemed sufficient for breast, colon, and prostate metastases, but ICC should be and usually is performed for confirmation. These experts, however, proposed that esophageal, gastric, and non-small-cell lung cancer (NSCLC) metastases cannot be definitively confirmed by cytomorphology alone. In most but not all cases, the comparison of cytology from a pancreatic metastasis to a previous cytology or histology specimen was believed to be sufficient for a cytodiagnosis of a metastasis even in the absence of ICC. When EUS-FNA with or without ICC is nondiagnostic, histology may be required to confirm a suspected diagnosis of suspected pancreatic metastases. In these patients, EUS-TCB (Cook Endoscopy, Winston-Salem, NC) with a 19-gauge needle may be helpful (Figures 16–15 - 16–18).

In conclusion, pancreatic metastases represent an important cause of pancreatic masses. The two most common primary tumors are renal and lung cancers. However, a wide variety of other primary sites have also been implicated. Obtaining a detailed medical history for previous malignancy may raise suspicion for this diagnosis. These lesions usually have well-rounded margins, but otherwise distinguishing these

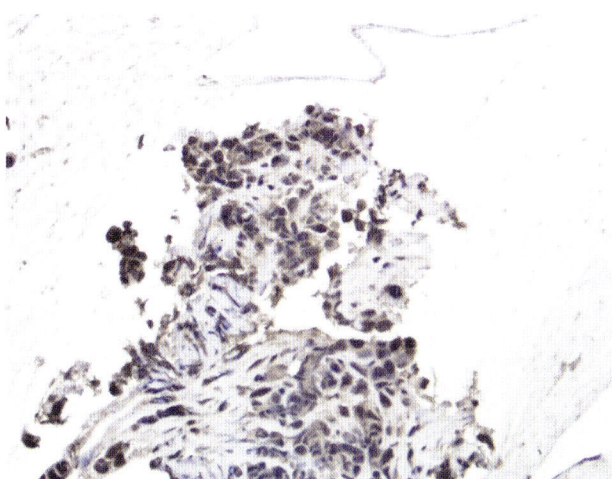

FIGURE 16–14. Immunocytochemistry of same cell block specimen is also positive for S-100 consistent with melanoma (original magnification 100x).

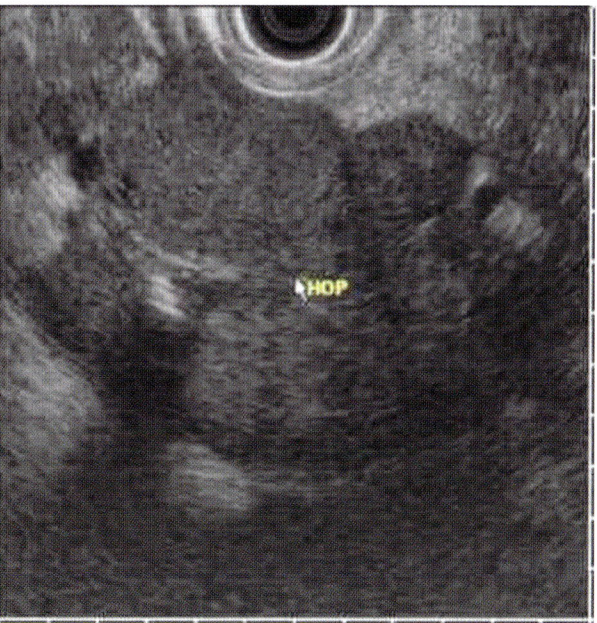

FIGURE 16–15. Radial EUS (7.5 MHz) of a 72-year-old male who had a left RCC resected fifteen years prior to EUS. The patient had metastatic RCC to the cervical spine discovered thirteen years after nephrectomy, and this recurrence was treated successfully with laminectomy and subsequent radiation therapy. He developed diabetes, which prompted a CT scan just prior to EUS. It showed bile duct dilation and diffuse pancreatic enlargement without a definite mass. EUS demonstrated multiple, round, well-defined masses in the head of the pancreas completely replacing the normal gland.

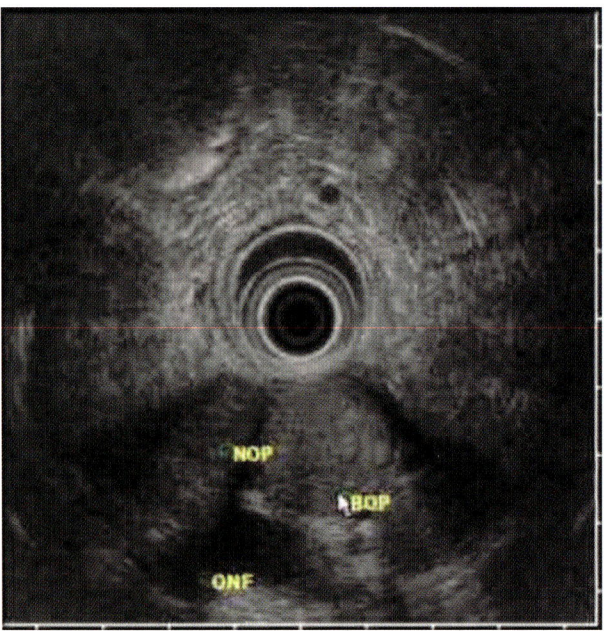

FIGURE 16–16. Radial EUS (7.5 MHz) image of the neck and downstream body of the pancreas adjacent to the confluence of the splenic and portal veins similarly in the same patient showing complete replacement of the pancreas by multiple, round masses suggestive of metastases.

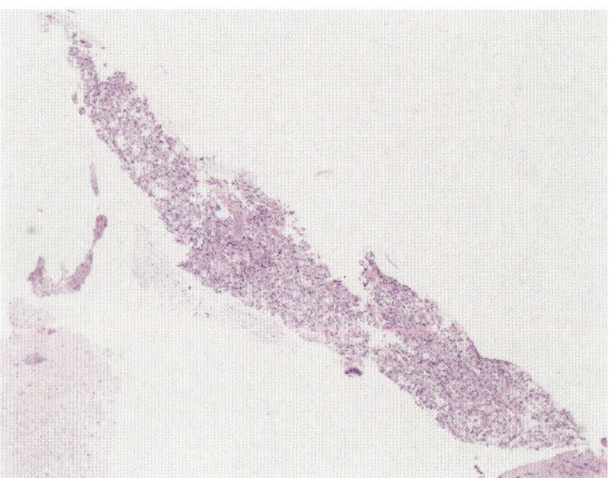

FIGURE 16–17. Photomicrograph of a 4 mm surgical pathology specimen from EUS-guided Tru-cut biopsy (EUS-TCB) of the pancreatic body in the patient described in Figures 16–14 and 16–15 (H&E; 40x). EUS-TCB was performed because the rapid interpretation and the final pathology report from EUS-FNA of the pancreatic body and a celiac lymph node in this patient were both nondiagnostic, demonstrating only blood.

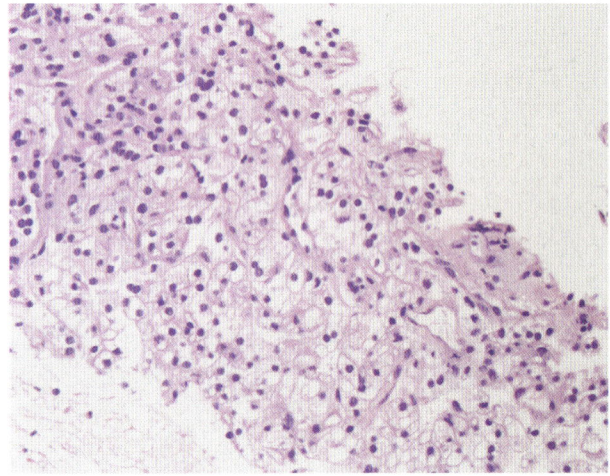

FIGURE 16–18. Higher power view of the same specimen from Figure 16–16, demonstrating clear cells consistent with metastatic RCC (H&E; 200x).

lesions from primary pancreatic cancer by imaging alone is often difficult. EUS-FNA or EUS-TCB may be used to help diagnose these lesions. Communication with the pathologist and the preparation of a cell block for immunocytochemistry are essential to obtain a correct diagnosis.

Video: Available at www.pmph-usa.com/bhutani
Video 16–1: Linear array EUS evaluation and FNA of a mass in the pancreas that was ultimately shown to be metastatic renal cell carcinoma.

References

1. Roland, C. F., van Heerden, J. A.: Nonpancreatic primary tumors with metastasis to the pancreas. Surg Gynecol Obstet 1989;168:345–347.
2. Nakeeb, A., Lillemoe, K. D., Cameron, J. L.: The role of pancreaticoduodenectomy for locally recurrent or metastatic carcinoma to the periampullary region. J Am Coll Surg 1995;180:180–192.
3. Sperti, C., Pasquali, C., Liessi, G., et al.: Pancreatic Resection for Metastatic Tumors. J Surg Oncol 2003;83:161–166.

4. Z'graggen, K., Fernandez-del Castillo, C., Rattner, D. W., et al.: Metastases to the pancreas and their surgical extirpation. Arch Surg 1998;133:413–419.
5. Ghavamian, R., Klein, K. A., Stephens, D. H., et al.: Renal cell carcinoma metastatic to the pancreas: clinical and radiological features. Mayo Clin Proc 2000;75:581–585.
6. Faure, J. P., Tuech, J. J., Richer, J. P., Pessaux, P., et al.: Pancreatic metastasis of renal cell carcinoma: presentation, treatment and survival. J Urol 2001;165:20–22.
7. Minni, F., Casadei, R., Perenze, B., et al.: Pancreatic metastases: observations of three cases and review of the literature. Pancreatology 2004;4:509–520.
8. Mesa, H., Stelow, E. B., Stanley, M. W., et al.: Diagnosis of nonprimary pancreatic neoplasms by endoscopic ultrasound-guided fine-needle aspiration. Diagn Cytopathol 2004;31:313–318.
9. Ferrozzi, F., Bova, D., Campodonico, F., et al.: Pancreatic metastases: CT assessment. Eur Radiol 1997;7:241–245.
10. Charnsangavej, C., Whitley, N. O.: Metastases to the pancreas and peripancreatic lymph nodes from carcinoma of the right side of the colon: CT findings in 12 patients. AJR Am J Roentgenol 1993;160:49–52.
11. Ng, C. S., Loyer, E. M., Iyer, R. B., et al.: Metastases to the pancreas from renal cell carcinoma: findings on three-phase contrast-enhanced helical CT. AJR Am J Roentgenol 1999;172:1555–1559.
12. Klein, K. A., Stephens, D. H., Welch, T. J.: CT characteristics of metastatic disease of the pancreas. Radiographics 1998;18:369–378.
13. Wiersema, M. J., Vilmann, P., Giovannini, M., et al.: Endosonography-guided fine-needle aspiration biopsy: diagnostic accuracy and complication assessment. Gastroenterology 1997;112:1087–1095.
14. Williams, D. B., Sahai, A. V., Aabakken, L., et al.: Endoscopic ultrasound guided fine needle aspiration biopsy: a large single centre experience. Gut 1999;44:720–726.
15. Gress, F., Gottlieb, K., Sherman, S., et al.: Endoscopic ultrasonography-guided fine-needle aspiration biopsy of suspected pancreatic cancer. Ann Intern Med 2001;134:459–464.
16. Harewood, G. C., Wiersema, M. J.: Endosonography-guided fine needle aspiration biopsy in the evaluation of pancreatic masses. Am J Gastroenterol 2002;97:1386–1391.
17. Raut, C. P., Grau, A. M., Staerkel, G. A., et al.: Diagnostic accuracy of endoscopic ultrasound-guided fine-needle aspiration in patients with presumed pancreatic cancer. J Gastrointest Surg 2003;7:118-128.
18. Eloubeidi, M. A., Chen, V. K., Eltoum, I. A., et al.: Endoscopic ultrasound-guided fine needle aspiration biopsy of patients with suspected pancreatic cancer: diagnostic accuracy and acute and 30-day complications. Am J Gastroenterol 2003;98:2663–2668.
19. Gress, F., Michael, H., Gelrud, D., et al.: EUS-guided fine-needle aspiration of the pancreas: evaluation of pancreatitis as a complication. Gastrointest Endosc 2002;56:864–867.
20. Palazzo, L., Borotto, E., Cellier, C., et al.: Endosonographic features of pancreatic metastases. Gastrointest Endosc 1996;44:433–436.
21. Fritscher-Ravens, A., Sriram, P. V., Krause, C., et al.: Detection of pancreatic metastases by EUS-guided fine-needle aspiration. Gastrointest Endosc 2001;53:65–70.
22. Béchade, D., Palazzo, L., Fabre, M., Algayres, J. P.: EUS-guided FNA of pancreatic metastasis from renal cell carcinoma. Gastrointest Endosc 2003; 58:784–788.
23. Moussa, A., Mitry, E., Hammel, P., et al.: Pancreatic metastases: a multicentric study of 22 patients. Gastroenterol Clin Biol 2004;28:872–876.
24. DeWitt, J., Jowell, P., LeBlanc, J., et al.: EUS-FNA of Pancreatic Metastases: A Multicenter Experience. Gastrointest Endosc 2005; 61:689–696.
25. Eloubeidi, M. A., Jhala, D., Chhieng, D. C., et al.: Multiple late asymptomatic pancreatic metastases from renal cell carcinoma: diagnosis by endoscopic ultrasound-guided fine needle aspiration biopsy with immunocytochemical correlation. Dig Dis Sci 2002;47:1839–1842.
26. Sweeney, J. T., Crabtree, D. K., Tassin, R., Somogyi, L.: Metastatic uterine leiomyosarcoma involving the pancreas diagnosed by EUS with fine-needle aspiration. Gastrointest Endosc 2002;56:596–597.
27. DeWitt, J. M., Chappo, J., Sherman, S.: EUS-FNA of Metastatic Malignant Melanoma to the Pancreas: Report of Two Cases and Review. Endoscopy 2003; 35:219–222.
28. Rengen, M. R., De, J., Kott, M. M., Adler, D. G.: Endoscopic ultrasound diagnosis of colon cancer metastatic to the pancreas. Endoscopy 2006;38:853.
29. Siddiqui, A. A., Olansky, L., Ravindranauth, N. S., Tierney, W. M.: Pancreatic Metastasis of Tall Cell Variant of Papillary Thyroid Carcinoma: Diagnosis by Endoscopic Ultrasound-Guided Fine Needle Aspiration. JOP 2006;7:417–422.
30. Silva, R. G., Dahmoush, L., Gerke, H.: Pancreatic Metastasis of an Ovarian Malignant Mixed Mullerian Tumor Identified by EUS-Guided Fine Needle Aspiration and Tru-cut Needle Biopsy. JOP 2006;7:66–69.
31. Klapman, J. B., Logrono, R., Dye, C. E., Waxman, I.: Clinical impact of on-site cytopathology interpretation on endoscopic ultrasound-guided fine needle aspiration. Am J Gastroenterol 2003;98:1289–1294.

CHAPTER 17

Cystic Pancreatic Lesions

Dr. Kunal Jajoo
Dr. William R. Brugge

The frequent utilization of cross-sectional radiographic imaging has lead to an increase in the identification of cystic lesions of the pancreas. Many of these lesions are inflammatory fluid collections or pseudocysts and may be diagnosed by a characteristic antecedent history of acute pancreatitis and radiographic features.[1] However, an increasing proportion of pancreatic cystic lesions are found incidentally, with no history of pancreatitis or other attributable symptoms. Such cysts very likely represent cystic neoplasms, ranging from benign to pre-malignant, to malignant. Certainly, the distinction of benign from neoplastic cyst is crucial in the management of such patients. Endoscopic ultrasound (EUS) with fine needle aspiration (FNA) can provide critical findings in this diagnostic delineation.

In the initial phase of evaluation, the radiographic imaging exams that lead to the diagnosis of a pancreatic cyst should be reviewed. The size, morphology, and location of the lesion should be confirmed. EUS is very sensitive to the presence of cystic lesions, particularly in the pancreas, and the EUS findings may vary from the cross-sectional exam. Cyst fluid projects as anechoic against the "salt and pepper" background of the pancreatic parenchyma. Care should be taken to examine the entire gland and surrounding structures in a systematic fashion, even if the cyst is identified early in the examination. EUS can provide details of the structural characteristics of the cyst, pancreatic parenchyma, pancreatic duct as well as surrounding structures, but it is not sufficient to distinguish malignant from benign lesions.[2] The key morphologic findings that should be noted include the presence of : 1) microcystic morphology 2) adjacent mass 3) dilated main pancreatic duct 4) mural nodule 5) adenopathy.

FNA of the cyst fluid and analysis of cellular material, amylase level, and tumor markers, such as carcinoembryonic antigen (CEA), have been shown to assist in narrowing the differential diagnosis and improving the diagnostic capability of EUS. In studies where surgical correlation is available, EUS with FNA and cytopathology has an accuracy of 55–91%.[3,4] In particular, a cyst fluid CEA concentration of greater than 192 ng/mL is predictive of a mucinous lesion with 79% accuracy.[5] High amylase levels in the cyst fluid are generally indicative of pseudocyst, but can also be seen with IPMN.[6] Novel diagnostic techniques, including Tru-cut biopsy of the cyst wall and molecular analysis of cyst fluid for DNA mutations, have been developed for use with EUS guidance.[7,8] These promising procedures require further investigation and will hopefully add to the clinician's armamentarium of methods to distinguish neoplastic from non-neoplastic cysts. (Table 17–1)

The diagnostic techniques described previously are particularly pertinent in those patients who are not surgical candidates or do not have symptoms attributable to the cyst. EUS with FNA should be reserved for those cases in which the results would alter clinical management. If a cyst is found in the setting of recurrent acute pancreatitis in a patient who is fit for surgery, resection should be considered, and EUS is not indicated. Low operative mortality in specialized centers, the malignant potential of mucinous pancreatic cysts, and the excellent prognosis of completely resected mucinous lesions justify surgical resection in appropriately selected patients.

Table 17–1 Demographics and Characteristics of Pancreatic Cystic Neoplasms

Cyst Type	Age of Onset	Gender Distribution	Morphology	Malignant Potential
Serous cystadenoma	Seventh decade	Female	Microcystic with honeycombing, minority are macrocystic	Very low
Mucinous cystic neoplasm	Fifth decade	Strongly female	Macrocystic, can be septated	High
Intraductal papillary mucious neoplasm	Sixth to Seventh decade	Equal	Main branch - dilated duct, mixed macro, microcystic Brach duct – cluster of grapes	High
Solid pseudopapillary neoplasm	Fourth decade	Strongly female	Encapsulated, mixed-solid and cystic	Moderate
Cystic endocrine tumor	Fifth to Sixth decade	Equal	Variable	Variable based on type

Pseudocysts

Pancreatic pseudocysts occur as a result of inflammation and necrosis, which in turn develop into fluid-filled structures surrounded by granulation tissue. There is no epithelial lining within pseudocysts, and surrounding structures including the stomach, transverse mesocolon, and the pancreas itself form the borders of pseudocysts. Pseudocysts typically require more than four weeks to form and most often occur after severe acute pancreatitis.[9] Less frequently, pseudocysts occur in conjunction with chronic pancreatitis. Imaging findings of chronic pancreatitis, including parenchymal calcifications, increase the likelihood that a cystic lesion is a pseudocyst.[10]

The EUS features of pseudocysts can overlap with those of mucinous cystic lesions (Figure 17–1). A pseudocyst can be unilocular or contain several compartments with intervening septations. Echogenic debris may be present within a pseudocyst, representing remains of necrotic tissue or coagulated blood. Relative to a mucinous cystic neoplasm, a pseudocyst typically has a thick wall adherent to adjacent structures.[11] Aspiration of a pseudocyst demonstrates thin, brown, amylase-rich fluid. Microscopic examination reveals inflammatory cells and occasionally necrotic debris.[12] In patients with symptomatic pseudocysts, EUS-guided drainage and catheter placement via the transgastric approach have been shown to be effective in small studies.[13,14] In this setting, EUS can confirm the absence of intervening vessels, such as gastric varices, and can be used to assure that the distance between the cyst lumen and the gastric wall is less than one centimeter. In these ways, EUS is useful in both the diagnosis and management of pancreatic pseudocysts.

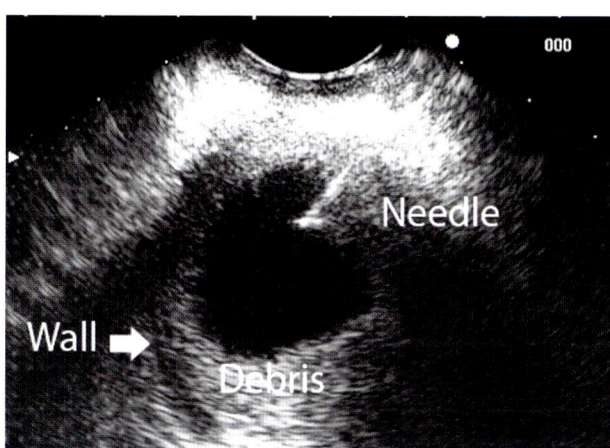

FIGURE 17–1. Thick-walled unilocular cystic lesion undergoing FNA. The lesion was resected and was a pseudocyst.

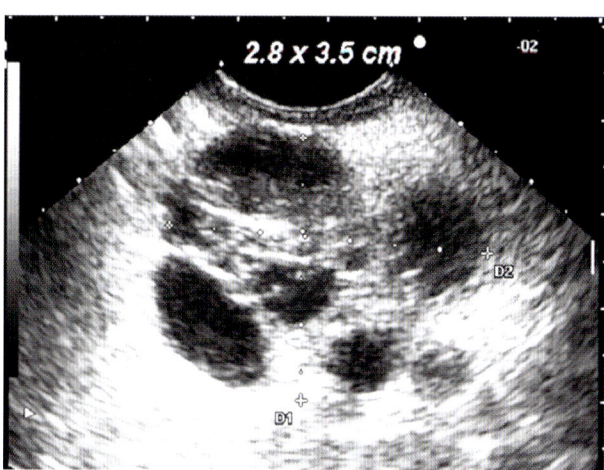

FIGURE 17–2. Serous cystadenoma. Multicystic lesion in the body of the pancreas with microcystic and macrocystic components and a central scar. Total size 2.8 cm x 3.5 cm

 ## Serous Lesions

Serous cystadenomas (Figure 17–2) are the most commonly encountered cystic tumors of the pancreas, comprising approximately one-third of cystic tumors.[15] These lesions typically have a microcystic morphology, creating a honeycomb appearance. The microcysts are divided by thin septations that can become fibrotic and form the classic central stellate scar. Macrocystic morphology is seen in a minority of serous cystadenoma. Microscopically, the cyst lining is composed of cuboidal cells with glycogen-rich cytoplasm and dense chromatin.[16] The peak age of diagnosis is the seventh decade with a female-to-male ratio of 3 to 1. Serous cystadenocarcinoma is extremely rare, therefore clinical observation of asymptomatic serous cystadenoma is recommended if pre-operative diagnosis is possible.

 ## Mucinous Lesions

Mucinous cystic neoplasms (MCNs) account for 10–45% of cystic neoplasms of the pancreas. MCNs are predominantly found in women, with a male-to-female ratio that was previously reported to range from 1 in 5 to 1 in 9, and an incidence that peaks in the fifth decade of life.[17,18] Recent studies have demonstrated that MCNs occur almost exclusively in women when they are defined by the presence of ovarian stroma.[19] These tumors are principally located in the tail of the pancreas, can be uni- or multilocular,

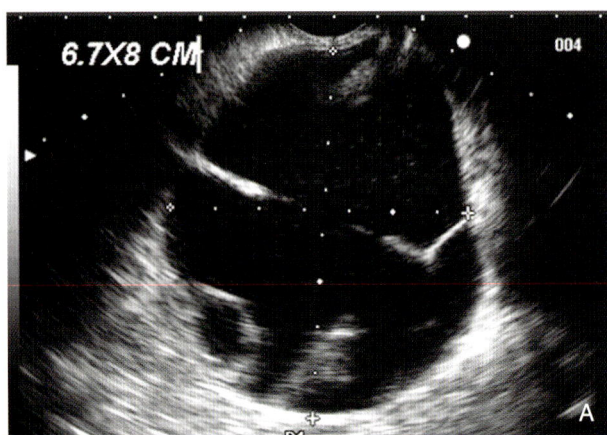

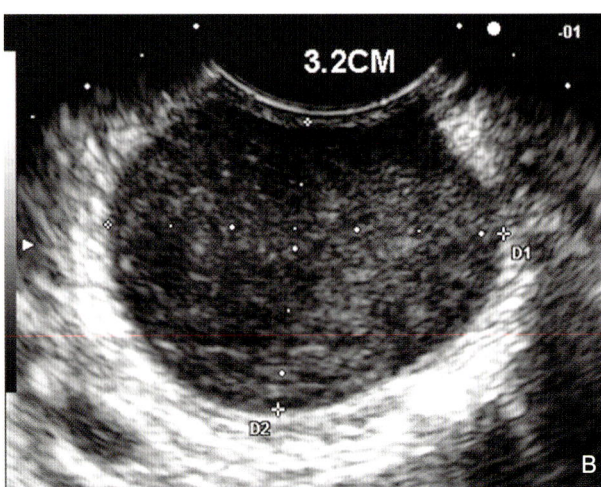

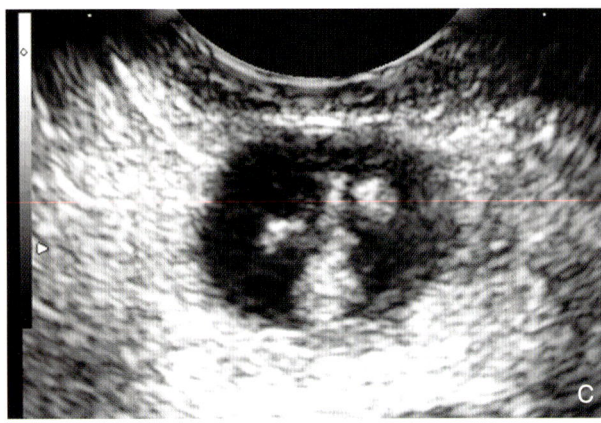

FIGURES 17–3. *A to C* (A) Benign mucinous cystic neoplasm with multiple septations (B) Mucinous cystic neoplasm with mucin visible as echoic material within the cyst (C) 1.5cm malignant mucinous cystic neoplasm with thick and irregular septations

and can range in size from 2 to 35 cm in diameter (Figure 17–3A). MCNs are defined by a lining of mucus secreting epithelial cells surrounded by an ovarian-like stroma (Figure 17–3B). Depending on the degree of cellular atypia, MCNs are classified as adenomas, borderline tumors, or carcinomas (Figure 17–3C). The cysts do not communicate with the pancreatic ductal system, and the cyst fluid generally contains mucin and a high concentration of CEA. The female predominance and ovarian stromal elements of MCNs have lead to the postulation that their pathogenesis involves hormonal elements.[20] En bloc resection is recommended, given the latent potential of these cysts to become malignant.

Intraductal papillary mucinous neoplasms (IPMNs) are seen equally in males and females, and generally present in the seventh decade of life. The diagnosis of IPMNs has been increasing in incidence in recent years, likely a result of increased recognition of this diagnosis and increased use of imaging.[21] The World Health Organization put forth the diagnostic criteria for IPMNs in 1996: intraductal mucin-producing neoplasm with tall, columnar, mucin-containing epithelium, with or without papillary projections.[22] IPMNs can be divided into morphologic subtypes: main-duct IPMNs, branch-duct IPMNs, and mixed. Main-duct IPMNs carry a much greater likelihood of malignancy than branch-duct IPMNs.[23] The characteristic imaging features of branch-duct IPMNs include multilocular appearance with a cluster of grapes configuration, communication with the pancreatic duct, and dilated ductal structures with filling defects representing mucus (Figures 17–4B and 17–4C).[24] In addition, a dilated main pancreatic duct, cyst size greater than 3.0 cm, and mural nodularity are features of IPMNs that predict an increased likelihood of malignancy.[25,26]

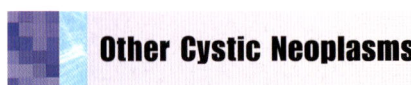

Other Cystic Neoplasms

Solid pseudopapillary epithelial neoplasms (SPENs) demonstrate a strong female predilection and the earliest age of onset among cystic lesions of the pancreas. Though these lesions are rare, recognition is important given their malignant potential and very high cure rate with surgical resection.[27] SPENs are typically large, encapsulated, and well defined with

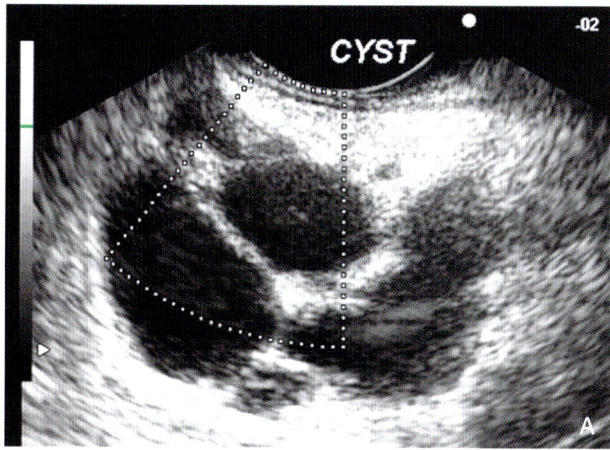
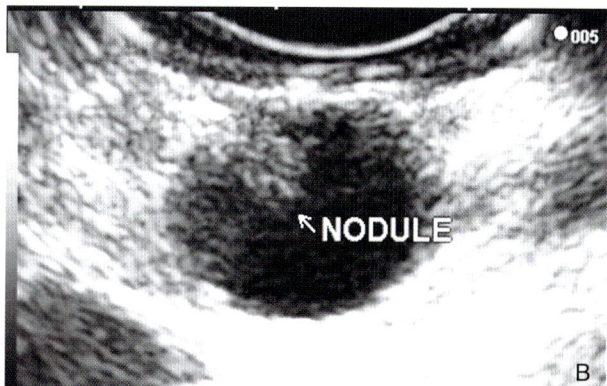
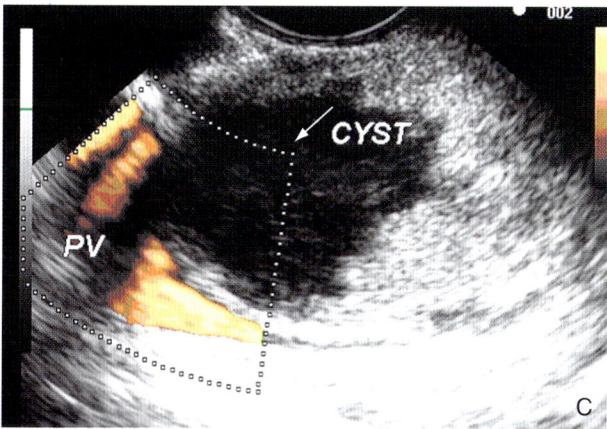

FIGURES 17–4. *A to C* (A) Thinly septated IPMN in the head of the pancreas (B) IPMN with mural nodule suggestive of malignancy (C) Malignant IPMN with a thick wall (see arrow)

solid and cystic features. The majority of patients with these lesions present with abdominal pain. FNA cytopathology may demonstrate branching papillae and myxoid stroma.[28]

Pancreatic endocrine tumors (Figure 17–5A) can present with cystic degeneration and are classified as either functional or nonfunctional, dependent on their ability to secrete hormones, and thereby produce classic clinical symptoms. Endocrine tumors of the pancreas have a male-to-female ratio of 1 to 1, with a peak incidence in the fifth and sixth decades.[29] Given their vascularity, EUS with color-flow Doppler may demonstrate increased blood flow within these lesions (Figure 17–5B). Other rare cystic malignancies, such

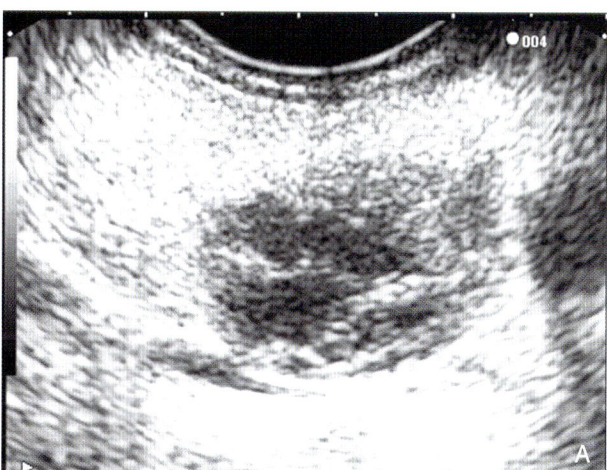
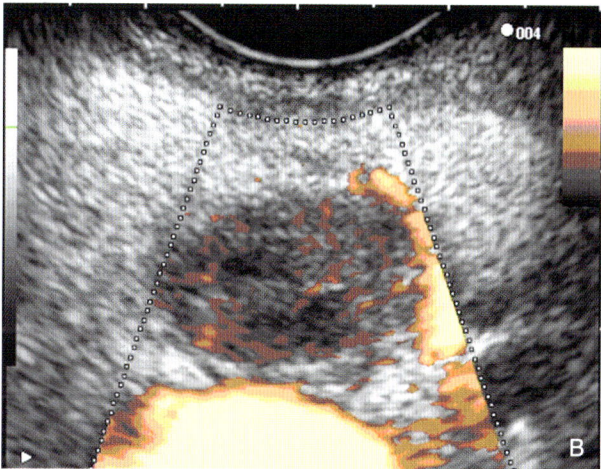

FIGURES 17–5. *A and B* (A) Pancreatic cystic endocrine tumor (B) Pancreatic endocrine tumor. Color-flow Doppler demonstrates hypervascularity within the solid portions of the mass

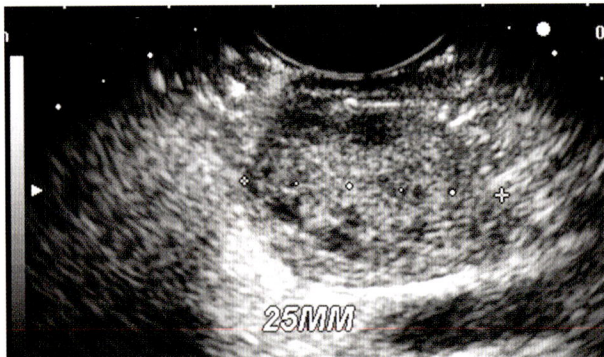

FIGURE 17-6. Lymphoepithelial cyst of the body of the pancreas

as lymphoepithelial cysts, may mimic cystic neuroendocrine malignancies. (Figure 17–6).

Ductal adenocarcinoma can present with cystic morphology either due to mucin production or cystic degeneration. As with solid adenocarcinoma of the pancreas, there is a male predominance, and the typical age of onset is late 60s to early 70s. EUS may demonstrate mixed solid-cystic mass with resultant ductal obstruction and possible invasion of adjacent structures.

Summary

Cystic lesions of the pancreas are a challenging and frequently encountered clinical diagnosis. The differentiation of cystic neoplasms of the pancreas from pseudocysts is critical given the malignant potential of such lesions, particularly IPMNs and MCNs. In the setting of a symptomatic surgically fit patient, the indication for surgical resection is clear. In the case of uncertain cyst type or medical co-morbidity, EUS with FNA for chemical, cytological, and molecular analysis is valuable in the diagnosis and management of cystic lesions of the pancreas.

References

1. Brugge, W. R., Lauwers, G. Y., Sahani, D., et al.: Current concepts: cystic neoplasms of the pancreas. N Engl J Med 2004;351:1218–1226.
2. Ahmad, N. A., Kochman, M. L., Lewis, J. D., et al.: Can EUS alone differentiate between malignant and benign cystic lesions of the pancreas? Am J Gastroenterol 2001;96:3295–300.
3. Sedlack, R., Affi, A., Vazquez-Sequeiros, E., et al.: Utility of EUS in the evaluation of cystic pancreatic lesions. Gastrointest Endosc 2002;56:543–547.
4. Moparty, B., Logroño, R., Nealon, W. H., et al.: The role of endoscopic ultrasound and endoscopic ultrasound-guided fine-needle aspiration in distinguishing pancreatic cystic lesions. Diagn Cytopathol 2007;35:18–25.
5. Brugge, W. R., Lewandrowski, K., Lee-Lewandrowski, E., et al.: Diagnosis of pancreatic cystic neoplasms: a report of the cooperative pancreatic cyst study. Gastroenterology 2004;126:1330–1336.
6. Ryu, J. K., Woo, S. M., Hwang, J. H., et al.: Cyst fluid analysis for the differential diagnosis of pancreatic cysts. Diagn Cytopathol 2004;31:100–105.
7. Levy, M. J., Smyrk, T. C., Reddy, R. P., et al.: Endoscopic Ultrasound–Guided Tru-cut Biopsy of the Cyst Wall for Diagnosing Cystic Pancreatic Tumors. Clin Gastroenterol Hepatol 2005;3:974–979.
8. Khalid, A., McGrath, K. M., Zahid, M., et al.: The role of pancreatic cyst fluid molecular analysis in predicting cyst pathology. Clin Gastroenterol Hepatol 2005;3:\967–973.
9. Sonnenday, C. J., Lillemoe, K. D., Yeo, C. J.: Pseudocysts and other complications of pancreatitis. In Zuideme, G. D., Yeo, C. J., editors. Shackelford's Surgery of the Alimentary Tract. Vol III. 5th ed. Philadelphia: WB Saunders; 2002. p. 36.
10. Sand, J. A., Hyöty, M. K., Matilla, J., et al.: Clinical assessment compared with cyst fluid analysis in the differential diagnosis of cystic lesions in the pancreas. Surgery 1996;119:275–280.
11. Brugge, W. R., Lewandrowski, K., Lee-Lewandrowski, E., Centeno, B. A., Szydlo, T., Regan, S., del Castillo, C. F., Warshaw, A. L.: Diagnosis of pancreatic cystic neoplasms: a report of the cooperative pancreatic cyst study. Gastroenterol 2004;126:1330.6.
12. Nguyen, G. K., Suen, K. C., Villanueva, R. R.: Needle aspiration cytology of pancreatic cystic lesions. Diagn Cytopathol 1997;17:177–182.
13. Azar, R. R., Oh, Y. S., Janec, E. M., et al.: Wire-guided pancreatic pseudocyst drainage by using a modified needle knife and therapeutic echoendoscope. Gastrointest Endosc 2006;63:688–692.
14. Antillon, M. R., Shah, R. J., Steigmann, G., et al.: Single-step EUS-guided transmural drainage of simple and complicated pancreatic pseudocysts. Gastrointest Endosc 2006;63:797–803.
15. Compton, C. C.: Serous cystic tumors of the pancreas. Semin Diagn Pathol 2000;17:43–56.
16. Klimstra, D. S., Adsay, N. V.: Benign and malignant tumors of the pancreas. In: Odze, R. D., Goldblum, J. R., Crawford, J. M.: Surgical Pathology of the GI Tract, Liver, Biliary Tract, and Pancreas. 1st ed. Philadelphia: Saunders; 2004. p. 709–711.
17. Klöppel, G., Kosmahl, M.: Cystic lesions and neoplasms of the pancreas: The features are becoming clearer. Pancreatology 2001 1:648–655.
18. Yamaguchi, K., Tanaka, M.: Atlas of cystic neoplasms of the pancreas. Fukuoka, Japan: Kyushu University Press/Karger AG, 2000. pp. 45–51.
19. Reddy, R. P., Smyrk, T. C., Zapiach, M., et al.: Pancreatic mucinous cystic neoplasm defined by ovarian stroma: demographics, clinical features, and prevalence of cancer. Clin Gastroenterol Hepatol 2004;2:1026–1031.
20. Yeh, T. S., Jan, Y. Y., Chiu, C. T., et al.: Characterisation of oestrogen receptor, progesterone receptor, trefoil factor 1, and epidermal growth factor and its receptor in pancreatic cystic neoplasms and pancreatic ductal adenocarcinoma. Gut 2002;51:712–716.
21. Sohn, T. A., Yeo, C. J., Cameron, J. L., et al. : Intraductal papillary mucinous neoplasms of the pancreas: an updated experience. Annals of Surgery. 2004;239: 788–797.

22. Klöppel, G., Solcia, E., Longnecker, D. S., et al.: Histological typing of tumors of the exocrine pancreas. In: World Health Organization International Classification of Tumors, 2nd ed. Berlin: Springer, 1996. pp. 11–20.
23. Serikawa, M., Sasaki, T., Fujimoto, Y., et al.: Management of intraductal papillary-mucinous neoplasm of the pancreas: treatment strategy based on morphologic classification. J Clin Gastroenterol 2006;40:856–862.
24. Itoh, S., Ishiguchi, T., Ishigaki, T., et al.: Mucin-producing pancreatic tumor: CT findings and histopathologic correlation. Radiology 1992;183:81–86.
25. Sugiyama, M., Izumisato, Y., Abe, N., et al.: Predictive factors for malignancy in intraductal papillary-mucinous tumors of the pancreas. Br J Surg 2003; 90:1244–1249.
26. Sugiyama, M., Atomi, Y., Saito, M.: Intraductal papillary tumors of the pancreas: evaluation with endoscopic ultrasonography. Gastrointest Endosc 1998;48:164–171.
27. Klimstra, D. S., Wenig, B. M., Heffess, C. S.: Solid-pseudopapillary tumor of the pancreas: a typically cystic carcinoma of low malignant potential. Semin Diagn Pathol 2000;17:66–80.
28. Bardales, R. H., Centeno, B., Mallery, J. Ss, et al.: Endoscopic ultrasound-guided fine-needle aspiration cytology diagnosis of solid-pseudopapillary tumor of the pancreas: a rare neoplasm of elusive origin but characteristic cytomorphologic features. Am J Clin Pathol 2004;121:654–662.
29. Ferrari, L., Seregni, E., Bajetta, E., et al.: The biological characteristics of chromogranin A and its role as a circulating marker in neuroendocrine tumors. Anticancer Research. 1999;19:3415–3427.

CHAPTER 18

Endoscopic Ultrasonography in Intraductal Papillary Mucinous Tumors of the Pancreas

Dr. Assaad M. Soweid
Dr. Assaad M. Skoury

Introduction

Intraductal papillary mucinous tumors (IPMTs), first described in 1982[1] are characterized by a dilated main pancreatic duct, patulous ampullary orifice, and mucus secretion (Figure 18–1). In 1996, the World Health Organization proposed a clear definition of this entity, differentiating it from other mucinous cystic tumors of the pancreas.[2] IPMTs should always be considered as a precancerous condition, as the progression along the adenoma to carcinoma line has been well described.[3] Although the exact etiology of these tumors remains unclear, several abnormalities have been described on the molecular level including: K-ras mutation (50%), p-53 overexpression, DPC4 expression (100%), MUC2 mucin and MUC5 overexpression, MUC1 mucin absence, and 14-3-3 sigma protein overexpression.[3–9] Reaching an accurate diagnosis of IPMTs most often requires the use of two or more imaging modalities. Traditional transabdominal ultrasound (US) and computed tomography (CT) have always denoted nonspecific abnormalities in patients with IPMTs,[10] often leading to overlooking of the diagnosis for long periods. Endoscopic ultrasound (EUS) has been increasingly used since 1987 to evaluate patients with cystic lesions of the pancreas. EUS is minimally invasive and it has demonstrated high accuracy in diagnosing IPMTs and defining their location in addition to features of malignancy

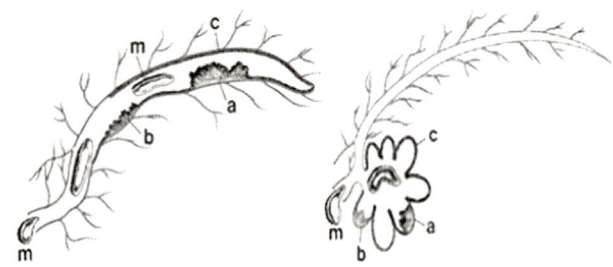

Main duct type   Branch duct type

FIGURE 18–2. A schematic representation of the two main types of IPMTs (A) mural nodule containing adenocarcinoma; (B) mural nodule containing adenoma; (C) hyperplasia of ductal cells causing cystic dilatation; m: mucin. Reproduced with permission from Lim, J. H.[52]

and invasiveness.[11] EUS coupling with fine needle aspiration/biopsy (FNA-B) has resulted in a further increase in its diagnostic accuracy, which is essential prior to surgical intervention.[12]

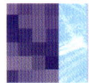 ## Classification

Based on the anatomic involvement of the pancreatic duct, IPMTs are classified as main duct type (MDT-IPMTs) or branch duct type (BDT-IPMTs) (Figure 18–2). Recently, a third type has been described, which is a combination of main duct and branch duct involvement (combined-type IPMTs). MDT-IPMTs comprise 75% of all IPMTs, and mainly arise in the head of the pancreas progressing distally. The tumors occur predominantly within the dilated main pancreatic duct (MPD), and their involvement may be focal, segmental, or diffuse. They are usually more aggressive on histopathological examination than other types of IPMTs. In contrast, BDT-IPMTs mainly arise in the uncinate process or the tail of the pancreas and carry a lower risk of malignant transformation on histopathological examination. The cystic tumors reside within the dilated branch duct and may cause secondary compressive effects.

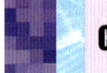 ## Clinical Manifestations

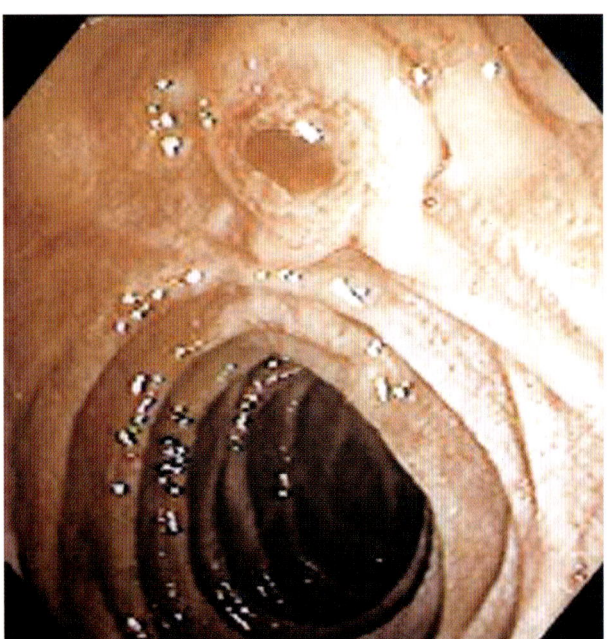

FIGURE 18–1. Endoscopic image of mucin oozing from the gaping orifice of the ampulla of Vater. Reproduced with permission from Aithal, G. P.[11]

IPMT is described mostly in male patients, 60–70 years of age, who present with symptoms of recurrent acute pancreatitis or chronic pancreatitis due to obstruction of the pancreatic ducts by mucus plugs and/or by intraductal tumorous growth.[13] However, many of these lesions may be incidentally detected during the performance of imaging studies. In some patients, there are associated elevations in the levels of liver and pancreatic enzymes or tumor markers, such as CA 19-9 and CEA[13,14] nevertheless, the elevations in tumor markers are not always indicative of malignant transformation. The median delay from first symptoms to making the diagnosis is estimated at one to two years. As though, these tumors usually course indolently and have a slow rate of transforming into malignancy.[15,16] Less frequently, patients may present with back pain, jaundice, and weight loss. Chronic obstruction of the pancreatic duct may also cause exocrine and endocrine insufficiency leading to steatorrhea and diabetes mellitus.[13,17,18]

maintain macroscopic communication with the MPD.[13,18] Histopathologically, the mucin-producing epithelial cells of the pancreatic ducts proliferate in a papillary fashion, with or without excessive mucus production and/or cystic dilatation of the pancreatic ducts in a diffuse or segmental fashion (Figure 18–3). Fibro-atrophic changes of chronic, obstructive pancreatitis due to long-standing ductal obstruction are commonly seen in the background.[13] A single lesion might often have multiple foci of gradations of histopathological aggressiveness, from simple epithelial hyperplasia, to atypical hyperplasia, to carcinoma in situ to invasive carcinoma.[19] Due to that, IPMTs are classified into three categories: benign, borderline, and malignant.[20] MDT-IPMTs commonly manifest more aggressive pathologic changes when compared with BDT-IPMTs.[21]

Pathology

Differential Diagnosis

Grossly, MDT-IPMTs are described as multilocular cystic and papillary lesions with a markedly dilated pancreatic duct, mucin-filled, that are usually located in the head of the pancreas. The BDT-IPMTs are, on the other hand, well circumscribed cystic lesions that

Cystic lesions of the pancreas can be divided into either pancreatic pseudocysts (PPCs), serous cyst adenomas (SCAs), mucinous cystic tumors (MCTs) or IPMTs.[22,23] Accurate distinction between these lesions is paramount to successful medical therapy. This can

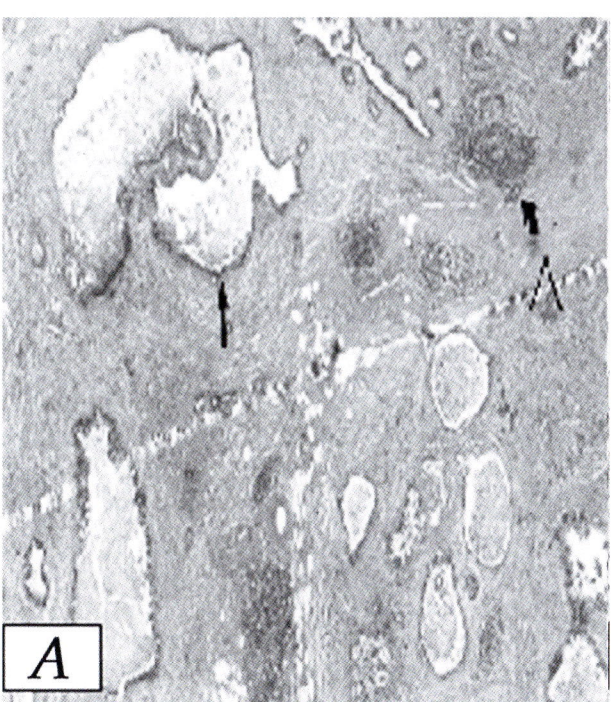
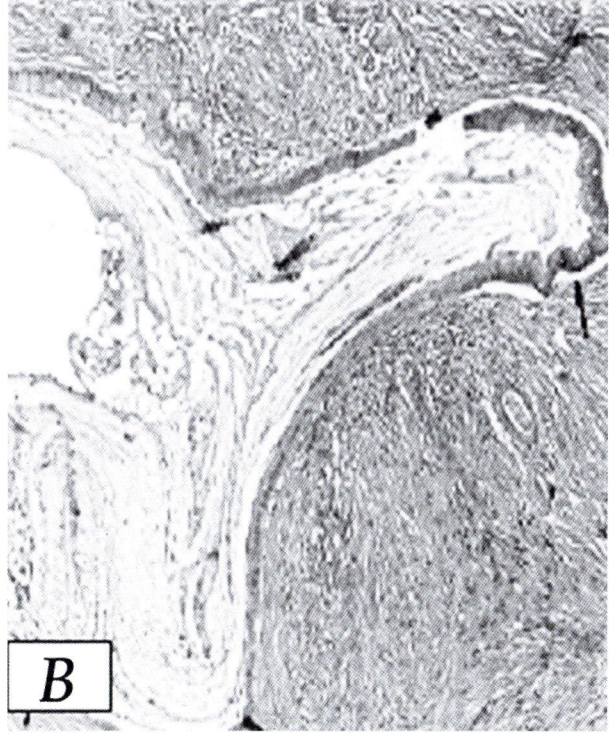

FIGURES 18–3. *A and B* Histopathological study of IPMTs. (A) Characteristic histopathology of IPMTs: dilated mucin-filled ducts (*arrow*) against the background of atrophied glandular elements with periglandular inflammatory changes (*curved arrow*). (B) Magnified view of a mucin-filled, ectatic duct lined by epithelium (*arrow*).

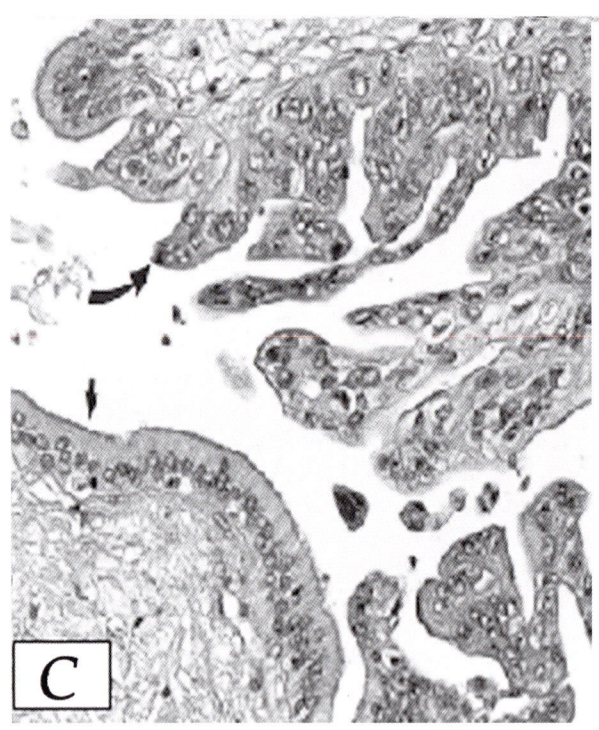

FIGURE 18–3. *C* (C) Magnified view of microscopic papillary projections (*curved arrow*). Note the normal ductal epithelium (*straight arrow*). Reproduced with permission from Prasad, S. R.[53]

usually be achieved through careful history, and the use of various biochemical, pathological, and imaging modalities that characterize these lesions.[22,24] (Table 18–1).

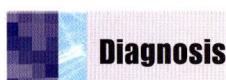 **Diagnosis**

There are different imaging modalities that can be used in the diagnosis of IPMTs. As previously mentioned, usually two or more tests are needed to reach a more accurate diagnosis. Commonly used modalities such as US and CT may demonstrate nonspecific abnormalities (Figures 18–4A, 18–4B). Representative anatomy from the Visible Human Data Base is shown in Figures 18–4C, and 18–4D. In addition, these modalities used alone cannot differentiate IPMTs from diseases like MCT of the pancreas, chronic obstructive pancreatitis, and pancreatic ductal adenocarcinoma. Endoscopic retrograde cholangio-pancreatography (ERCP) is an invasive, yet accurate imaging modality to evaluate patients with suspected IPMT. It often shows segmental or diffuse dilatation of the pancreatic duct, commonly with filling defects from mucus plugs[25] (Figure 18–5, Figure 18–6). ERCP also allows tissue sampling as well as performing therapeutic maneuvers. During ERCP, a common finding is oozing of mucin from the gaping orifice of the ampulla of Vater (Figure 18–1).

Magnetic resonance cholangio-pancreatography (MRCP) (Figures 18–7, 18–8) has a high diagnostic accuracy for IPMTs and can reveal the full extent of ductal involvement, particularly when obstructing mucus prevents full opacification of the MPD.[26]

Role of Endoscopic Ultrasonography

EUS is an extremely valuable tool for the evaluation of cystic lesions of the pancreas. It is minimally invasive and can provide detailed imaging of pancreatic lesions due to the ability to place the high-frequency ultrasound transducer in close proximity to the pancreas. Furthermore, the use of different frequencies and various scanning windows (gastric or duodenal) may further contribute to an enhanced, detailed image quality of the target lesion.

Aithal et al demonstrated that EUS, when performed by an experienced endosonographer, can accurately identify IPMT. When compared to ERCP for the detection of IPMT, EUS had an excellent accuracy (sensitivity of 86%, specificity of 99%, positive predictive value of 78%, and negative predictive value of 99%).[11]

EUS findings for IPMTs include dilatation (segmental or diffuse) of the MPD (Figure 18–9) with the presence of intraductal (mural) nodules in MDT-IPMTs (Figure 18–10), or multiple cysts in BDT-IPMTs (Figures 18–11, 18–12). Pancreatic parenchymal atrophy is also noted on EUS. However, the paucity of

Table 18-1 Clinical, Laboratory, and Endosonographic Features Differentiating Cystic Lesions of the Pancreas.

	SCA	MCT	IPMT	PPC
Gender	F>M	F>M	M>F	M>F
Mean Age (years)	~60	~60	~60	Variable
History of Pancreatitis	Uncommon	Uncommon	Common	Common
Malignant Potential	Very Low	High	High	No
Location	Even	Body/Tail	Head	Head
Presence of Septae	Yes	Yes	Rare	Variable
Locularity	Multiple small	Multilocular	Multilocular	Unilocular
Aspirated Fluid				
Viscocity	Low	High	High	Low
Amylase	Variable	Variable	High	High
CA 15-3	Low	High	Variable	Low
CEA	Low	High	Variable	Low
CA 19-9	Variable	Variable	Variable	Variable
Cytology	Glycogen	Mucinous	Mucinous	Histiocytes

SCA: Serous Cyst Adenoma; MCT: Mucinous Cystic Tumors; IPMT: Intraductal Papillary Mucinous Tumors; PPC: Pancreatic Pseudocysts; CEA: Carcinoembryonic Antigen; CA: Carbohydrate Antigen

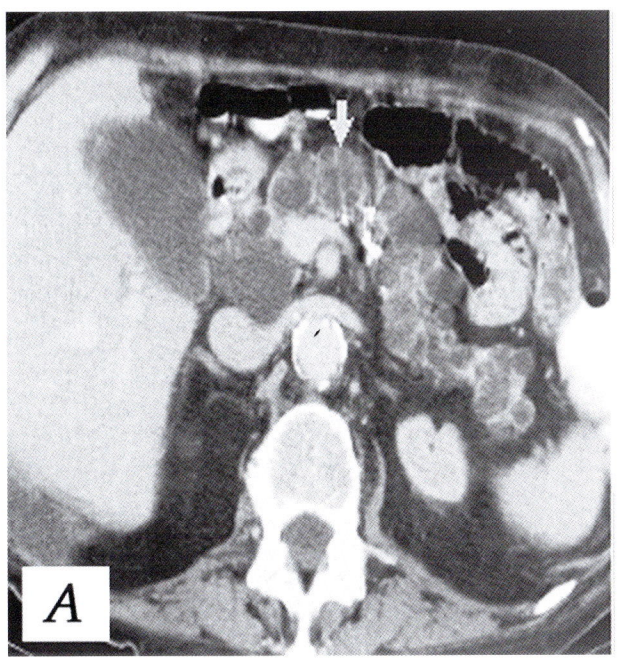
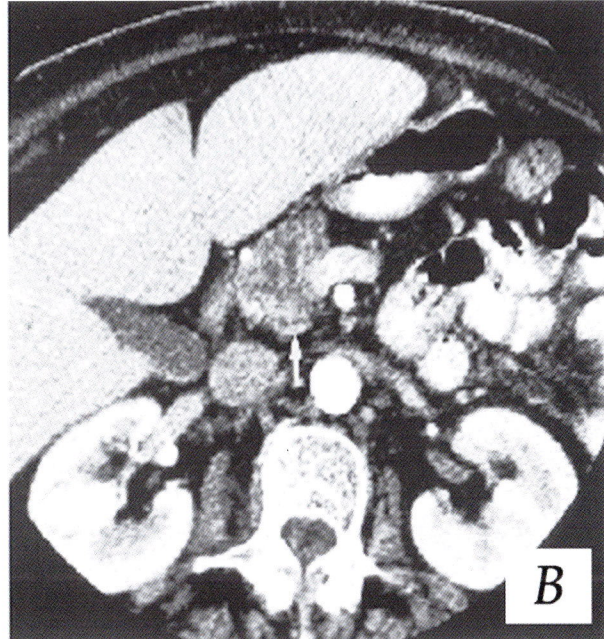

FIGURES 18-4. *A and B* Contrast-enhanced CT of MDT-IPMTs. (A) Diffuse pancreatic ductal dilatation (*arrow*) without a pancreatic mass. (B) A rare microcystic variant of IPMT resembling a microcystic serous cystadenoma (*arrow*). Reproduced with permission from Prasad, S. R.[53] Axial cross-section from Visible Human female

196   EUS Pathology with Digital Anatomy Correlation

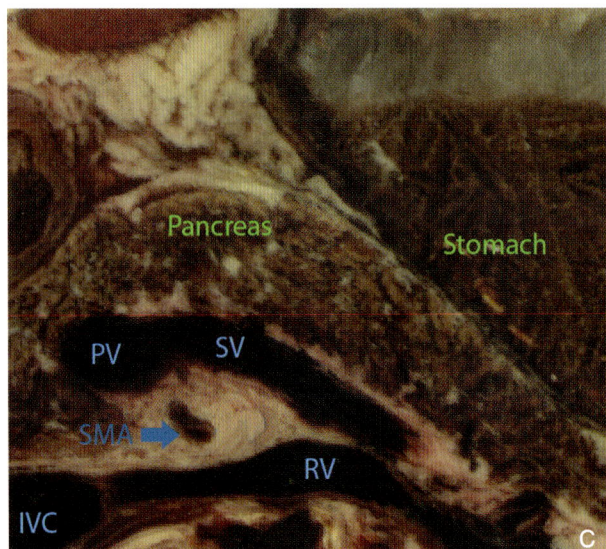

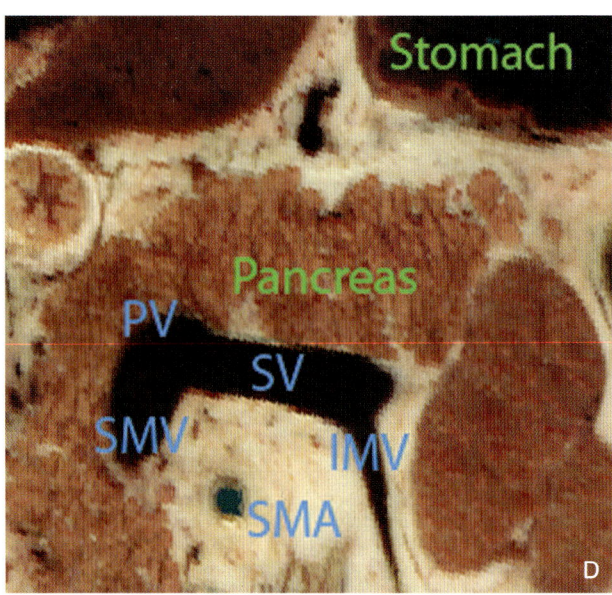

FIGURES 18–4. C and D   (C) and Visible Human male (D) at a level that corresponds to Figure 18–4A. PV=portal vein, SV=splenic vein, IVC=inferior vena cava, RV=left renal vein. SMA=superior mesenteric artery, SMV= superior mesenteric vein, IMV=inferior mesenteric vein.

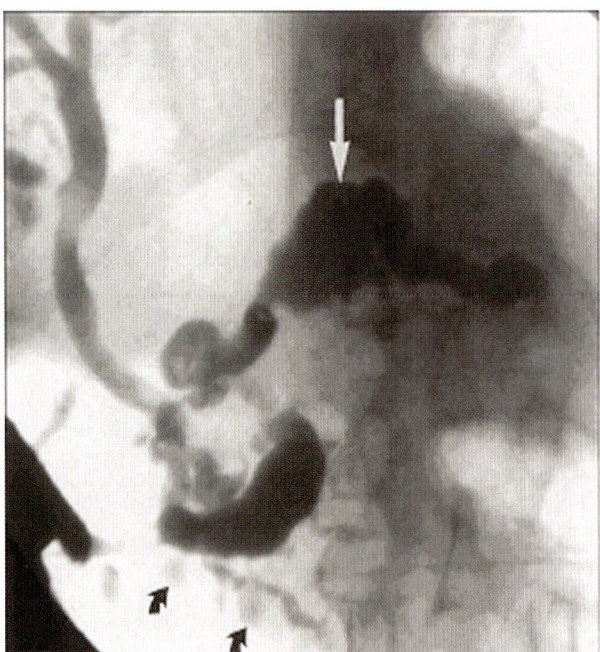

FIGURE 18–5.   Combined-type IPMT. ERCP demonstrates diffuse dilatation of the MPD (*straight arrow*) and ectatic branch ducts (*curved arrows*). Reproduced with permission from Prasad, S. R.[53]

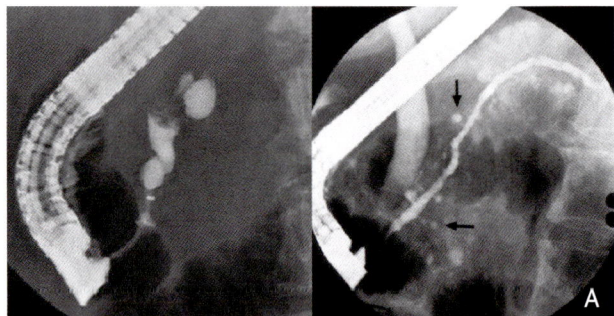

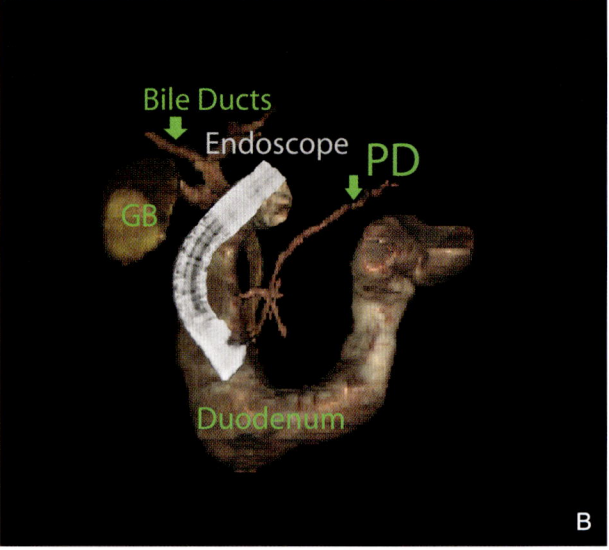

FIGURES 18–6. A and B   (A) ERCP view of a MDT-IPMT lesion with diffuse dilatation of the MPD and filling defects due to mucinous plugs (left), and normal-caliber MPD duct with few dilated side-branch ducts (*arrows*) denoting a BDT-IPMT (right). (B) Visible Human Model of the relevant anatomy. GB = gall bladder, PD = pancreatic duct.

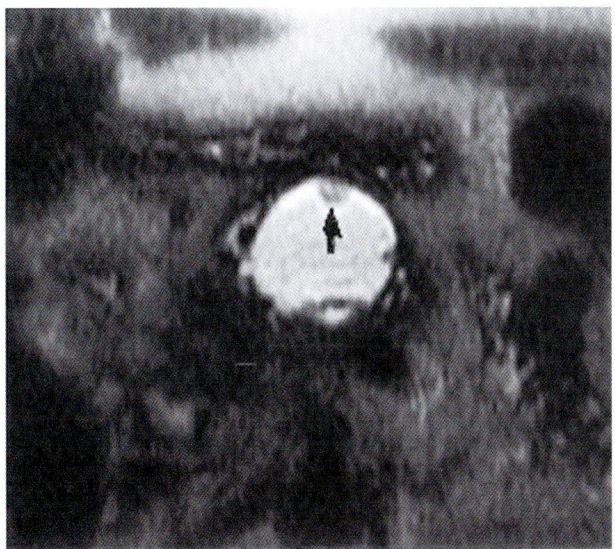

FIGURE 18-7. Cystic dilatation of the MPD with a hypointense area on T2 weighted MRI demonstrating an intramural nodule (arrow). Reproduced with permission from Prasad, S. R.[53]

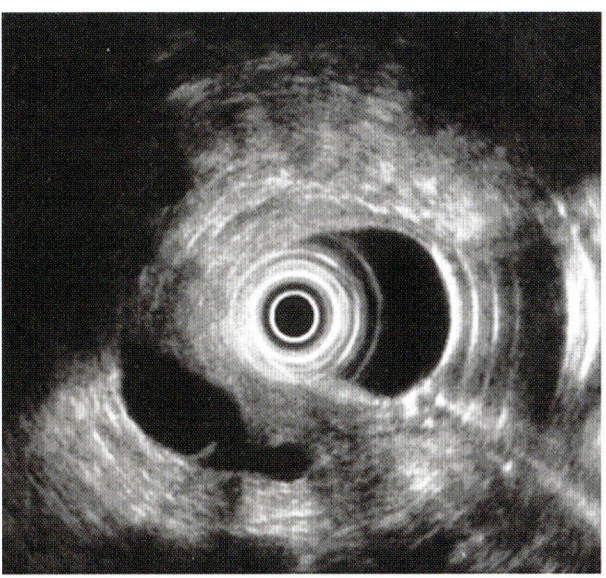

FIGURE 18-9. Radial EUS image of diffuse dilatation of the MPD in MDT-IPMT.

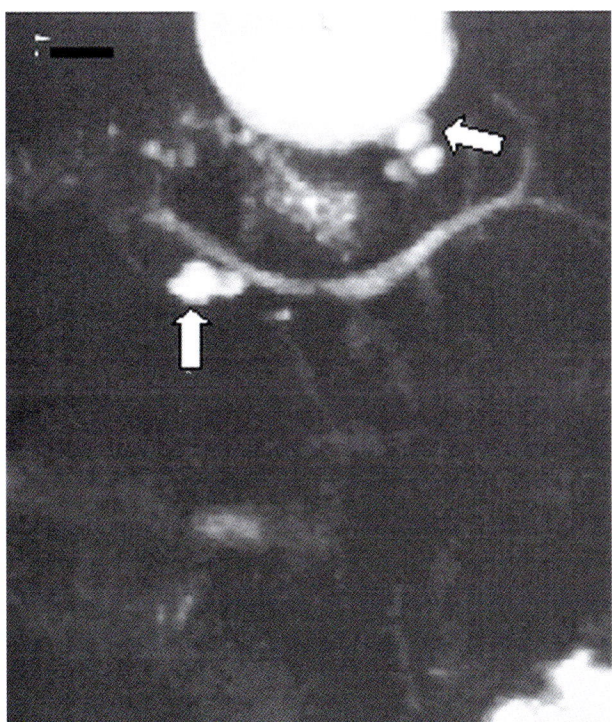

FIGURE 18-8. MRCP image in a patient with BDT-IPMT showing normal MPD with cystic dilatation of branch pancreatic ducts (arrows). Reproduced with permission from Irie, H.[54]

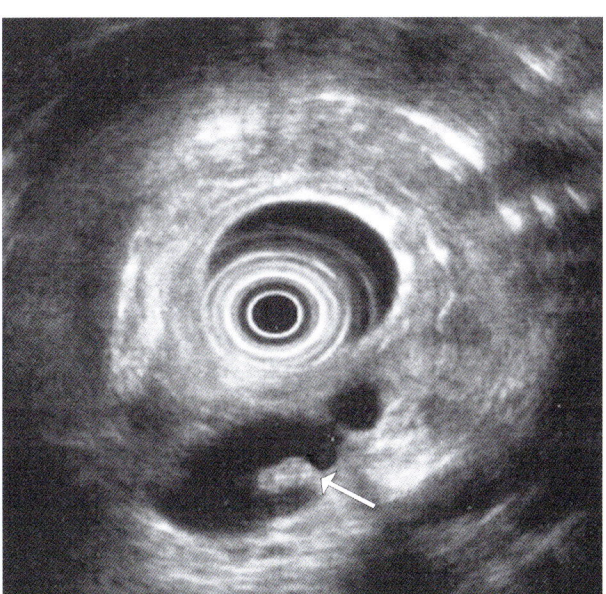

FIGURE 18-10. EUS appearance of a hyperechoeic intraductal (mural) nodule in MDT-IPMT *(straight arrow)*.

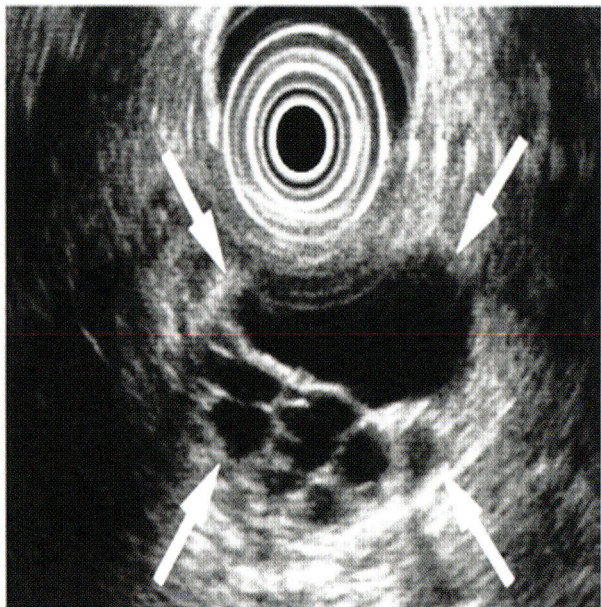

FIGURE 18–11. EUS view showing a cluster of multiple cystic dilatations *(arrows)* separated by thick septae in a lesion demonstrating a BDT-IPMT. Reproduced with permission from Kubo, H.[29]

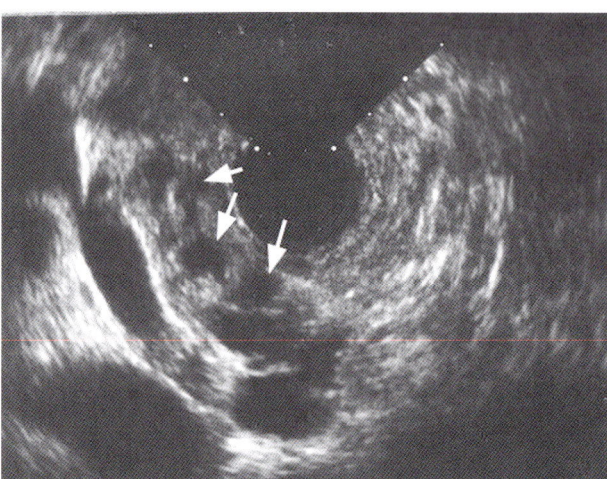

FIGURE 18–12. EUS image of multiple cysts *(arrows)* in BDT-IPMT

endosonographic parenchymal features of chronic pancreatitis (one or less) carries high odds in differentiating IPMT from other causes of chronic pancreatitis. EUS features of dilated pancreatic duct, presence of cysts, and presence of pancreatic atrophy are significantly more common in patients with IPMTs as compared to those with chronic pancreatitis.[11] Comparative studies have demonstrated that EUS was superior to US and ERCP in the diagnosis of IPMTs [27] and as accurate as CT and ERCP in distinguishing between invasive and noninvasive tumors.[28]

Certain EUS features suggestive of malignancy include the presence of mural nodules (especially greater than 4 mm) (Figure 18–13) and dilated MPD (usually greater than 10 mm) in MDT-IPMTs (Figure 13–14); a large tumor size (greater than 30 mm) with irregular, thick septum in BDT-IPMTs (Figure 18–15).[22,27,29–33]

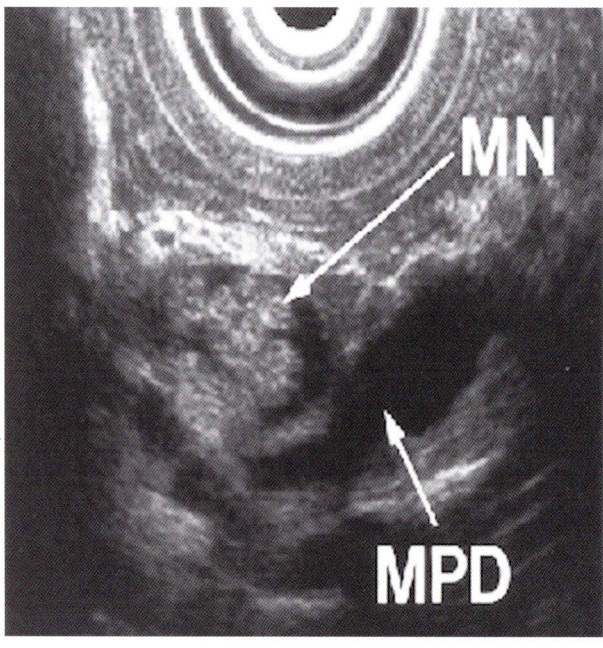

FIGURE 18–13. EUS view of a large mural nodule (MN) suggestive of malignant transformation. Reproduced with permission from Kubo, H.[29]

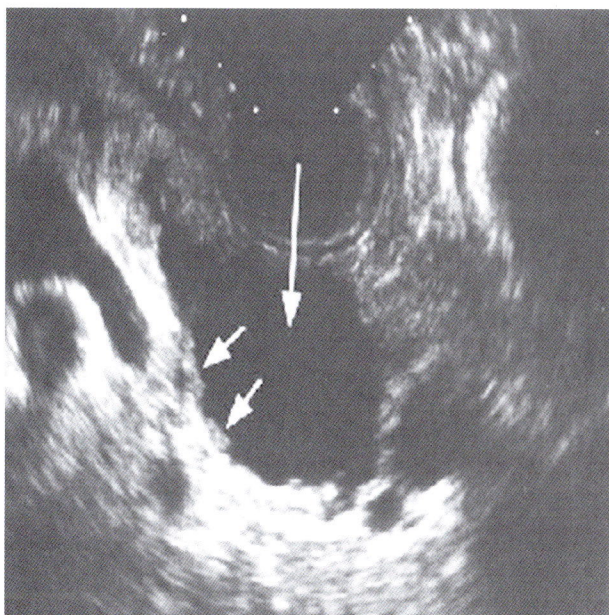

FIGURE 18–14. EUS image obtained with a radial echoendoscope showing features of MDT-IPMT. There is MPD dilatation *(large arrows)* with small intraductal nodules *(small arrows)*.

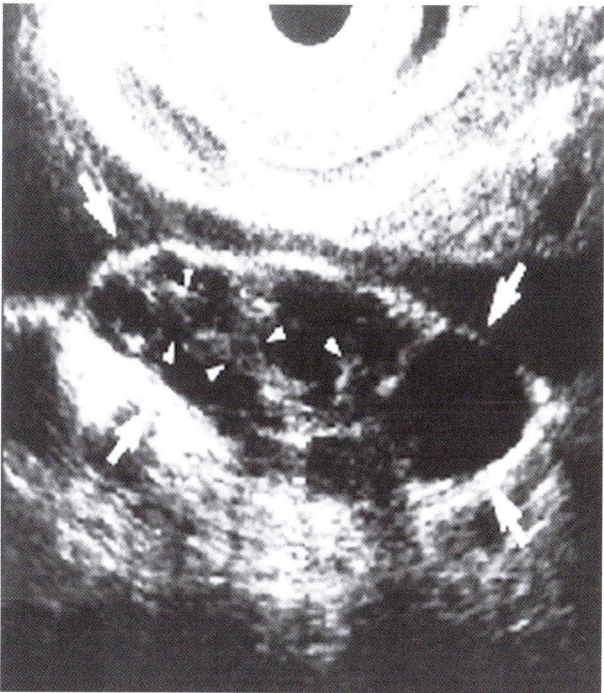

FIGURE 18–15. An EUS examination demonstrating a BDT-IPMT with a large (45 mm) multicystic lesion (arrows) with thick septae (arrow heads) suggestive of malignancy. Reproduced with permission from Kubo, H.[29]

Role of EUS with Fine Needle Aspiration

EUS also offers the possibility of guided FNA of mural nodules and pancreatic juice. Aspirated samples can be sent for cytological evaluation, tumor markers, and possibly, determination of K-ras mutation and telomerase activity. EUS-FNA was found to be superior to EUS alone for diagnosing malignancy in IPMTs[3,8,34,35] (Figure 18–16).

IPMTs possess distinctive cytopathological features, which can be used to distinguish them from other cystic pancreatic lesions.[36] The most common features of IPMTs were the presence of extracellular mucin

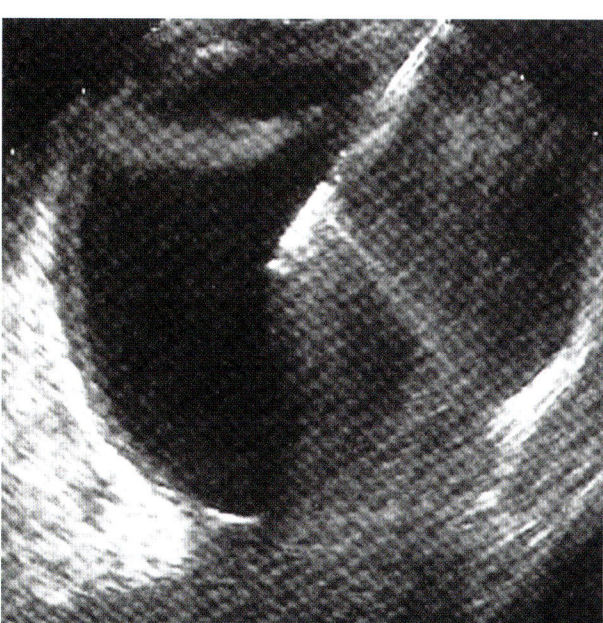

FIGURE 18–16. EUS-guided introduction of a fine needle into a pancreatic cystic lesion

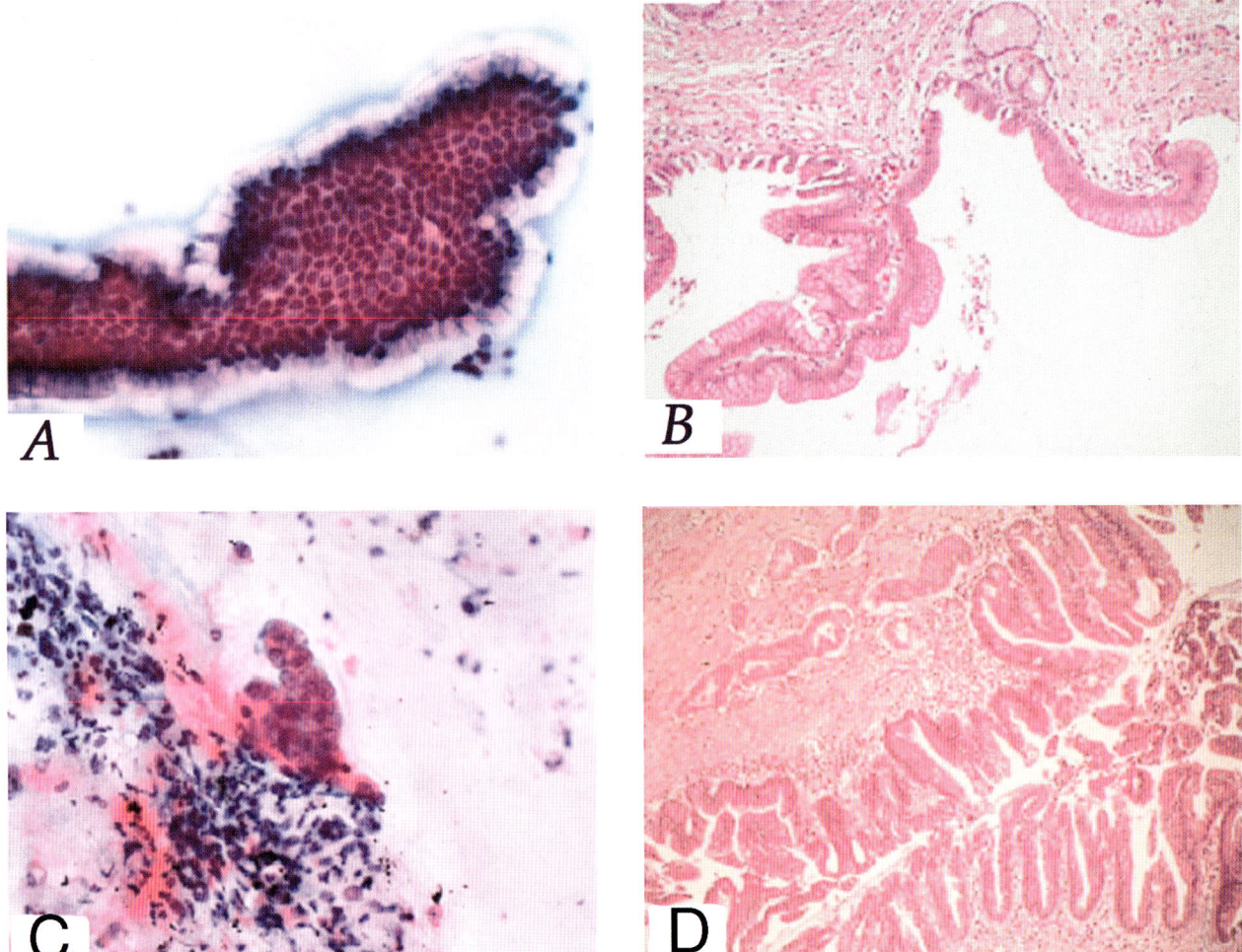

FIGURES 18-17. A to D Fine needle aspirate specimen with counterpart surgical specimen. (A) Mucinous epithelium without atypia from a benign IPMT lesion. (B) The counterpart surgical specimen of the papillary tumor in A. (C) Micropapillary cluster of highly atypical cells on a mucinous background in an EUS-FNA of an IPMT lesion with invasive ductal carcinoma. (D) A papillary intraductal proliferation lined with eosinophilic epithelium containing goblet cells, as the surgical counterpart specimen of the tumor aspirated in C. (**A and C**: Papanicolaou stain, Original Magnification X 400; **B and D**: H & E stain, Original Magnification X 200 and X 100 respectively). Reproduced with permission from Sole, M.[37]

and sheets of mucinous epithelium. Nonmucinous epithelium, severe atypia, single atypical cells, and irregular clusters indicated a high probability of malignant transformation[37,38] (Figure 18-17). The sensitivity of histopathological analysis of EUS-guided biopsy specimens was 91% for positive diagnosis of IPMTs with solid components.[39] The integration of clinical, endosonographic, and cytological information may be the best way to obtain the most accurate diagnosis possible.[40] Furthermore, EUS-guided FNA appears to be a safe procedure.[41]

Role of Intraductal Ultrasound and 3-Dimentional EUS

The standard echoendoscopes are limited by their large diameter and resultant inability to gain access to ductal systems or stenoses. They are also limited by their relatively low scanning frequencies (7.5/12 MHz), and thus, inadequate image resolution. Ultrasound miniprobes were developed to offer access to narrow intraluminal spaces and to the pancreaticobiliary system (Figure 18-18). Intraductal ultrasonography (IDUS) involves the use of high-frequency miniprobes with the advantages of enhanced image resolution and access to strictures. The use of IDUS had a significant impact on the management in many patients with various gastrointestinal and pancreaticobiliary diseases.[42]

IDUS has been reported as a reliable method for more detailed evaluation of IPMT (Figure 15-19).[43] It was also found useful in the preoperative localization and prediction of extension of IPMTs, which is valuable in selecting pancreatic resection methods.[44] Combined use of IDUS with peroral pancreatoscopy

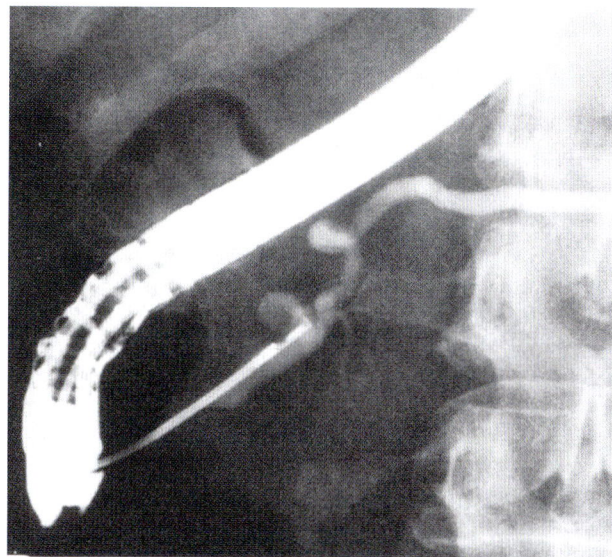

FIGURE 18–18. Image of miniprobe introduction into the MPD during ERCP

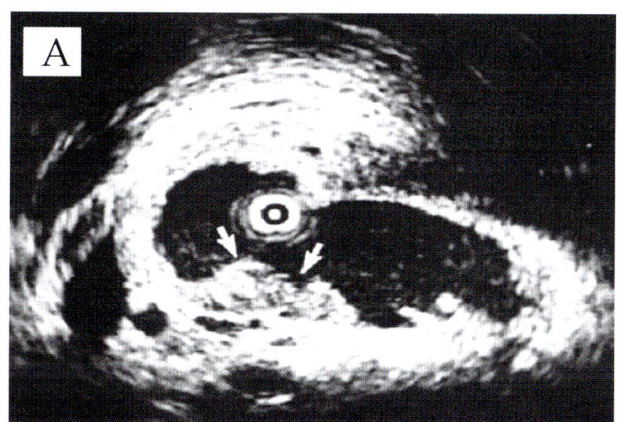
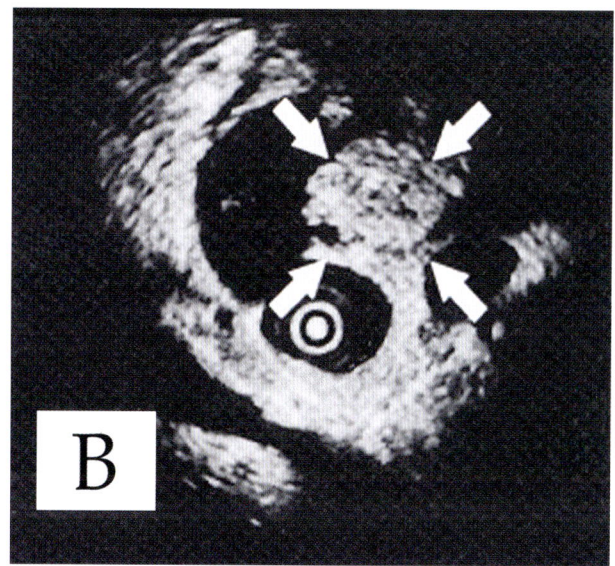
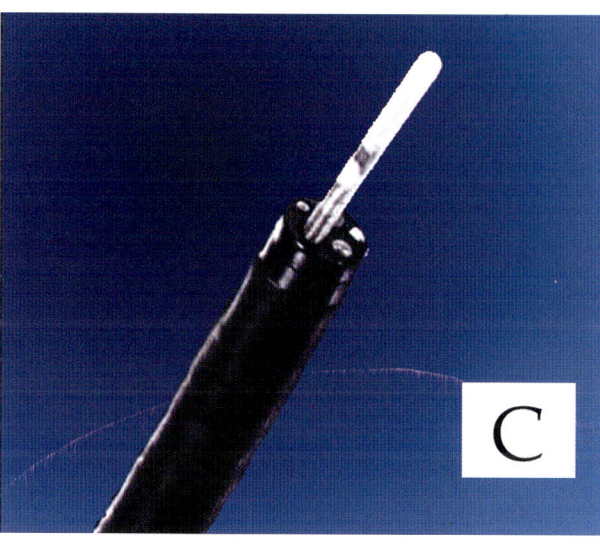

FIGURES 18–19. *A to C* Intraductal ultrasound (IDUS). (A) IDUS image demonstrating a hyperechoic nodule (arrows) in the MPD. (B) IDUS view of intraductal lesion (arrows) protruding into the dilated pancreatic duct. (C) A photograph of the ultrasound miniprobe.

resulted in improvement of the differential diagnosis between benign and malignant IPMTs and was useful in determining an effective therapeutic approach.[33,45] Combination of EUS and IDUS showed a high accuracy rate in the diagnosis of invasive IPMTs.[46]

Three-dimensional EUS is another novel imaging modality that was found accurate in the assessment of pancreatic tumor extension into surrounding structures in a reduced period of exam time.[47] It can clearly display the papillary structures of IPMTs and, with more sophisticated software and hardware developments, is expected to evaluate more accurately tumor extension and invasion into surrounding structures.[48]

Outcome and Therapy

The five-year survival rate for patients with IPMTs is 98–100% in adenoma to noninvasive carcinoma cases, 89% in minimally invasive carcinoma cases, and 58% in invasive carcinoma cases.[22] The therapeutic modality of choice remains surgical resection, including partial or total pancreatectomy, depending on the extent of ductal involvement and regardless of MDT-IPMTs or BDT-IPMTs.[30] Survival data showed improved five-year survival following surgical resection, even in invasive carcinoma when compared to cases of ductal adenocarcinoma.[4] Long-term surveillance is of critical importance because of the risk of recurrent disease in cases of partial pancreatectomy.[30,49–51]

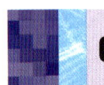

Conclusion

EUS is an increasingly used, accurate modality for the diagnosis of IPMTs. Certain endosonographic features are highly indicative of a malignancy. The addition of FNA further enhances diagnostic capability through sampling of the mural nodules or aspiration of the pancreatic juice for cytology and tumor markers determination. IDUS provides high-resolution imaging of the pancreatic duct and can be used for the localization and prediction of extension of IPMTs. IDUS can be used in conjunction with other modalities (like EUS or pancreatoscopy) to further improve the diagnostic yield.

References

1. Ohhashi, K., Murakami, Y., Maruyama, M., et al.: Four cases of mucous secreting pancreatic cancer. Prog Dig Endosc 1982;20:348–51.
2. Kloppel, G., Solcia, E., Longnecker, D. S., et al.: Histological typing of tumors of the exocrine pancreas. In World Health Organization international histological classification of tumors. Second ed. Berlin: Springer; 1996. pp. 1–61.
3. Sessa, F., Solica, E., Capella, C., et al.: Intraductal papillay-mucinous tumors represent a distinct group of pancreatic neoplasms: an investigation of tumor cell differentiation and K-ras, p-53, c-erbB-2 abnormalities in 26 patients. Virchows Arch 1994;425:357–567.
4. Raimondo, M., Tachibana, I., Urrutia, R., et al.: Invasive cancer and survival of intraductal papillary mucinous tumors of the pancreas. Am J Gastroenterol 2002; 97:2553–2558.
5. Moore, P. S., Orlandini, S., Zamboni, G., et al.: Pancreatic tumors: molecular pathways implicated in ductal cancer are involved in ampullary but not in exocrine nonductal or endocrine tumorogenesis. Br J Cancer 2001;84:253–262.
6. Yonezawa, S., Sato, E.: Expression of mucin antigens in human cancers and its relationship with malignancy potential. Pathol Int 1997;47:813–830.
7. Okada, T., Masuda, N., Fukai, Y., et al.: Immunohistochemical expression of 14-3-3 sigma protein in intraductal papillary-mucinous tumor and invasive ductal carcinoma of the pancreas. Anticancer Res. 2006; 26:3105–110.
8. Ito, H., Endo, T., Oka, T., et al.: Mucin expression profile is related to biological and clinical characteristics of intraductal papillary-mucinous tumors of the pancreas. Pancreas 2005;30:96–102.
9. Soldini, D., Gugger, M., Burckhardt, E., et al.: Progressive genomic alterations in intraductal papillary mucinous tumors of the pancreas and morphologically similar lesions of the pancreatic ducts. J Pathol 2003;199:453–461.
10. McDowell, R. K., Gazelle, G. S., Murphy, B. L., et al.: Mucinous ductal ectasia of the pancreas. J Comput Assist Tomogr 1997;21:383–288.
11. Aithal, G. P., Chen, R., Cunningham, J., et al.: Accuracy of EUS for detection of intraductal papillary-mucinous tumors of the pancreas. Gastrintest Endosc 2002; 56:701–707.
12. Bounds, B. C.: Diagnosis and fine needle aspiration of intraductal papillary mucinous tumors by endoscopic ultrasound. Gastrointest Endosc Clin N Am. 2002;12:735–745.
13. Bassi, C., Procacci, C., Zamboni, G., et al.: Intraductal papillary mucinous tumors of the pancreas. Verona University Pancreatic Team. Int J Pancreatol 2000; 27:181–193.
14. Tanaka, M., Sawai, H., Okada, Y., et al.: Clinicopathological study of intraductal papillary mucinous tumors and mucinous cystic tumors of the pancreas. Hepatogastroenterology. 2006;53:783–787.
15. Paal, E., Thompson, L. D., Przygodzki, R. M., et al.: A clinicopathologic and immunohistochemical study of 22 intraductal papillary mucinous neoplasms of the pancreas, with a review of the literature. Mod Pathol 1999;12:518–528.
16. Warshaw, A. L.: Mucinous cystic tumors and mucinous ductal ectasia of the pancreas. Gastrointest Endosc 1991;37:199–201.
17. Kobari, M., Egawa, S., Shibuya, K., et al.: Intraductal papillary mucinous tumors of the pancreas comprise 2 clinical subtypes: differences in clinical characteristics and surgical management. Arch Surg 1999;134: 1131–1136

18. Taouli, B., Vilgrain, V., Vullierme, M. P., et al. Intraductal papillary mucinous tumors of the pancreas: helical CT with histopathological correlation. Radiology 2000;217:757–764.
19. Nagai, E., Ueki, T., Chijiiwa, K., et al.: Intraductal papillary mucinous neoplasms of the pancreas associated with so-called "mucinous duct ectasia": histochemical and immunohistochemical analysis of 29 cases. Am J Surg Pathol 1995;19:576–589.
20. Solcia, E., Capella, C., Kloppel, G.: Tumors of the pancreas. In: Atlas of tumor pathology. Washington, D. C. Armed Forces Institute of Pathology; 1997. pp. 53–64.
21. Terris, B., Ponssot, P., Pave, F., et al.: Intraductal papillary mucinous tumors of the pancreas confined to secondary ducts show less aggressive pathologic features as compared with those involving the main pancreatic duct. Am J Surg Pathol 2000;24:1372–1377.
22. Suzuki, Y., Atomi, Y., Sugiyama, M., et al.: Cystic neoplasm of the pancreas: a Japanese multiinstitutional study of intraductal papillary mucinous tumor and mucinous cystic tumor. Pancreas 2004;28:241–246.
23. Goh, B. K., Tan, Y. M., Cheow, P. C., et al.: Cystic neoplasms of the pancreas with mucin production. Eur J Surg Oncol 2005;31:282–287.
24. Levy, M. J., Wiesema, M. J.: Pancreatic neoplasms. Gastrointest Endoscopy Clin N Am. 2005;15:117–142.
25. Raijman, I., Kortan, P., Walden, D., et al.: Mucinous ductal ectasia: cholangiopancreatographic and endoscopic findings. Endoscopy 1994;26:303–307.
26. Farrell, J. J., Brugge, W. R.: Intraductal papillary mucinous tumor of the pancreas. Gastrointest Endosc 2002;55:701–714.
27. Sugiyama, M., Atomi, Y., Saito, M.: Intraductal papillary tumors of the pancreas: Evaluation with endoscopic ultrasonography. Gastrointest Endosc 1998;48:164–171.
28. Cellier, C., Cuillerier, E., Palazzo, L., et al.: Intraductal papillary and mucinous tumors of the pancreas: accuracy of preoperative computed tomography, endoscopic retrograde pancreatography and endoscopic ultrasonography, and long-term outcome in a large surgical series. Gastrointest Endosc 1998;47:42–49.
29. Kubo, H., Chijiiwa, Y., Akahoshi, K., et al.: Intraductal papillary-mucinous tumors of the pancreas: differential diagnosis between benign and malignant tumors by endoscopic ultrasonography. Am J Gastroenterol 2001;96:1429–1434.
30. Jang, J. Y., Kim, S. W., Ahn, Y. J., et al.: Multicenter analysis of clinicopathologic features of intraductal papillary mucinous tumor of the pancreas: is it possible to predict the malignancy before surgery? Ann Surg Oncol 2005;12:124–132.
31. Sugiyama, M., Izumisato, Y., Abe, N., et al.: Predictive factors for malignancy in intraductal papillary–mucinous tumors of the pancreas. Br J Surg 2003; 90:1244–1249.
32. Kawai, M., Uchiyama, K., Tani, M., et al.: Clinicopathological features of malignant intraductal papillary mucinous tumors of the pancreas: the differential diagnosis from benign entities. Arch Surg. 2004; 139:188–192.
33. Hara, T., Yamaguchi, T., Ishihara, T., et al. : Diagnosis and patient management of intraductal papillary-mucinous tumor of the pancreas by using peroral pancreatoscopy and intraductal ultrasonography. Gastroenterology 2002;122:34–43.
34. Inoue, H., Tsuchida, A., Kawasaki, Y., et al.: Preoperative diagnosis of intraductal papillary-mucinous tumors of the pancreas with attention to telomerase activity. Cancer 2001;91:35–41.
35. Brandwein, S. L., Farell, J. J., Centeno, B. A., et al.: Detection and tumor staging of malignancy in cystic, intraductal and solid tumors of the pancreas by EUS. Gastrointest Endosc 2001;53:722–727.
36. Recine, M., Kaw, M., Evans, D. B., et al.: Fine-needle aspiration cytology of mucinous tumors of the pancreas. Cancer 2004;102:92–99.
37. Sole, M., Iglesias, C., Fernandez-Esparrach, G., et al.: Fine-needle aspiration cytology of intraductal papillary mucinous tumors of the pancreas. Cancer 2005;105: 298–303.
38. Stelow, E. B., Stanley, M. W., Bardales, R. H., et al.: Intraductal papillary-mucinous neoplasm of the pancreas. The findings and limitations of cytologic samples obtained by endoscopic ultrasound-guided fine-needle aspiration. Am J Clin Pathol 2003;120: 398–404.
39. Maire, F., Couvelard, A., Hammel, P., et al. : Intraductal papillary mucinous tumors of the pancreas: the preoperative value of cytologic and histopathologic diagnosis. Gastrointest Endosc 2003;58:701–706.
40. Soweid, A., Azar, C., Labban, B.: Endoscopic evaluation of intraductal papillary mucinous tumors of the pancreas. J Pancreas 2004;5:258–265.
41. Lai, R., Stanley, M. W., Bardales, R., et al.: Endoscopic ultrasound-guided pancreatic duct aspiration: diagnostic yield and safety. Endoscopy 2002;4:715–720.
42. Chak, A., Soweid, A., Hoffman, B., et al.: Clinical implications of endoluminal ultrasonography using through-the-scope catheter probes. Gastrintest Endosc 1998;48: 485–490.
43. Taki, T., Goto, H., Naitoh, Y., et al. : Diagnosis of mucin-producing tumor of the pancreas with an intraductal ultrasonographic system. J Ultrasound Med 1997;16: 1–6.
44. Moon, J. H., Cho, Y. D., Cheon, Y. K., et al.: Wire-guided intraductal US in the assessment of bile duct strictures with Mirizzi syndrome-like features at ERCP. Gastrointest Endosc 2002;56:873–879.
45. Yamaguchi, T., Hara, T., Tsuyguchi, T., et al.: Peroral pacreatoscopy in the diagnosis of mucin-producing tumors of the pancreas. Gastrointest Endosc 2000; 52:67–73.
46. Yamao, K., Ohashi, K., Nakamura, T., et al.: Evaluation of various imaging methods in the differential diagnosis of intraductal papillary-mucinous tumor (IPMT) of the pancreas. Hepatogastroenterology. 2001;48: 962–966.
47. Kanemaki, N., Nakazawa, S., Inui, K., et al.: Three-dimensional intraductal ultrasonography: preliminary results of a new technique for the diagnosis of diseases of the pancreaticobiliary system. Endoscopy 1997; 29:726–731.
48. Ishikawa, H., Hirooka, Y., Itoh, A., et al.: A comparison of image quality between tissue harmonic imaging and fundamental imaging with an electronic radial scanning echoendoscope in the diagnosis of pancreatic diseases. Gastrintest Endosc 2003;57: 931–936.
49. Sohn, T. A., Yeo, C. J., Cameron, J. L., et al.: Intraductal papillary mucinous neoplasm of the pancreas: an updated experience. Ann Surg 2004;239:788–799.
50. Lee, S. Y., Lee, K. T., Lee, J. K., et al.: Long-term follow-up results of intraductal papillary mucinous tumors of the pancreas. Journal Gastroenterol Hepatol 2005; 20;1379–1384.

51. Maire, F., Hammel, P., Terris, B., et al.: Prognosis of malignant intraductal papillary mucinous tumors of the pancreas after surgical resection: comparison with pancreatic ductal adenocarcinoma. Gut 2002;51: 717–722.
52. Lim, J. H., Lee, G., Oh, Y. L.: Radiologic spectrum of intraductal papillary mucinous tumors of the pancreas. Radiographics 2001;21:323–337.
53. Prasad, S. R., Sahani, D., Nasser, S., et al.: Pictorial essay: intraductal papillary mucinous tumors of the pancreas. Abdom Imaging 2003;28:357–365.
54. Irie, H., Yoshimitsu, K., Aibe, H., et al.: Natural history of intraductal papillary mucinous tumors of branch duct type: follow-up study by magnetic retrograde cholangiopancreatography. J Comput Assist Tomogr 2004;28:117–122.

CHAPTER 19

Chronic Pancreatitis

Dr. Lyndon V. Hernandez
Dr. Marc F. Catalano
Dr. Manoop S. Bhutani

EUS Features of Chronic Pancreatitis

According to the Marseilles conference, chronic pancreatitis (CP) is defined as an inflammatory disease characterized by permanent and progressive morphologic or functional damage in the pancreas.[1] Several years later, the Cambridge criteria was established as a severity index using pancreatography, CT scan, and transabdominal ultrasound to define pancreatic ductal abnormalities as well as other features, such as cavity and filling defects.[2]

The advancement of EUS over the past two decades has made it possible to assess the gross structure of the pancreas in a relatively less invasive manner than ERCP. More importantly, it has revealed reproducible parenchymal features that were not appreciated in previous imaging modalities. A patient is sent for EUS evaluation of the pancreas to detect the presence of CP when there is a suspicion of CP based on clinical findings, or when there is a need to assess the extent of disease in cases of established CP. In the former group of patients, the indications for EUS include assessing patients with idiopathic acute pancreatitis (one or more episodes).

In reality an endosonographer is left in a difficult situation knowing that the gold standard in diagnosing CP is quite elusive. Pancreatic function tests are performed in only a handful of centers in the United States and are not readily available to many clinicians. On the other hand, there are no established histological criteria for CP (chronic inflammation, fibrosis, and acinar atrophy) that are universally agreed upon among pathologists.[3] Apart from the inherent difficulty in obtaining an adequate specimen, the patchy nature of CP can lead to sampling error. EUS and all other imaging methods, such as ERCP, are obviously not 100% accurate. Although EUS appears to be a "benign" diagnostic test, it is subject to operator bias and can lead to false-positive results that carry important clinical consequences to a patient's emotional, financial, and physical well-being. ERCP, particularly in those with subtle imaging abnormalities, has become inconsequential, in light of inconclusive findings that it often leads to and the unnecessary risk of acute pancreatitis.

Several EUS features of CP that have been described (Table 19–1).[4,5,6,9,12] Wiersema et al[5] validated 11 EUS criteria comprising parenchymal and ductal abnormalities representing chronic pancreatitis. ROC curve showed that three or more criteria gave a sensitivity, specificity, and accuracy of 80%, 86%, and 86%, respectively. EUS has also been compared with ERCP and secretin test.[6] ERCP had excellent agreement with normal, moderate, and severe CP by EUS criteria, but poor (17%) for mild disease. Moreover, secretin tests had excellent agreement with normal and severe CP by EUS criteria, but poor for mild (13%) and moderate disease (50%). Chowdhury et al[7] produced similar results with EUS and secretin tests leading to discordant results among patients with minimal change chronic pancreatitis, which is a loosely defined term to describe a condition presenting with pancreatic-type pain but inconclusive imaging tests. It appears that EUS is accurate and useful in assessing opposite ends of the spectrum: healthy pancreas as well as severe CP. On the other hand, the diagnosis of CP remains difficult among those with mild or moderate disease, which is quite commonly encountered in clinical practice. Thus in the absence of an acceptable gold standard, it is not known whether EUS features of early CP truly represent mild disease or if they merely overestimate a normal pancreas.

In a retrospective cohort study,[8] our group followed patients with minimal change chronic pancreatitis by EUS for at least 6 years (mean 8.5 years). Of the 37 patients with minimal criteria for CP, 20 developed worse CP by EUS, including 14 moderate and 6 severe disease cases. Based on this preliminary data, subtle abnormalities detected by EUS in patients with typical epigastric pain radiating to the back appear to be significant and could progress over several years. We need prospective long-term follow-up of these patients using multiple modalities including newer generation EUS for precise benchmarking of the natural history of early CP.

The reliability of EUS features of CP have also been evaluated from a study[9] of 11 expert endosonographers' interpretation of videotaped EUS examinations of 45 patients. There was good agreement for main pancreatic duct (MPD) dilation (kappa=0.61) and lobularity (kappa=0.51), but poor for 7 other features including stones (kappa=0.38) and hyperechoic duct margins (kappa=0.36). With regard to importance of each EUS feature, the presence of stones was regarded as the most predictive of CP by the endosonographers, followed by visible side branches, and lobularity, while the least important feature was MPD dilation.

The clinical utility of each EUS feature is unclear. It is interesting that, although MPD dilation garnered the highest kappa score in the study by Wallace et al,[9] it was also deemed the least predictive of CP. Thus an objective criterion such as MPD diameter may have little clinical significance, especially because pancreatic duct size appear to increase with age, as discussed below. Also, visible side branches that is presumed to be a marker of periductal fibrosis, display no significant difference in diameter when patients with CP are compared with normal volunteers.[2]

Table 19-1 Comparison of EUS features of chronic pancreatitis used by various authors: Wiersema (1993), Catalano (1998), Sahai (1998), Wallace (2001), and DeWitt (2005) and colleagues (gray areas, no corresponding feature in the study). Ductal features refer to main pancreatic duct unless specified. When available, descriptors for each feature are shown in parenthesis.

	Wiersema et al	Catalano et al	Sahai et al	Wallace et al	DeWitt et al
Ductal Features					
	Dilation	Dilation more than 3 mm	Dilation (more than 3 mm in the head, more than 2 mm in the body, more than 1 mm in the tail)	Dilation (more than 2 mm in the body or more than 1mm in the tail)	Dilation more than 3 mm (for at least half the distance of its entire course)
	Irregularity Hyperechoic wall	Irregularity Hyperechoic wall	Irregularity Hyperechoic wall	Irregularity Hyperechoic wall	Irregularity Hyperechoic wall
	Calculi	Calculi		Calculi	Calculi (with or without shadowing)
	Side branch dilation	Side branch dilation	Side branch visible (anechoic structure budding from the main PD)	Side branch visible	Side branch visible
		Narrowing			
Parenchymal Features					
	Hypoechoic foci	Hypoechoic foci (1–3 mm)			Hypoechoic foci (1–3 mm)
	Hyperechoic Foci (more than 3 mm)	Hyperechoic foci	Hyperechoic foci (1–2 mm)	Hyperechoic foci	Hyperechoic foci
	Cysts (more than 3 mm)	Cysts (more than 5 mm)	Cysts (thin walled anechoic structures more than 2 mm)	Cysts	Cysts (more than 5 mm)
	Lobularity	Lobularity	Lobularity (2-5 mm lobules)	Lobularity	Lobularity
		Prominent interlobular septae Heterogenous			
			Hyperechoic strands (irregular lines of varied length) Shadowing calcifications	Hyperechoic strands	Hyperechoic strands
Total # of Features	10	11	9	9	10

Table 19-2. Selected EUS features of chronic pancreatitis with the corresponding official definitions from the Minimal Standard Terminology in Gastrointestinal Endosonography,[5] and the implied histologic correlates

EUS Features	Minimum Standard Definition[17]	Histologic Implication
Ductal Changes		
Dilated	Abnormal increase in caliber	Ductal dilation more than 3 mm in the head, more than 2 mm in the body, more than 1 mm in the tail
Irregular contour	Coarse, uneven outline of the duct	Ductal irregularity
Visible side branches	No standard definition	Periductal fibrosis
Stone (or calculi)	Hyperechoic lesion with acoustic shadowing within a duct	Calcified stone
Hyperechoic wall	No standard definition	Periductal fibrosis
Parenchymal changes		
Hyperechoic foci	Small, distinct reflectors	Calcifications
Calcification	Hyperechoic lesion with acoustic shadow within a parenchyma	Calcifications
Hyperechoic strands	Small string-like hyperechoic structures	Fibrosis
Lobularity	Containing lobules that are rounded, homogenous areas separated by strands of another echogenicity	Fibrosis
Cysts	Well-demarcated anechoic areas	Pseudocyst

Histologic correlates of each EUS feature of CP have also been described (Table 19-2). It should be emphasized that these correlates are proposed implications that have not been studied formally. It is inherently difficult to directly compare gross EUS findings with microscopic histologic features. In the largest study[10] comparing EUS features with histopathology, a retrospective cohort of 71 patients who underwent pancreatic surgery for presumed CP were analyzed. Twenty-eight out of 30 patients (93%) with calcifications detected by EUS turned out to have abnormal histology (93% positive predictive value, 95% CI 78%-99%). On the other hand, 36 out of the 41 patients (88%) without calcifications on EUS had an abnormal histology. There was a low but statistically significant correlation ($P = 0.01$) between fibrosis score and EUS criteria. The role of EUS to guide tissue sampling for the diagnosis CP has also been investigated.[11,12] DeWitt et al evaluated the utility and safety of EUS-guided transgastric Tru-cut biopsy among 16 patients with suspected nonfocal CP. Six were nondiagnostic and one had device malfunction. With regards to procedure-related complications, one had acute pancreatitis and another had abdominal pain without pancreatitis. Thus, because of the limited diagnostic yield and potential complications, the authors did not recommend performing this technique in this setting.

Another dilemma arises because there is no agreement among institutions and individuals with regard to EUS terminology and criteria for CP, and there is quite a wide variation with image interpretation. For example, how does one differentiate between hyperechoic foci and hyperchoic strands? Irregular pancreatic duct margins can be subjective as well. Do we put more clinical significance on beaded pancreatic duct margins over mutliple undulations? How does one objectively define parenchymal lobularity to a student of EUS without being misunderstood? What is the minimum cutoff for diagnosing CP? Is finding a pancreatic duct stone alone without accompanying features enough to diagnose CP? In addition, many experts utilize a varying number of terminologies (Table 19-1), while others subjectively observe the pancreas via an overall *gestalt* approach.

Recently, a consensus conference among expert endosonographers was convened in Rosemont, Illinois, to address these issues. Our collection of EUS images follows, depicting features of chronic pancreatitis (Figures 19-1 - 19-8, 7.5-MHz, Olympus GF-UE160, Olympus America, Melville, NY), accompanied

Chronic Pancreatitis 209

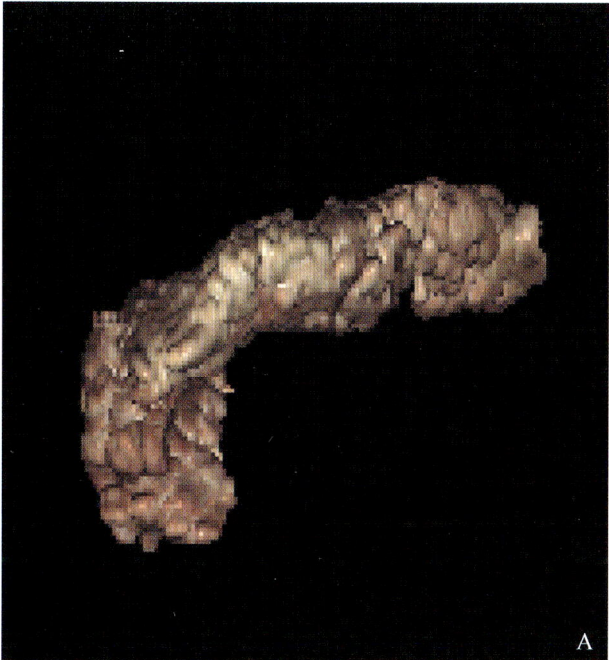
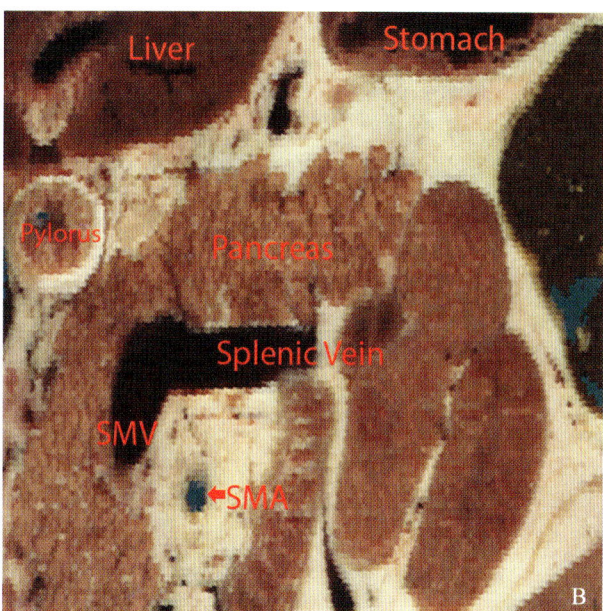

FIGURES 19–1. *A* and *B* (A) Coronal Model of the pancreas from the Visible Human Data Set. (B) Coronal cross-sectional anatomy of the pancreas at the level of the confluence of the splenic vein and superior mesenteric vein (SMV). Superior mesenteric artery (SMA)

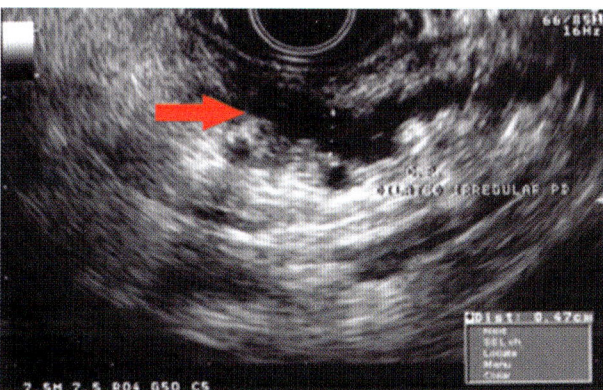

FIGURE 19–2. Radial EUS image of dilated, tortuous main pancreatic duct in the body of the pancreas (red arrow). In general, pancreatic duct dilation in EUS is defined as diameter more than 3 mm in the head, more than 2 mm in the body, and more than 1 mm in the tail of the pancreas.

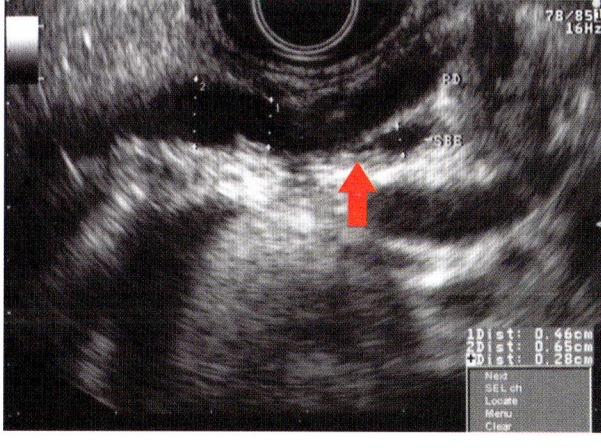

FIGURE 19–3. Radial EUS image of the body of the pancreas with a dilated main pancreatic duct with visible side branch (red arrow)

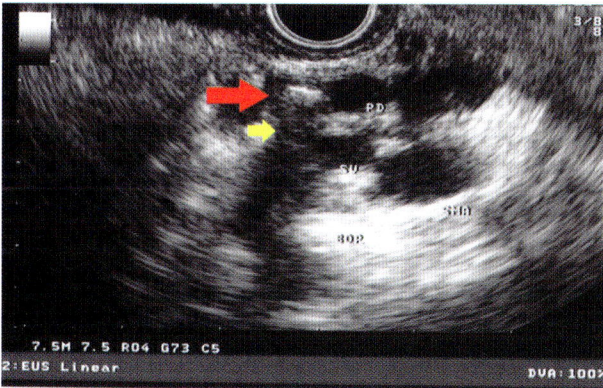

FIGURE 19–4. Linear EUS image of a pancreatic duct (PD) stone (red arrow) with acoustic shadowing (yellow arrow)

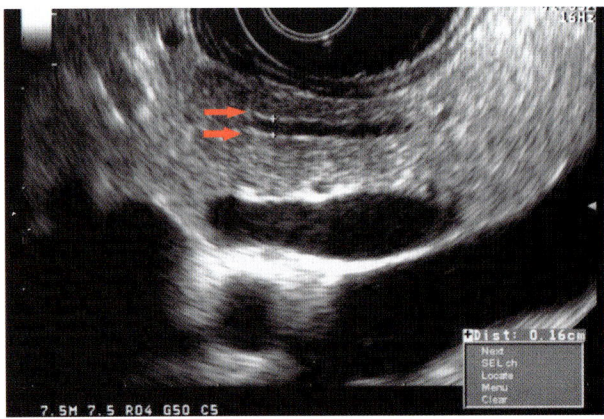

FIGURE 19–5. Radial EUS image of hyperechoic pancreatic duct wall (red arrow) in the body of the pancreas

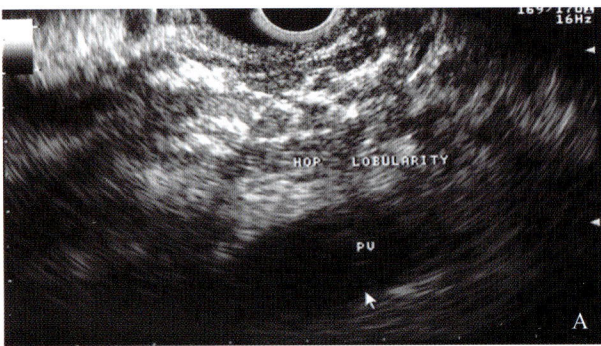 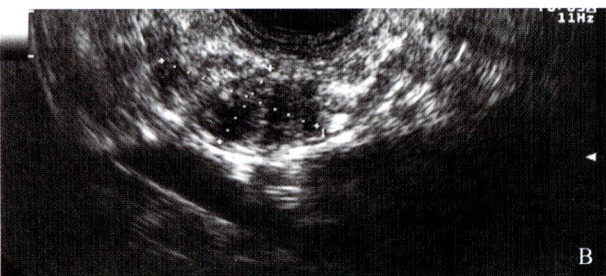

FIGURES 19–6. *A and B* Radial EUS images of pancreatic body demonstrating lobularity. Adjacent to the pancreas in Figure 19–5-A is the portal vein (PV). A normal-looking pancreas by EUS in Figure 19–6C is homogenous and has a "salt-and-pepper" appearance.

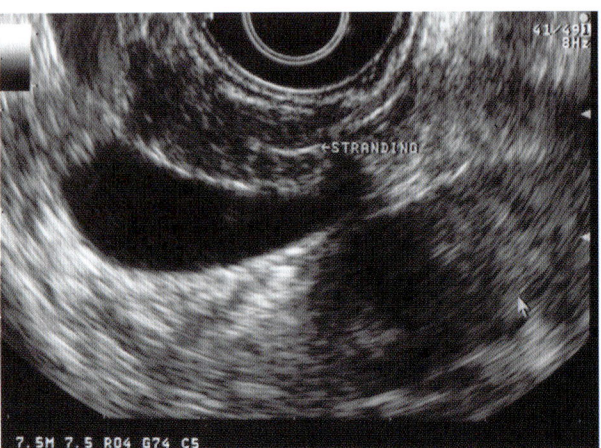 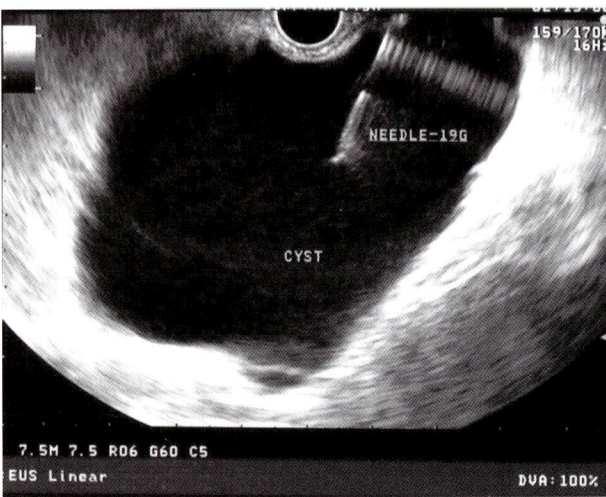

FIGURE 19–7. Linear EUS image of the pancreas with hyperechoic strands

FIGURE 19–8. Linear EUS image of EUS-guided FNA of a pancreatic cyst

by a brief description of each feature reflecting some of the preliminary information that we have learned from this meeting. Prior to imaging the pancreas, it is necessary to pay attention to technical parameters of ultrasound and adjust the grain control to make known anechoic structures, such as adjacent major blood vessels, appear completely black. This is done in order to appropriately assess the echogenicity of pancreatic duct and parenchyma. Figure 19–1 shows a coronal model of the pancreas with a coronal cross-section to help orient the reader to the general pancreas relational anatomy.

Ductal Features of Chronic Pancreatitis

Figure 19–2 shows a dilated, irregular pancreatic duct in the body of the pancreas. Experts generally agree on the "*3-2-1 rule*" for the upper limits of normal pancreatic duct diameter (3 mm in the head, 2 mm in the body, and 1 mm in the tail of the pancreas). Data obtained from screening 130,951 subjects have shown that pancreatic duct diameter appears to increase with age.[13] In another study[14] of 120 patients without clinical evidence for pancreatic disease, over a quarter of patients had at least one parenchymal and/or ductal abnormality with an age-dependent increase in number of abnormal features: more than 40 years (23%), 40 to 60 years (25%), and more than 60 years (39%); $p = 0.13$. Another group of patients to consider are those with significant alcohol history. EUS has been shown to detect three or more features of CP in 58% of asymptomatic alcoholics and in 89% of alcoholics with pancreatic type pain.[15] Whether or not we should adjust our threshold according to age or alcohol use remains a subject of further studies.

Visible side branches, which are small anechoic tubular structures budding from the main pancreatic duct (Figure 19–3) thought to represent periductal fibrosis, are easier to appreciate in newer generation echoendoscopes with an electronic transducer. However, side branches are not pathognomonic for chronic pancreatitis. The majority of the control group in our study[8] had these structures visible. On the other hand, few experts would disagree that main pancreatic duct calculi (Figure 19–4) with shadowing is an indispensable criterion of chronic pancreatitis. Hyperechoic pancreatic duct walls (Figure 19–5) are identified as visible hyperechoic distinct structures compared to the surrounding parenchyma. To account for acoustic reverberation artifacts, hyperechoic pancreatic duct walls should be circumferential (i.e., involving both walls on cross-sectional imaging) and involve at least 50% of the entire main pancreatic duct in the body and tail of the pancreas to increase the likelihood for detecting a significant finding.

Parenchymal Features of Chronic Pancreatitis

Lobularity is defined as round heterogenous structures encircled by echogenic enhancement (Figure 19–6). It can be seen in the central or peripheral portions of the parenchyma, and may or may not be associated with glandular atrophy. Hyperechoic strands are echogenic lines of variable length that run in multiple directions (Figure 19–7). Cysts are circular anechoic structures greater than 2 mm in diameter (Figure 19–8).

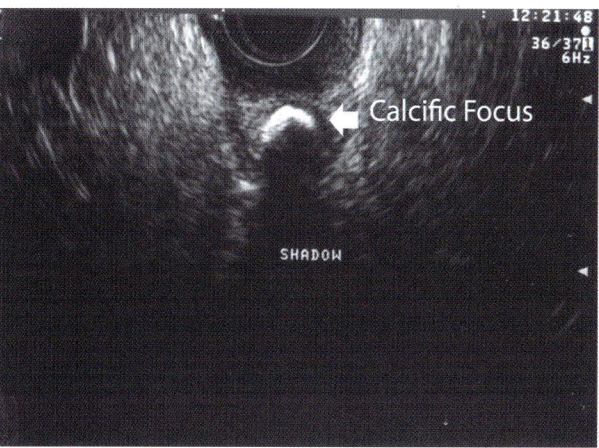

FIGURE 19–9. Radial EUS image of a hyperechoic focus with shadowing. This parenchymal calcification (arrow) is characterized by a crescent-shaped hyperechoic structure with acoustic shadowing. Some authors consider hyperechoic foci with shadowing as a ductal criterion because they are presumed to be located in an unseen side-branch.

Hyperechoic foci, with or without shadowing (also called a calcification or calcific foci by some when shadowing is present), are echogenic structures of variable size and shape (Figure 19–9). When hyperechoic foci with our without shadowing are seen within the main pancreatic duct (Figure 19–10), they are labeled as pancreatic duct stones. Some authors[10] consider parenchymal hyperechoic foci with shadowing as a ductal criterion because they are presumed to be located in an unseen side-branch. Hyperechoic foci should also not be used in context when examining the area of the ventral anlage in the uncinate process, due to its lower fat content and hypoechoic appearance compared to the dorsal pancreas. Thus, for purposes of documentation, it is essential to take note of the location of the EUS features of CP, whether it is in the head, body, or tail of the pancreas to account for normal variations in echogenicity.

Conclusion

Endosonographers are not exempt from facing difficulties in diagnosing and assessing the degree of CP. However, EUS has the advantage of providing unique and reproducible ductal and parenchymal features of CP not found in other imaging modalities. Only time will tell if minimal EUS changes are the forerunner of a debilitating disease such as CP. Meanwhile, in the absence of large prospective long-term studies that can

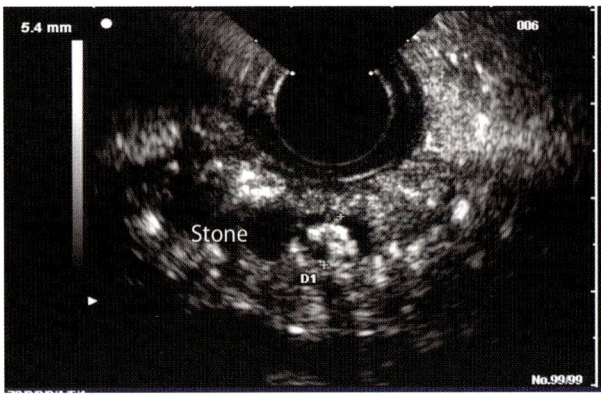

FIGURE 19–10. EUS of pancreatic body in CP showing hyperechoic foci without shadowing in the parenchyma with a 5 mm hyperechoic focus in the dilated main pancreatic duct (pancreatic duct stone).

validate these features, experts need to form a consensus on 1) standard terminology and descriptors; 2) minimal EUS criteria or grading system for CP; 3) prioritizing research work to improve diagnostic accuracy and to reduce interobserver variability (for example, computer-assisted analysis of EUS images[16]).

As mentioned before, recently 32 internationally recognized endosonographers anonymously voted on EUS features of CP and agreed on the following: Major criteria for CP were (1) hyperechoic foci with shadowing and main pancreatic duct (PD) calculi and (2) lobularity with honeycombing. Minor criteria for CP were cysts, dilated ducts > or =3.5 mm, irregular PD contour, dilated side branches > or =1 mm, hyperechoic duct wall, strands, nonshadowing hyperechoic foci, and lobularity with noncontiguous lobules. The authors have called this as "Rosemont criteria" for the EUS diagnosis of CP[18].

Acknowledgments:

The authors wish to thank Dr Vivek Kaul for digitally storing and providing the EUS images presented in this chapter.

References

1. Gyr, K. E., Singer, M. V., Sarles, H.: Revised classification of pancreatitis. In Gyr, K. E., Singer, M. V., Sarles, H., eds.: Pancreatitis: concepts and classification, Amsterdam: Elsevier, 1984:xxiii.
2. Sarner, M., Cotton, P. B.: Classification of pancreatitis. Gut. 1984 Jul;25(7):756–759.
3. Shimizu, M., Hirokawa, M., Manabe, T.: Histological assessment of chronic pancreatitis at necropsy. J. Clin. Pathol. 1996 Nov;49(11):913–915.
4. Sahai, A. V., Zimmerman, M., Aabakken, L., Tarnasky, P. R., Cunningham, J. T., van Velse, A., Hawes, R. H., Hoffman, B. J.: Prospective assessment of the ability of endoscopic ultrasound to diagnose, exclude, or establish the severity of chronic pancreatitis found by endoscopic retrograde cholangiopancreatography. Gastrointest Endosc. 1998 Jul;48(1):18–25.
5. Wiersema, M. J., Hawes, R. H., Lehman, G. A., Kochman, M. L., Sherman, S., Kopecky, K. K.: Prospective evaluation of endoscopic ultrasonography and endoscopic retrograde cholangiopancreatography in patients with chronic abdominal pain of suspected pancreatic origin. Endoscopy. 1993 Nov;25(9):555–564.
6. Catalano, M. F., Lahoti, A., Geenen, J. E., Hogan, W. J.: Prospective evaluation of endoscopic ultrasonography, endoscopic retrograde pancreatography, and secretin test in the diagnosis of chronic pancreatitis. Gastrointest Endosc. 1998 Jul;48(1):11–17.
7. Chowdhury, R., Bhutani, M. S., Mishra, G., Toskes, P. P., Forsmark, C. E.: Comparative analysis of direct pancreatic function testing versus morphological assessment by endoscopic ultrasonography for the evaluation of chronic unexplained abdominal pain of presumed pancreatic origin. Pancreas. 2005 Jul;31(1):63–68.
8. Catalano, M. F., Kaul, V., Pezanoski, J., Guda, N., Geenen, N.: Long-term outcome of endosonographically detected minimum criteria for chronic pancreatitis (MCCP) when conventional imaging and functional testing are normal. Gastrointestinal Endosc. 2007 April 65(5): AB120.
9. Wallace, M. B., Hawes, R. H., Durkalski, V., Chak, A., Mallery, S., Catalano, M. F., Wiersema, M. J., Bhutani, M. S., Ciaccia, D., Kochman, M. L., Gress, F. G., Van Velse, A., Hoffman, B. J.: The reliability of EUS for the diagnosis of chronic pancreatitis: interobserver agreement among experienced endosonographers. Gastrointestinal Endosc. 2001 Mar;53(3):294–299.
10. Chong, A. K., Hawes, R. H., Hoffman, B. J., Adams, D. B., Lewin, D. N., Romagnuolo, J.: Diagnostic performance of EUS for chronic pancreatitis: a comparison with histopathology. Gastrointest. Endosc. 2007 May;65(6):808–814.
11. Hollerbach, S., Klamann, A., Topalidis, T., Schmiegel, W. H.: Endoscopic ultrasonography (EUS) and fine-needle aspiration (FNA) cytology for diagnosis of chronic pancreatitis. Endoscopy. 2001 Oct;33(10):824–831.
12. DeWitt, J., McGreevy, K., LeBlanc, J., McHenry, L., Cummings, O., Sherman, S.: EUS-guided Tru-cut biopsy of suspected nonfocal chronic pancreatitis. Gastrointest Endosc. 2005 Jul;62(1):76–84.
13. Ikeda, M., Sato, T., Morozumi, A., Fujino, M. A., Yoda, Y., Ochiai, M., Kobayashi, K.: Morphologic changes in the pancreas detected by screening ultrasonography in a mass survey, with special reference to main duct dilatation, cyst formation, and calcification. Pancreas 1994 Jul;9(4):508–512.
14. Rajan, E., Clain, J. E., Levy, M. J., Norton, I. D., Wang, K. K., Wiersema, M. J., Vazquez-Sequeiros, E., Nelson, B. J., Jondal, M. L., Kendall, R. K., Harmsen, W. S., Zinsmeister, A. R.: Age-related changes in the pancreas identified by EUS: a prospective evaluation. Gastrointest Endosc 2005 Mar;61(3):401–406.
15. Bhutani, M. S.: Endoscopic ultrasonography: changes of chronic pancreatitis in asymptomatic and symptomatic alcoholic patients. J Ultrasound Med. 1999 Jul;18(7):455–462.
16. Irisawa, A., Mishra, G., Hernandez, L.V., Bhutani, M. S.: Quantitative analysis of endosonographic parenchymal echogenicity in patients with chronic pancreatitis. J. Gastroenterol. Hepatol. 2004 Oct;19(10):1199–1205.
17. Minimum Standard Terminology version 1.0. Dig Endosc 1998;10:158–184.
18. Catalano MF, Sahai A, Levy M, Romagnuolo J, Wiersema M, Brugge W, Freeman M, Yamao K, Canto M, Hernandez LV. EUS-based criteria for the diagnosis of chronic pancreatitis: the Rosemont classification. Gastrointest Endosc. 2009 Jun;69(7):1251-61. Epub 2009 Feb 24.

CHAPTER 20

Autoimmune Pancreatitis

Dr. Michael J. Levy
Dr. Naoki Takahashi
Dr. Thomas C. Smyrk
Dr. Suresh T. Chari

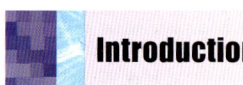

Introduction

Autoimmune pancreatitis (AIP) is a form of chronic pancreatitis with often distinct clinical, serological, histological, and imaging features. AIP is part of a systemic fibro-inflammatory process that afflicts not only the pancreas, but also other organs including the bile duct, retroperitoneum, lymph nodes, salivary glands, and kidneys. Affected organs demonstrate a lymphoplasmacytic infiltrate containing IgG4-positive cells. The initially described finding is the presence of a pancreatic head mass that mimics pancreatic ductal adenocarcinoma. However, emerging data indicate that patients with AIP present with a much wider spectrum of clinical disease and imaging findings than previously noted. The diagnosis is often delayed many months or years following symptom onset, with many patients having undergone prior pancreatic resection for presumed malignancy. Most patients present with obstructive jaundice—with or without a pancreatic mass. While vague abdominal pain is common, it is usually of insufficient intensity to require narcotics, and despite the term AIP, few patients develop pancreatitis. Other presenting manifestations include an isolated pancreatic mass, new-onset diabetes, steatorrhea, and pancreatic atrophy. A hallmark of this disorder is a rapid and dramatic response to steroid therapy.

The purpose of this chapter is to review the breadth of EUS findings associated with AIP, and to consider the EUS features in the context of clinical, imaging, histological, and laboratory findings. We will also discuss the utility and suggest a role for EUS-guided tissue sampling. The ultimate goal is to employ each diagnostic criterion in a manner that optimizes diagnostic accuracy, management, and clinical outcomes for patients with AIP.

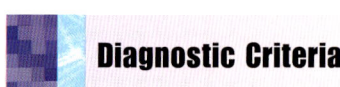

Diagnostic Criteria

Prospectively evaluated criteria do not exist for establishing the presence of AIP and most rely on a combination of clinical, laboratory, and imaging findings to make the diagnosis.[1-4] Two classification schemes have been established that rely on a spectrum of findings to establish the diagnosis. The Japan Pancreas Society established the first set of criteria (Table 20–1) that in order to diagnose AIP requires: 1) diffuse pancreatic enlargement, and 2) diffuse, irregular main pancreatic duct narrowing. Diagnosis also requires any of the following: 1) increased immunoglobulin G (IgG) level, 2) presence of autoantibodies

Table 20–1 Japan Pancreas Society Criteria for Diagnosing Autoimmune Pancreatitis

Mandatory Criteria

1. Diffuse pancreatic enlargement
2. Diffusely irregular MPD narrowing

Additional Criteria (at least 1)

3. Increased IgG (total) or increased titers of atoantibodies (antinuclear antibody or rheumatoid factor)
4. Fibrosis and lymphoplasmacytic infiltration

(antinuclear antibody or rheumatoid factor), and/or 3) fibrosis and lymphoplasmacytic infiltration within tissue specimens. Creation of the Japanese criteria was an important step in the diagnosis and management of patients with AIP.

The Japan Pancreas Society criteria require that certain procedures be performed that are often unnecessary and potentially risky, including mandatory pancreatography. In addition, there is emerging evidence for the presence and/or value of histological criteria[3] atypical imaging findings[5] specific elevation of IgG4 subclass[6] other organ involvement[7] and steroid response[8] that are not considered by the Japanese criteria. As such, their criteria are insufficient to recognize the full disease spectrum thereby restricting diagnosis to a narrow subgroup of patients. These limitations have led the Japan Pancreas Society to modify its initial criteria to include focal pancreatic enlargement and focal pancreatic duct stricture, which are often seen in AIP.[9] Chari and colleagues[4] incorporated other cardinal features of AIP to establish the Mayo Clinic **HISORt** Criteria that rely on **H**istology, **I**maging, **S**erology, other **O**rgan involvement, and **R**esponse to steroid therapy. Incorporation of these criteria into a diagnostic algorithm has been shown to enhance diagnostic sensitivity without sacrificing specificity.

Histological Findings

The classic cluster of histological findings in AIP is termed lymphoplasmacytic sclerosing pancreatitis (LPSP), which consists of: 1) a lymphoplasmacytic infiltrate that surrounds, a.) medium and large size interlobular pancreatic ducts, and b.) pancreatic venules (obliterative phlebitis) while sparing arterioles;

and 2) swirling fibrosis centered around pancreatic ducts (storiform fibrosis).[10,11] Histology accurately distinguishes AIP from other causes of chronic pancreatitis and pancreatic carcinoma.[12–14] More recently, IgG4 immunostaining of tissue samples has been performed to identify IgG4-positive plasma cells. The finding of either moderate (11-30 cells/HPF) or severe (more than 30 cells/HPF) is considered diagnostic.[15,16] These findings distinguish AIP from alcohol-induced pancreatitis and the peri-tumoral inflammation associated with ductal carcinoma.[16] The systemic nature of this disease allows immunostaining of affected distant sites providing information that can be used in support of the diagnosis. While traditionally, histopathologic diagnosis required review of resected pancreatic specimens, the recent introduction of EUS-guided Tru-cut biopsy has simplified the diagnosis.[17]

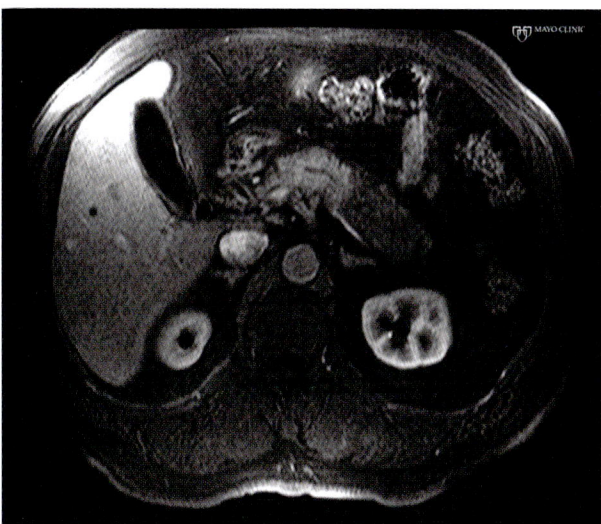

FIGURE 20–2. Magnetic resonance imaging (MRI) reveals a diffusely enlarged sausage-shaped gland with capsule-like rim enhancement.

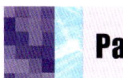
Pancreatic Imaging

Computed Tomography (CT) and Magnetic Resonance Imaging (MRI)

The characteristic CT and MRI findings of AIP are a diffusely enlarged, sausage-shaped gland with a capsule-like rim. (Figures 20–1 and 20–2; Videos 20–1 and 20–2). The capsule-like rim is the most pathognomonic finding and it appears as a low-attenuation rim of soft tissue surrounding the pancreas on contrast-enhanced CT. On MRI, it appears hypointense on both T1- and T2-weighted images, and shows delayed enhancement.[18] However, the capsule-like rim is present only in 12 to 30% of patients.[19,20]

Diagnostic confusion, particularly between pancreatic carcinoma, may occur with the findings of less common manifestations, such as focal or asymmetrical enlargement of the pancreas. This pattern of pancreatic manifestation is not uncommon and is seen in 28 to 41% of patients with AIP.[5,19] On CT, the enlarged segment of the pancreas is typically iso-attenuation to the uninvolved pancreatic parenchyma.[19] However, in a small number of cases, the enlarged segment is low-attenuation compared to the uninvolved pancreatic parenchyma on CT and may be indistinguishable from pancreatic carcinoma.[5,19] Soft tissue infiltration around the major vessels can be seen approximately 15% of the time; this should not be interpreted as a sign of malignancy. Other atypical findings that may cause diagnostic confusion with other types of pancreatitis include pancreatic atrophy, pancreatic calcifications, pseudocyst formation, and stranding around the pancreas.

The second-most-pathognomonic finding is the presence of other organ involvement including biliary involvement (68–90%),[19–22] retroperitoneal fibrosis (3–11%),[19,21,23,24] and renal involvement (30%).[24] Biliary involvement typically involves the distal CBD, but it may involve the intrahepatic bile duct. It appears as PSC-like strictures on MRCP, or thickening and abnormal enhancement of the bile duct on contrast-enhanced CT or MRI. Retroperitoneal fibrosis appears as a rim of soft tissue surrounding the abdominal aorta. Renal involvement may appear as wedge-shaped or round low-attenuation lesions on contrast-enhanced CT or MRI.[24] Such findings in the

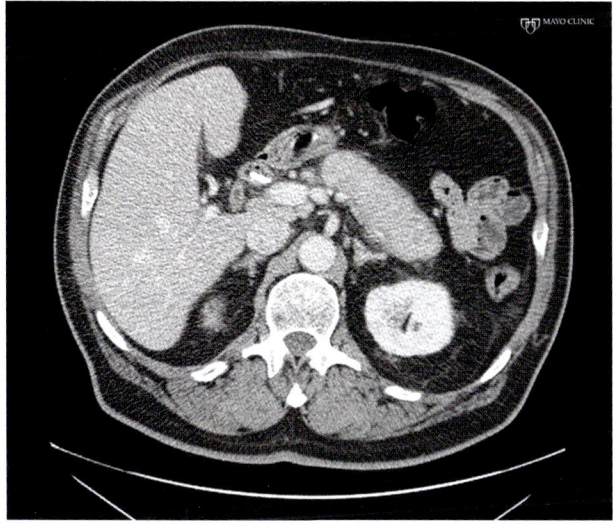

FIGURE 20–1. The classic AIP finding of a diffusely enlarged sausage-shaped gland seen on computed tomography.

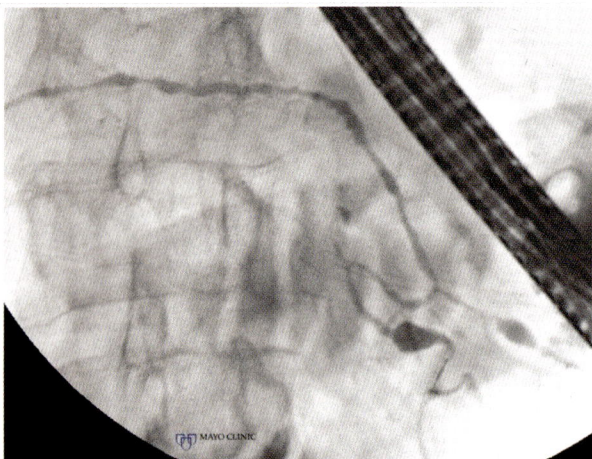

FIGURE 20–3. Endoscopic retrograde pancreatography revealing the classic finding in patients with AIP of a diffusely (more than one-third of gland), irregularly narrowed main pancreatic duct.

presence of atypical pancreatic findings should raise the possibility of AIP.

Endoscopic Retrograde Cholangiopancreatography (ERCP)

The classic pancreatographic finding in patients with AIP is the presence of a diffusely (more than 1/3 of gland), and irregularly narrowed main pancreatic duct (Figure 20–3). While most classic, this appearance is uncommonly seen. Instead, patients often present with focal pancreatic duct strictures (with or without proximal dilatation), ductal dilatation (focal or narrow, with or without a stricture), or may have a normal appearing pancreatic duct. Similarly, variable cholangiographic abnormalities are found in patients with AIP. While the classic appearance is a distal (intrapancreatic) bile duct stricture, strictures can develop in any portion of the extrahepatic and/or intrahepatic biliary tree. The bile duct strictures that develop with AIP can mimic strictures seen in pancreatic carcinoma, cholangiocarcinoma, "benign" primary sclerosing cholangitis, chronic pancreatitis, and nearly any cause of obstructive jaundice (Figures 20–4 and 20–5). More helpful than the location or appearance of the strictures, is the development of migrating and/or fleeting strictures, which is uncommon for most types of pancreatobiliary disease.

Endoscopic Ultrasound (EUS) and Tissue Sampling

There are emerging data supporting the utility of EUS imaging and tissue acquisition for addressing these

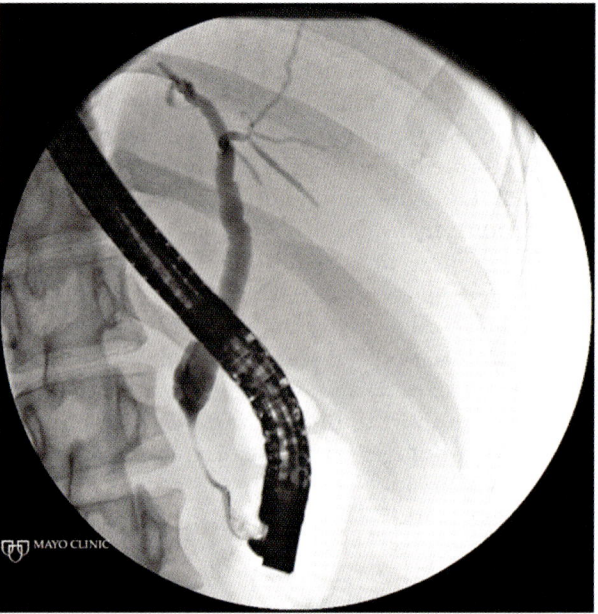

FIGURE 20–4. Endoscopic retrograde cholangiography demonstrating a distal bile duct stricture that can be mistaken for a pancreatic carcinoma.

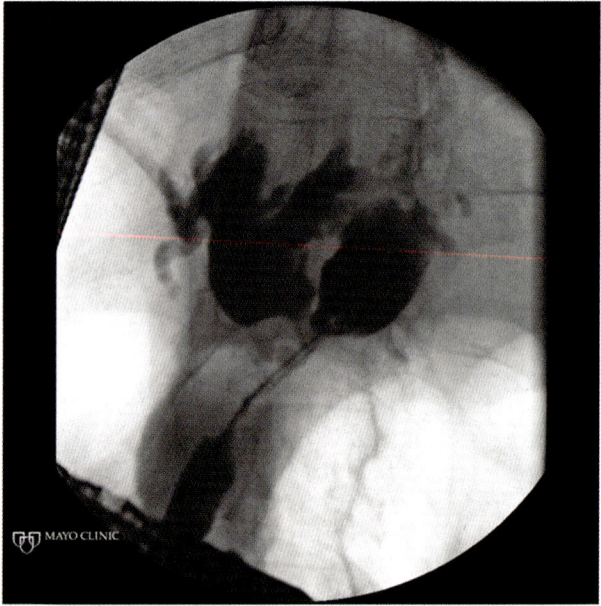

FIGURE 20–5. Endoscopic retrograde cholangiography showing a proximal (hilar) bile duct stricture that can be mistaken for cholangiocarcinoma.

new criteria to aid AIP diagnosis.[16,17] The most characteristic EUS finding is diffuse (sausage-shaped) pancreatic enlargement with a hypoechoic, coarse, patchy, heterogeneous appearance (Figure 20–6A; Videos 20–3 and 20–4). Corresponding Visible Human Anatomy is shown in Figure 20–6B. However, there may be significant overlap between the appearance

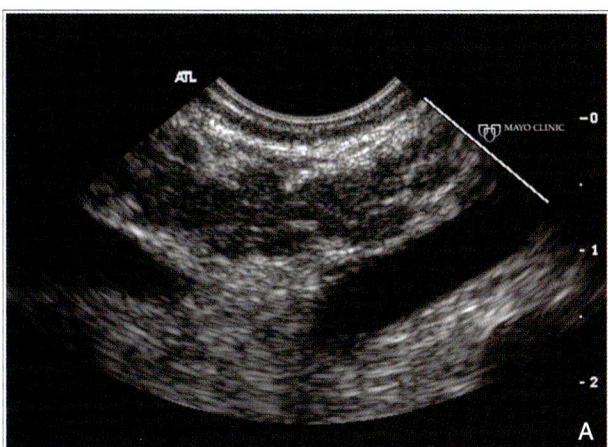
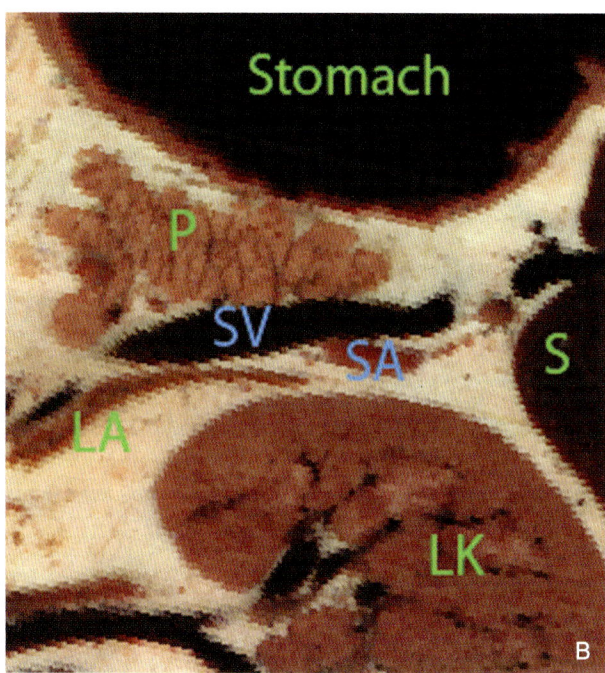

FIGURES 20–6. *A and B* (A) Classic EUS appearance of AIP including hypoechoic diffuse (sausage-shape) pancreatic enlargement with hypoechoic, coarse, patchy, heterogeneous parenchyma. (B) Corresponding Visible Human anatomy is shown. P=pancreas, LA=left adrenal, S=spleen, LK=left kidney, SV=splenic vein, SA=splenic artery.

of AIP and other pancreatic disorders. EUS may also reveal an isolated lesion or multiple mass lesions that can mimic "unresectable" ductal carcinoma. (Figure 7A). Corresponding Visible Human Anatomy is shown in Figure 20–7B. Other less common EUS features include glandular atrophy, calcification, cystic spaces, features of nonspecific chronic pancreatitis, (Figure 20–8) or even a normal gland. Unfortunately, there are no pathognomonic EUS findings for AIP. Furthermore, while there are a few characteristic features of AIP, none have proven useful in isolation to diagnose AIP, and presence in other pancreatic disorders is common. The lack of pathognomonic features and diverse spectrum of EUS findings limits the utility of EUS imaging alone. This has driven the pursuit of safe methods for obtaining tissue to enhance diagnostic accuracy.

Despite reports of the diagnosis of AIP by FNA alone, there are no broadly accepted criteria for cytologic diagnosis, and there is a great reluctance by most pathologists for reliance on FNA diagnosis. FNA commonly yields a diminutive tissue sample and results in a loss of tissue architecture, thereby prohibiting histologic evaluation. To overcome limitations of FNA needles that only allow cytologic review, large-caliber cutting biopsy needles have been developed that acquire samples to allow preservation of tissue architecture and histologic examination.[25-32] (Figure 20–9) The Tru-cut biopsy device operates with echoendoscopes (Quick-Core, Wilson-Cook, Winston-Salem, North Carolina) and incorporates a disposable 19-gauge needle with a tissue tray and sliding sheath that permits a histologic core to be obtained. A standard spring-loaded mechanism is employed within the handle to permit automated procurement of biopsy specimens. We previously reported our EUS TCB experience and find the device particularly useful for diagnosing stromal tumors, lymphoma, and well-differentiated, desmoplastic and/or vascular tumors that are often difficult to diagnose by cytology alone.[33-37] Although characteristic histologic findings exist, until recently it has been impractical to use histology to definitively establish the diagnosis preoperatively. We more recently demonstrated that EUS TCB acquires core specimens, preserves tissue architecture, and permits histologic review and preoperative diagnosis of AIP.[17]

In updating our initial report, to date, 16 patients with a final diagnosis of AIP have undergone EUS TCB with a disposable 19-gauge Tru-cut needle (QuikCore, Wilson-Cook, Winston-Salem, NC), 10 of whom also underwent EUS FNA. The criteria for the diagnosis of AIP were based on a previously established combination of clinical presentation, patient outcome, laboratory findings, and imaging studies.[1-3] The mean age was 63 years (range 29–85) and 12 were males. A total of 43 TCBs (2.7 biopsies/patient, range 1–4) were obtained from the pancreatic neck, body, and/or tail

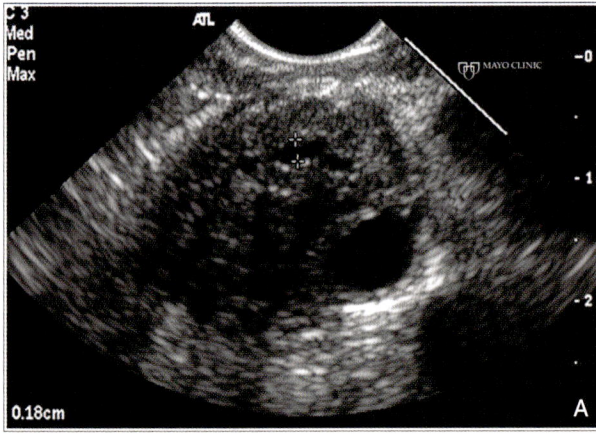

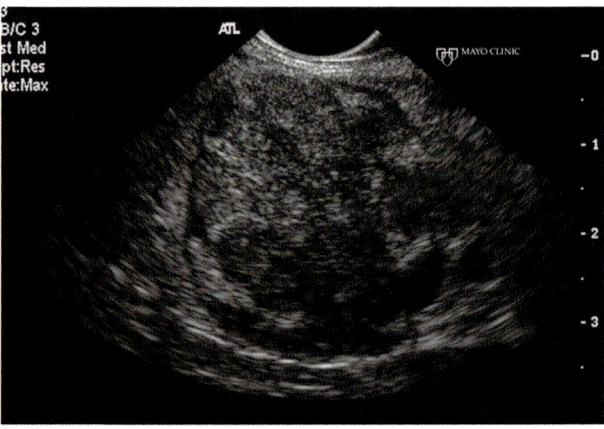

FIGURE 20–8. EUS features of nonspecific chronic pancreatitis in a patient with AIP.

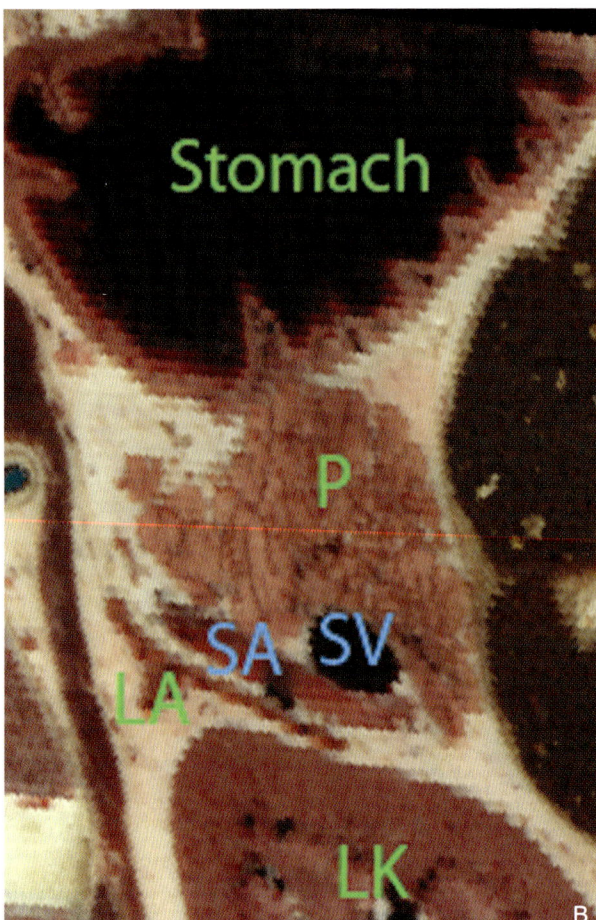

FIGURES 20–7. A and B (A) EUS finding of a mass-like lesion in a patient with AIP that may be confused with an "unresectable" pancreatic ductal carcinoma. (B) Corresponding Visible Human Anatomy is shown. P=pancreas, LA=left adrenal, LK=left kidney, SV=splenic vein, SA=splenic artery

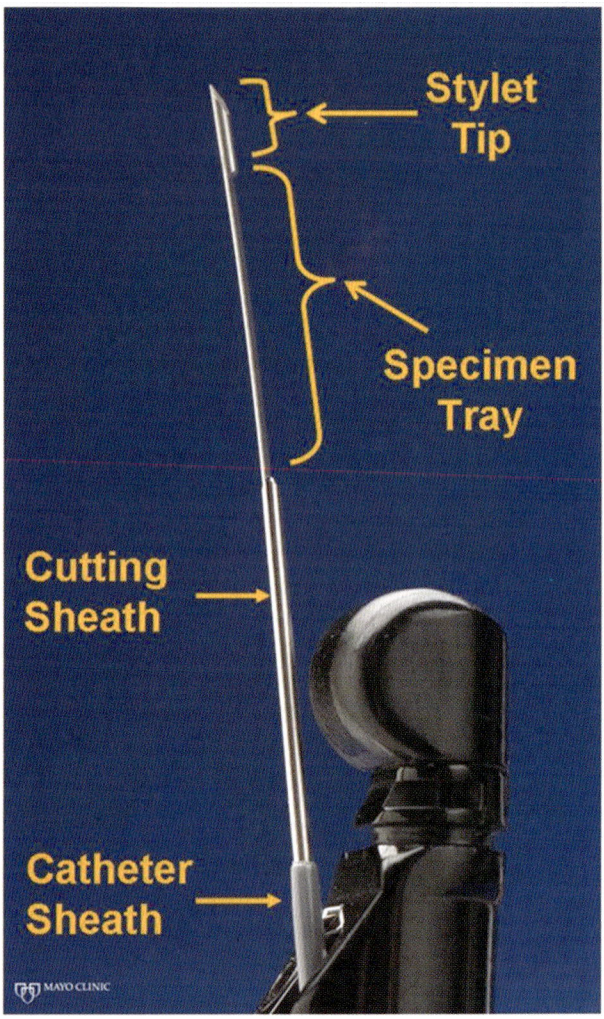

FIGURE 20–9. Endoscopic ultrasound-guided Tru-cut biopsy (TCB) needle that acquires samples allowing preservation of tissue architecture and histologic examination

region. In addition 53 FNAs (5.3 passes/patient, range 2–12) were obtained from 10 of the patients. In none of the 10 patients undergoing EUS FNA was the diagnosis of AIP possible with FNA alone. FNA was not performed in all patients due to the earlier experience of failed diagnosis following FNA. The findings of TCB were considered "diagnostic" when either: 1) histologic review identified an intense lymphoplasmacytic infiltrate surrounding both pancreatic duct branches and venules, or 2) IgG4 staining detected moderate (10–30 cells/hpf) or severe (more than 30 cells/hpf) staining of plasma cells. The findings of TCB were considered "strongly suggestive" when either: 1) histologic review identified an intense lymphoplasmacytic infiltrate without focal involvement of the pancreatic duct branches and venules, (Figures 20–10 and 20–11) or 2) IgG4 staining detected mild (less than 10 cells/hpf) staining of plasma cells (Figure 20–12). Using these TCB criteria, specimens were considered "diagnostic" (n=12) or "strongly suggestive" (n=4), respectively. Other than mild transient abdominal pain (n=1), no complications were identified.

The inability to exclude malignancy led to initial consideration of pancreatic resection in 9 patients. In this group, EUS TCB findings alone led to histologic confirmation of AIP thereby avoiding unnecessary resection. EUS TCB and pathologic examination revealed findings strongly suggestive of AIP in 4 patients that when considered along with the HISORt criteria led to medical management. In two patients, although the EUS TCB was not diagnostic of AIP, it did demonstrate the non-specific finding of chronic pancreatitis. In the latter patients, other features were present that led to close observation and medical therapy. All patients were initially treated with Prednisone

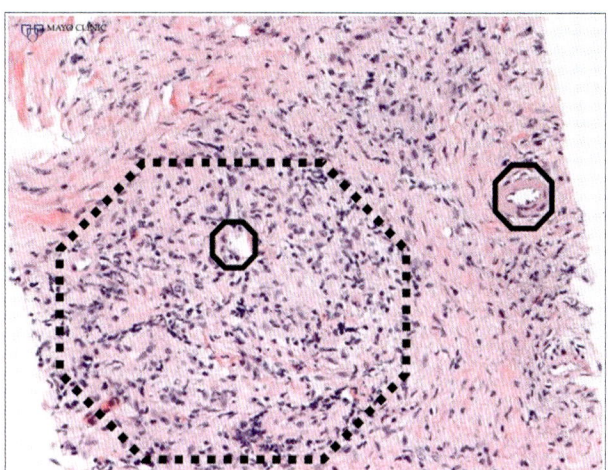

FIGURE 20–11. An intact artery is seen at the right of the image (single solid marker). In addition, an intense infiltration by lymphocytes and histiocytes results in near complete obliteration of the vein (obliterative phlebitis) shown at the left of the image (dashed marker surrounding solid marker). (H&E, orig. mag. x300).

40 mg/d for 3 months (1-5 months) with clinical resolution and normalization of liver chemistries. Three patients are in the initial phase of steroid therapy. All patients have experienced a benign course without evidence of malignancy.

Serology

AIP is associated with serologic abnormalities that include elevated titers of γ-globulins, rheumatoid

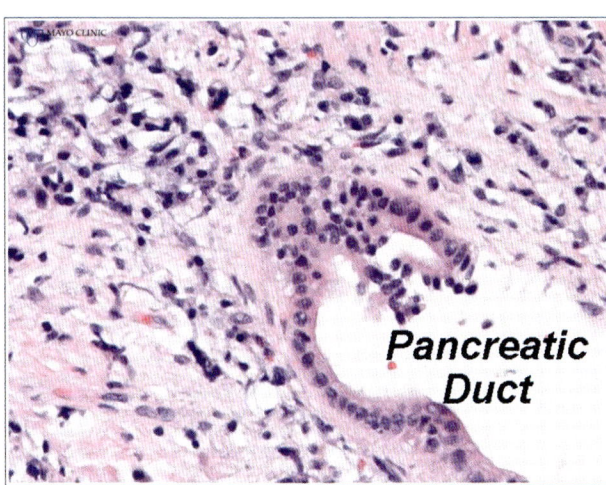

FIGURE 20–10. Histologic examination of EUS TCB specimen reveals an intense lymphoplasmacytic infiltrate surrounding a pancreatic duct. (H&E, orig. mag. x400).

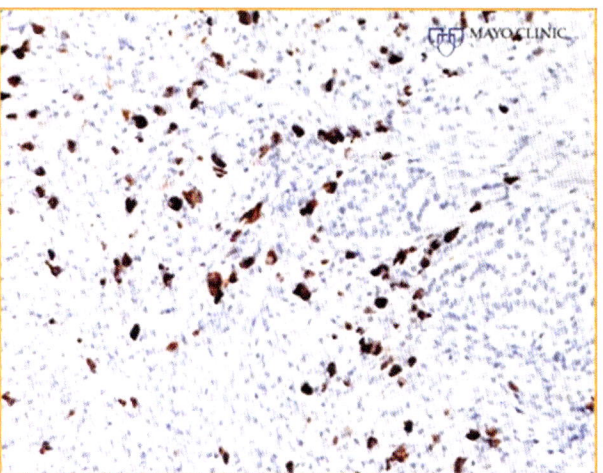

FIGURE 20–12. IgG4 staining of the Tru-cut biopsy specimen reveals more than 30 plasma cells/hpf, which establishes the diagnosis of AIP.

factor, and antinuclear, anti-carbonic anhydrase, and antilactoferrin antibodies.[38-40] The low diagnostic accuracy of these serologic markers limits their clinical utility. Elevated serum IgG4 levels are characteristic of AIP.[6,41] However, in a recent study of 510 patients, including 45 with AIP and 135 with pancreatic cancer, we found that mild (less than 2-fold) elevations in serum IgG4 are seen in up to 10% of subjects without AIP, including pancreatic cancer, and cannot be used alone to distinguish AIP from pancreatic cancer. Since AIP is uncommon, IgG4 elevations in patients with low pretest probability of having AIP are likely to represent false positives.

Other Organ Involvement

The systemic nature of this disease is demonstrated by the common occurrence of other organ involvement that is reported in the majority of patients (if you include distal bile duct strictures).[41] The most common sites of involvement include the distal common bile duct leading to strictures that mimic pancreatic ductal carcinoma. Focal strictures of the common hepatic duct and/or intrahepatic bile duct raise suspicion of cholangiocarcinoma, while diffuse strictures produce a PSC-like pattern.[41] A Sjogren's-like syndrome is manifest by parotid and lacrimal gland involvement. In addition, retroperitoneal fibrosis, aortitis, mediastinal lymphadenopathy, and renal involvement are reported as well.[41]

Contrary to prior thinking that these extra-pancreatic findings represent associated disorders, it is now believed that they instead signify systemic manifestations of a diffuse process. This theory is supported by the finding of IgG4-positive plasma cells in extra-pancreatic sites of involvement that is not seen in the diseases they mimic.[15,42] In addition, extra-pancreatic manifestations usually respond to steroid therapy.[8,22]

Response to Steroids

Pancreatic and extra-pancreatic manifestations of AIP commonly demonstrate a dramatic and rapid response to steroid therapy. While there is no standard regimen, most administer 30–40mg/day for approximately four weeks followed by an eight-week taper (5mg/week). Most patients have a complete and enduring response to steroid therapy. However, it is important to note that only the inflammatory component responds to steroid therapy and the fibrotic component persists and can progress, likely accounting for many of the failed therapeutic steroid trials. In addition, a subgroup of patients who initially respond, require repeat therapy often leading to lasting resolution. Immunosuppressants are occasionally required for those unable to tolerate steroid withdrawal or failing multiple steroid trials.

It is important to emphasize that steroid should be administration only after an exhaustive and negative work-up for known etiologies for pancreatic disease. A steroid trial is not an appropriate substitute for a thorough diagnostic evaluation. Furthermore, steroid therapy is only useful in persons in whom a response to a particular manifestation can be objectively assessed, such as those with a persisting pancreatic mass or enlargement, biliary strictures causing obstructive jaundice or leading to uncertain presence of cholangiocarcinoma or pancreatic carcinoma, pancreatic strictures without a mass with suspicion of neoplasia, and uncontrolled diabetes or weight loss.

Discussion

Autoimmune pancreatitis has historically been considered a rare disorder, but is increasingly being recognized due to an evolving understanding of the diverse nature of this protean disorder. It is now realized that the pancreatic manifestations are but one of often many manifestations of a systemic fibro-inflammatory process. However, the underlying pathogenesis and pathophysiology are unknown. AIP is otherwise referred to as chronic inflammatory sclerosis of the pancreas, sclerosing pancreatitis, pancreatitis showing the narrowing appearance of the pancreatic duct (PNPD), sclerosing pancreatocholangitis, duct destructive chronic pancreatitis, and lymphoplasmacytic sclerosing pancreatitis. Although most patients are 55–65 years of age at the time of diagnosis, the diagnosis may be made at the age extremes.[1,2] There is a male predominance (2 to 1) except in patients with other nonpancreatic autoimmune manifestations.[1,2]

A low threshold is needed and the diagnosis should be considered in patients presenting with unexplained pancreatic disease, especially those with a current or prior history of obstructive jaundice. The diagnosis should also be entertained in patients with a pancreatic mass or enlargement, pancreatic atrophy, or exocrine insufficiency. AIP is seldom the cause of pancreatitis. And while many patients with AIP present with vague abdominal pain, routinely searching for AIP in patients predominantly complaining of abdominal pain is of low yield.

However, even when the diagnosis is considered, diagnostic uncertainty often exists, in particular for patients with "tumefactive" autoimmune pancreatitis in which the disease is manifested by a mass-like lesion that may lead to biliary obstruction when in the pancreatic head and can be mistaken for pancreatic cancer.[12,43,44] As a result, incomplete or inadequate evaluation risks unnecessary surgical intervention for a benign lesion that tends to have a fluctuating course, often with complete resolution of all manifestations, including jaundice, with or without immunosuppressive therapy.[2,8]

Limitations of the Japan Pancreas Society's minimal consensus criteria led to development of the Mayo Clinic's HISORt criteria that enhance diagnostic sensitivity.[41] (Table 20–2) Given the limitations of imaging features alone, including EUS, safe and reliable methods for tissue sampling are needed to facilitate diagnosis. There are few data concerning the use of EUS FNA for establishing the diagnosis of AIP and most consider FNA and cytology inadequate for diagnosis. While cytologic specimens can be examined for lymphocytes and plasma cells, their presence in other disorders limits specificity risking mismanagement of an unrecognized pancreatic carcinoma. Tissue samples collected via FNA lack preservation of tissue architecture, which most pathologists consider necessary for diagnosis. As such, until data show otherwise, we strongly discourage reliance on FNA to establish the diagnosis of AIP opting instead for TCB. However, we and others have shown that optimization of diagnostic accuracy using TCB requires both histologic evaluation and IgG4 immunostaining.[13,41] Unfortunately, it may not be possible to obtain pancreatic core biopsies due to technical, anatomical, or personnel limitations. In such patients, it is necessary to consider all HISORt criteria in a manner that often allows diagnosis even in the absence of histologic evaluation. (Table 20–3)

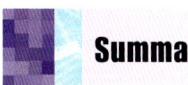

Summary

The lack of pathognomonic imaging features, considerable variation in pancreatic imaging, and diverse spectrum of clinical disease highlight the need for safe measures for acquiring core tissue specimens to enhance the diagnostic accuracy of AIP. As such, in patients with AIP, we perform ERCP only when otherwise indicated and not solely to satisfy diagnostic criteria. On the other hand, our initial experience supports the assumption that tissue obtained with EUS TCB is sufficient to allow adequate histologic review to diagnose AIP. We perform EUS TCB for

Table 20–2 Mayo Clinic HISORt Criteria for Diagnosing Autoimmune Pancreatitis

Category	Criteria

A. **H**istology	1. Diagnostic (any one):
	  a) Pancreatic histology showing periductal lymphoplasmacytic infiltrate with obliterative phlebitis (LPSP)
	  b) Lymphoplasmacytic infiltrate with abundant (>10 cells/hpf) IgG4 positive cells in the pancreas
	2. Supportive (any one)
	  a) Lymphoplasmacytic infiltrate with abundant (>10 cells/hpf) IgG4 positive cells in involved extra-pancreatic organ
	  b) Lymphoplasmacytic infiltrate with fibrosis in the pancreas

B. **I**maging	Typical imaging features: 1. CT/MR : diffusely enlarged gland with delayed (rim) enhancement 2. ERCP: Diffusely irregular, attenuated main pancreatic duct Atypical Imaging Features* : Pancreatitis, focal pancreatic mass, focal pancreatic duct stricture, pancreatic atrophy, pancreatic calcification
C. **S**erology	Elevated serum IgG4 level (normal 8-140 mg/dl)
D. **O**ther **O**rgan Involvement	Hilar/intrahepatic biliary strictures, persistent distal biliary stricture, Parotid/lacrimal gland involvement, Mediastinal lymphadenopathy, Retroperitoneal fibrosis
E. **R**esponse to Steroid **T**herapy	Resolution/marked improvement of pancreatic/extrapancreatic manifestation with steroid therapy

Table 20-3 Diagnosis of AIP: Patients Meeting Criteria for More Than One of the Following Groups*

Group A: Diagnostic Pancreas Histology (one or both, based on surgical specimen or core biopsy)

1. Full spectrum of LPSP
   a) Periductal lymphoplasmacytic infiltrate, and
   b) Obliterative phlebitis with storiform fibrosis
2. Immunostain demonstrating ≥10 IgG4-positive cells/HPF

Group B: Characteristic Imaging and Serology (all the following)

1. CT or MRI showing both
   a) Diffusely enlarged pancreas, and
   b) Delayed and "rim" enhancement
2. Pancreatogram showing diffusely irregular pancreatic duct
3. Elevated serum IgG4 levels

Group C: IgG4 (serum or tissue) and Response to Steroids (both of the following)

1. Elevated serum IgG4 level and/or other organ involvement (>10 IgG4-positive cells/HPF) †
2. Resolution/marked improvement in pancreatic/extrapancreatic manifestations with steroids ‡

* Assumes negative work-up for known etiologies for pancreatic disease, especially cancer

† Evidence of other organ involvement can be confirmed by biopsy showing lymphoplasmacytic infiltrate with abundant IgG4-positive cells or by resolution or marked improvement with steroid therapy.

‡ Steroid administration should be restricted to patients with a negative work-up for known etiologies for pancreatic disease and to persons in whom a response to the particular manifestation can be objectively assessed. A steroid trial is not an appropriate substitute for a thorough diagnostic evaluation.

patients with a compatible clinical presentation in whom there is diagnostic uncertainty and when the finds are likely to alter management. Doing so may prevent misdiagnosis of pancreatic carcinoma risking lost opportunity for potentially curative resection while avoiding unnecessary surgical interventions for those with AIP. While these findings clearly indicate the ability of EUS TCB to establish the diagnosis of AIP, the limited number of patients evaluated prohibits any determination of sensitivity, specificity, or safety in this setting.

Videos: Available at www.pmph-usa.com/bhutani

Video 20–1: Characteristic computed tomography (CT) of AIP revealing a diffusely enlarged sausage-shaped gland.

Video 20–2: In the same patient, magnetic resonance imaging (MRI) also reveals a diffusely enlarged sausage-shaped gland with capsule-like rim enhancement.

Video 20–3: Radial EUS image in a patient with AIP highlighting diffuse (sausage-shape) pancreatic enlargement with a hypoechoic, coarse, patchy, heterogeneous appearance.

Video 20–4: The same features are noted during the linear EUS examination.

References

1. Pearson, R. K., Longnecker, D. S., Chari, S. T., Smyrk, T. C., Okazaki, K., Frulloni, L., Cavallini, G.: Controversies in clinical pancreatology: autoimmune pancreatitis: does it exist? Pancreas. 2003;27:1–13.
2. Okazaki, K., Chiba, T.: Autoimmune related pancreatitis. Gut. 2002;51:1–4.
3. Kloppel, G., Luttges, J., Lohr, M., Zamboni, G., Longnecker, D.: Autoimmune pancreatitis: pathological, clinical, and immunological features. Pancreas. 2003;27:14–19.
4. Chari, S. T., Smyrk, T. C., Levy, M. J., Topazian, M. D., Takahashi, N., Clain, J. E., Pearson, R. K., Petersen, B. T., Swaroop, V. S., Farnell, M. B.: Autoimmune pancreatitis: diagnosis using histology, imaging, serology, other organ involvement and response to steroids. Pancreas 2005 Nov. 31 (4):435-436.
5. Wakabayashi, T., Kawaura, Y., Satomura, Y., Watanabe, H., Motoo, Y., Okai, T., Sawabu, N.: Clinical and imaging features of autoimmune pancreatitis with focal pancreatic swelling or mass formation: comparison with so-called tumor-forming pancreatitis and pancreatic carcinoma. American Journal of Gastroenterology. 2003;98:2679–2687.
6. Hamano, H., Kawa, S., Horiuchi, A., Unno, H., Furuya, N., Akamatsu, T., Fukushima, M., Nikaido, T., Nakayama, K., Usuda, N., Kiyosawa, K.: High serum IgG4 concentrations in patients with sclerosing pancreatitis. New England Journal of Medicine 2001;344: 732–738.
7. Kamisawa, T., Egawa, N., Nakajima, H.: Autoimmune pancreatitis is a systemic autoimmune disease. American Journal of Gastroenterology. 2003;98:2811–2812.
8. Kojima, E., Kimura, K., Noda, Y., Kobayashi, G., Itoh, K., Fujita, N.: Autoimmune pancreatitis and multiple bile duct strictures treated effectively with steroid. Journal of Gastroenterology. 2003;38:603–607.
9. Okazaki, K., Kawa, S., Kamisawa, T., Naruse, S., Tanaka, S., Nishimori, I., Ohara, H., Ito, T., Kiriyama, S., Inui, K., Shimosegawa, T., Koizumi, M., Suda, K., Shiratori, K., Yamaguchi, K., Yamaguchi, T., Sugiyama, M., Otsuki, M.: Research Committee of Intractable Diseases of the P. Clinical diagnostic criteria of autoimmune pancreatitis: revised proposal. Journal of Gastroenterology 2006; 41:626–631.

10. Abraham. S. C., Wilentz, R. E., Yeo, C. J., Sohn, T. A., Cameron, J. L., Boitnott, J. K., Hruban, R. H.: Pancreaticoduodenectomy (Whipple resection) in patients without malignancy: are they all chronic pancreatitis? American Journal of Surgical Pathology 2003;27:110–120.
11. Kloppel, G., Luttges, J., Sipos, B., Capelli, P., Zamboni, G.: Autoimmune pancreatitis: pathological findings. Jop: Journal of the Pancreas [Electronic Resource] 2005;6:97–101.
12. Yadav, D., Notahara, K., Smyrk, T. C., Clain, J. E., Pearson, R. K., Farnell, M. B., Chari, S. T.: Idiopathic tumefactive chronic pancreatitis: clinical profile, histology, and natural history after resection. Clinical Gastroenterology & Hepatology. 2003;1:129–135.
13. Zamboni, G., Luttges, J., Capelli, P., Frulloni, L., Cavallini, G., Pederzoli, P., Leins, A., Longnecker, D., Kloppel, G.: Histopathological features of diagnostic and clinical relevance in autoimmune pancreatitis: a study on 53 resection specimens and 9 biopsy specimens. Virchows Archiv 2004;445:552–563.
14. Suda, K., Takase, M., Fukumura, Y., Ogura, K., Ueda, A., Matsuda, T., Suzuki, F.: Histopathologic characteristics of autoimmune pancreatitis based on comparison with chronic pancreatitis. Pancreas 2005;30:355–358.
15. Kamisawa, T.: IgG4-positive plasma cells specifically infiltrate various organs in autoimmune pancreatitis. Pancreas 2004;29:167–168.
16. Zhang, L., Chari, S. T., Levy, M. J., SMyrk, T. C.: Pancreatic IgG4 stain for diagnosing autoimmune pancreatitis (AIP) and for distinguishing AIP subtypes. Gastroenterology 2005;128:A474.
17. Levy, M. J., Reddy, R. P., Wiersema, M. J., Smyrk, T. C., Clain, J. E., Harewood, G. C., Pearson, R. K., Rajan, E., Topazian, M. D., Yusuf, T. E., Chari, S. T., Petersen, B. T.: EUS-guided Tru-cut biopsy in establishing autoimmune pancreatitis as the cause of obstructive jaundice. Gastrointestinal Endoscopy 2005;61:467–472.
18. Irie, H., Honda, H., Baba, S., Kuroiwa, T., Yoshimitsu, K., Tajima, T., Jimi, M., Sumii, T., Masuda, K.: Autoimmune pancreatitis: CT and MR characteristics. AJR. American Journal of Roentgenology. 1998;170: 1323–1327.
19. Sahani, D. V., Kalva, S. P., Farrell, J., Maher, M. M., Saini, S., Mueller, P. R., Lauwers, G. Y., Fernandez, C. D., Warshaw, A. L., Simeone, J. F.: Autoimmune pancreatitis: imaging features. Radiology 2004;233:345–352.
20. Yang, D. H., Kim, K. W., Kim, T. K., Park, S. H., Kim, S. H., Kim, M. H., Lee, S. K., Kim, A. Y., Kim, P. N., Ha, H. K., Lee, M. G.: Autoimmune pancreatitis: radiologic findings in 20 patients. Abdominal Imaging 2006;31: 94–102.
21. Kamisawa, T., Egawa, N., Nakajima, H., Tsuruta, K., Okamoto, A.: Extrapancreatic lesions in autoimmune pancreatitis. Journal of Clinical Gastroenterology 2005;39:904–907.
22. Nishino, T., Toki, F., Oyama, H., Oi, I., Kobayashi, M., Takasaki, K., Shiratori, K.: Biliary tract involvement in autoimmune pancreatitis. Pancreas 2005;30:76–82.
23. Ohara, H., Nakazawa, T., Sano, H., Ando, T., Okamoto, T., Takada, H., Hayashi, K., Kitajima, Y., Nakao, H., Joh, T.: Systemic extrapancreatic lesions associated with autoimmune pancreatitis. Pancreas 2005;31:232–237.
24. Takahashi, N., Kawashima, A., Fletcher, J. G., Chari, S. T.: Renal involvement in patients with atuoimmune pancreatitis: CT and MR imaging findings. Radiology 2007:Mar;242(3):791-801.
25. Piccinino, F., Sagnelli, E., Pasquale, G., Giusti, G.: Complications following percutaneous liver biopsy. A multicentre retrospective study on 68,276 biopsies. Journal of Hepatology 1986;2:165–173.
26. Kovalik, E. C., Schwab, S. J., Gunnells, J. C., Bowie, D., Smith, S. R.: No change in complication rate using spring-loaded gun compared to traditional percutaneous renal allograft biopsy techniques. Clinical Nephrology 1996;45:383–385.
27. Brandt, K. R., Charboneau, J. W., Stephens, D. H., Welch, T. J., Goellner, J. R.: CT- and US-guided biopsy of the pancreas. Radiology 1993;187:99–104.
28. Welch, T. J., Sheedy, P. F., 2nd, Johnson, C. D., Johnson, C. M., Stephens, D. H.: CT-guided biopsy: prospective analysis of 1,000 procedures. Radiology 1989;171: 493–496.
29. Harrison, B. D., Thorpe, R. S., Kitchener, P. G., McCann, B. G., Pilling, J. R.: Percutaneous Tru-cut lung biopsy in the diagnosis of localised pulmonary lesions. Thorax 1984;39:493–499.
30. Ingram, D. M., Sheiner, H. J., Shilkin, K. B.: Operative biopsy of the pancreas using the Tru-cut needle. Australian & New Zealand Journal of Surgery 1978;48:203–206.
31. Lavelle, M. A., O'Toole, A.: Tru-cut biopsy of the prostate. British Journal of Urology 1994;73:600.
32. Ball, A. B., Fisher, C., Pittam, M., Watkins, R. M., Westbury, G.: Diagnosis of soft tissue tumors by Tru-Cut biopsy. British Journal of Surgery 1990;77:756–758.
33. Wiersema, M. J., Levy, M. J., Harewood, G. C., Vazquez-Sequeiros, E., Jondal, M. L., Wiersema, L. M.: Initial experience with EUS-guided Tru-cut needle biopsies of perigastric organs. Gastrointestinal Endoscopy. 2002;56:275–278.
34. Levy, M. J., Jondal, M. L., Clain, J., Wiersema, M. J.: Preliminary experience with an EUS-guided Tru-cut biopsy needle compared with EUS-guided FNA. Gastrointestinal Endoscopy 2003;57:101–106.
35. Levy, M. J., Wiersema, M. J.: EUS-guided trucut biopsy. Gastrointestinal Endoscopy 2005;62:417–426.
36. Levy, M. J., Smyrk, T. C., Reddy, R. P., Clain, J. E., Harewood, G. C., Kendrick, M. L., Pearson, R. K., Petersen, B. T., Rajan, E., Topazian, M. D., Wang, K. K., Wiersema, M. J., Yusuf, T. E., Chari, S. T.: Endoscopic ultrasound-guided trucut biopsy of the cyst wall for diagnosing cystic pancreatic tumors. Clinical Gastroenterology & Hepatology 2005;3:974–979.
37. Gines, A., Wiersema, M. J., Clain, J. E., Pochron, N. L., Rajan, E., Levy, M. J.: Prospective study of a Tru-cut needle for performing EUS-guided biopsy with EUS-guided FNA rescue. Gastrointestinal Endoscopy 2005; 62:597–601.
38. Kino-Ohsaki, J., Nishimori, I., Morita, M., Okazaki, K., Yamamoto, Y., Onishi, S., Hollingsworth, M. A.: Serum antibodies to carbonic anhydrase I and II in patients with idiopathic chronic pancreatitis and Sjogren's syndrome. Gastroenterology 1996;110: 1579–1586.
39. Nishimori, I., Yamamoto, Y., Okazaki, K., Morita. M., Onodera, M., Kino, J., Tamura, S.: Identification of autoantibodies to a pancreatic antigen in patients with idiopathic chronic pancreatitis and Sjogren's syndrome. Pancreas 1994;9:374–9381.
40. Okazaki, K.: Autoimmune pancreatitis: etiology, pathogenesis, clinical findings and treatment. The Japanese experience. Jop: Journal of the Pancreas [Electronic Resource] 2005;6:89–96.

41. Chari, S. T., Smyrk, T. C., Levy, M. J., Topazian, M. D., Takahashi, N., Zhang, L., Clain, J. E., Pearson, R. K., Petersen, B. T., Vege, S. S., Farnell, M. B.: Diagnosis of autoimmune pancreatitis: the Mayo Clinic experience. Clinical Gastroenterology & Hepatology 2006;4:1010–1016; quiz 934.
42. Kamisawa, T., Funata, N., Hayashi, Y.: Lymphoplasmacytic sclerosing pancreatitis is a pancreatic lesion of IgG4-related systemic disease. American Journal of Surgical Pathology 2004;28.
43. Kamisawa, T., Egawa, N., Nakajima, H., Tsuruta, K., Okamoto, A., Kamata, N.: Clinical difficulties in the differentiation of autoimmune pancreatitis and pancreatic carcinoma. American Journal of Gastroenterology. 2003;98:2694–2699.
44. Taniguchi, T., Tanio, H., Seko, S., Nishida, O., Inoue, F., Okamoto, M., Ishigami, S., Kobayashi, H.: Autoimmune pancreatitis detected as a mass in the head of the pancreas without hypergammaglobulinemia, which relapsed after surgery: case report and review of the literature. Digestive Diseases & Sciences. 2003;48: 1465–1471.

CHAPTER 21

Pancreas Divisum and Other Pancreaticobiliary Anomalies

Dr. Kirk P. Bernadino
Dr. John C. Deutsch

Embryological development of the pancreas and biliary system is a complex phenomenon that begins with the development of the dorsal and ventral pancreatic buds at five weeks gestation. Differential growth leads to a larger dorsal pancreatic bud. The ventral pancreatic bud develops from a saculation that will eventually give rise to the biliary system. With rotation of the duodenum, at about eight weeks gestation, the smaller ventral bud passes around the duodenum posteriorly to join with the fixed dorsal bud. The ventral duct (Duct of Wirsung) then fuses with the dorsal duct (Duct of Santorini) establishing dorsal pancreatic drainage through the ventral duct and the major papilla. Most pancreaticobiliary anomalies, including pancreas divisum, anomalous pancreaticobiliary junction, biliary cysts, annular pancreas, and pancreatic agenesis are believed to result from a particular derangement of this embryologic process. In general, these anomalies are not threatening to the viability of the fetus and therefore persist after birth. They may become symptomatic anywhere from infancy to adulthood depending on the type of anomaly. Some may be discovered incidentally or not at all. Most are best visualized with ERCP or MRCP, but many can be demonstrated with endoscopic ultrasound (EUS) if the endosonographer is aware of the potential anomalies and their characteristic appearance.

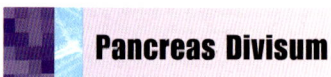

Pancreas Divisum

Pancreas divisum results from non- or incomplete fusion of the ventral and dorsal pancreatic ducts. It is subclassified into complete pancreas divisum if no communication exits between these ducts, and incomplete (or partial) pancreas divisum if a communication can be demonstrated. The normal pancreatic ductal anatomy is shown in a Visible Human Model in Figures 21–1A and 21–1B. A normal radial array EUS of the pancreatic head showing portal vein, common bile duct, and main pancreatic duct is shown in figure 21–1C. Various forms of pancreatic ductal anatomy are illustrated using Visible Human Models in figure 21–2. Generally, in incomplete divisum the narrow communication offers high resistance to flow, resulting in most of the pancreatic secretions draining through the dorsal duct and into the duodenum via the minor papilla. This drainage pattern is referred to as "dorsal duct syndrome." EUS images from a patient with suspected partial divisum are shown in Figures 21–3A and 21–3B. Acquired divisum, or pseudodivisum, results from post embryologic, usually malignant, strictures of the ventral duct often with resultant dorsal duct syndrome.

Pancreas divisum is the most common of the pancreatic ductal anomalies with an autopsy prevalence of 4–14%.[1-4] It is hypothesized, in pancreas divisum, that pancreatic outflow from the majority of the gland is impeded by the smaller-caliber minor papilla leading to higher intraductal pressures and subsequent pancreatitis. However, there is conflicting data about whether pancreas divisum actually increases one's risk of pancreatitis. Clearly most pancreas divisum is asymptomatic.

Pancreas divisum is best demonstrated on contrast pancreatogram from the major papilla at ERCP. EUS is also highly accurate in making the diagnosis. Using ERCP as the gold standard, the overall sensitivity and specificity of linear array EUS in detecting pancreas divisum are as high as 95% and 97%, respectively.[5] Other reports have been less optimistic, showing sensitivity of 50%.[6] Pancreas divisum may also be visible or suggested by CT if one can carefully follow the dorsal pancreatic duct to its duodenal insertion or by MRCP. Using intravenous secretin stimulation during MRCP can increase the yield of noninvasive test.[7]

ERCP is probably most sensitive for diagnosing pancreas divisum because it can best demonstrate small communications between the dorsal and ventral ducts. Pancreatogram typically shows arborization of the pancreatic duct limited to the region of the pancreatic head when the main duct is injected, while a complete distal pancreatogram can be obtained from the minor papilla (Figures 21–4A, 21–4B). No pancreatic duct is seen crossing the spine when the major duct is injected. A tapered or abrupt termination of the ventral duct suggests pseudodivisum and should raise suspicion for malignancy, stone, trauma, or other intraductal or extrinsic cause of obstruction.

Certain EUS findings can suggest or exclude the presence of pancreas divisum. A dilated dorsal pancreatic duct should raise one's suspicion for pancreas divisum as well as other causes of pancreatic outflow obstruction. Classically, the absence of a "stack sign" (stack sign seen in Figure 21–1C) as usually seen from the duodenum, has been described in pancreas divisum. Demonstrating a pancreatic duct duodenal insertion separate from and more proximal to the bile duct insertion is another suggestive EUS finding. Occasionally, the endosonographer will see a "crossed duct sign" in the pancreatic head (Figure 21-5). In this scenario, the dorsal pancreatic duct, normally further from the transducer in the "stack sign" crosses the distal common bile duct and becomes closer to the transducer as it courses toward its duodenal insertion.

If, when following the pancreatic duct from the major ampulla, the endosonographer can demonstrate that the duct maintains caliper and continuity around the portal vein (the usual location of the pancreatic head/body junction), pancreas divisum is

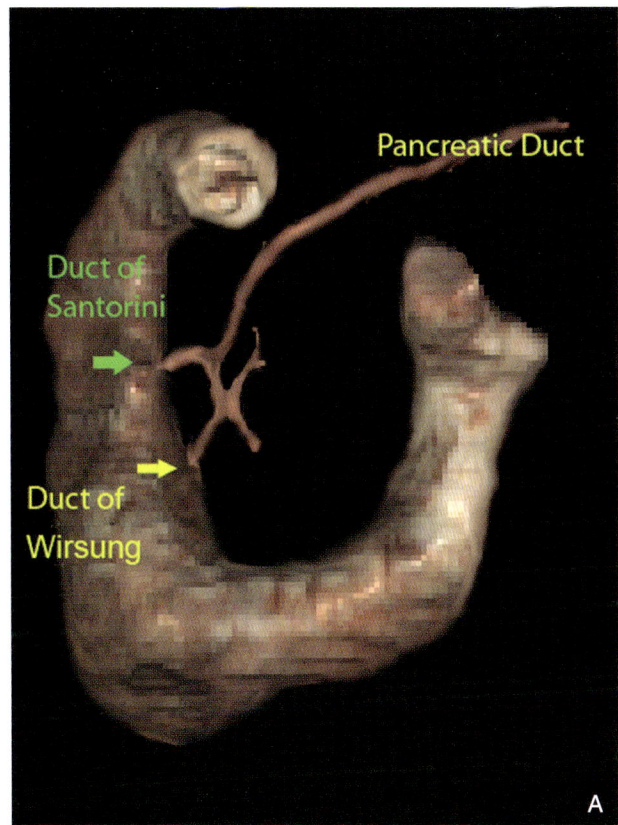
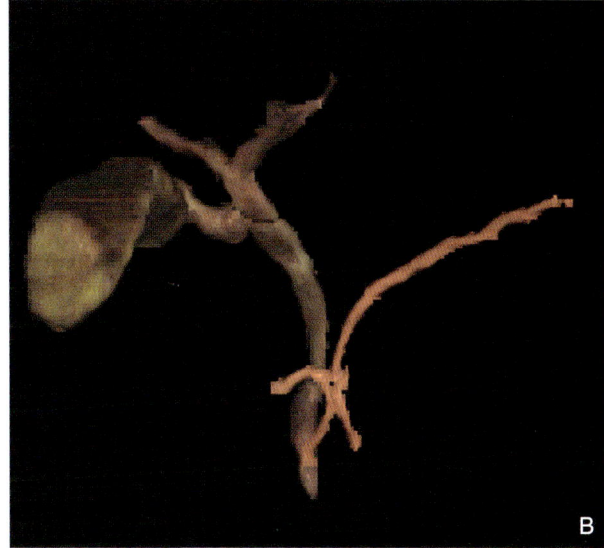
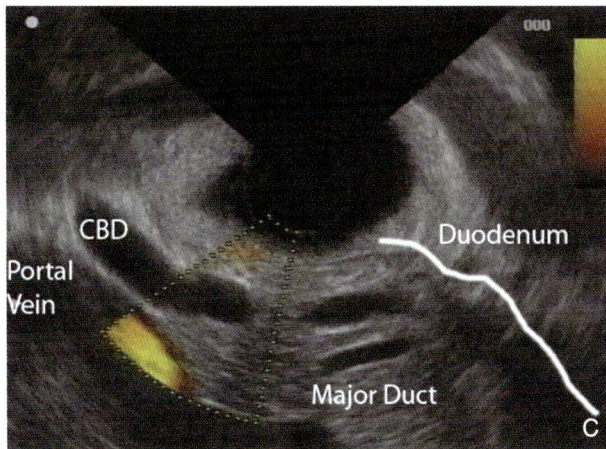

FIGURES 21-1. A to C (A) Visible Human Model derived from the VH Dissector Pro, showing the duodenum and normal pancreatic ductal anatomy. The duct of Wirsing and Santorini are shown. (B) Visible Human Model of the pancreatobiliary tree. (C) Radial array EUS showing the "stack sign, in which the portal vein, pancreatic duct and common bile duct are all visible on one image.

unlikely. (Video 21–1). Similarly, if the pancreatic duct is seen traversing the hypoechoic ventral anlage (visible dorsal/ventral pancreas demarcation), pancreas divisum is excluded.

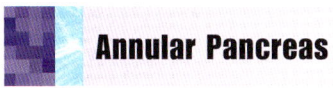

Annular Pancreas

Annular pancreas is a rare congenital pancreatic anomaly with a prevalence of 0.05%.[8] A Visible Human Model is shown in figure 21–6A. It presumably results from the ventral pancreatic bud partially or completely encircling the duodenum during duodenal rotation. When symptomatic, it usually presents as duodenal obstruction in infancy, but presentation in adulthood has also been reported.[9] Annular pancreas may have associations with duodenal diverticula, pancreatitis, or pancreatic cancer.

Annular pancreas can be diagnosed by CT, MRI/MRCP, EUS, or ERCP. Pancreatogram demonstrates the ventral pancreatic duct encircling the second portion of the duodenum (Figure 21–6B). EUS

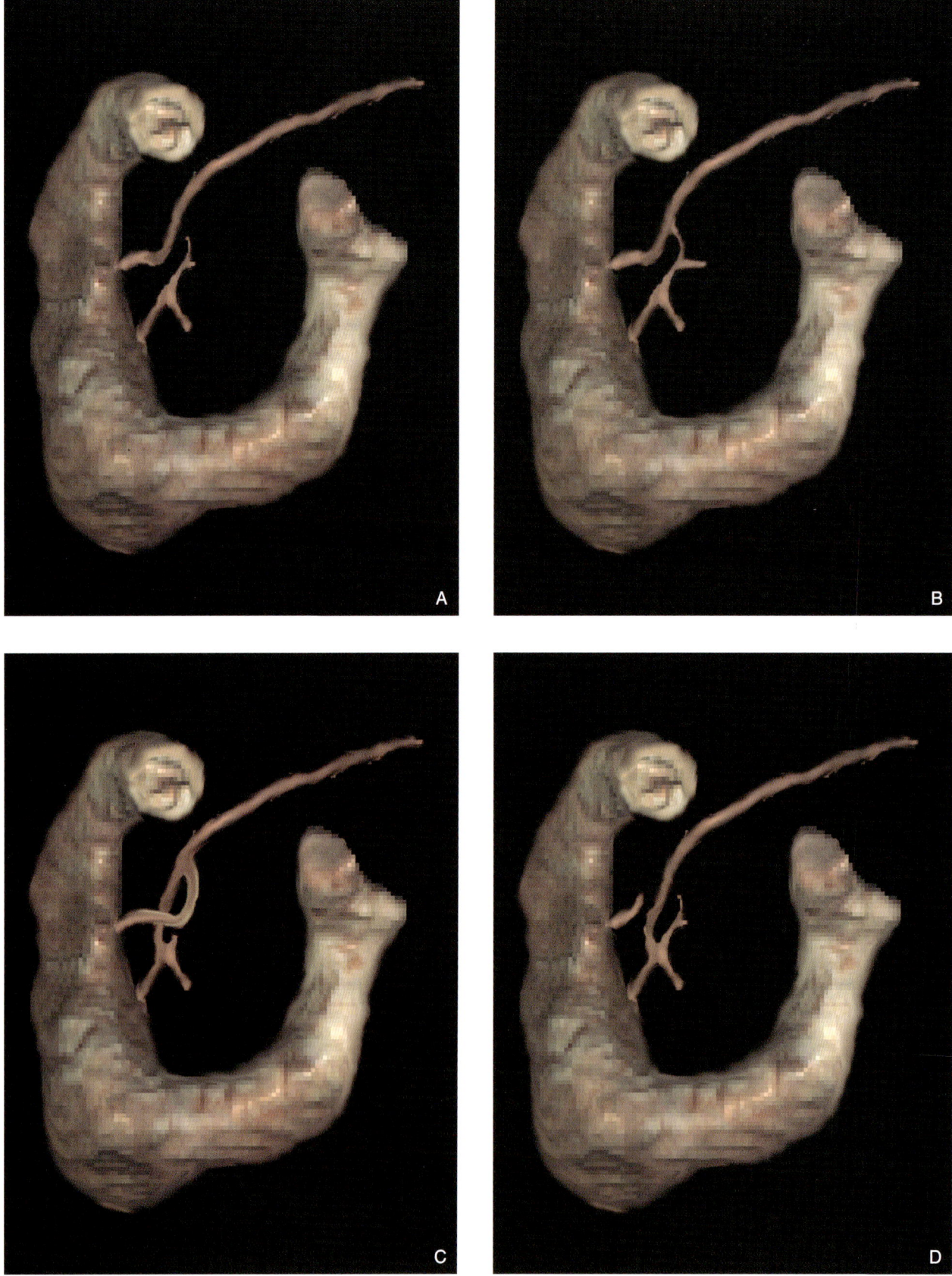

FIGURES 21-2. *A to D* Visible Human Models of the pancreatic duct and duodenum, which can be compared to figure 21-1A. (A) Pancreas divisum; (B and C) Variants of incomplete divisum; (D) Inverted divisum.

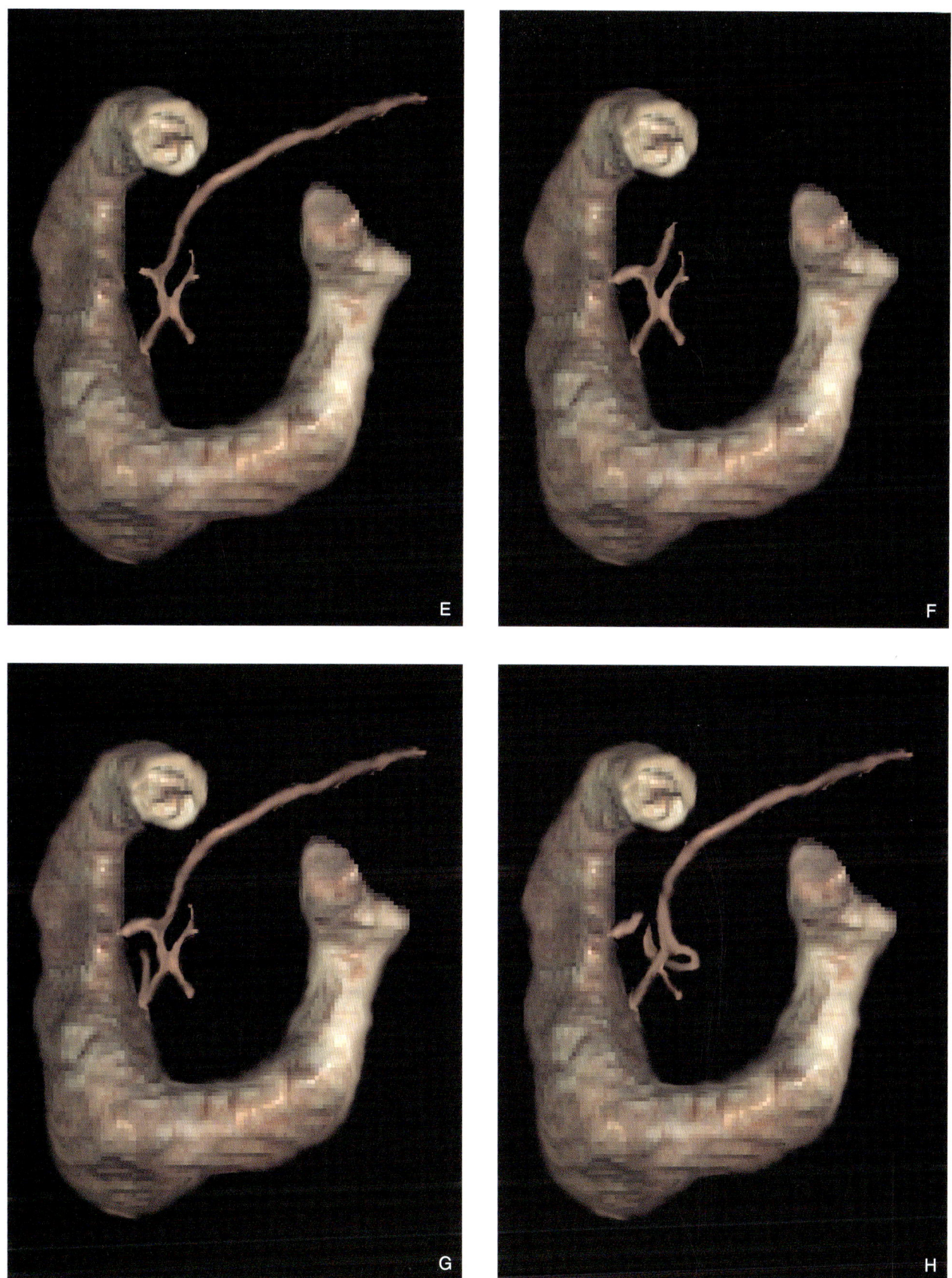

FIGURES 21–2. *E to H* (E) Obliterated minor duct; (F) Short pancreas; (G) Double ventral duct; (H) Ansa pancreatica

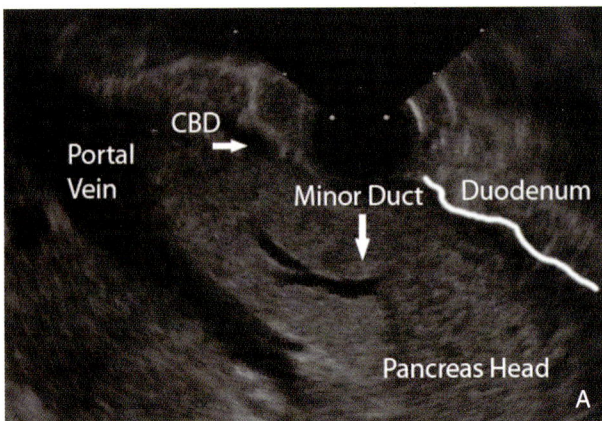 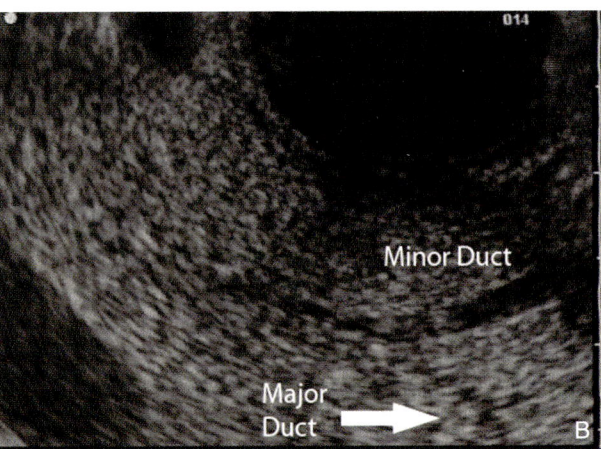

FIGURES 21–3. *A and B* (A) Radial array EUS image from the duodenum showing an enlarged minor pancreatic duct heading toward the duodenum. This suggests partial or complete divisum. (B) Radial EUS showing an enlarged minor duct and a diminutive connection toward the major duct, suggesting incomplete divisum.

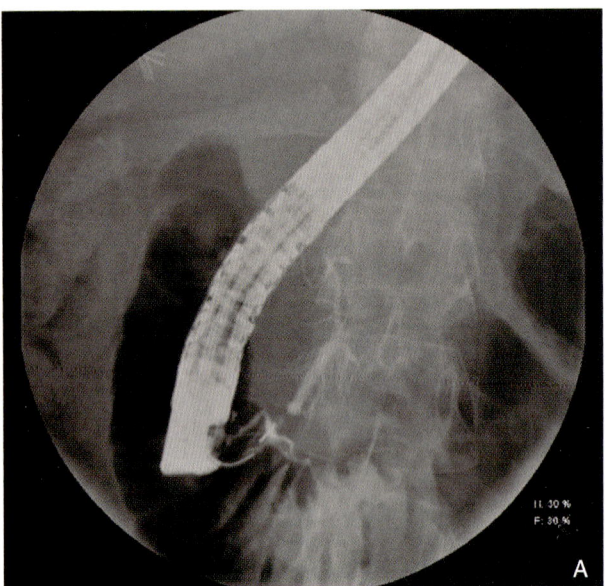 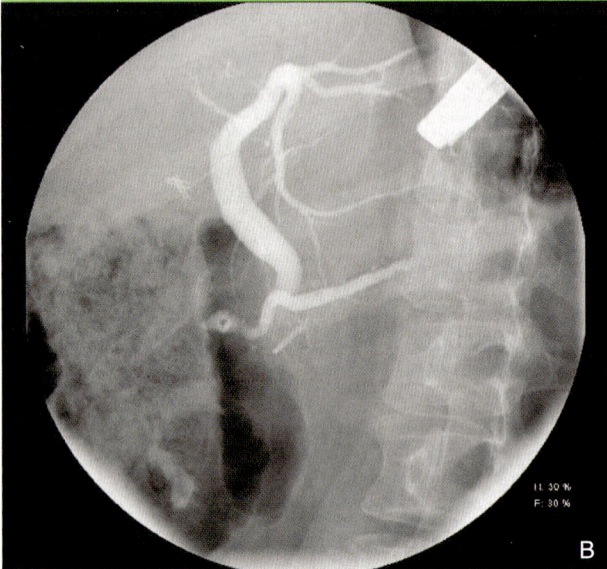

FIGURES 21–4. *A and B* (A) Injection of the main pancreatic duct during ERCP showing a blind end to the main duct and arborization in the head of the pancreas. (B) The same patient in 21–4A, but in this case the ERCP injection had been made through the minor papilla. Courtesy of Douglas A. Howell M. D.

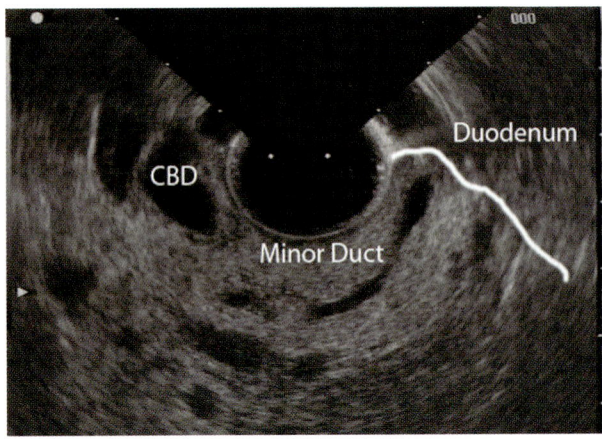

FIGURE 21–5. Radial EUS showing an enlarged minor duct. In real time, a "crossed stack sign" (see text) could be seen.

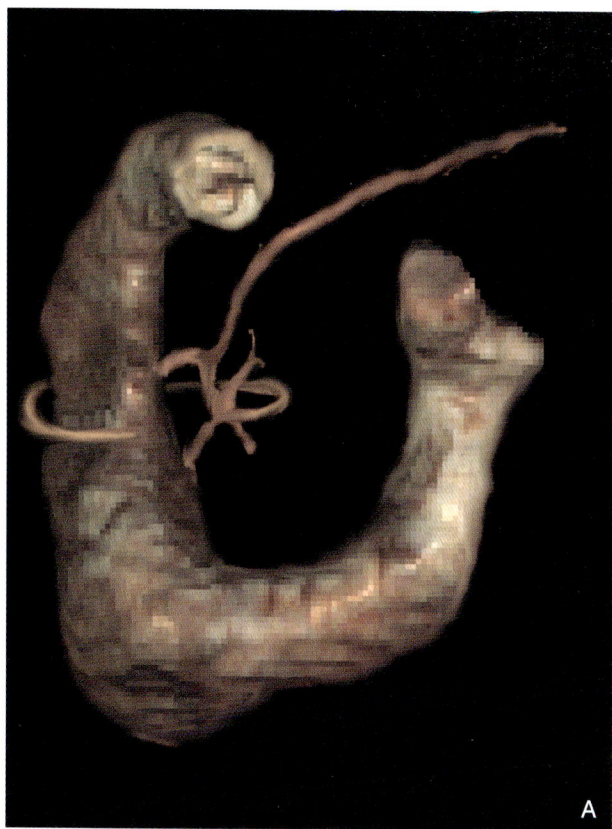

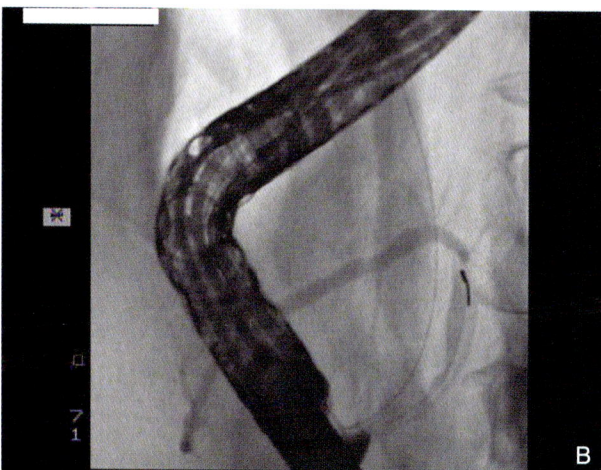

FIGURES 21–6. *A* and *B* (A) A Visible Human Model showing the pancreatic ducts in annular pancreas. (B) ERCP showing the pancreatic duct in annular pancreas. Courtesy of Douglas A. Howell M. D.

findings include a band of pancreatic tissue partially or completely encircling the duodenum proximal to the ampulla. The pancreatic parenchymal appearance of the annular portion is identical to that of the remainder of the gland.[10]

Santorinicele

A santorinicele is a sacular dilatation of the dorsal pancreatic duct duodenal terminus. It is generally visible endoscopically as bulging of the duodenal wall at the minor papilla and may be more obvious after intravenous secretin injection or contrast pancreatogram. It is unlikely of embryologic origin, but rather a result of chronic pancreatic outflow obstruction. It can occur in the presence or absence of pancreas divisum. ERCP best demonstrates santoriniceles as a contrast-filled dilation in the duodenal wall with upstream filling of the dorsal duct. When not decompressed, similar EUS findings can be seen (Figure 21–7).

Anomalous Pancreaticbiliary Junction

Anomalous pancreaticobiliary junction is a rare congenital anomaly. It describes an abnormally proximal junction of the ventral pancreatic and common bile ducts, usually greater than 1.5 cm from the ampulla.[11] It is also referred to as a long common channel. Visible Human Models of the normal and abnormal pancreatobiliary junction are shown in Figures 21-8A and 21-8B. The mechanism of its embryologic origin is unknown, but likely relates to a misarrangement of the pancreatic and biliary ductal system or an arrest of the normal migration of the common channel into the duodenal lumen.[12] The frequent coexistence with biliary cysts suggests a defect leading to weakening or abnormal elongation of the bile duct might be causative.

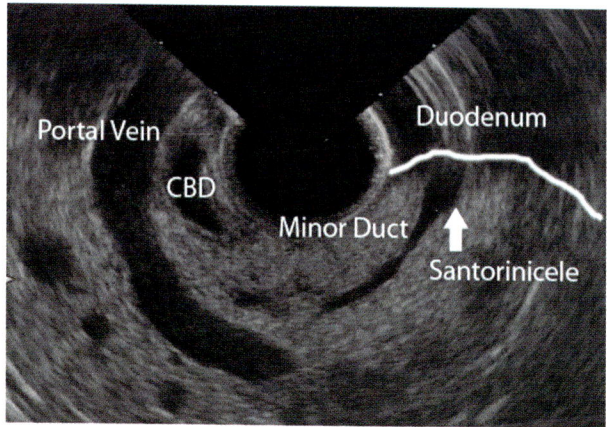

FIGURE 21–7. A small santorinicele in a patient with pancreas divisum (Same patient as in Figure 21–5).

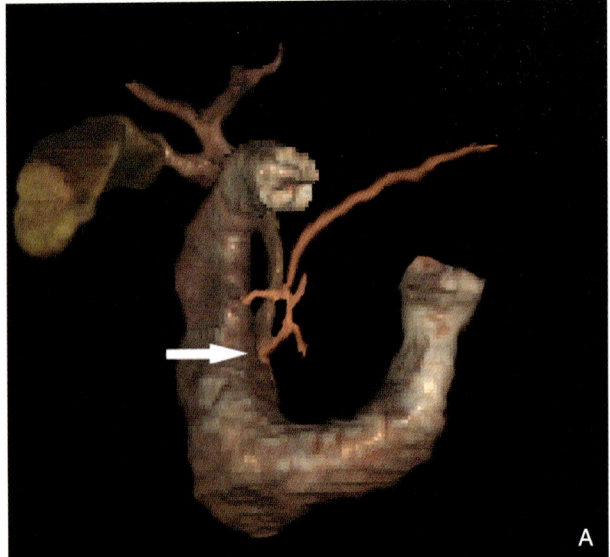
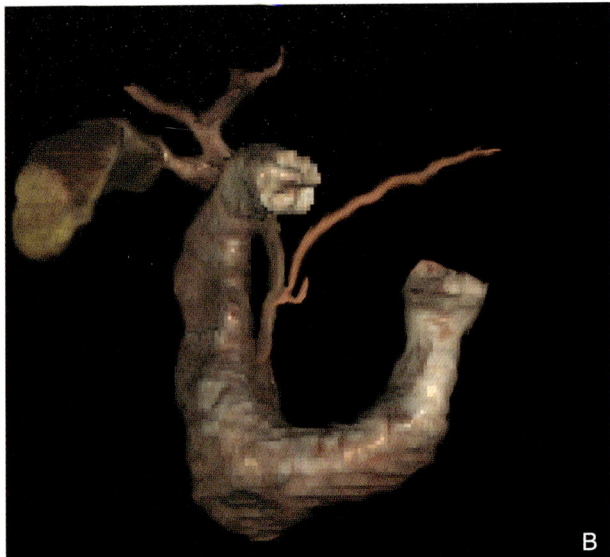
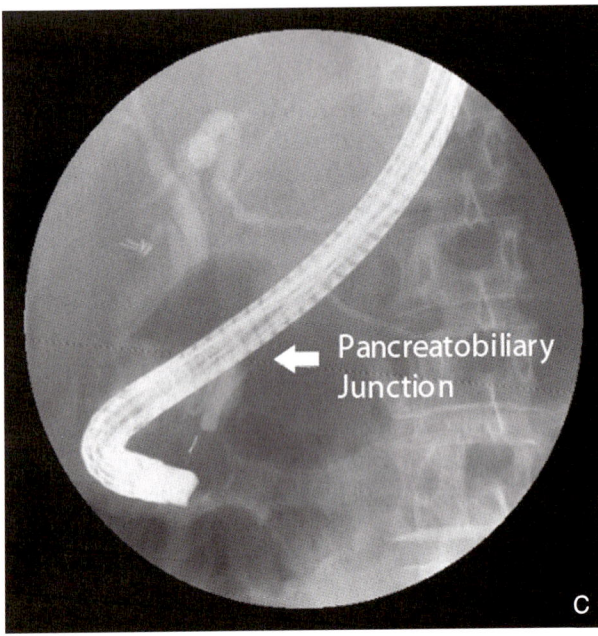

FIGURES 21–8. *A to C* (A) A Visible Human Model showing the normal pancreatobiliary junction (white arrow); (B) A Visible Human Model showing an anomalous pancreatobiliary junction; (C) ERCP showing anomalous pancreatobiliary junction.

Anomalous pancreaticobiliary junction is rare, but has a prevalence of 4–8% in some Asian reports.[13-14] Biliary cysts, further described in text that follows, are rare cystic dilations of the biliary system. Anomalous pancreaticobiliary junction has been demonstrated in 70–90% of patients with biliary cysts, and is therefore hypothesized to be causative. Whether the mechanism is reflux of pancreatic secretions into the biliary tree or an inherent bile duct defect is unknown.

Anomalous pancreaticobiliary junction is strongly associated with biliary malignancies. Sole anomalous pancreaticbiliary junctions increase the risk of gallbladder cancer, while anomalous pancreaticobiliary junction in association with biliary cysts increase the risk of malignancy in the biliary cyst. Anomalous pancreaticobiliary junction may also be associated with other pancreaticobiliary diseases including, gallbladder adenomyomatosis, biliary and nonbiliary pancreatitis, Sphincter of Oddi dysfunction, cholelithiasis, hilar cholangiocarcinoma, and pancreatic cancer.[15-20]

In anomalous pancreaticobiliary junction, ERCP demonstrates a long common channel from 1.5 cm to 5 cm (Figure 21-8c). Cholangiogram can demonstrate coexisting biliary cysts. Similarly, EUS can demonstrate a long (greater than 1 cm) common channel.[21-22] EUS can also be valuable in diagnosing extrapancreatic manifestations, including coexisting intra- or extrahepatic biliary cysts, gallstones, gallbladder carcinoma, or adenomyomatosis and cholangiocarcinoma.

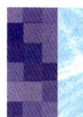

Partial or Complete Pancreatic Agenesis

Agenesis of part or all of the pancreas is exceedingly rare with only a handful of reports in the literature. Partial pancreatic agenesis generally involves the dorsal pancreas and can lead to long-term survival.[23-24] It has been associated with severe intrauterine grown retardation, infantile diabetes, recurrent acute and chronic pancreatitis, and pancreatic exocrine insufficiency. Complete pancreatic agenesis is universally fatal and associated with other extrapancreatic anomalies.

Truncation or diminished size of the pancreas may be evident on cross-sectional imaging or transabdominal ultrasound. In the case of dorsal agenesis, ERCP or MRCP pancreatogram may show pancreas divisum without a demonstrable dorsal pancreatic duct. EUS from the stomach can reveal an absence of pancreatic tissue and duct. The ventral gland is small, but remains visible from the duodenum.

Biliary Cysts

Biliary cysts, also referred to as choledochal cysts, are rare, congenital, or acquired cystic dilations of the intrahepatic and/or extrahepatic biliary tree. They are commonly described, using the Todani classification, according to their anatomic locations as follows:[25]

Type I: Common bile duct
    Ia: "common" type with sacular dilation of entire extrahepatic bile duct
    Ib: "segmental" dilation of the extrahepatic bile duct
    Ic: "diffuse" cylindrical dilation of the extrahepatic bile duct
Type II: Diverticulum of the extrahepatic bile duct.
Type III: Choledochocele – ampullary dilation
    IIIa: choledochocele with proximal biliary/pancreatic insertions
    IIIb: Intraduodenal bile duct dilation, "dilated common channel"
Type IV: multiple biliary cysts
    IVa: extrahepatic and intrahepatic cysts
    IVb: multiple extrahepatic cysts only
Type V: Intrahepatic cysts only, single or multiple

A normal Visible Human \Model of the biliary tree and the above anomalies are shown in Figure 21–9A – 21–9G. The mechanism of biliary cyst formation is not known. Various mechanisms likely exist. Congenital biliary cysts are thought to arise from focal structural weakness in the developing biliary tree. The high prevalence of anomalous pancreaticobiliary junction in people with biliary cysts suggests reflux of pancreatic secretions into the biliary tree can lead to chronic epithelial inflammation and subsequent formation of acquired biliary cysts. This chronic inflammation is also a postulated mechanism of malignant degeneration of biliary cysts. The presence of solitary or multiple biliary cysts increases one's risk of cholangiocarcinoma twenty- to thirty-fold over that of the general population.[26] It is unclear if choledochoceles impart an increased risk for cholangiocarcinoma; if so, it is likely of modest increase.

Biliary cysts can present at any age or may be discovered incidentally by CT (Figure 21–10A), MRCP, EUS or at ERCP (Figure 21–10B). Presenting symptoms range from jaundice or abdominal mass in neonates to abdominal pain, cholangitis, or pancreatitis in adults. Biliary cysts may be seen on cross-sectional imaging with CT or MRI as well as transabdominal ultrasound. ERCP can best delineate the cyst(s) and evaluate for concomitant anomalous pancreaticobiliary junction or biliary obstruction. Intraductal ultrasound at time of ERCP may be useful in detecting early cholangiocarcinoma in biliary cysts.[27] A Type III choledochocele may be evident endoscopically as a soft, compressible bulge behind or immediately proximal to the major ampulla. This bulging often displaces the ampulla inferiorly, pointing it in a downward direction toward the distal duodenum. In contrast, duodenal duplication cysts, having a somewhat similar endoscopic appearance, will arise from the duodenal wall immediately distal to the major ampulla, generally preserving the normal ampullary position.

MRCP is somewhat less reliable than ERCP for demonstrating cysts with a reported overall accuracy of 86%. MRCP may be limited in detecting small choledochoceles (Type III cysts).[28]

EUS evaluation for intrahepatic biliary cysts includes a careful examination of the hepatic parenchyma for ductal dilations. The left hepatic lobe being best visualized from the stomach, and the right from the duodenal bulb and second portion of the duodenum. Large field of view, low frequency and high gain may be necessary to adequately visualize the hepatic tissue most distant to the transducer. Intrahepatic biliary cysts appear as anechoic dilations

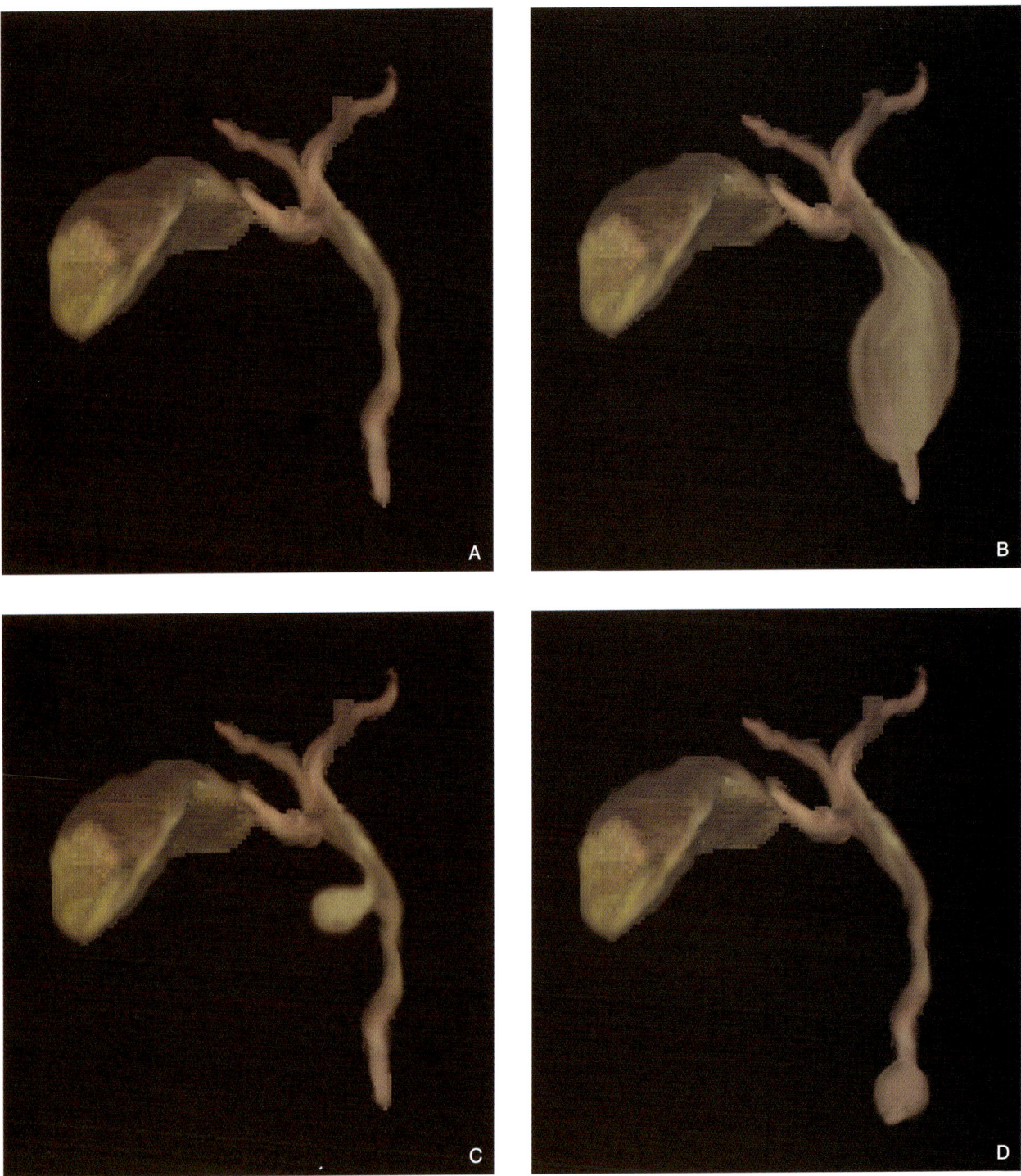

FIGURES 21–9. *A to D* Visible Human Models of biliary tree and various biliary cysts. (A) Normal; (B) Type I; (C) Type II; (D) Type III.

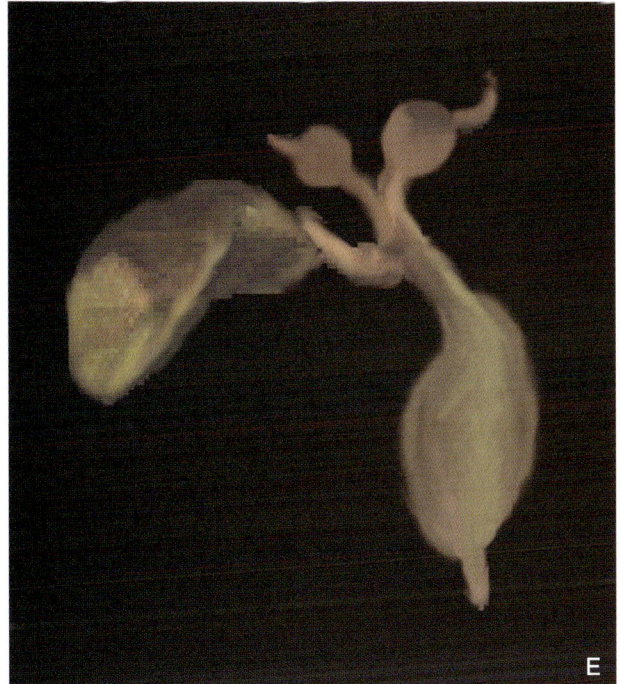
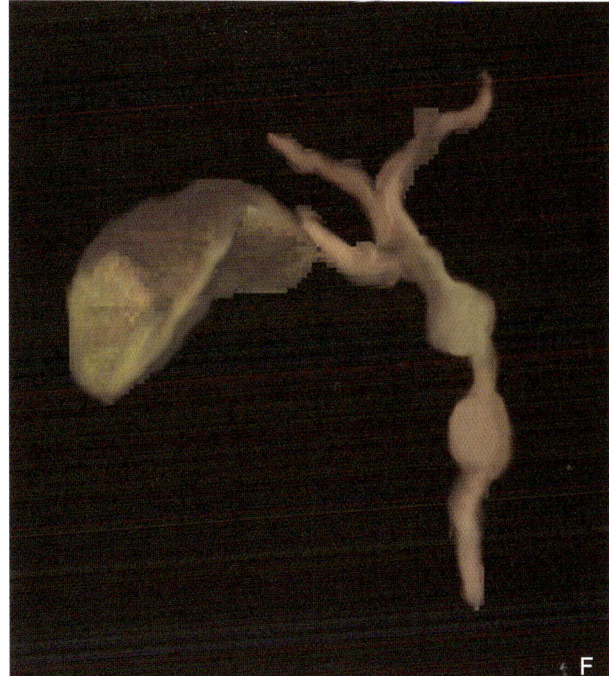
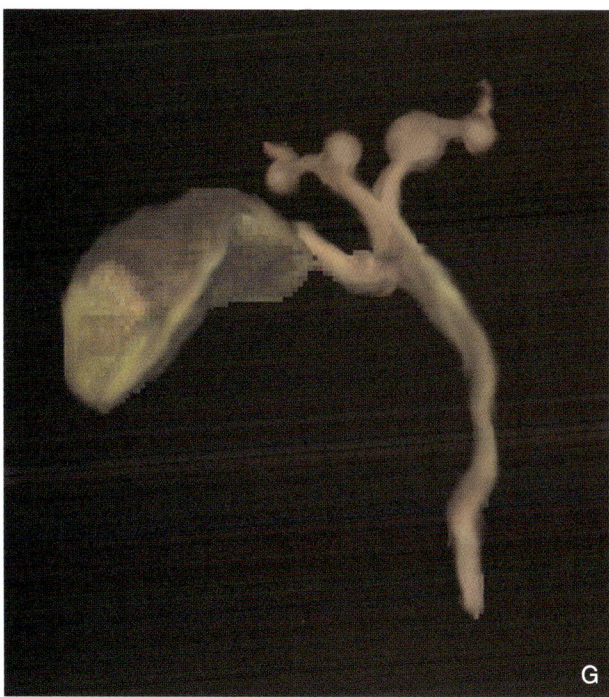

FIGURES 21-9. *E to G* (E) Type 4a; (F) Type IVb; (G) Type V

of the intrahepatic ducts. They do not posses a Doppler signal. EUS can demonstrate mural thickening or hyperechoic cyst contents with or without acoustic shadows, suggesting biliary sludge, cholangiocarcinoma, or other lesions within the cysts.[29]

The extrahepatic bile ducts, best seen from the duodenum, should be visualized completely. The common bile duct should be followed from its duodenal insertion to the common hepatic duct bifurcation. Large biliary cysts can be confused with the gallbladder. If the gallbladder is present, the endosonographer should trace the cystic duct to it to exclude a segmental or diffuse Type I choledochal cyst (Figure 21–11C). If the cystic duct can not be located another communication between the cyst and the extrahepatic bile duct should be sought. A Type III choledochocele will be located at the terminus of the bile duct, nearest the ampulla (Figures 21–11A-C). It can be differentiated

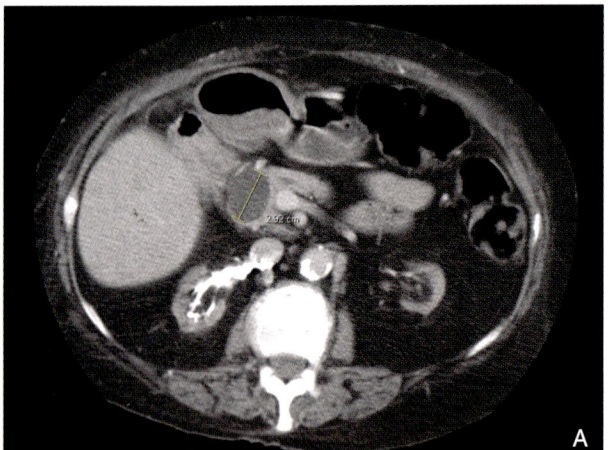
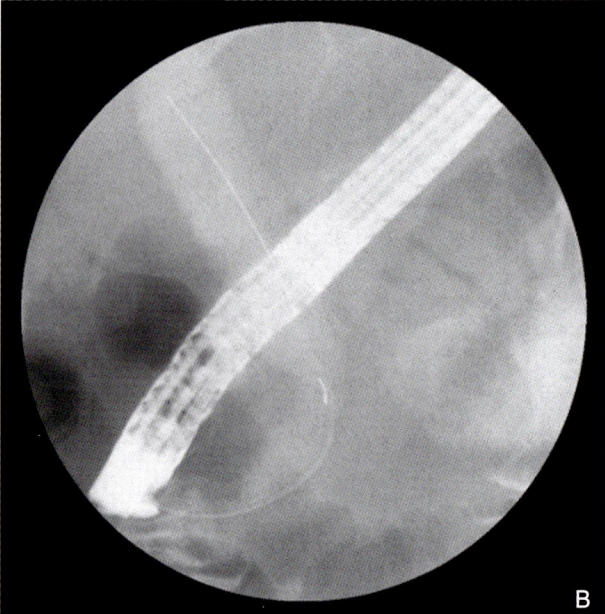
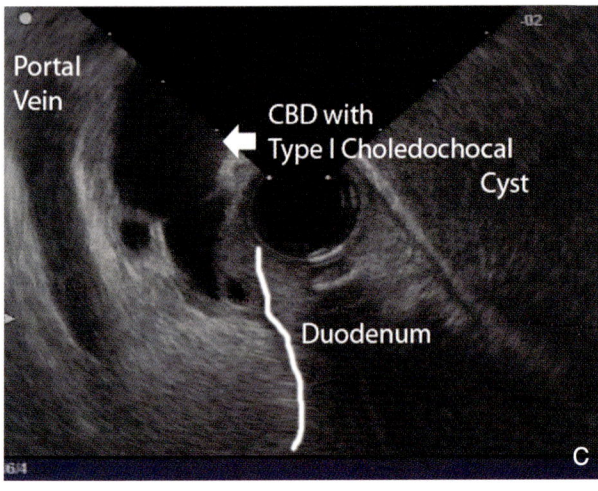

FIGURES 21–10. *A to C* (A) A CT scan in a patient with a Type I choledochocal/biliary cyst. (B) ERCP of a suspected Type I choledochocal cyst. (C) Radial Array EUS image of a Type I choledochocal/biliary cyst. The EUS image is from a similar location as that in figure 21–1C.

from a duodenal diverticulum by visualizing the structure while instilling water or saline through the echoendoscope accessory channel. If swirling bubbles are seen in the structure (Figure 21–12A) and the patient has an intact biliary sphincter, it is a diverticulum. A choledochocele will remain anechoic. The connection between the diverticulum and the duodenum can often be imaged by EUS (Figure 21–12B) or directly at endoscopy (Figure 21–12C).

Duodenal Duplication Cysts

Duodenal duplication cysts are rare congenital anomalies probably formed during the early weeks of gestation. These cysts, lined with duodenal mucosa, usually arise from the duodenal wall immediately distal to the major ampulla. Their presence does not directly alter biliary or pancreatic ductal anatomy. However, they may present with pancreatitis, presumably through predisposing to pancreatic outflow obstruction or bile reflux into the pancreatic duct. They may also present as duodenal obstruction in childhood, intermittent nausea, vomiting or abdominal pain as an adult or be incidentally discovered radiographically or at endoscopy. Although exceedingly rare, case reports of malignant transformation exist. Endoscopic marsupialization with endoscopic biopsy surveillance is the preferred management.[30]

On cross-sectional imaging duodenal duplication cysts can be confused with pancreatic or biliary cysts. The cyst is visible on MRCP although despite not communicating with the biliary or pancreatic ductal

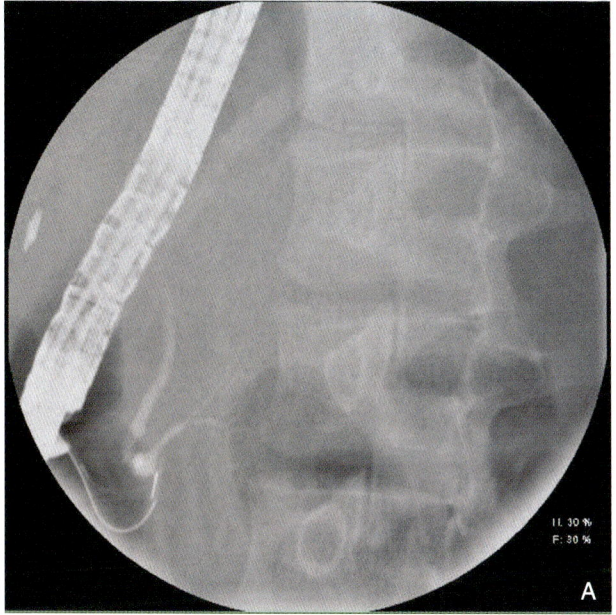
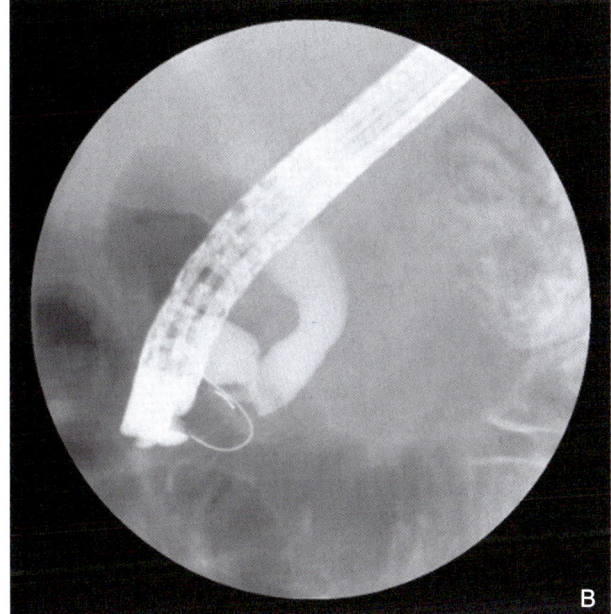
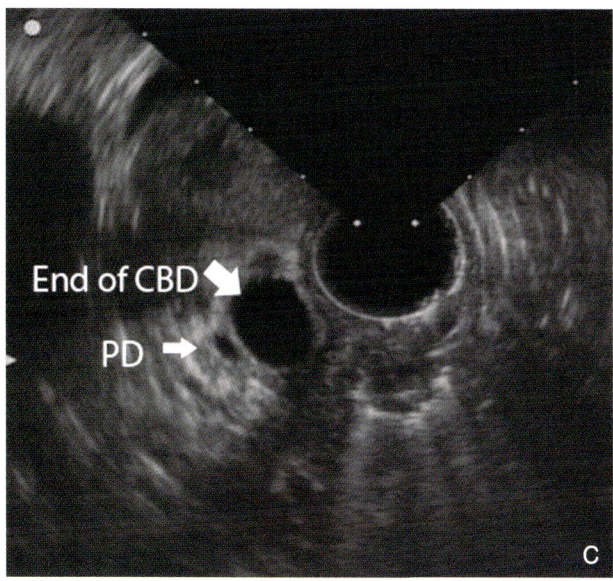

FIGURES 21–11. *A to C* (A) ERCP showing a Type IIIa choledochocele. (B) ERCP showing a prominent Type IIIA choledochocele with saccular dilation of the distal common bile duct. The pancreatic insertion is not visualized. (C) Radial EUS showing a type III choledochocele with bulbous end of the common bile duct (CBS) adjacent to the main pancreatic duct (PD. ERCP images courtesy of Dourglas A. Howell M. D.

systems. This noncommunication may not be evident on MRCP.

Endoscopically, duplication cysts resemble a windsock anchored on the distal aspect of the major ampulla. They are easily compressible and generally occupy the medial aspect of the duodenal lumen, extending distally for several centimeters. The proximal opening may range from a few millimeters in size to large enough to allow collection of food and debris. Although the distal aspect of the cyst resides with the duodenal lumen, it is a blind pouch and, thus, often filled with fluid or food debris. Rarely, duodenal duplication cysts communicate with the pancreatic duct or bile duct. In the latter case, the cyst may contain bilious fluid and possibly gallstones.

The vast majority of duodenal duplication cysts communicate only with the duodenum. In these cases, ERCP usually reveals a normal cholangiogram and pacreatogram. Often the cyst opening is visible edoscopically. Filling the cyst and duodenum with contrast may allow visualization of the entire cyst, confirming its short proximal duodenal attachment and "windsock" configuration.

Endoscopic ultrasound can demonstrate mucosa, submucosa, and muscularis mucosa layers within the cyst and absence of continuity with the bile duct differentiating it from a large, Type III choledochocele. Continuity with the duodenum may also be demonstrable using the "bubble test" described earlier in the section addressing biliary cysts.

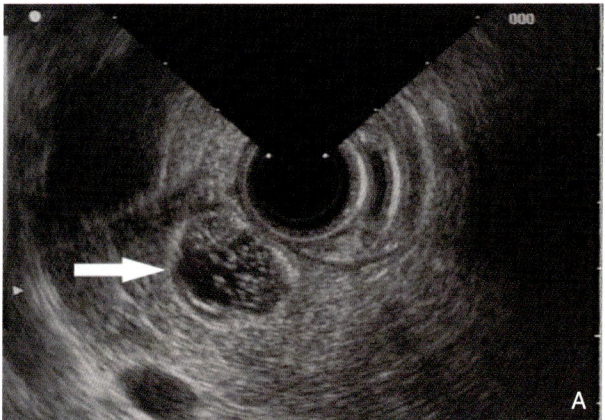
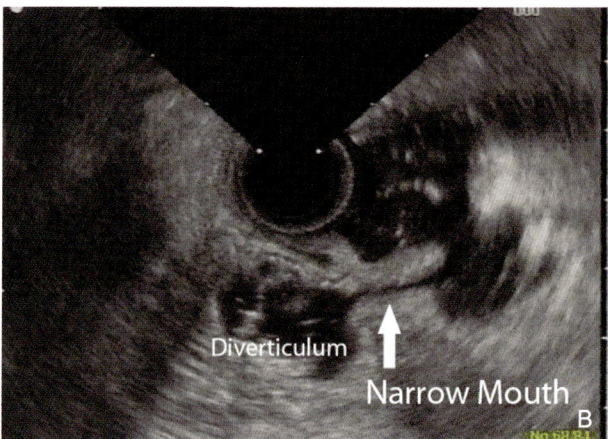
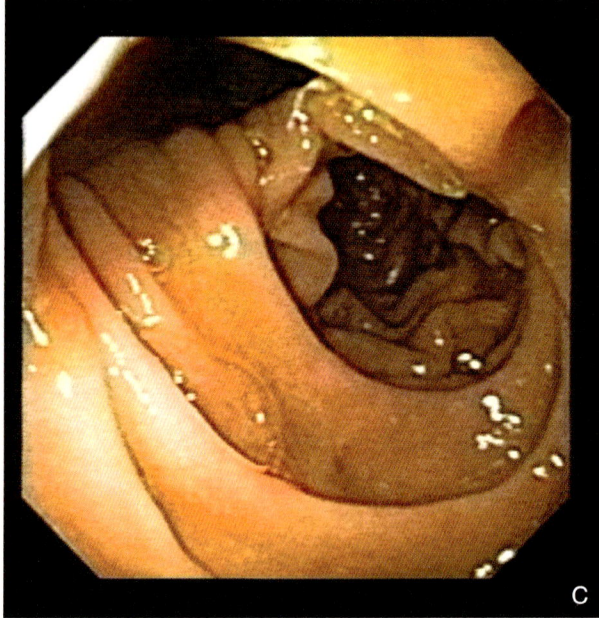

FIGURES 21–12. *A to C* (A) Duodenal diverticulum showing bubbles inside. (B) The same diverticulum showing a narrow mouth connecting it to the duodenal lumen. (C) Endoscopic view of a large periampullary duodenal diverticulum.

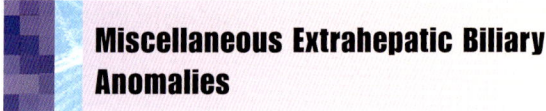

Miscellaneous Extrahepatic Biliary Anomalies

Variations in biliary confluence and cystic duct anatomy are common and, with the exceptions of impending biliary surgery or a postoperative bile leak, have little clinical significance. Ductal anomalies are most easily seen with ERCP or MRCP, but an observant endosonographer should be able to identify most.

Cystic duct anomalies, including low cystic duct take off (Figure 21-13A) and aberrant insertion, most commonly into the major ampulla or right hepatic duct, can be diagnosed with careful EUS examination of the extrahepatic bile ducts if particular attention is given to the site of cystic duct insertion. Evaluation from both the duodenal bulb and second portion stations may be necessary to visualize the entire cystic duct.

Short common bile duct refers to a low common hepatic duct bifurcation, possibly even within the pancreatic parenchyma (Figures 21-13B-D). Common pancreaticobiliary channel or "dilated common channel" (Figure 21–13E) as seen in anomalous pacreaticobiliary junctions and type III choledochoceles is described elsewhere in this chapter. An aberrant right hepatic duct describes an ectopic drainage of the right anterior or right posterior segmental hepatic duct into the common hepatic duct or, less commonly, the common bile or cystic duct. Again, the diagnosis is most obvious on ERCP (Figure 21–13F) or MRCP, but can be made with EUS. Endosonographic clues would include an abnormally low common hepatic duct bifurcation or identification of more than two ducts exiting the liver parenchyma. If either is present, each branch of the biliary confluence should be traced from its junction with hepatic parenchyma to the common hepatic duct.[31-32]

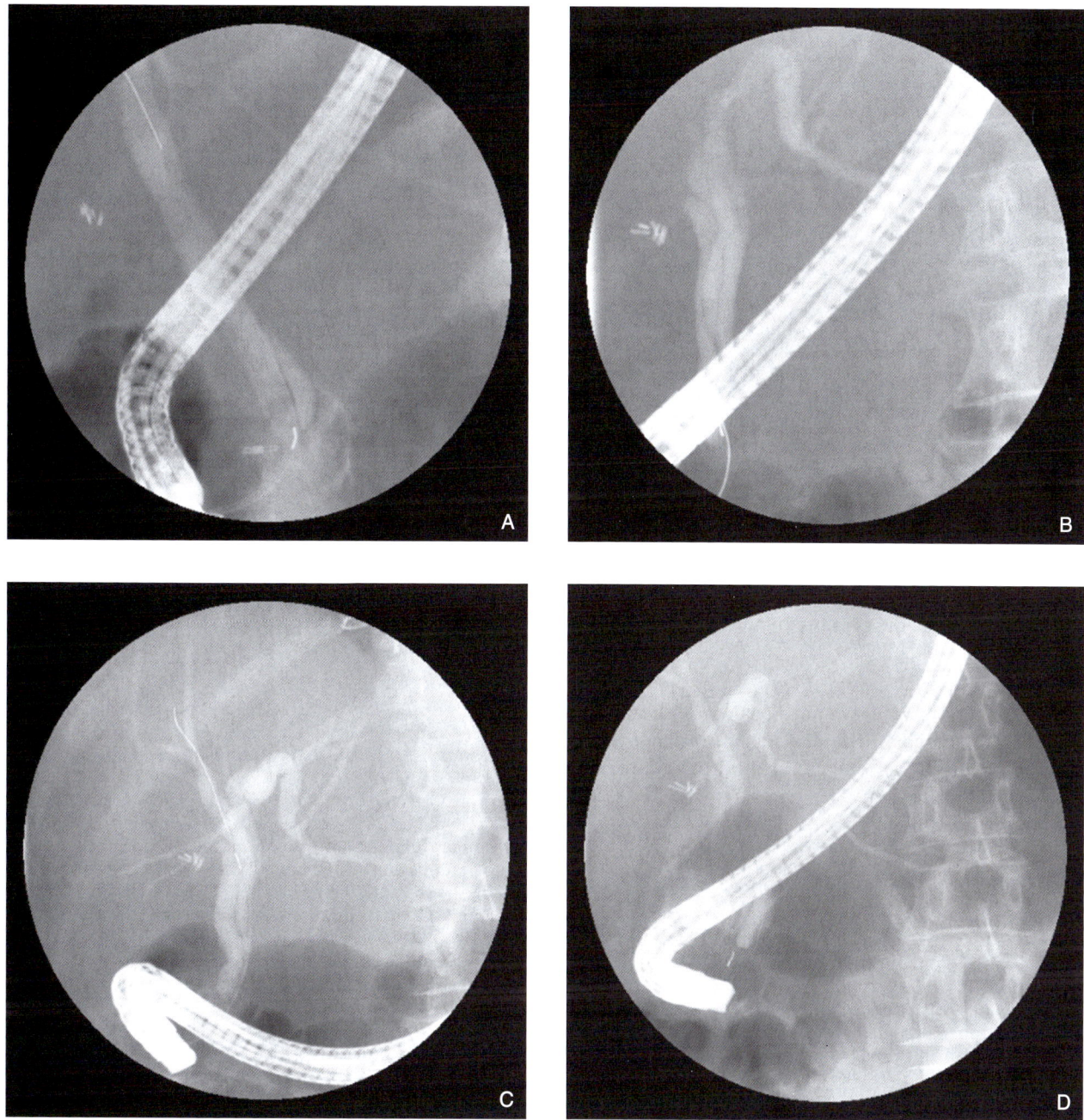

FIGURES 21–13. *A to D* ERCP of various extrahepatic biliary anomalies (A) Low cystic duct take-off. ERCP image showing abnormally distal location of cystic duct take-off nearly at the ampulla. (B) Short common bile duct. This cholangiogram initially shows a confusing swirling of ducts. (C) After advancing the duodenoscope and a small change in the fluoroscopic angle, the anatomy untangles revealing a low hepatic bifurcation and cystic duct take-off. (D) This patient also has an anomalous pancreaticobiliary junction. Courtesy of Douglas A. Howell M. D.

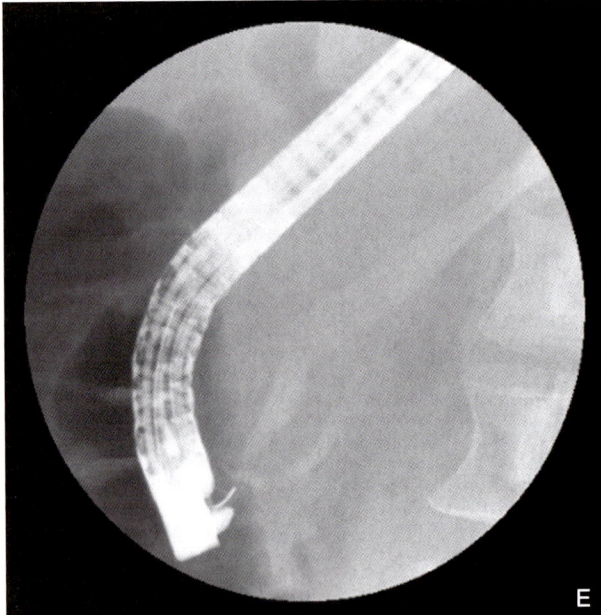
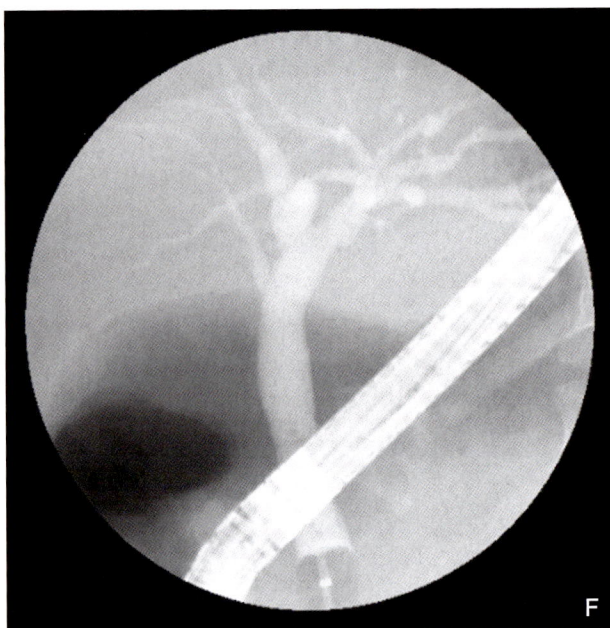

FIGURES 21–13. *E to F* (E) Common pancreaticobiliary channel. ERCP demonstrating a subtle, short common channel through which the common bile and main pancreatic ducts drain. (F) Aberrant right hepatic duct. Small segmental hepatic duct inserting into the common bile duct, rather than the right main hepatic duct. Courtesy of Douglas A. Howell M. D.

Video: Available at www.pmph-usa.com/bhutani

Video 21–1: Radial ERCP showing a normal pancreatic duct from the ampulla to around the genu. This exam excludes divisum.

References

1. Kleitsch, W. Anatomy of the pancreas; a study with special reference to the duct system.: AMA Arch Surg 1955; 71(6):795–802.
2. Berman, L. G., Prior, J., Abramow, S., Ziegler, D.: A study of the pancreatic duct system in man by the use of vinyl acetate casts of postmortem preparations. Surg gynecol obstet 1960; 110:391–403.
3. Dawson, W., Langman, J.: An anatomical-radiological study on the pancreatic duct pattern in man. Anat rec 1961; 139:59–68.
4. Smanio, T.: Proposed nomenclature and classification of the human pancreatic ducts and duodenal papillae. Study based on 200 post mortems. Int Surg 1969; 52(2):125–141
5. Lai, R., Freeman, M. L., Cass, O. W., Mallery, S.: Accurate diagnosis of pancreas divisum by linear-array endoscopic ultrasonography. Endoscopy 2004; 36(8):705–709.
6. Vaughan, R., Mainie, I., Hoffman, B., Hawes, R., Romagnuolo, J.: Accuracy of endoscopic ultrasound in the diagnosis of pancreas divisum in a busy clinical setting. Gastrointest.Endosc. 63[5], AB 263. 2006
7. Matos, C., Metens, T., Deviere, J., Delhaye, M., LeMoine, O., Cremer, M.: Pancreas divisum: evaluation with secretin-enhanced magnetic resonance cholangiopancreatography Gastrointest Endosc. 2001 Jun;53(7): 728–733
8. Georgios, I. Papachristou, Mark D. Topazian, Ferga C. Gleeson, Michael J. Levy: EUS features of annular pancreas Gastrointestinal Endoscopy, February 2007 (Vol. 65, Issue 2, pp. 340–344).
9. Nancy L. Harthun, James H. Morse, Hubert A. Shaffer, John S. Minasi: Duodenal obstruction caused by intraluminal duodenal diverticulum and annular pancreas in an adult, Gastrointestinal Endoscopy, June 2002 (Vol. 55, Issue 7, pp. 940–943).
10. Frank Gress, Anusak Yiengpruksawan, Stuart Sherman, Steven Ikenberry, Steven Kaster, Richard Y. Ng, Maurice A. Cerulli, Glen A. Lehman: Diagnosis of annular pancreas by endoscopic ultrasound, Gastrointestinal Endoscopy, October 1996 (Vol. 44, Issue 4, pp. 485–489).
11. Tatsuya Nomura, Yoshio Shirai, Norimasa Sandoh, Shigenori Nagakura, Katsuyoshi Hatakeyama: Cholangiographic criteria for anomalous union of the pancreatic and biliary ducts, Gastrointestinal Endoscopy, February 2002 (Vol. 55, Issue 2, pp. 204–208).
12. Yoshiro Matsumoto, Hideki Fujii, Jun Itakura, Masatoshi Mogaki, Masanori Matsuda, Atsuro Morozumi, Masayuki A. Fujino, Koichi Suda, Pancreaticobiliary maljunction: Etiologic concepts based on radiologic aspects, Gastrointestinal Endoscopy, May 2001 (Vol. 53, Issue 6, pp. 614-619).
13. Hsiu-Po Wang, Ming-Shiang Wu, Chun-Che Lin, Li-Ying Chang, Ai-Wen Kao, Hsih-Hsi Wang, Jaw-Town Lin: Pancreaticobiliary diseases associated with anomalous pancreaticobiliary ductal union, Gastrointestinal Endoscopy, August 1998 (Vol. 48, Issue 2, pp. 184–189)
14. Hong-Ja Kim, Myung-Hwan Kim, Sung-Koo Lee, Dong-Wan Seo, Yong-Tae Kim, Dong-Ki Lee, Si-Young Song, Im-Hwan Roe, Jin-Hong Kim, Jae-Bock Chung, Chang-Duck Kim, Chan-Sup Shim, Yong-Bum Yoon, Ung-Suk Yang, Jin-Kyung Kang, Young-Il Min: Normal structure, variations, and anomalies of the pancreaticobiliary

ducts of Koreans: A nationwide cooperative prospective study, Gastrointestinal Endoscopy, June 2002 (Vol. 55, Issue 7, pp. 889–896)
15. Satoshi Tanno, Takeshi Obara, Hiroyuki Maguchi, Yusuke Mizukami, Ryushi Shudo, Tsuneshi Fujii, Kuniyuki Takahashi, Noriyuki Nishino, Satoshi Arisato, Yusuke Saitoh, Hitoshi Ura, Yutaka Kohgo: Thickened inner hypoechoic layer of the gallbladder wall in the diagnosis of anomalous pancreaticobiliary ductal union with endosonography, Gastrointestinal Endoscopy December 1997 (Vol. 46, Issue 6, pp. 520–526).
16. Ming-Shiang Wu, Hsiu-Po Wang, Chia-Tung Shun, Sen-Chang Yu, Teh-Hong Wang, Jaw-Town Lin: Coexistence of anomalous pancreaticobiliary ductal union with adenomyomatosis of the gallbladder, Gastrointestinal Endoscopy, September 1995 (Vol. 42, Issue 3, pp. 265-269).
17. Matsumoto, S, Tanaka, M, Ikeda, S, Yoshimoto, H.: Sphincter of Oddi motor activity in patients with anomalous pancreaticobiliary junction, Am J Gastroenterol. 1991 Jul;86(7):831–834.
18. Bing Hu, Biao Gong, Dai-yun Zhou: Association of anomalous pancreaticobiliary ductal junction with gallbladder carcinoma in Chinese patients: an ERCP study, Gastrointestinal Endoscopy, April 2003 (Vol. 57, Issue 4, pp. 541–545).
19. Shyam S. Sharma, Pancreaticobiliary ductal union in cholangiocarcinoma, Gastrointestinal Endoscopy, March 1994 (Vol. 40, Issue 2, pp. 171–173).
20. Sugiyama, M., Abe, N., Tokuhara, M., Masaki, T., Mori, T., Atomi, Y.: Pancreatic carcinoma associated with anomalous pancreaticobiliary junction, Hepatogastroenterology. 2001 Nov-Dec;48(42):1767–1769.
21. Sugiyama, M., Atomi, Y., Kuroda, A.: Pancreatic disorders associated with anomalous pancreaticobiliary junction, Surgery. 1999 Sep;126(3):492–497.
22. Masanori Sugiyama, Yutaka Atomi: Endoscopic ultrasonography for diagnosing anomalous pancreaticobiliary junction, Gastrointestinal Endoscopy, March 1997 (Vol. 45, Issue 3, pp. 261–267).
23. Uygur-Bayramiçli, O., Dabak, R., Kiliçoglu, G., Dolapçioglu, C., Oztas, D.: Dorsal pancreatic agenesis, JOP. 2007 Jul 9;8(4):450–452.
24. Madeline Pokorney, John C. Deutsch, James Wise: Agenesis of Dorsal Pancreashttp: www.vhjoe.org/Volume6Issue1/6-1-5.htm.
25. Todani, T.; Watanabe, Y., Narusue, M., Tabuchi, K., Okajima, K.: Congenital bile duct cysts: Classification, operative procedures, and review of thirty-seven cases including cancer arising from choledochal cyst. Am J Surg 1977 Aug;134(2):263–269.
26. Soreide, K., Soreide, J. A.: Bile duct cyst as precursor to biliary tract cancer. Ann Surg Oncol. 2007 Mar;14(3): 1200–1211. Epub 2006 Dec 23.
27. Yazumi, S., Takahashi, R., Tojo, M., Watanabe, N., Imamura, M., Chiba, T., Intraductal US aids detection of carcinoma in situ in a patient with a choledochal cyst. Gastrointest Endosc 2001 Feb;53(2):233–236.
28. Park, D. H.; Kim, M. H., Lee, S. K., Lee, S. S., Choi, J. S., Lee, Y. S., Seo, D. W., Won, H. J., Kim, M. Y.: Can MRCP replace the diagnostic role of ERCP for patients with choledochal cysts? Gastrointest Endosc. 2005 Sep;62(3):360–366.
29. Hiroshi, Kawakami, Masaki, Kuwatani, Manabu, Onodera, Masahiro, Asaka, Satoshi, Hirano, Satoshi, Kondo: Villous adenoma arising in choledochocele, Gastrointestinal Endoscopy, December 2007 (Vol. 66, Issue 6, pp. 1231-1232).
30. Fadi Antaki, Andrea Tringali, Pierre Deprez, Vu Kwan, Guido Costamagna, Olivier Le Moine, Myriam Delhaye, Michel Cremer, Jacques Devière: A case series of symptomatic intraluminal duodenal duplication cysts: presentation, endoscopic therapy, and long-term outcome, Gastrointestinal Endoscopy, January 2008 (Vol. 67, Issue 1, pp. 163-168).
31. Michael Häfner, Rainer Schöfl, Alfred Gangl: A rare anomaly of the biliary tree: the interhepatic duct Gastrointestinal Endoscopy, June 1997 (Vol. 45, Issue 6, pp. 523–525)
32. Mitsunobu Matsushita, Kiyoshi Hajiro, Hiroshi Takakuwa, Akiyoshi Nishio Interhepatic duct accompanied by cholestasis Gastrointestinal Endoscopy, April 2000 (Vol. 51, Issue 4, pp. 503–504).

CHAPTER 22

Choledocholithiasis and Other Benign Bile Duct Lesions

Dr. Max A. Shapiro
Dr. Nadim G. Haddad

Introduction

Endoscopic ultrasound (EUS) is an advanced technique combining endoscopy with ultrasonography to yield high-resolution images of the gastrointesintal (GI) tract and surrounding structures. This allows for assessment of many different disease processes, and the use of fine needle aspiration and Doppler technology has further broadened the diagnostic capabilities.[1] EUS evaluations have consistently shown benefit to patients by aiding in establishing their diagnoses and often guiding their management. In this chapter we will explore the role of EUS in the evaluation of choledocholithiasis.

Instruments and Techniques

There are now three commonly used echoendoscopes. The first is a radial array echoendoscope, which allows evaluation of a field perpendicular to the endoscope 270–360 degrees. The frequencies used are typically 7.5 and 12 MHz to scan at a depth of 3–100mm. The linear or curvilinear array echoendoscopes provide a parallel scanning direction (100–180 degrees). These echoendoscopes are usually operated at a frequency of 5 and 7.5 MHz and again allow a 3–100mm depth of field. This design enables the use of guidance of a needle for aspiration, biopsy, or injection. Doppler is generally available on both of these scopes to assess flow and differentiate between vascular and other tubular structures. Finally, ultrasound catheter probes can be passed through the therapeutic channel of a standard endoscope. These scan circumfirentially (360 degrees) and use a higher frequency with more limited depth of field. This set-up is most appropriate for the evaluation of small mucosal or submucosal lesions and for intraductal imaging.

Uses of EUS

As mentioned earlier, EUS has a broad range of diagnostic utility.[1] The wall of the GI tract is normally visible by EUS as a series of definable layers. This is utilized in the staging of GI malignancies and in the evaluation of subepithelial lesions. Also, many organs and structures surrounding the GI tract can be well seen with EUS. These include the pancreas, the biliary tree, and gallbladder, and even mediastinal structures, such as lymph nodes. The common bile duct can be visualized, and EUS can be useful in evaluating causes of obstruction and dilation, including stones, as will be reviewed here.

When evaluating the common bile duct by radial array EUS, it is important to realize that images are generated from a posterior-to-anterior view (Figures 22–1 - 22–3). Figure 22–1 shows a Visible Human Model of the duodenum and biliary tree in the anterior to posterior view. This is similar to images

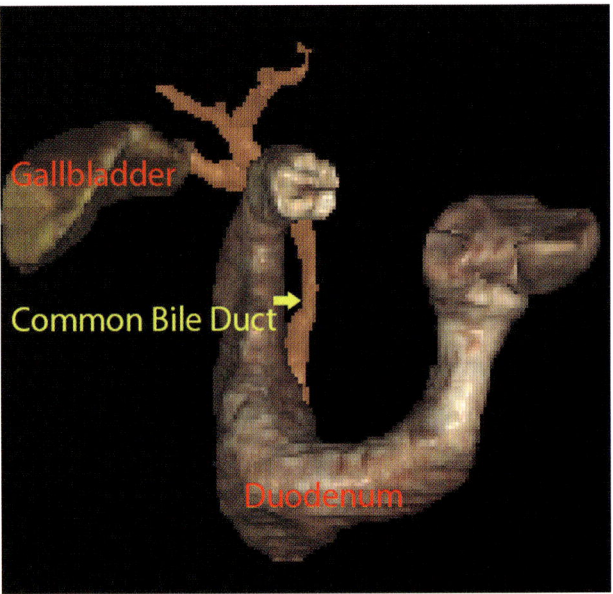

FIGURE 22–1. Visible Human Model of duodenum and biliary tree from the anterior-to-posterior orientation

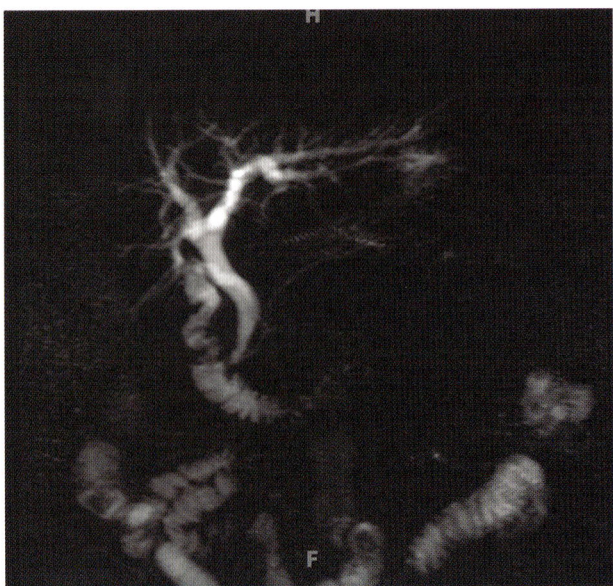

FIGURE 22–2. MRCP showing biliary tree in an anterior-to-posterior orientation.

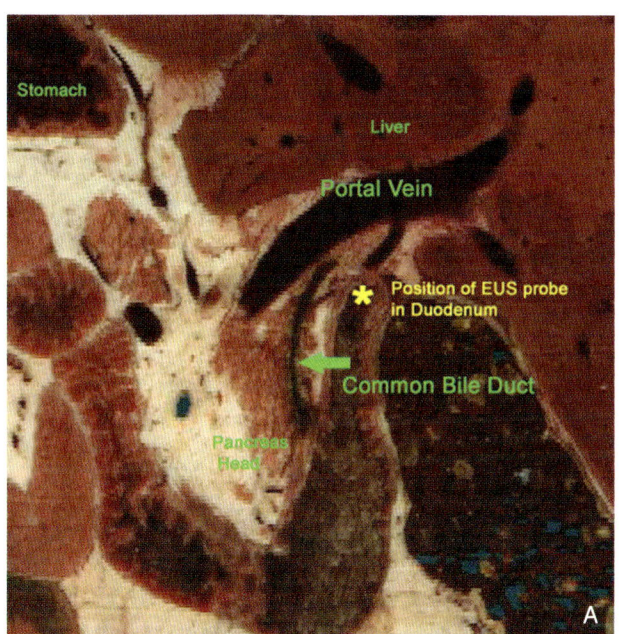

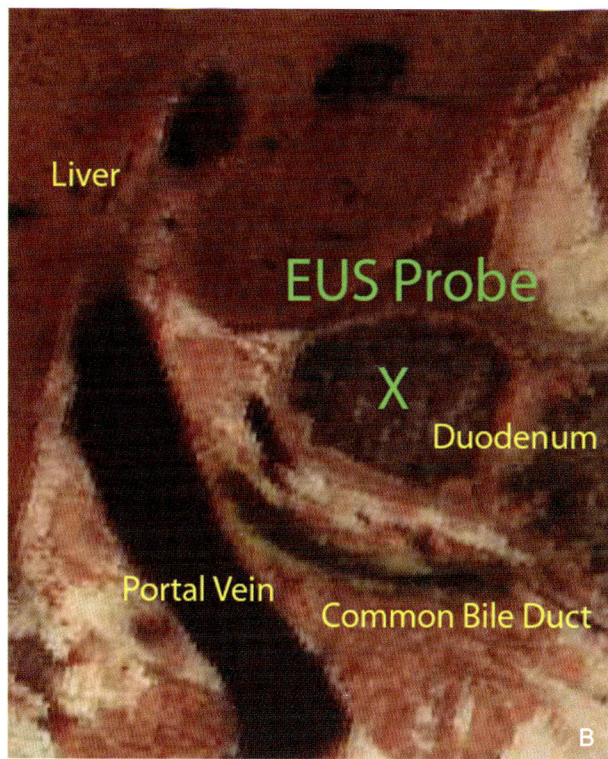

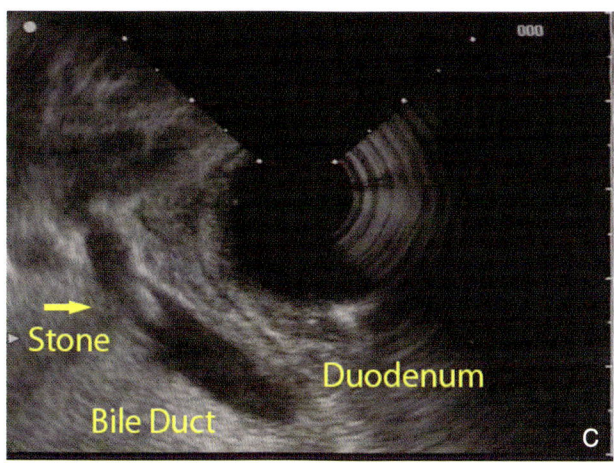

FIGURES 22–3A. *A to C* (A) Visible Human Anatomy showing a cross-section of the bile duct in the posterior-to-anterior orientation, as is often seen during radial array EUS. (B) Magnification of the Visible Human Anatomy showing more typical images, as often seen during Radial Array EUS. (C) Radial Array EUS of the common bile duct showing a CBD stone.

obtained during MRCP (Figure 22–2) or ERCP. During EUS, particularly with radial array devices, the anatomy is seen in the posterior-to-anterior view (Figure 22–3A), which is sometimes slightly rotated in the counterclockwise position (Figures 22–3B, 22–3C).

The Problem of Choledocholithiasis

Approximately 10–15% of the United States (U.S.) population has gallstones.[2] In addition to cystic duct obstruction leading to cholecystitis, stones can often migrate into the common bile duct and cause significant morbidity. Choledocholithiasis is the cause of 35% of attacks of pancreatitis in the US[3] and together with acute cholangitis, they account for the most severe complications of retained common bile duct stones. In such cases, the stone should be removed with an endoscopic retrograde chloangio-pancreatogram (ERCP). It is generally accepted that asymptomatic stones should be removed as well, due to the risk of developing one of the earlier-mentioned complications.

Unfortunately, the diagnosis of choledocholithiasis is not always straightforward. Biochemical analysis can be confounded by multiple other processes, and the accuracy of the most common radiographic modalities (transabdominal ultrasound and CT) is limited. ERCP is generally considered the "gold standard" for diagnosis, and therapeutic interventions can be performed, as noted previously. However, this procedure is invasive and is associated with procedure-related complications. Therefore, it would ideally be reserved for therapeutic indications, and multiple noninvasive imaging modalities, including EUS are now available.

EUS for CBD Stones

As mentioned, the EUS evaluation of the common bile duct is noninvasive with a complication rate comparable to standard upper endoscopy.[4] The EUS probe can be positioned endoscopically in the descending duodenum to allow close proximity scanning of the common bile duct without interference from abdominal fat or gas (Figure 22–3). Once the duct is identified, stones are easily recognizable as hyperechoic, mobile lesions usually with acoustic shadowing within the duct (Figures 22–4 - 22–6). EUS may also reveal other debris within the common bile duct. This includes microlithiasis (echogenic, nonshadowing foci measuring 3 mm or less (Figure 22–7), or sludge (echogenic, nonshadowing material that layers in the dependent portion of the duct). The sensitivity for identifying common bile duct stones and/or debris has been reported in multiple series as ranging from 93% to 100%.[5–9] Because of the high negative predictive value of this test, many unnecessary ERCPs can be avoided. In three series, the strategy of first performing EUS in patients with suspected choledocholithiasis was shown to reduce complications and was cost effective compared with initial ERCP.[5,10,11]

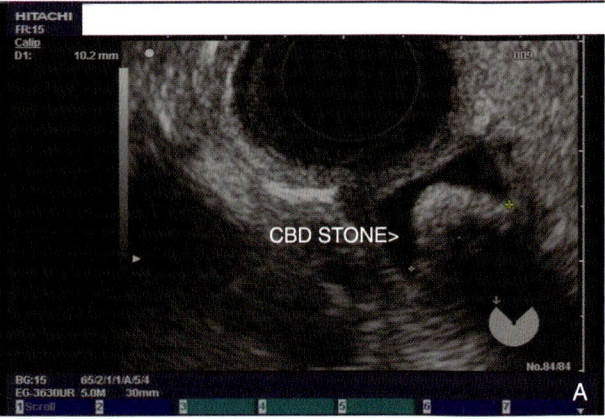

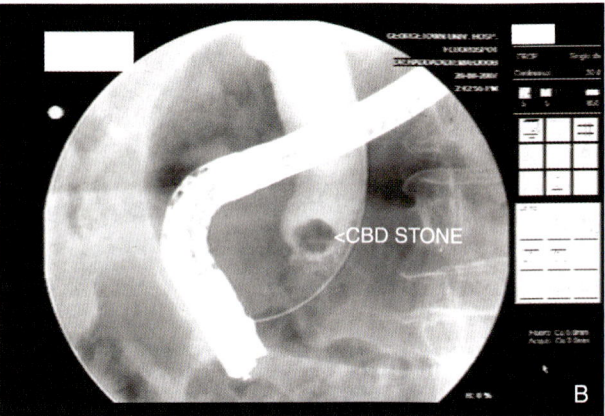

FIGURES 22–5. *A and B* (EUS, ERCP): A large (greater than 1cm) echogenic, shadowing lesion is seen within the common bile duct by EUS (A) and corresponding ERCP image (B).

EUS Compared to Other Imaging

EUS has been compared to the other imaging modalities in several studies. It appears to significantly outperform the TUS and CT. Sugiyama, et al, in a prospective series of 155 patients, found that the sensitivity of EUS for the detection of choledocholithiasis of 96% was significantly superior to TUS (63%) and CT (71%). The difference was most apparent in patients with small stones (3–10 mm) and those with a nondilated or mildly dilated (4–14 mm) common duct.[7] Another study found that CT correctly detected choledocholithiasis in 21 of 24 (sensitivity 88%) patients, where EUS detected all 24. All 3 stones missed by CT were less than 5 mm in size.[9]

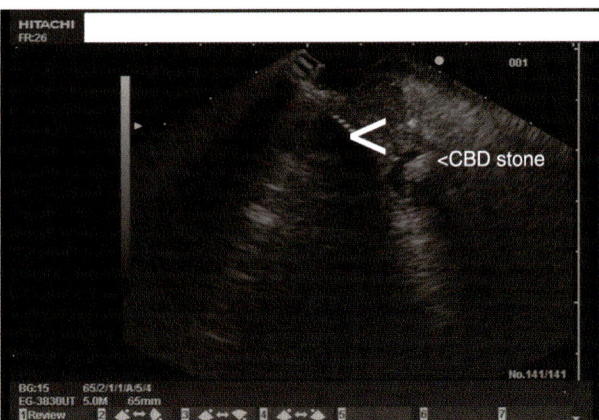

FIGURE 22–4. (EUS): An echogenic, shadowing lesion within the common bile duct. Also seen is linear, echogenic material from a previously placed CBD stent.

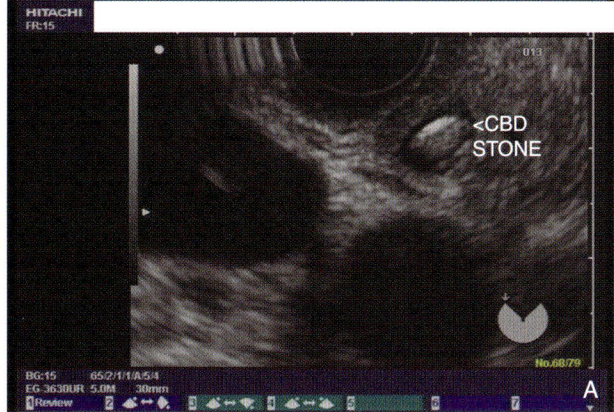
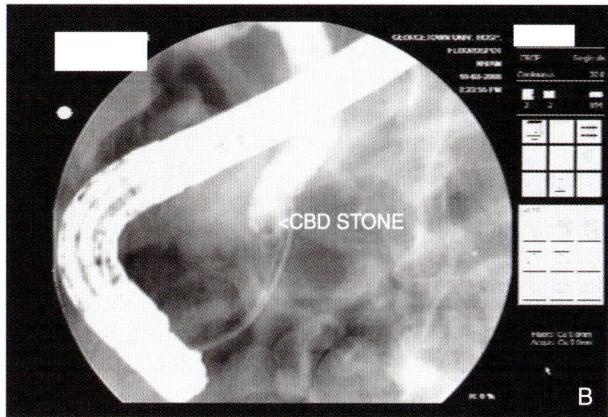
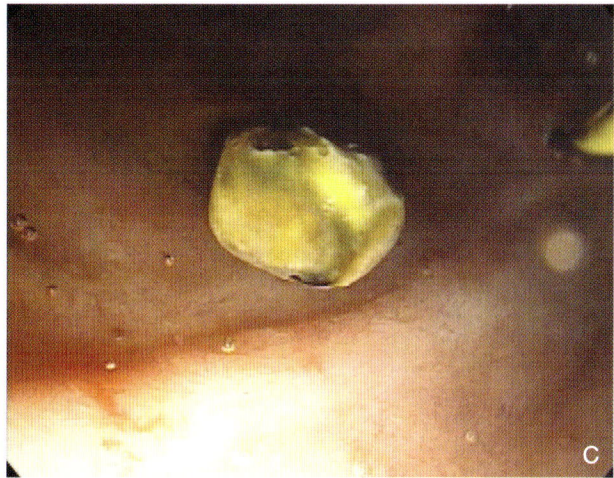

FIGURES 22–6. *A to C* (EUS, ERCP, Endo): An echogenic lesion in the common bile duct is seen on EUS (A) and corresponding ERCP image (B). Endoscopic view of stone after retrieval (C).

MRCP (Figure 22–2) is another rapidly evolving, noninvasive imaging modality, which can accurately evaluate the biliary tree. MRCP and EUS for the evaluation of choledocholithiasis have been compared in several recent publications. Many of these were reviewed by Verma et al in 2006. In their pooled data of five randomized trials, the aggregated sensitivities for the detection of choledocholithiasis by EUS and MRCP were 93% and 85% respectively. Moreover, their specificities were 96% and 93% respectively. However, no statistically significant differences were found between the tests. The authors conclude that both modalities have a high diagnostic performance in the evaluation of suspected choledocholithiasis.

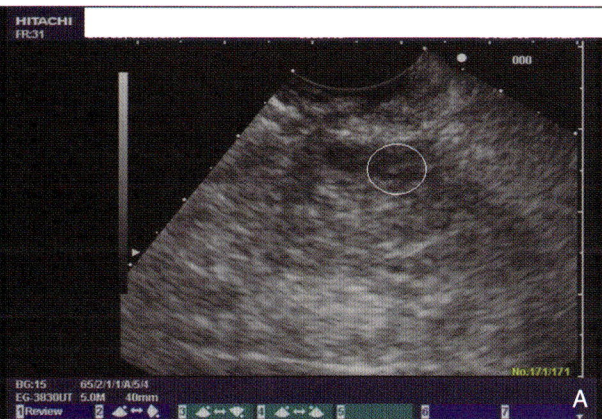
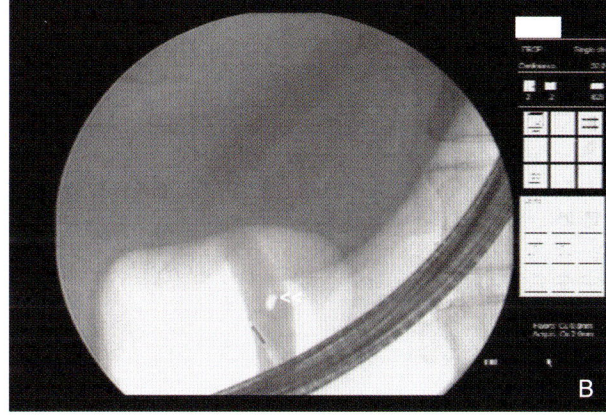

FIGURES 22–7. *A and B* (EUS, ERCP): A less than 3 mm echogenic lesion, consistent with microlithiasis, is seen (circled) on EUS (A) and corresponding ERCP image (B).

Therefore, other factors such as resource availability, experience, and cost considerations should guide the clinician between the two tests.[8]

Intraductal US and ERCP

Finally, intraductal ultrasound (IDUS) performed during ERCP has emerged as a way to differentiate stones or sludge from air bubbles, tumor, or artifact. In a study by Das et al, 62 patients with suspected choledocholithiasis underwent ERCP with IDUS. The overall accuracy of diagnosing common bile duct stones or sludge improved from 87% to 97% with the addition of the IDUS evaluation. Also, IDUS provided additional information in eight patients, including identification of cystic duct stones in five, choledochal varices in one, and characterization of bile duct strictures in two.[12]

Conclusion

Choledocholithiasis is a relatively common condition, which can have significant complications and in many cases can be a diagnostic challenge. Avoiding unnecessary ERCPs should be a goal in patients with low-to-moderate suspicion of CBD stones. Endoscopic ultrasound is generally safe and its accuracy is comparable, if not superior, to MRCP in these situations. Both tests may spare patients from the risks and costs associated with ERCP, and the decision of which to obtain should depend on local availability and expertise, predicted costs, and the patient's risk of undergoing an endoscopic procedure. In addition, intraductal EUS may be a useful adjunct to ERCP in patients with a high suspicion of CBD stones. In these settings, EUS is an excellent choice for the evaluation of choledocholithiasis.

References

1. ASGE Standards of Practice Committee, Gan, S. I., Rajan, E., Adler, D. G., et al.: Role of EUS. Gastrointest Endosc. 2007; 66:425–434.
2. NIH Consensus conference. Gallstones and laparoscopic cholecystectomy. JAMA 1993; 269:1018–1024.
3. Riela, A., Zinsmeister, A. R., Melton, L. J., et al.: Etiology, incidence, and survival of acute pancreatitis in Olmsted County, Minnesota. Gastroenterology 1991; 100:A296.
4. Yusuf, T. E., Bhutani, M. S.: Role of endoscopic ultrasonography in diseases of the extrahepatic biliary system. J Gastroenterol Hepatol. 2004; 19:243–250.
5. Buscarini, E., Tansini, P., Vallisa, D., et al.: EUS for suspected choledocholithiasis: do benefits outweigh costs? A prospective, controlled study. Gastrointest Endosc. 2003; 57:510–518.
6. Kohut, M., Nowakowska-Dulawa, E., Marek, T., et al.: Accuracy of linear endoscopic ultrasonography in the evaluation of patients with suspected common bile duct stones. Endoscopy. 2002; 34:299–303.
7. Sugiyama, M., Atomi, Y.: Endoscopic ultrasonography for diagnosing choledocholithiasis: a prospective comparative study with ultrasonography and computed tomography. Gastrointest Endosc. 1997; 45:143–146.
8. Verma, D., Kapadia, A., Eisen, G. M., et al.: EUS vs MRCP for detection of choledocholithiasis. Gastrointest Endosc. 2006; 64:248–254.
9. Kondo, S., Isayama, H., Akahane, M., et al.: Detection of common bile duct stones: comparison between endoscopic ultrasonography, magnetic resonance cholangiography, and helical-computed-tomographic cholangiography. Eur J Radiol. 2005; 54:271–275.
10. Scheiman, J. M., Carlos, R. C., Barnett, J. L., et al.: Can endoscopic ultrasound or magnetic resonance cholangiopancreatography replace ERCP in patients with suspected biliary disease? A prospective trial and cost analysis. Am J Gastroenterol. 2001; 96:2900–2904.
11. Polkowski, M., Regula, J., Tilszer, A., et al.: Endoscopic ultrasound versus endoscopic retrograde cholangiography for patients with intermediate probability of bile duct stones: a randomized trial comparing two management strategies. Endoscopy. 2007; 39:296–303.
12. Das, A., Isenberg, G., Wong, R. C., et al.: Wire-guided intraductal US: an adjunct to ERCP in the management of bile duct stones. Gastrointest Endosc 2001; 54:31–36.

CHAPTER 23

Malignant Bile Duct Lesions: Cholangiocarcinoma

Dr. Mohamad A. Eloubeidi
Dr. C. Mel Wilcox
Dr. Shyam Varadarajulu

Introduction

Cholangiocarcinoma remains a very difficult neoplasm to diagnose nonoperatively. Advances in imaging with computer tomography (CT), magnetic resonance cholangiopancreatography (MRCP), endoscopic ultrasound (EUS), endoscopic ultrasound fine needle aspiration (EUS-FNA) and intraductal ultrasound (IDUS) made it possible to further characterize common bile duct (CBD) strictures more accurately. The purpose of this review is to examine the role of EUS, EUS-FNA, and IDUS in imaging, staging, and diagnosing cholangiocarcinoma.

EUS Equipment and Techniques

Recent advances in endoscopic ultrasound (EUS) allowed expansion of its role to include staging and tissue diagnosis of complex extrahepatic strictures and hilar cholangiocarcinoma. The basic anatomy of the region is shown in the Visible Human Models in Figure 23–1. Equipment available includes the radial echoendoscope, the electronic radial array (ERA), the curvilinear array (CLA), echoendoscope, and the intraductal probes. In the authors' practice, and upon careful review of outside records, we prefer to use the radial echoendoscope (or the ERA) to provide cross-sectional imaging and to identify small bile duct lesions when cholangiocarcinoma is suspected. These lesions are more readily identified when a stent is in place. Small bile duct lesions can be easily missed with EUS, particularly with the CL A echoendoscope in the absence of a stent. Distal CBD lesions closer to the ampulla are particularly illusive to CL A echoendoscope detection. It is crucial to follow the bile duct all the way to its insertion in the ampulla to ensure adequate imaging. Filling the duodenum with water to enhance acoustic coupling and imaging of the ampulla is very useful in full evaluation of the distal bile duct (Figure 23–2).

EUS and EUS-FNA Technique

EUS is performed initially with the radial echoendoscope in all patients, unless prior cross-sectional imaging identifies an obvious mass along the extrahepatic bile duct or the hilum.[1] The echoendoscope is positioned at the apex of the duodenum. The bile duct and biliary stent (if present) traversing the head of the pancreas are identified. With a subtle counterclockwise maneuver, the path of the stent is followed. Visualization of the bile duct to the proximal region is possible by gradually withdrawing and rotating the instrument counterclockwise into the duodenal bulb and the pyloric region. The bile duct is followed to the perihilar region until the substance of the liver is

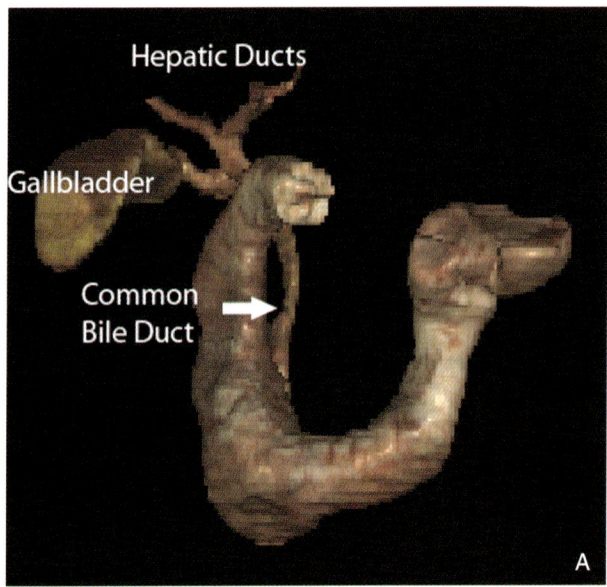
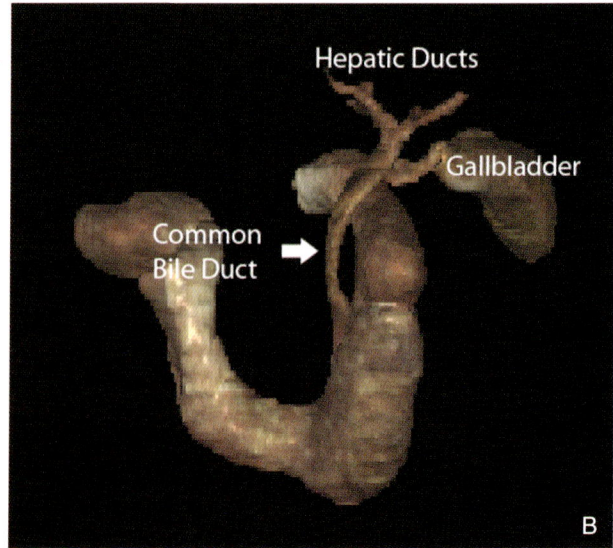

FIGURES 23–1. *A and B* Visible Human Models of the duodenum and biliary tree. (A) shows an anterior view, which is similar to images obtained at ERCP. (B) shows a posterior view, which is similar to images obtained during radial array EUS.

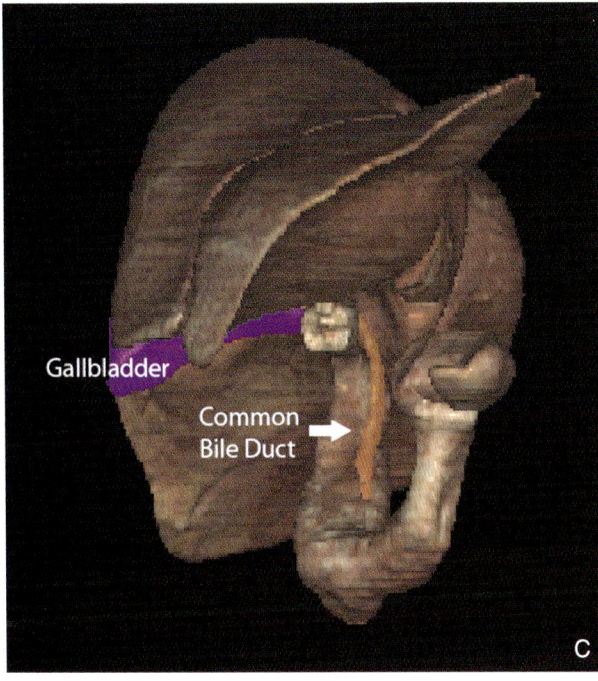
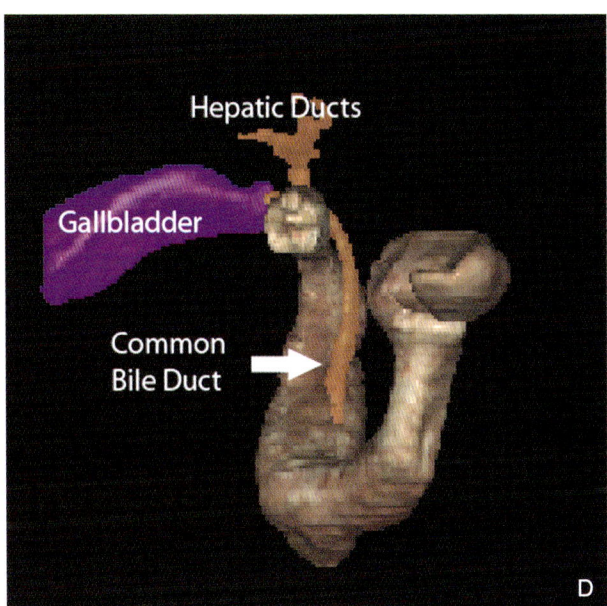

FIGURES 23–1. *C and D* (C) shows left lateral view with the liver. (D) shows left lateral view without the liver.

apparent (until the bile duct is no longer visualized.) Tumor appears as an echo-poor transductal lesion (Figure 23–3). The tumor size is usually documented, and an assessment for vascular invasion of the portal vein and the hepatic artery are performed. In addition, the presence of any lymphadenopathy is documented.[1] Absence of pancreatic duct dilation is a reliable sign of the absence of pancreatic cancer in patients presenting with obstructive jaundice.

Intraductal Ultrasound

If we have EUS or ERCP findings suspicious for cholangiocarcinoma, and for indeterminate strictures, we resort to intraductal ultrasound for further characterization of the stricture. IDUS is easily performed in the ERCP suite because its apparatus is easily movable from one room to another in the EUS suite. The IDUS probe used for local staging of biliary

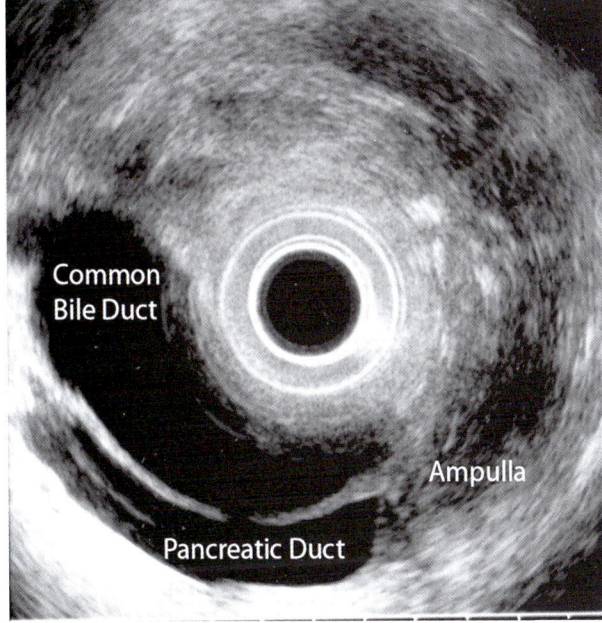

FIGURE 23–2. Complete evaluation of the ampulla with visualization of the distal common bile duct (CBD) and pancreatic duct (PD) to rule out mass lesion (Olympus GG-UM-160 imaging at 7.5 Mhz).

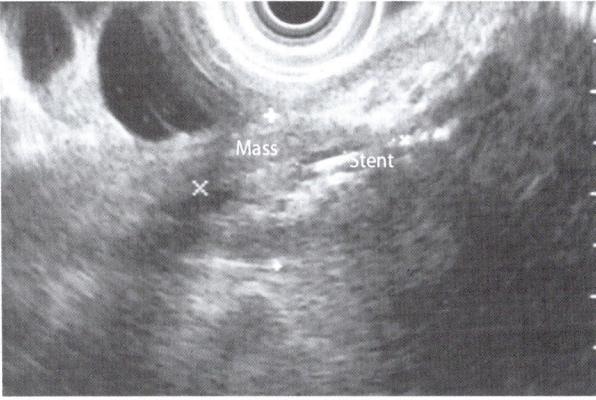

FIGURE 23–3. Radial EUS reveals a 22 × 15 mm echo-poor mass traversed by a stent (Olympus GF-UM-130).

strictures can be inserted into the bile duct at ERCP over a guide wire. Although initial studies suggested a need for biliary sphincterotomy, a new small-diameter IDUS probe has been developed that obviates the need for sphincterotomy.[2,3] Its small diameter and monorail design allows insertion over a 0.035-inch guidewire and greatly simplifies IDUS. The IDUS image of the normal bile duct wall comprises two or three sonographic layers: An outer hyperechoic layer represents the adipose layer of the subserosa, the serosa, and the interface echo between serosa and surrounding organs. Occasionally a third inner hyperechoic layer will be identified and represents an interface echo.

IDUS criteria that suggest malignancy include a hypoechoic mass, especially if it is infiltrating surrounding tissues, heterogeneity of the internal echo pattern, notching or irregularity of the outer border, a papillary surface, and disruption of the normal sonographic structure of the duct.[2,3]

EUS-FNA Technique

Once a tumor is identified, the radial echoendoscope is removed and the curvilinear echoendoscope is inserted (we use Olympus UC 30P or the UCT 140). EUS-guided fine needle aspiration biopsy is carried out using a 22-gauge needle (we use Wilson-Cook, Winston-Salem, North Carolina, or the Olympus Ezshot needle). Color flow and Doppler imaging is performed to identify vascular structures, which would exclude safe passage of the needle.[1] Slides are usually prepared for rapid onsite interpretation as we previously described.[4] Due to smaller sizes, desmoplastic reaction, and location, cholangiocarcinoma FNAs are more difficult to perform compared to pancreatic lesions or other peri-intestinal targets (Figures 23–4 - 23–7).

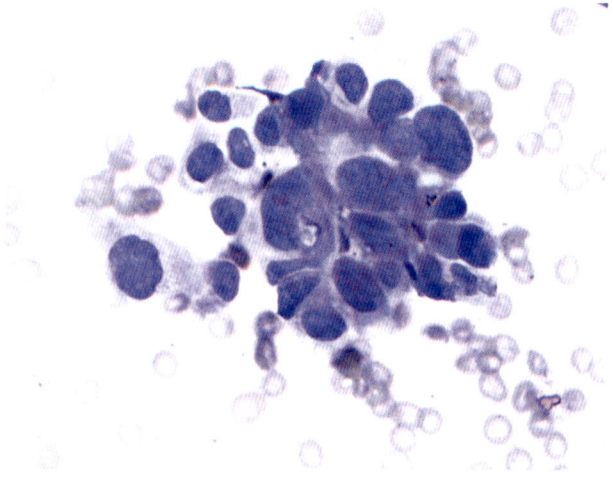

FIGURE 23–5. Photomicrograph of Diff-Quik-stained, air-dried smear reveals characteristic features of carcinoma, including loosely cohesive cell groups with nucleomegaly, marked variation in nuclear size, and dyscohesive single cells (Diff-Quik X400).

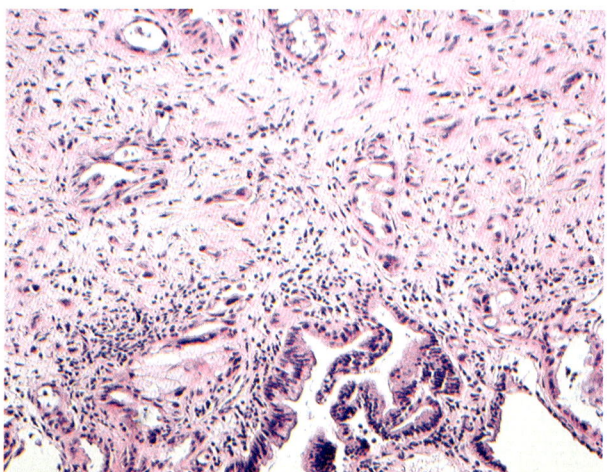

FIGURE 23–6. Photomicrograph of Hematoxylin and Eosin-stained histologic section of the bile duct and surrounding parenchyma shows classical histological changes of cholangiocarcinoma: moderately to poorly differentiated carcinoma with extensive fibrosis. (X200)

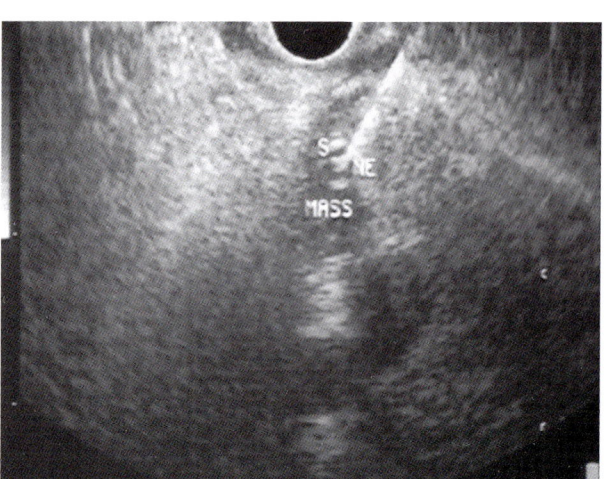

FIGURE 23–4. EUS reveals an echo-poor mass traversed by a stent (S). EUS-FNA with linear EUS (Olympus UC- 30P) was performed next to the stent and revealed malignant-appearing cells compatible with cholangiocarcinoma. NE denotes needle.

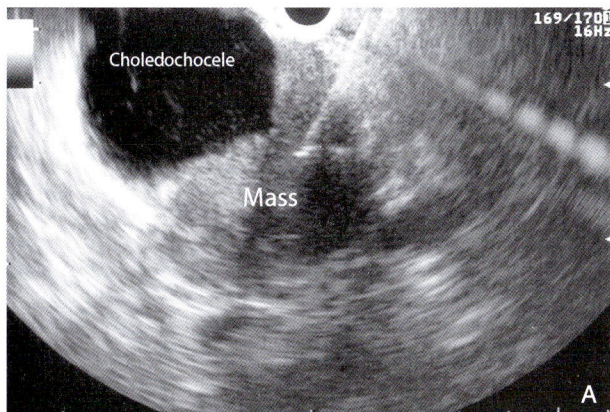
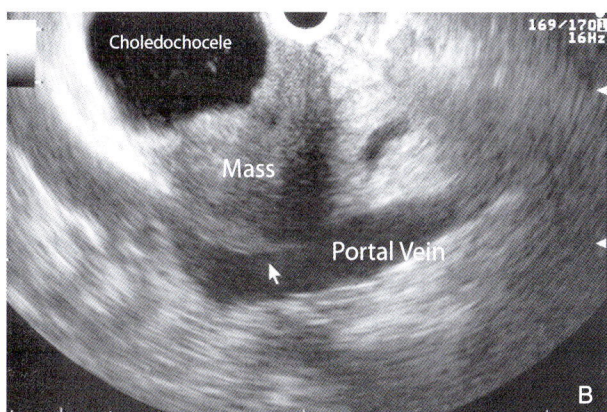

FIGURES 23-7. *A and B* (A) EUS-guided FNA of cholangiocarcinoma arising in Type I choledochocele. EUS-FNA (Olympus UC-30P). (B) Imaging also identified vascular invasion of the portal vein. Please note dilation of CBD (labeled choledochocele) should not be confused with the gallbladder.

 Role of EUS and IDUS

One study[5] examined the role of ERCP, EUS, and MRCP for characterization of CBD strictures in 50 patients. The sensitivity and specificity for diagnosis of malignancy in the 50 patients were as follows: 85% and 75% respectively for ERCP/PTC; 85% and 71% respectively for MRCP; 77% and 63% respectively for CT; and 79% and 62% respectively for EUS, with similar values in the 40 patients who underwent all four imaging methods. The combination of MRCP and EUS improved specificity. The authors concluded that, although MRCP provides the same imaging information as direct cholangiography, it has limited specificity for the diagnosis of malignant strictures.[5] Another study[6] compared the impact of endoscopic retrograde cholangiopancreatography (ERCP), intraductal ultrasonography (IDUS), and magnetic resonance cholangiopancreatography (MRCP) with regard to diagnosing bile duct strictures in 33 patients. ERCP and MRCP allowed correct differentiation of malignant from benign lesions in 76% and 58% of cases (p= 0.057), respectively. By supplementing ERCP with IDUS, the accuracy of correct differentiation of malignant from benign lesions increased significantly to 88%. ERCP supplemented by IDUS gives more reliable and precise information about differentiation of malignant and benign lesions than MRCP alone.[6] (Figures 23-8A and 23-8B) In another study that included 56 consecutive patients with bile

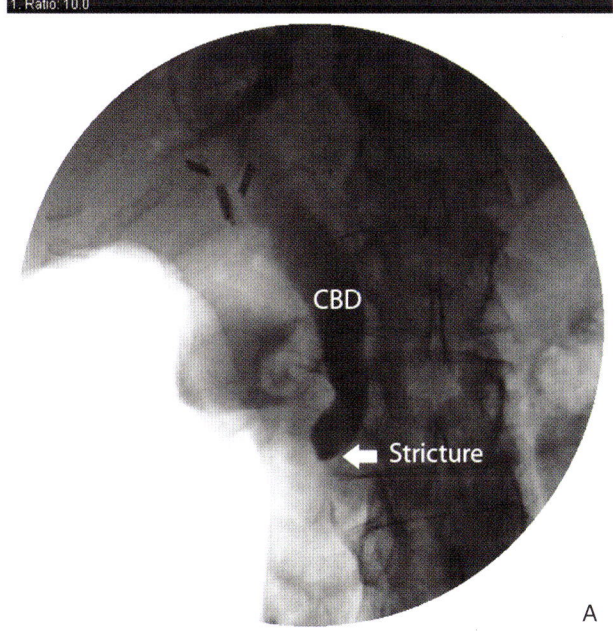
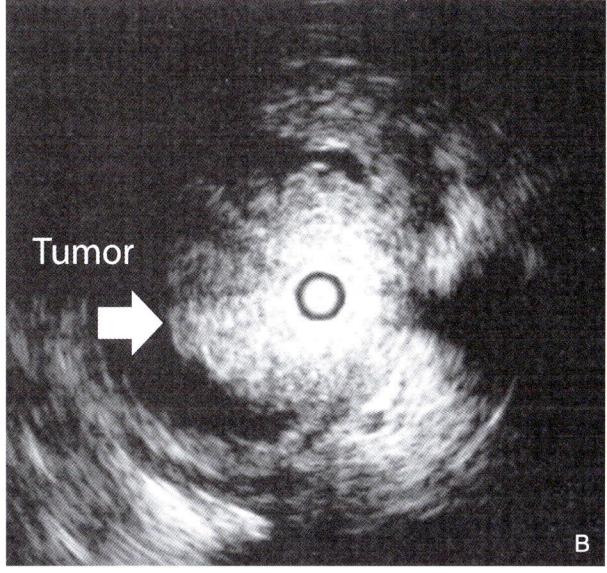

FIGURES 23-8. *A and B* (A) ERCP shows a common bile duct stricture and a cutoff in the distal bile duct. (B) IDUS reveals a distal bile duct mass that on surgery was found to be carcinoma.

duct strictures and obstructive jaundice,[2] IDUS was more accurate than EUS (89% versus 76%, p less than 0.002) for determining the nature of the bile duct strictures. IDUS was also better for determining the resectability of bile duct tumors (82% versus 76%, p less than 0.0002) and T stage (78% versus 54%, p less than 0.001). Although IDUS does not reliably determine the nature of a stricture in all cases, the findings may be useful in directing management. As suggested by another study, when IDUS identifies disruption of the wall layers by a protruding tumor, surgical exploration is indicated, even in the absence of tissue confirmation of malignancy.[3] IDUS improves the accuracy of local tumor staging of bile duct carcinomas. When compared with operative findings, one study found that local tumor staging by IDUS was accurate in 77% of patients compared with 54% for staging by EUS.[2] The benefit of IDUS over EUS may be even greater for tumors arising from mid-duct to bifurcation. The limited depth of penetration restricts the value of IDUS for assessing tumor extension outside the hepatic-duodenal ligament and precludes assessment of distant metastasis (M-stage). The utility of IDUS for lymph node assessment (N-stage) is uncertain and likely limited by the inability to perform fine needle aspiration.

Role of EUS-FNA in Cholangiocarcinoma

While EUS can identify biliary strictures, tissue diagnosis is crucial for differentiation of malignant versus benign lesions. Two prospective studies have evaluated the role of EUS-FNA in biliary strictures.[1,7] In the first study from Germany,[7] of 44 patients with strictures at the liver hilum who underwent EUS-FNA, the accuracy, sensitivity, and specificity for diagnosis of cholangiocarcinoma were 91%, 89%, and 100%, respectively. EUS and EUS-FNA changed preplanned surgical approach in 27 of 44 patients.[7] In the second study from the United States, 28 patients with previously failed tissue diagnosis underwent EUS-FNA of biliary strictures.[1] The sensitivity, specificity, positive predictive value, negative predictive value, and accuracy of EUS-FNA were 86%, 100%, 100%, 57% and 88% respectively. EUS-FNA had a positive impact on patient management in 84% of patients: preventing surgery for tissue diagnosis in patients with inoperable disease (n=10), facilitating surgery in patients with unidentifiable cancer by other modalities (n=8), and avoiding surgery in benign disease (n=4).[1] No major complications were reported in both studies. Both studies were done at tertiary referral centers by expert endosonographers. It remains to be seen whether these results can be replicated and reproduced in other settings. EUS is most optimal for lesions in the mid- or distal bile duct. Hilar lesions, when not visualized by EUS, can usually be seen using the IDUS probes with the caveat that tissue procurement is not possible. Two additional studies reported from tertiary medical centers reported similar success and limitations in sampling cholangiocarcinoma.[8,9]

Two cases are presented (Figures 23–9, 23–10) that illustrate various imaging modalities used in the

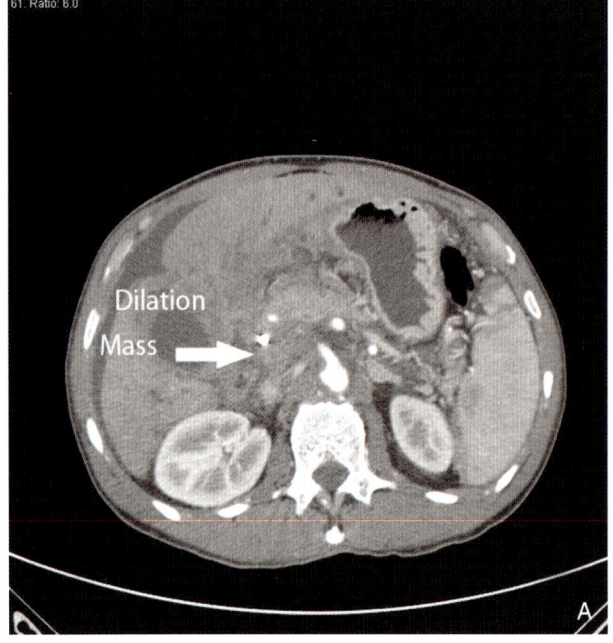
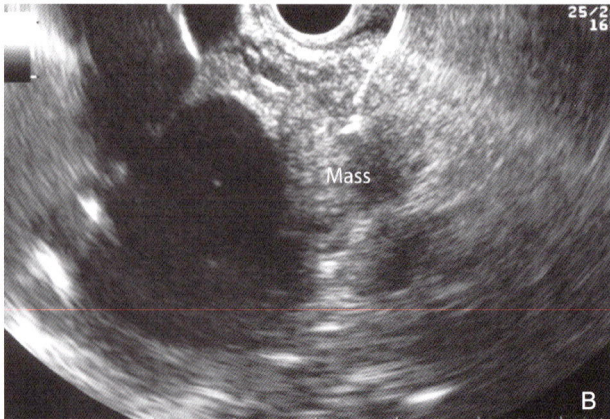

FIGURES 23–9. *A and B* A 65-year-old patient presents with obstructive jaundice, worsening upper abdominal and back pain, intermittent pruritus, and weight loss of more than 10 pounds. (A) CT shows moderate-to-severe intrahepatic biliary ductal dilation. Extensive infiltration of the porta hepatic by a neoplasm with liver metastasis and carcinomatosis. (B) EUS-guided FNA porta hepatic mass was consistent with carcinoma

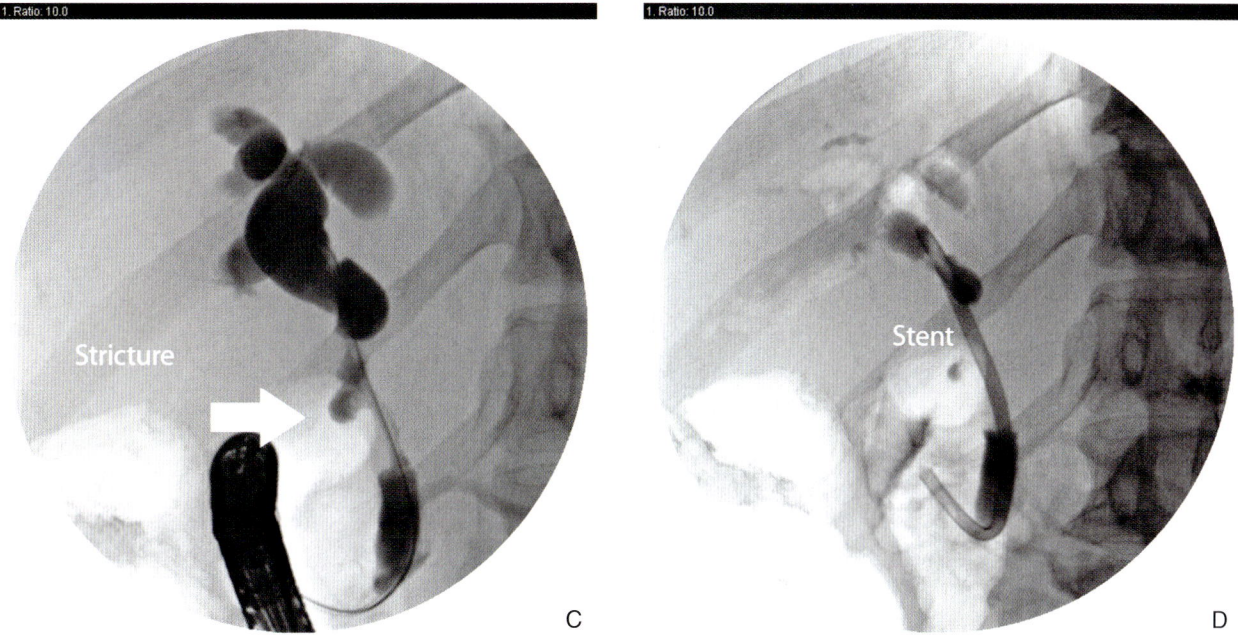

FIGURES 23–9. *C and D* (C) ERCP shows a hilar common bile duct stricture. (D) Palliative stent insertion.

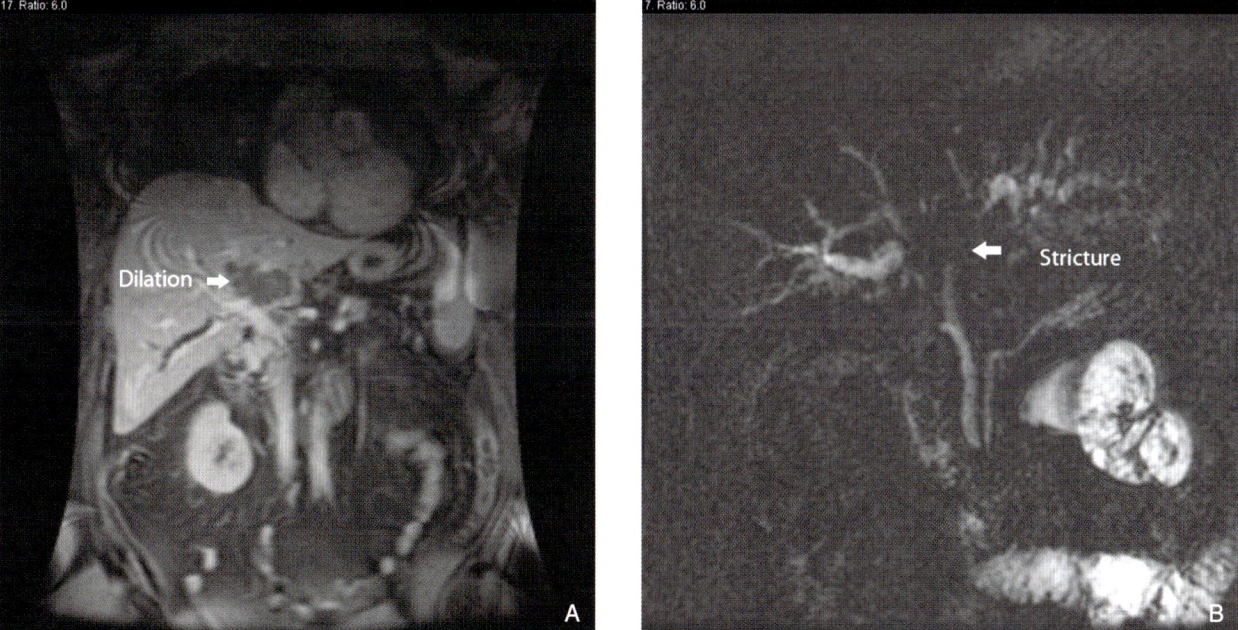

FIGURES 23–10. *A and B* A 57-year-old woman with jaundice. (B) MRI/MRCP shows intrahepatic ductal dilation with a transition point in the hilum consistent with cholangiocarcinoma.

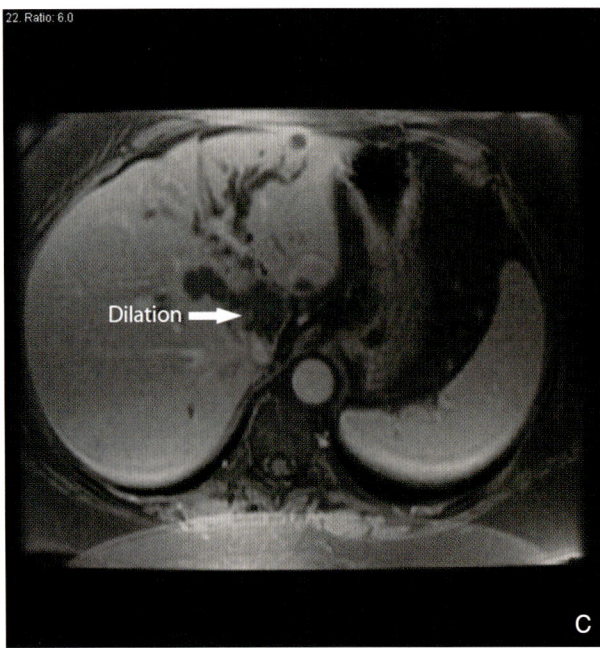 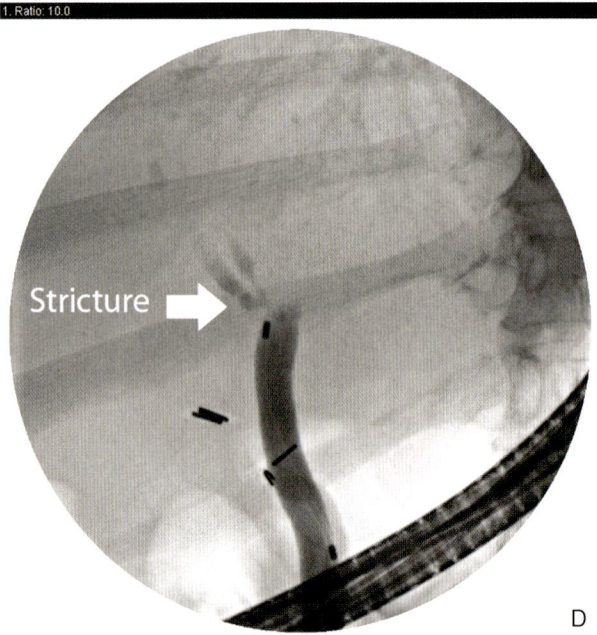

FIGURES 23–10. *C and D* (C) MRI/MRCP shows intrahepatic ductal dilation with a transition point in the hilum consistent with cholangiocarcinoma. (D) ERCP confirmed the presence of a hilar stricture. Tissue diagnosis was obtained with EUS-FNA from a metastatic liver lesion.

evaluation of patients with potentially malignant biliary strictures.

Conclusion

EUS, IDUS, and EUS-FNA play an important role in the management of patients with cholangiocarcinoma. In conjunction with ERCP, the information obtained can guide patient management. While other technologies such as cholangioscopy and spyglass continue to evolve, more comparative studies are needed.

References

1. Eloubeidi, M. A., Chen, V. K., Jhala, N. C., Eltoum, I. E., Jhala, D., Chhieng, D. C., Syed, S. A., Vickers, S. M., Mel, W. C.: Endoscopic ultrasound-guided fine needle aspiration biopsy of suspected cholangiocarcinoma. Clinical Gastroenterology & Hepatology 2004;2:209–213.
2. Menzel, J., Poremba, C., Dietl, K. H., Domschke, W.: Preoperative diagnosis of bile duct strictures—comparison of intraductal ultrasonography with conventional endosonography. Scand J Gastroenterol 2000;35:77–82.
3. Tamada, K., Ueno, N., Tomiyama, T., Oohashi, A., Wada, S., Nishizono, T., Tano, S., Aizawa, T., Ido, K., Kimura, K.: Characterization of biliary strictures using intraductal ultrasonography: comparison with percutaneous cholangioscopic biopsy. Gastrointest Endosc 1998;47:341–349.
4. Eloubeidi, M. A., Tamhane, A., Jhala, N., Chhieng, D., Jhala, D., Crowe, D. R., Eltoum, I. A.: Agreement between rapid onsite and final cytologic interpretations of EUS-guided FNA specimens: implications for the endosonographer and patient management. Am J Gastroenterol 2006;101:2841–2847.
5. Rosch, T., Meining, A., Fruhmorgen, S., Zillinger, C., Schusdziarra, V., Hellerhoff, K., Classen, M., Helmberger, H.: A prospective comparison of the diagnostic accuracy of ERCP, MRCP, CT, and EUS in biliary strictures. Gastrointest Endosc 2002;55:870–876.
6. Domagk, D., Wessling, J., Reimer, P., Hertel, L., Poremba, C., Senninger, N., Heinecke, A., Domschke, W., Menzel, J.: Endoscopic retrograde cholangiopancreatography, intraductal ultrasonography, and magnetic resonance cholangiopancreatography in bile duct strictures: a prospective comparison of imaging diagnostics with histopathological correlation. Am J Gastroenterol 2004; 99:1684–1689.
7. Fritscher-Ravens, A., Broering, D. C., Knoefel, W. T., Rogiers, X., Swain, P., Thonke, F., Bobrowski, C., Topalidis, T., Soehendra, N.: EUS-guided fine-needle aspiration of suspected hilar cholangiocarcinoma in potentially operable patients with negative brush cytology. Am J Gastroenterol 2004;99:45–51.
8. Byrne, M. F., Gerke, H., Mitchell, R. M., Stiffler, H. L., McGrath, K., Branch, M. S., Baillie, J., Jowell, P. S.: Yield of endoscopic ultrasound-guided fine-needle aspiration of bile duct lesions. Endoscopy 2004;36:715–719.
9. Dewitt, J., Misra, V. L., Leblanc, J. K., McHenry, L., Sherman, S.: EUS-guided FNA of proximal biliary strictures after negative ERCP brush cytology results. Gastrointest Endosc 2006;64:325–333.

CHAPTER 24

Benign and Malignant Lesions of the Gallbladder

Dr. Norio Fukami
Dr. Takao Itoi
Dr. Akio Katanuma

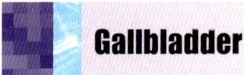
Gallbladder

The gallbladder (GB) is a reservoir for bile that is produced in the liver. Traditionally, the GB has been best imaged by transabdominal ultrasound or other radiologic imaging modalities. With endoscopic ultrasound (EUS), the GB is examined with better detail due to its close proximity to the gut wall and the use of higher frequencies. Small lesions can be seen in detail with EUS. However, EUS is more challenging due to variations in individual anatomy and the need for a skilled operator. In addition, unfamiliarity with the disease process and its representative imaging may hinder correct diagnosis of gallbladder pathology. We will describe the EUS images of gallbladder pathology with corresponding images in this chapter.

Visible Human Models of the gallbladder and its relation to the stomach, duodenum, and liver are shown in Figures 24–1A - 24–1C. The gallbladder can be examined from the gastric antrum, from the duodenal bulb, and from the second part of the duodenum. The cystic duct to neck of the gallbladder is best examined from duodenal bulb. The body and the fundus of the gallbladder can be seen from the gastric antrum, duodenal bulb, and from the descending portion of duodenum. However, there are considerable anatomical variations in the position of the gallbladder in relation to the liver and duodenum. Therefore, it is important to keep in mind the difficulty of thorough examination of the gallbladder. It may, at times, not be possible to confirm a complete examination. Nevertheless, the proximity to the gallbladder and the higher resolution of endoscopic ultrasound images makes EUS the superior modality for examining lesions of the gallbladder.

Abnormalities in the gallbladder are commonly found initially by transabdominal ultrasound or computed tomography (CT). The abnormalities are largely classified into the thickening of the wall and protruded lesions. The main differential diagnoses are listed in Table 24–1.

A normal gallbladder wall is imaged as two to three layers by EUS. It is less than 3 mm in thickness. The first layer is the interface echo (hyperechoic layer) starting from the inner surface of the GB; the second is the hypoechoic layer; the third is the hyperechoic layer. First, the hyperechoic layer may not be clearly seen making a two-layer structure. The first layer represents interface echo and mucosa, the second represents muscular layer and fibrous connective tissue, including the superficial part of subserosa. (In a two-layer structure, the first hypoechoic layer represents mucosa, muscular layer, and fibrous connective tissue). The third (or second for a two-layer structure) layer represents subserosal connective tissue and serosa.

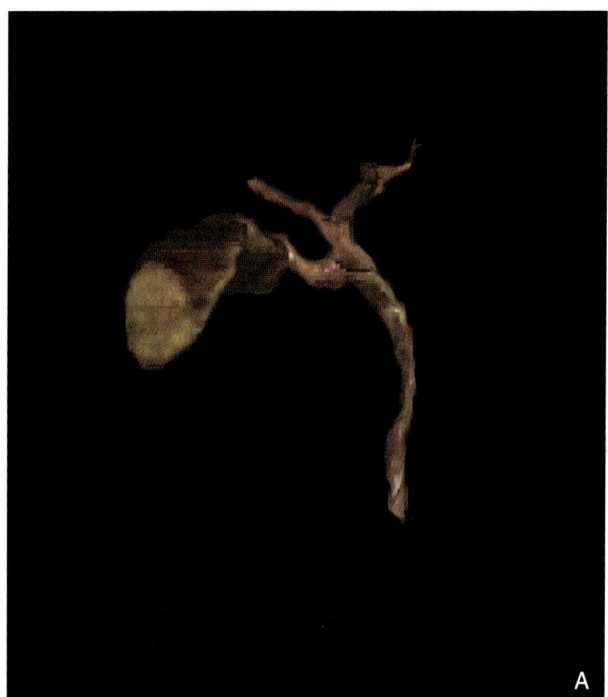
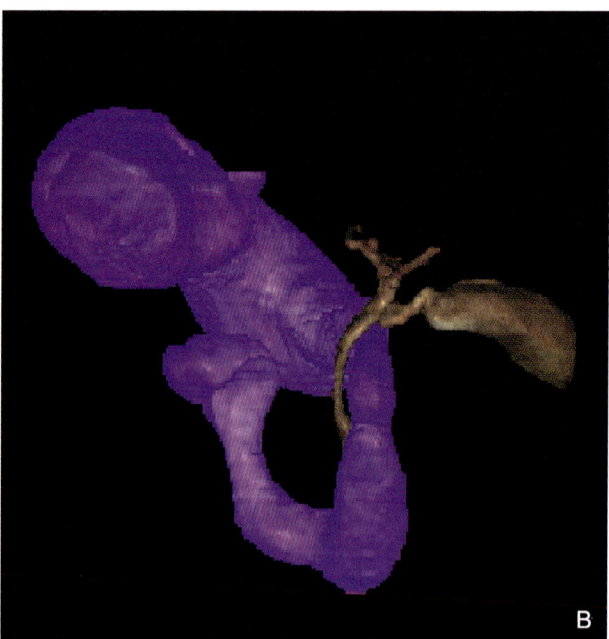

FIGURES 24–1. *A and B* Visible Human Models (A) The gallbladder and bile ducts (B) The biliary tree as it relates to the stomach (purple) and duodenum (purple)

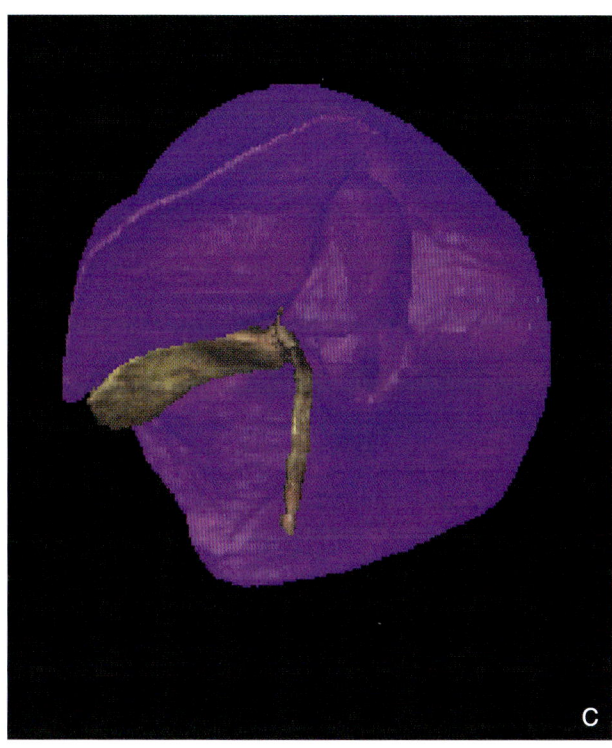

FIGURE 24–1. C (C) The biliary tree as it relates to the liver (purple)

Table 24–1 Differential Diagnosis of Common Gallbladder Abnormalities

Thickening of the Wall vs. Broad-Based Protruded Lesion

Segmental abnormality
  Adenomyomatosis; fundal and segmental type
  Adenocarcinoma
Diffuse abnormality
  Adenomyomatosis, diffuse type
  Cholecystitis; acute, chronic, xanthogranulomatous
  Cholesterolosis
  Mucosal hyperplasia associated with pancreaticobiliary maljunction
  Adenocarcinoma

Protruded lesion: polypoid lesion with stalk or sessile lesion

  Cholesterol polyp
  Hyperplastic/inflammatory polyp
  Adenomyomatosis, localized type
  Adenoma
  Adenocarcinoma
  Rare neoplastic lesions (squamous cell carcinoma, melanoma, carcinoid, sarcoma etc.)

Pathologic Findings

Cholesterolosis/Cholesterol Polyp

Cholesterolosis is an acquired condition resulting in an excessive accumulation of cholesterol esters and triglyceride within epithelial macrophages.[1] Excessive accumulation results in the formation of polypoid configuration, which is a cholesterol polyp. This condition usually does not cause symptoms, and only large cholesterol polyps present the diagnostic challenge to differentiate them from neoplastic polyps. EUS images are characterized by granular appearance, spotty hyperechogenecities (clustered hyperechoic foci) within the lesion, and a separation from the wall of the GB (as it is a polyp with a stalk). A cholesterol polyp can be enhanced by intravenous contrast on CT. (Figures 24–2A - 24–2C, cholesterolosis, Figures 24–3A - 24–3D, cholesterol polyps).

Adenomyomatosis

Adenomyomatosis (ADM) of the gallbladder is a hyperplastic lesion that is characterized by proliferation of the mucosal epithelium and hypertrophy of

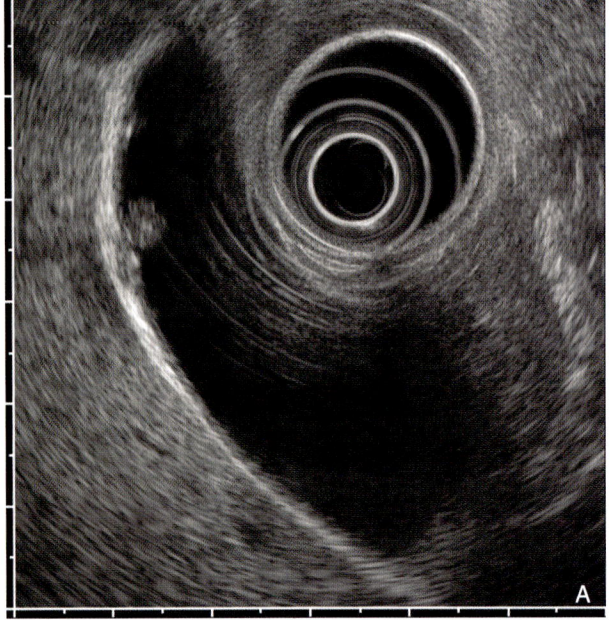
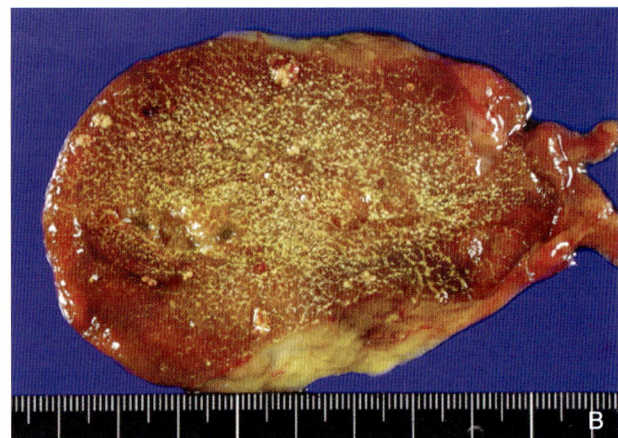
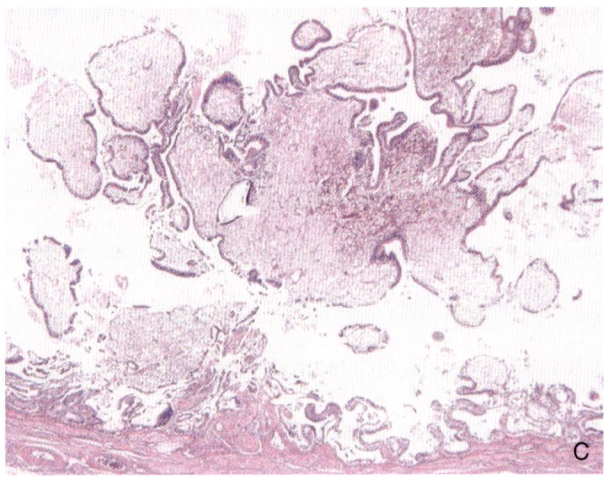

FIGURES 24–2. *A to C* Cholesterolosis (A) EUS image: One small GB polyp is imaged as a cluster of hyperechoic foci. An area of several echogenic foci are seen within the first layer of GB (cholesterolosis) (B) Gross appearance of resected GB: Multiple yellow linear streaks are seen; *strawberry gallbladder* (C) Photomicrograph (H&E): Cholesterolosis and cholesterol polyp: Elongated villi with abundant macrophages are seen adjacent to the cholesterol polyp

the muscularis layer with invagination of the mucosa through the hypertrophied muscularis forming intramural diverticula (Rokitansky-Aschoff sinuses; RAS).[1] Ultrasonographically, this is seen as a thickening of the wall characterized by the cystic area (the representation of RAS) within. This lesion is considered not to have potential for malignant transformation. Nevertheless, there are reports of coexisting adenocarcinoma within an area of adenomyomatosis, and the adenocarcinoma may contain a cystic area due to dilated neoplastic glands or mucin production.[2-6]

This condition is classified into three types, depending on the distribution of the lesion: diffuse, segmental, or localized types. EUS images are characterized by hypoechoic thickening (hypertrophic muscularis) of the wall with cystic anechoic areas (RAS) within the thickened area. Echogenic foci can be seen within the wall representing intramural stone or concentrated bile. (Figures 24–4A - 24–4C, segmental ADM, Figure 24–5, localized ADM, Figures 24–6A - 24–6E, ADM with adenocarcinoma)

Cholecystitis

Chronic cholecystitis is recognized as a diffuse thickening of the gallbladder wall and is often accompanied by gallstones. It can mimic neoplastic wall thickening and it is sometimes difficult to differentiate an inflammatory change from a neoplastic one. As a rule, inflammatory wall thickening shows preserved echo layers. This is most accurately shown by EUS.[7]

Benign and Malignant Lesions of the Gallbladder 261

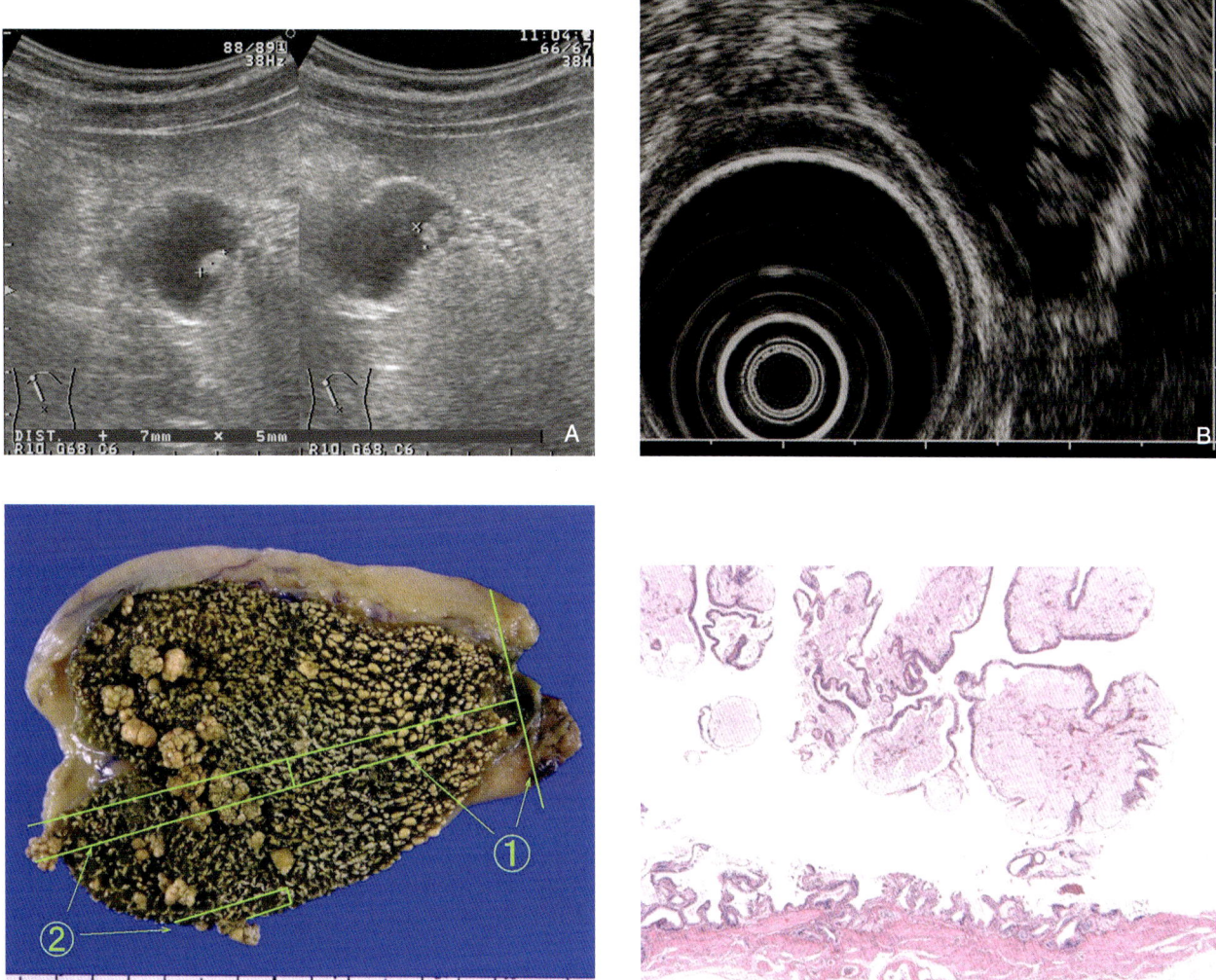

FIGURE 24–3. *A to D* Cholesterol polyps (A) Transabdominal US: Several hypoechoic polyps adherent to the wall are seen, measured as 9 mm. It shows slight hyperechoic foci within rather homogeneous internal hypoechoic pattern. (B) EUS image: The polyps are seen as lobulated echogenic nodules with clusters of hyperechoic foci. They appear separated from the wall of GB. (C) Gross appearance after fixation with formalin: Multiple yellowish lobulated polyps are seen with multiple linear streaks (cholesterolosis). (D) Photomicrograph (H&E); Cholesterol polyp: Enlarged lipid layden macrophage filled villi has formed lobulated polypoid configuration accompanied by hyperplasia of mucosa.

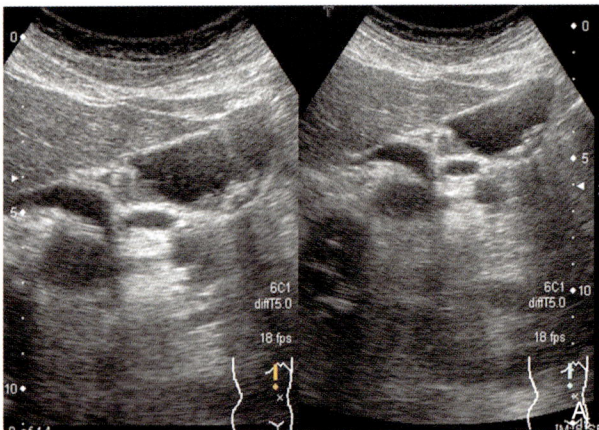

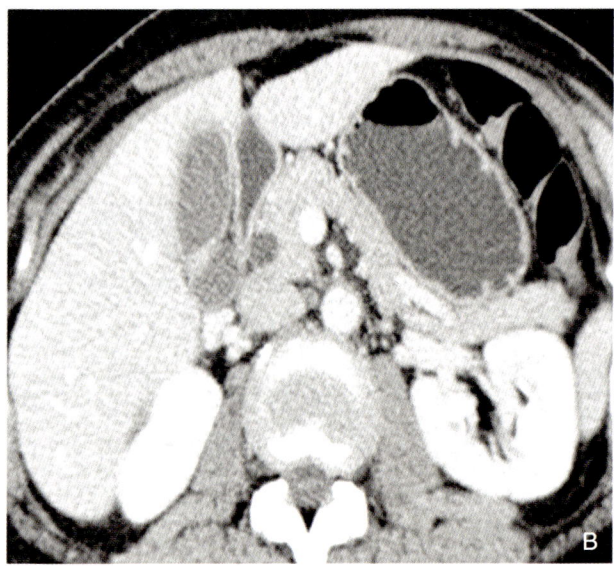

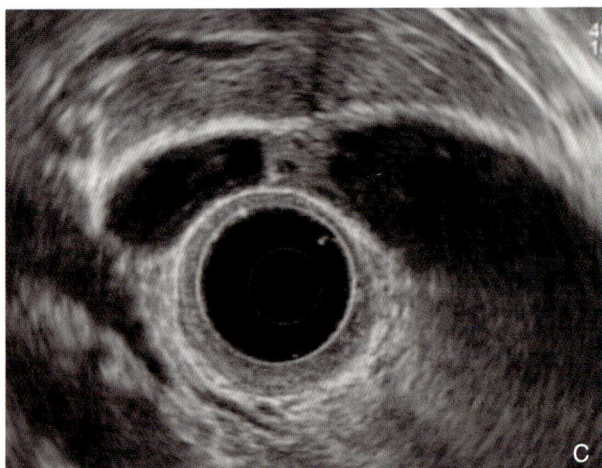

FIGURES 24–4. *A to C* Segmental ADM (A) Transabdominal US: Localized thickened wall is recognized in the body of GB. Small cystic area and comet-tail artifacts are barely seen in these images. Several echogenic stones are seen in the fundus with faint acoustic shadow. (B) CT image with contrast: There is a smooth, thick wall separating the fundus and the neck of GB. Thick wall at this site is homogeneously enhanced as the same level as the adjacent wall. Cystic structure is suspected, but not readily discerned. (C) EUS image: A focus of thickened wall appeared to separate the neck and the fundus of GB. Several anechoic areas (Rokitansky-Aschoff sinuses: RAS) are well seen within the thickened wall. Outer hyperechoic layer is smooth and clear. This is a case of typical segmental ADM.

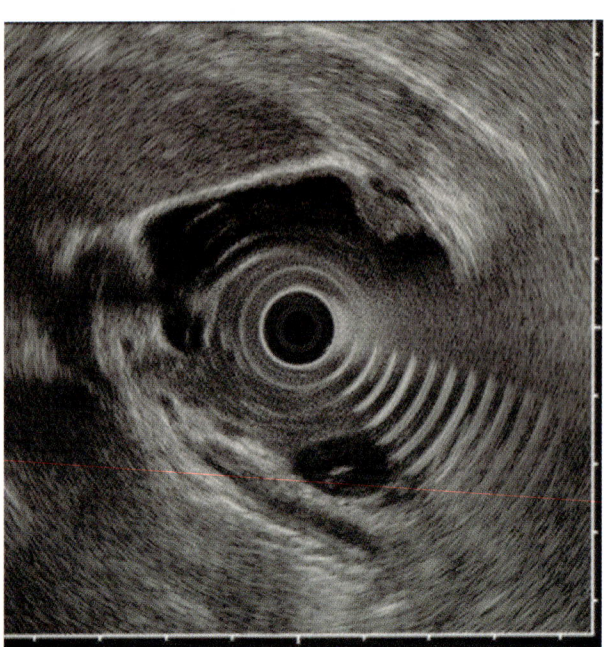

FIGURE 24–5. Localized ADM; EUS image: Focal hypoechoic thickening is seen in the body to the fundus of the GB. The surface is rather smooth. Please note two anechoic foci (Rokitansky-Aschoff sinuses) seen deep to this hypoechoic thickening (hypertrophic muscularis layer) consistent with localized adenomyomatosis.

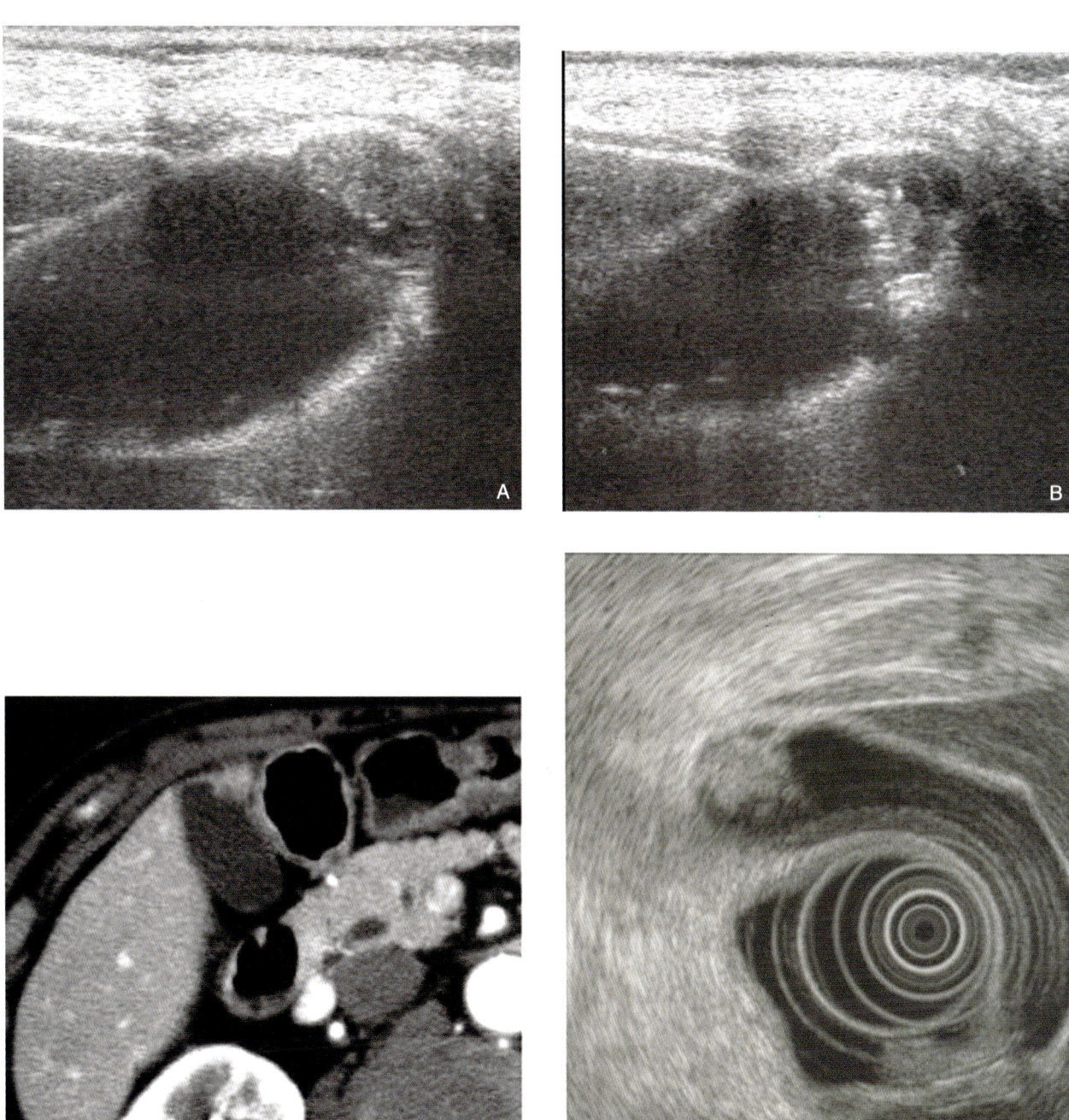

FIGURES 24–6. A to D1 ADM and cancer (a rare case presentation) (A) Transabdominal US: Incidental finding of focal thickening at the fundus of the GB. (B) Transabdominal US: Anechoic foci (RAS) are seen. Surface of this thickening is rather rough and irregular. (C) CT image with contrast: Well-enhanced focal wall thickening is seen in the fundus of the GB. (D1) EUS image 1: Focal thickening of the fundus is seen. This lesion is homogeneously hypoechoic and it appears protruded with irregular surface—somewhat unusual for adenomyomatosis. There are anechoic areas deep to this lesion. Outer hyperechoic layer of the GB is well preserved.

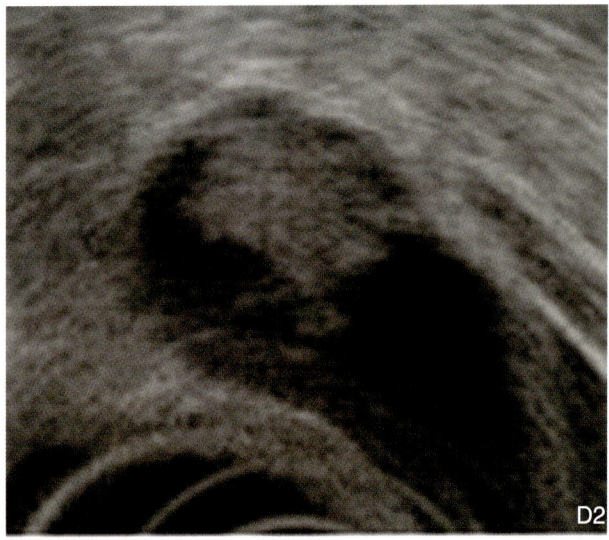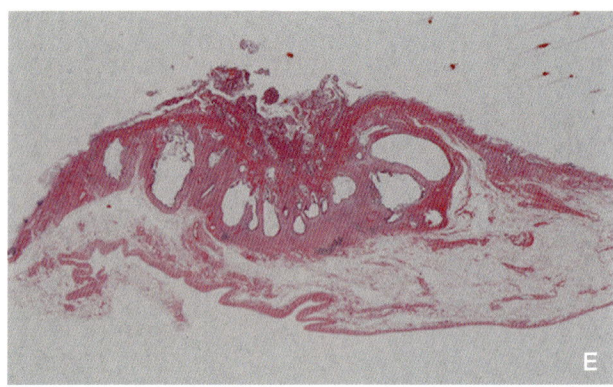

FIGURES 24–6. *D2 and E* (D1) EUS image 2 (magnified): It is seen as a broad-based polypoid lesion with irregular surface. Anechoic foci are still evident above the outer hyperechoic layer. (E) Photomicrograph (H&E): Hypertrophic muscularis layer with invagination of the mucosa (RAS) is confirmed. There is moderately differentiated adenocarcinoma arising from the surface of adenomyomatosis. Adenocarcinoma is seen within the wall of deeply invaginated mucosa (T2 stage).

Xanthogranulomatous cholecystitis is an uncommon lesion characterized by fibroblast proliferation, inflammatory cell infiltration, and foamy cell accumulation that mimics a gallbladder tumor. EUS findings are irregular hypertrophy of the wall with preserved layers containing small anechoic areas and hyperechoic nodules.[8]

(Figures 24–7A - 24–7D, chronic cholecystitis, Figures 24–8A - 24–9E, xanthogranulomatous cholecystitis)

Inflammatory Polyp

An inflammatory polyp is a rare gallbladder polyp that is considered to be reactive to gallstones or chronic inflammation. Large inflammatory polyps show iso-hypoechogenicity with increased vasculature (enhancement during contrast CT or positive flow by Doppler study) similar to adenoma/adenocarcinoma. They are often multiple, small in size, and accompanied by cholelithiasis. Solitary large inflammatory polyps cannot be reliably differentiated from adenoma/adenocarcinoma.[9] (Figures 24–9A - 24–9E, inflammatory polyp)

Adenoma

Adenoma of the gallbladder is most commonly found as a protruded lesion on the wall. The main differential diagnoses are cholesterol polyps and inflammatory polyps. The key finding of an adenomatous polyp is homogenous echogenicity within the lesion without cystic areas (different from benign polyp), but an adenomatous polyp can be heterogeneous as it enlarges. The surface is rather nodular in appearance compared to lobulation seen in cholesterol, inflammatory, and hyperplastic polyps. Adenomas are usually enhanced by intravenous contrast on CT. (Figures 24–10A - 24–10D, adenoma of gallbladder)

Adenocarcinoma

Adenocarcinoma of the gallbladder is often found as wall thickening with relative hypo-echogenicity and granular or nodular surface. Gallbladder adenocarcinoma is enhanced with intravenous contrast on CT and with Doppler study during EUS. It is often found at an advanced stage due to the lack of symptoms. To determine the proper course of therapy, staging of the tumor is important. Early stage of gallbladder cancer is defined as tumor invading lamina propria and muscularis layer (T1 and T2), and is often treated surgically with radical resection.[10] T-stage is evaluated by the examination of layered structures. If the polypoid lesion is attached to the wall that shows normal layers of the gallbladder, this is considered adenoma or carcinoma in situ. In the presence of a neoplastic process in the gallbladder wall, if a well-preserved hyperechoic outer layer is seen, the tumor is judged to be either T1 or T2. Attenuation of the third hyperechoic layer signifies invasion of the tumor beyond

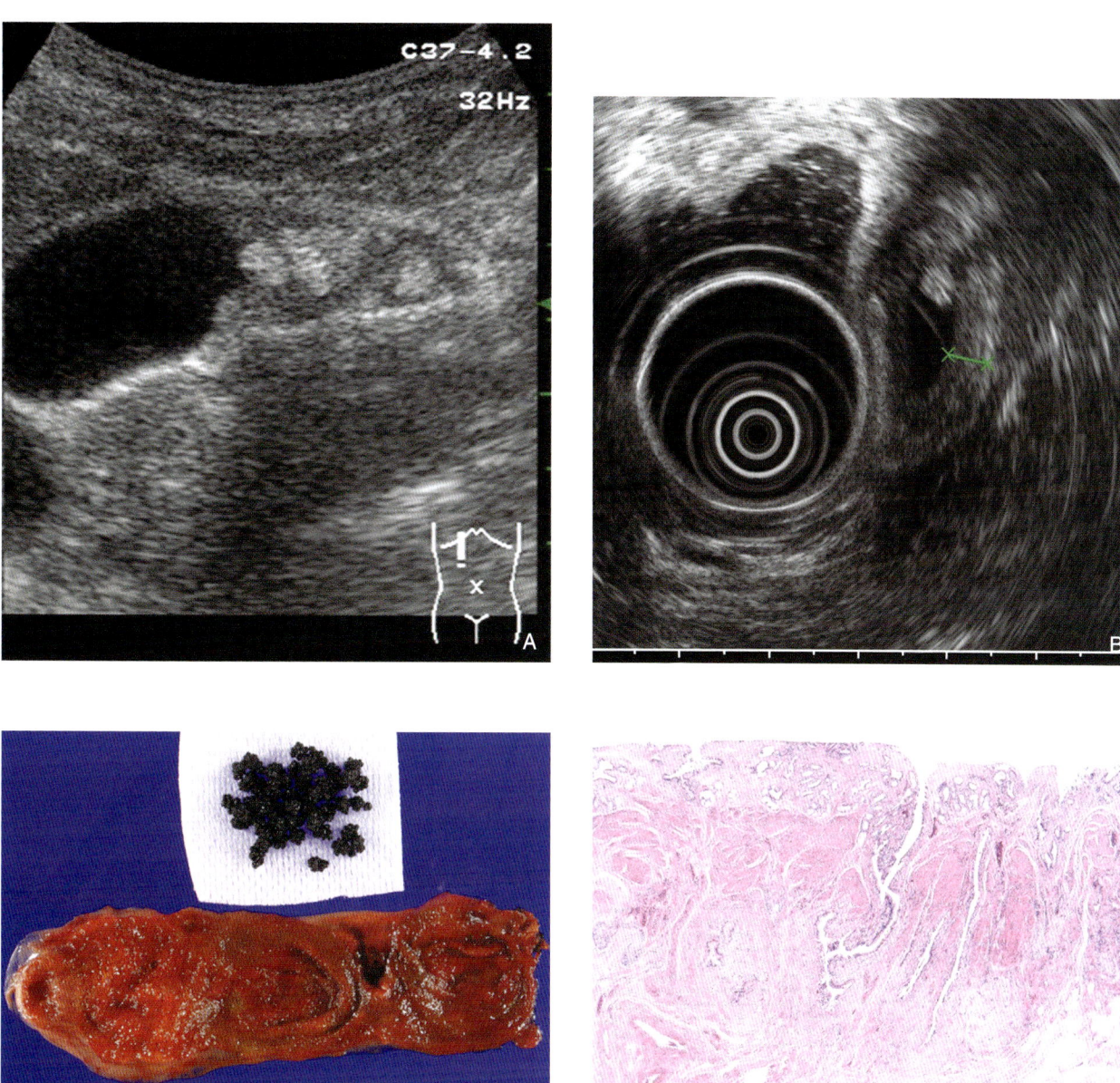

FIGURES 24–7. A to D Chronic cholecystitis (A) Transabdominal US: Thickened wall of the body to the fundus of gallbladder is seen with smooth and intact outer layer. There are many echogenic foci within the lumen representing gallstones. (B) EUS image: Thickened wall is seen as multi-layered wall measured as 4.7 mm. Echogenic focus accompanied by acoutic shadow is seen within the lumen. No anechoic area is seen within the thickened wall. (C) Gross appearance of resected GB: Thickened wall of fundus is seen without protruded lesion. Multiple pigment stones are placed aside. (D) Photomicrograph (H&E): Hypertrophic muscular layer is seen with abundant fibrosis and chronic inflammatory cell infiltration. No evidence of dysplastic mucosa.

muscularis layer but not through the serosa (T2). The disruption of the third hyperechoic layer signifies infiltration of the tumor through the serosa (T3 or T4).[11] Degree and extension of invasion outside of the gallbladder wall will determine T3 and T4 stages. N1 stage represents advanced stage with poor prognosis even after the surgery. Thus, careful examination for lymph nodes (LNs) at peri-cystic duct, peri-portal, peri-pancreatic, along the hepatic artery to the celiac artery, and para-aortic areas is extremely important. EUS-guided fine-needle aspiration of those LNs is often helpful. (Figures 24–11A - 24–11D, T1 stage GB cancer, Figures 24–12A Figure 24–12D, T2-3 stage GB cancer).

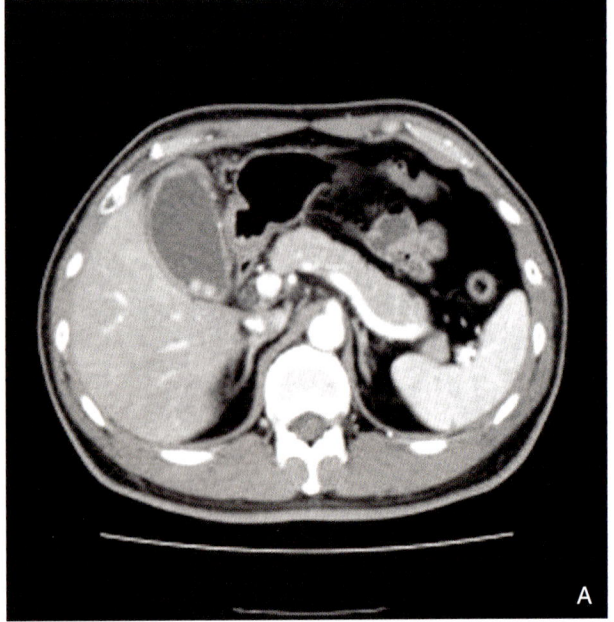
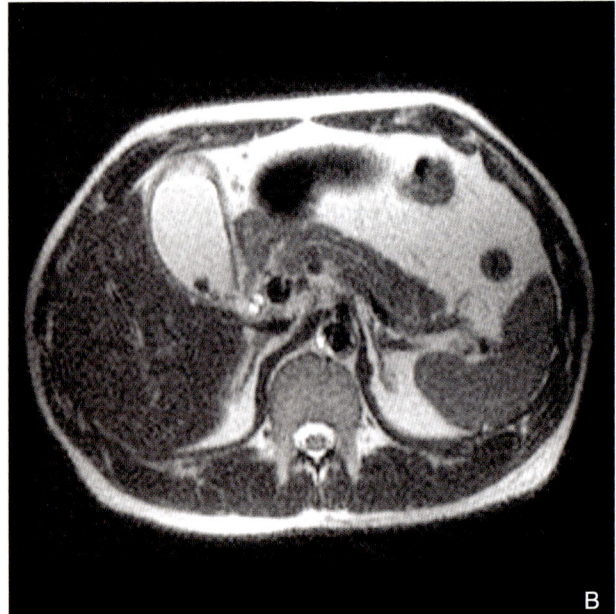
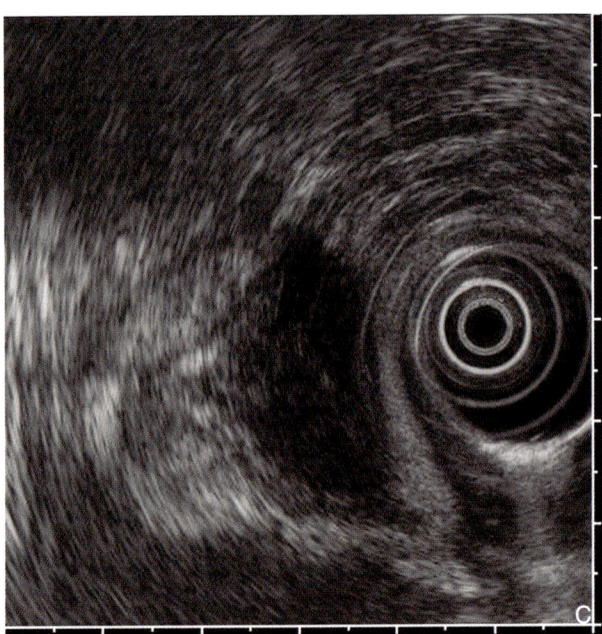
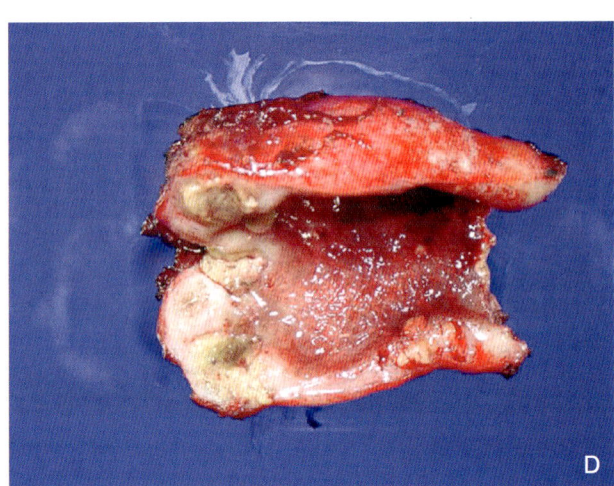
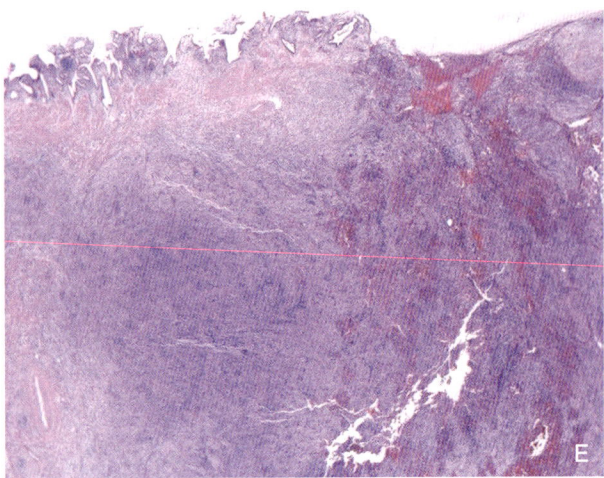

FIGURES 24–8. *A to E* Xanthogranulomatous cholecystitis (A) CT image: Slight thickening of the fundus of the GB with small calcified gallstones are seen. Outer wall is slightly irregular. (B) MRI image: T2-weighted image shows thickened wall of GB with areas of slightly high signal intensity within the wall. (C) EUS image: The wall of the fundus of GB is significantly thickened with nodular hyperechoic area (corresponds to xanthogranuloma). Notably, the wall layer is preserved. (D) Gross appearance of resected GB: Diffuse thickening of the wall is seen, especially at fundus. Yellowish nodules within the thickened wall correspond to xanthogranulomas. Gallstones were present (removed). (E) Photomicrograph (H&E): Marked thickening of wall is seen with infiltrating mixed chronic inflammatory cells (including giant cell and foamy cell), fibrosis and hemorrhage.

Benign and Malignant Lesions of the Gallbladder

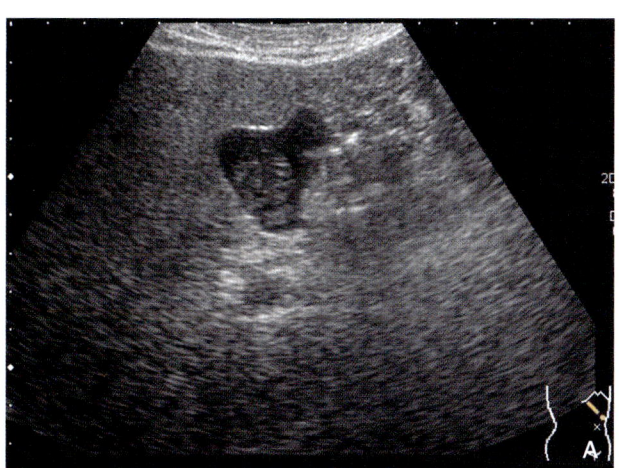
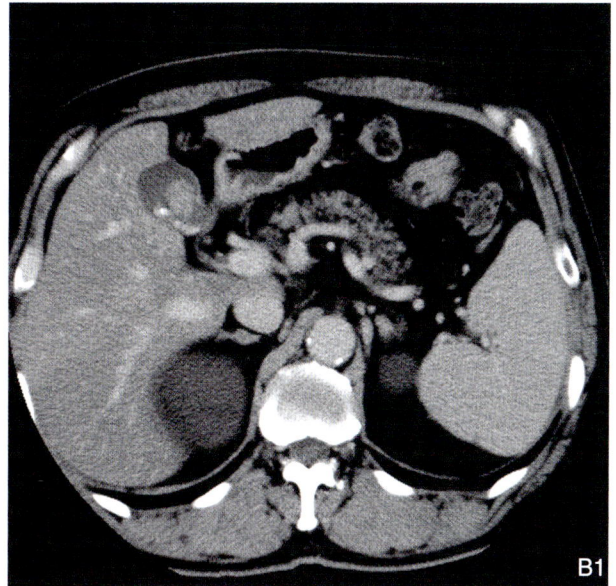
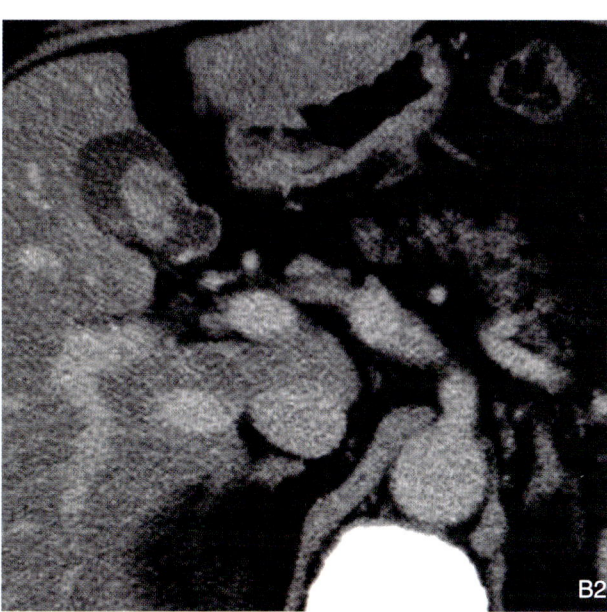
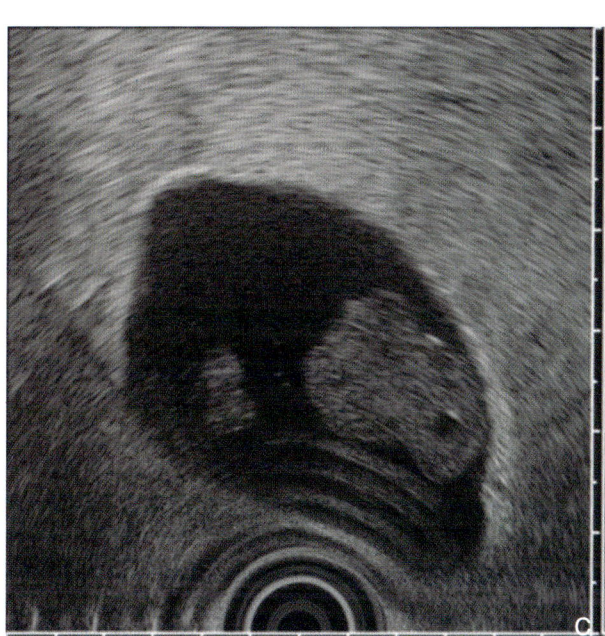
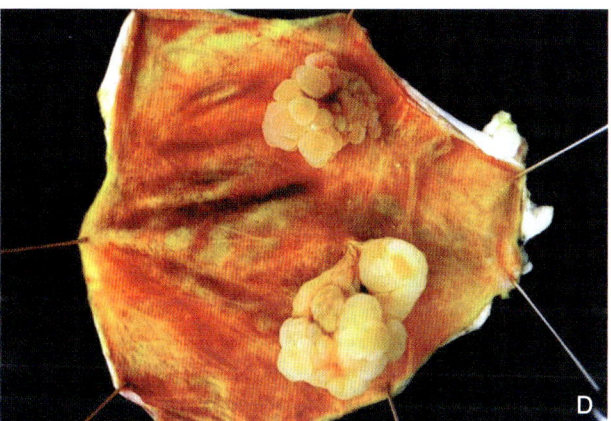

FIGURES 24–9. *A to D* Inflammatory polyp (A) Transabdominal US image: A 20 mm isoechoic polypoid lesion is seen within the gallbladder. Spotty anechoic areas are seen within the lesion. Echogenic gallstones were also seen. (B) CT image (1,2): Protruded lesion showed marked enhancement by intravenous contrast. Outer wall of GB is smooth without thickening. (C) EUS image: Homogeneous isoechoic mass is seen separated from the normal GB wall. Surface is smooth and slightly nodular. It is difficult to differentiate from adenoma but small anechoic areas are seen unusual for adenoma. (D) Gross appearance of resected GB: Smooth lobulated protruded polyps are seen.

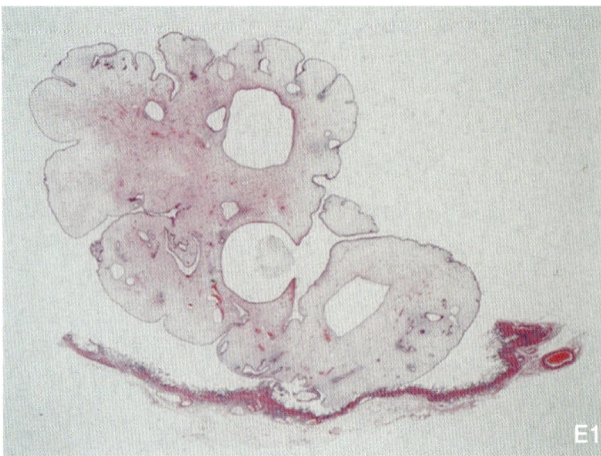

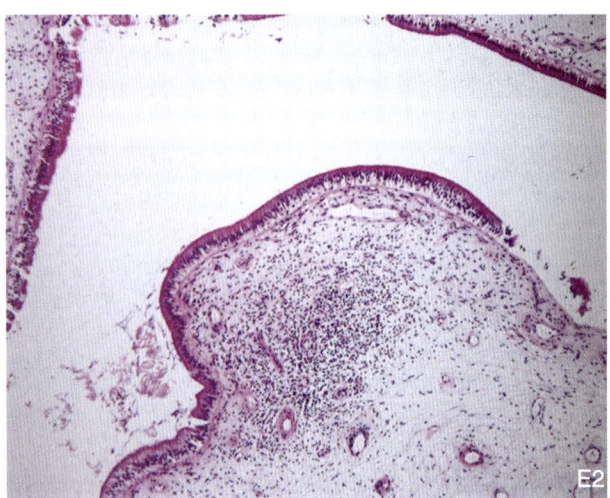

FIGURES 24–9. *E1 and E2* (E) Photomicrograph (H&E, 1,2): The large polyp is a nodular lesion with a short stalk containing cystic areas. The polyp has abundant vascular stroma with chronic inflammatory cell infiltrate, lined with hyperplastic epithelium.

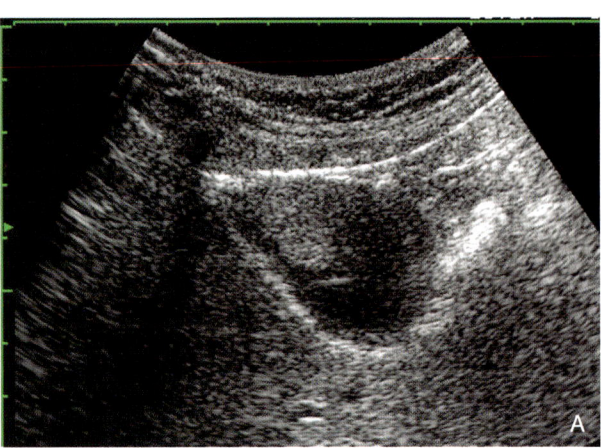

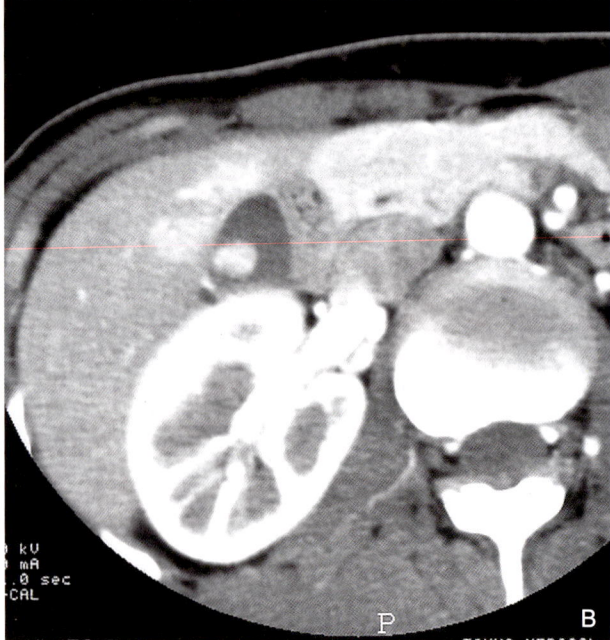

FIGURES 24–10. *A and B* Adenoma of gallbladder (A) Transabdominal US: Pedunculated hypoechoic polypoid lesion is visualized in the GB. (B) CT image: Well-enhanced polypoid lesion is seen within the GB. Gallbladder wall is smooth and intact.

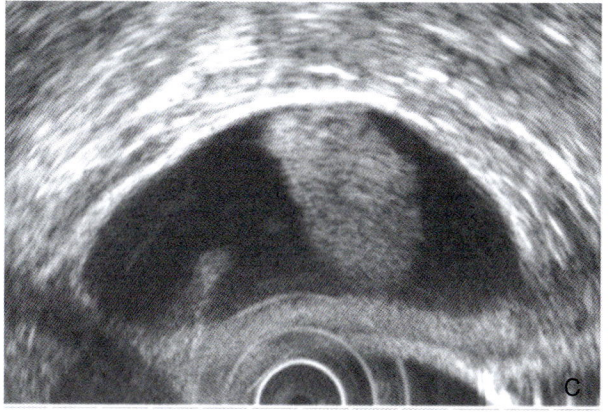
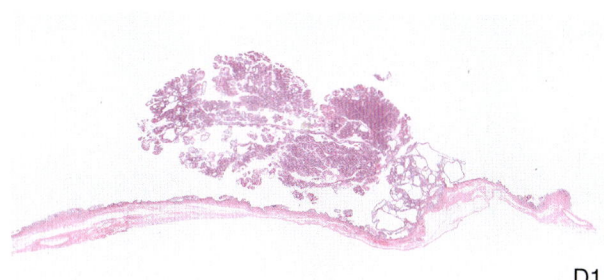
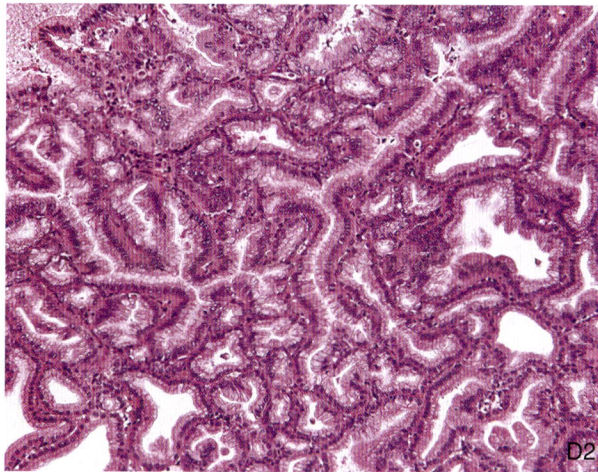

FIGURES 24–10. *C and D* (C) EUS image: Homogenously hypoechoic protruded lesion with smooth surface border is seen. Internal anechoic area is absent. (D) Photomicrograph (H&E, 1,2): Pedunculated lesion is confirmed to be adenoma with moderate atypia.

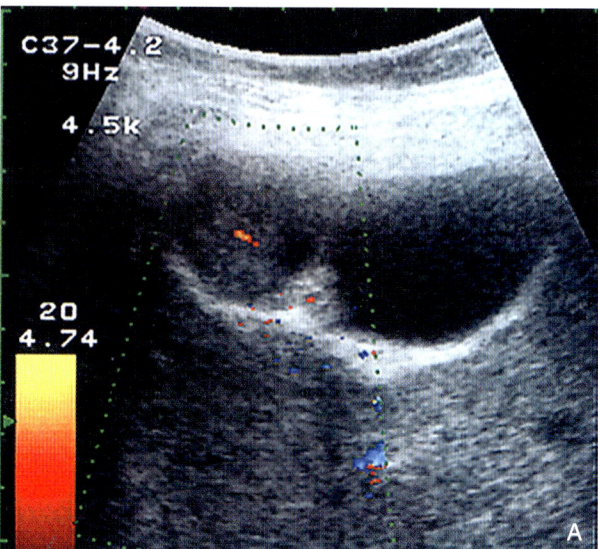
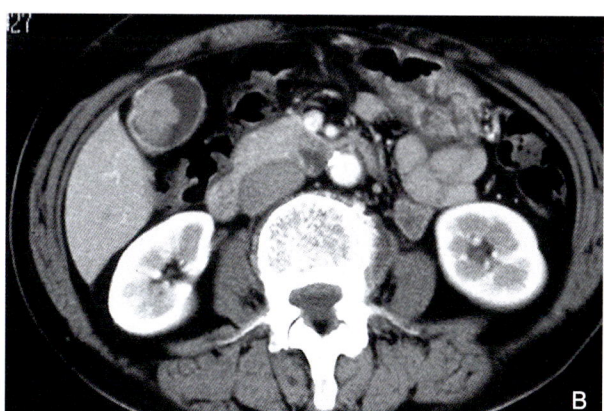

FIGURES 24–11. *A and B* T1-stage gallbladder cancer (A) Transabdominal US: Isoechoic polypoid lesion in the fundus of the GB is seen with internal vascular flow on Doppler study. (B) CT image: Large protruded lesion is demonstrated with moderate homogenous enhancement. Outer border is nodular.

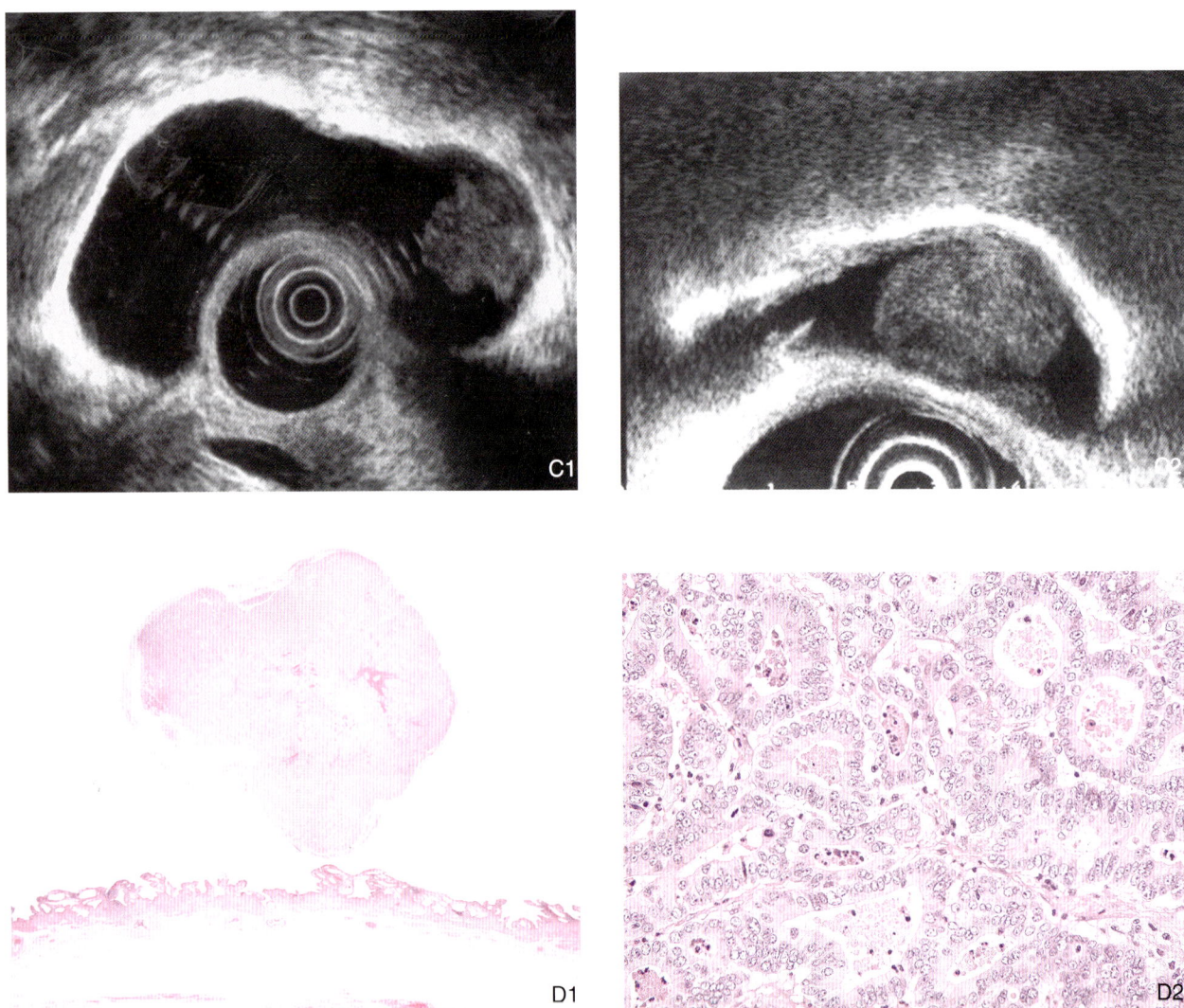

FIGURES 24–11. *C1 to D2* (C) EUS image (1,2): Hypoechoic protruded lesion is imaged in the fundus of the GB. Mixed internal echogenicity (heterogeneity) of the lesion is noted with nodular surface border. Outer layer of GB is well preserved. (D) Photomicrograph (H&E, 1,2): Pedunculated polypoid lesion was diagnosed as well differentiated adenocarcinoma, papillary type. It was invading into but not through muscularis layer (T1b).

Benign and Malignant Lesions of the Gallbladder 271

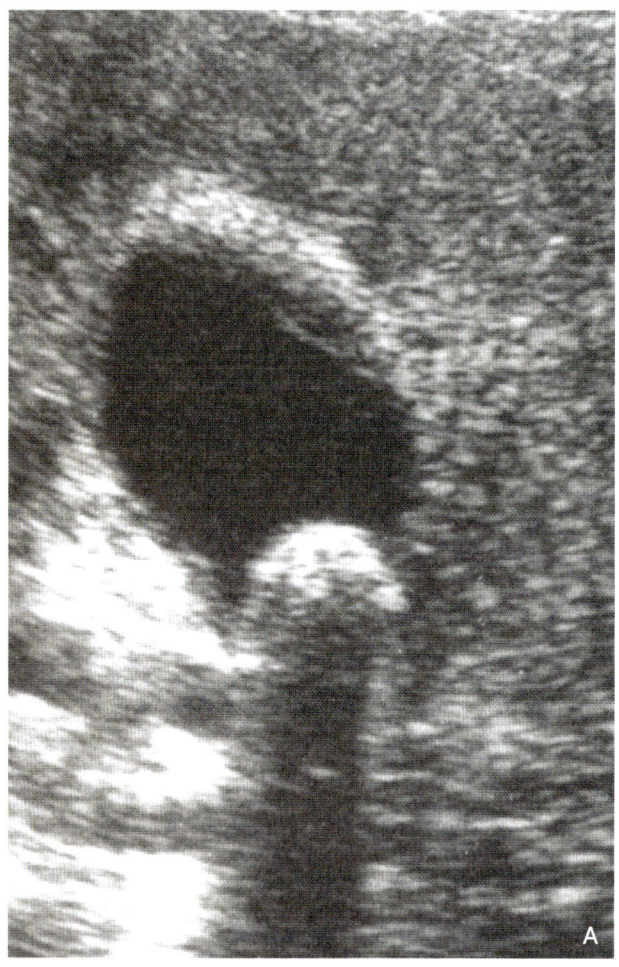

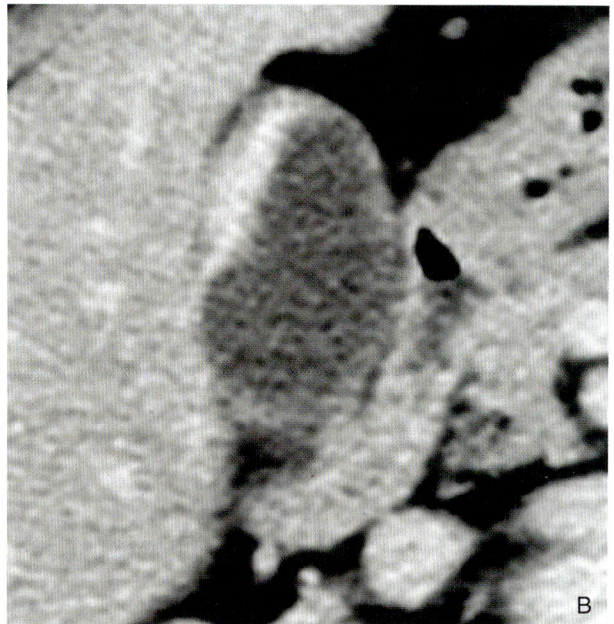

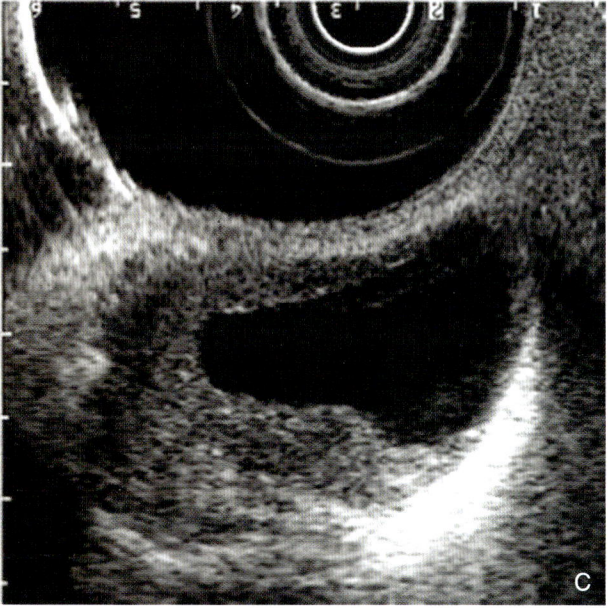

FIGURES 24–12. *A to C* T2-3 stage gallbladder cancer (A) Transabdominal US: Thickened wall is evident in the fundus of the GB. Outer hyperechoic layer is preserved in this sectional image. Echogenic focus with acoustic shadow is seen representing a gallstone. (B) CT image: There is an asymmetric thickening of the GB on hepatic side with marked contrast enhancement. (C) EUS image: Hypoechoic thickening of GB wall is demonstrated with mixed internal echogenesity. Hyperechoic outer layer is significantly attenuated by the hypoechoic process suggesting tumor invasion through muscularis layer.

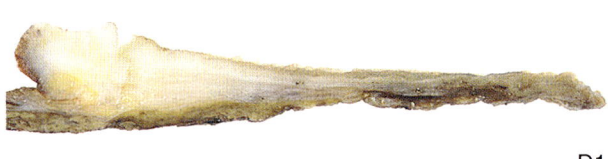

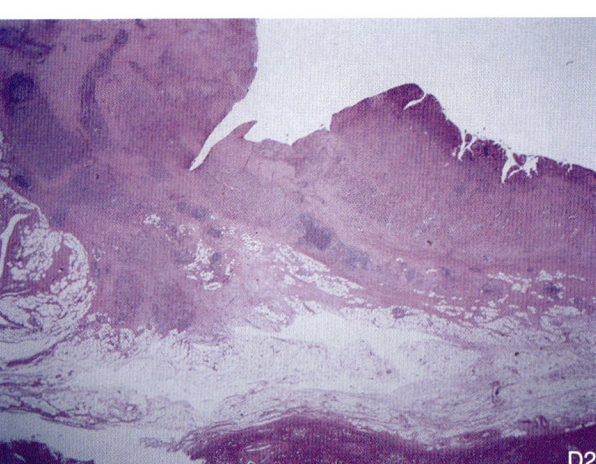

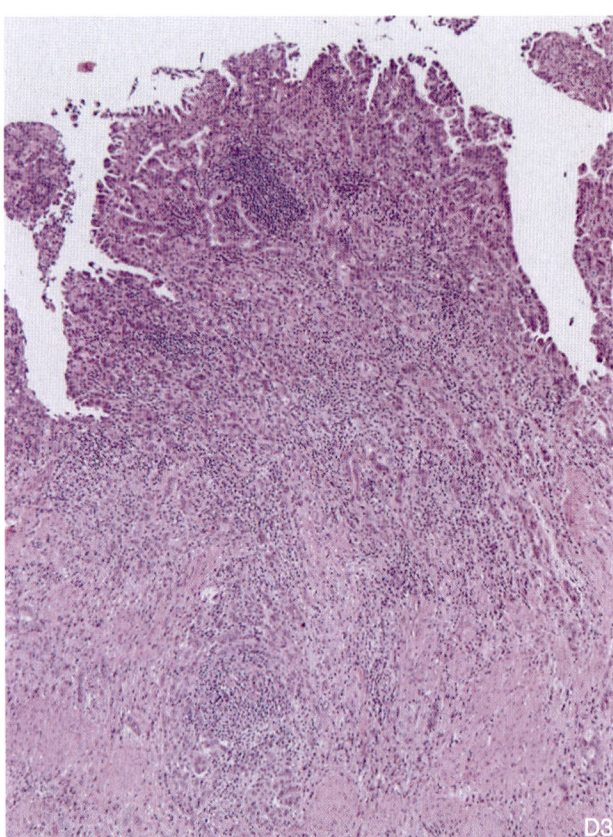

FIGURES 24–12. *D1 to D3* (D) Photomicrograph (H&E, 1,2,3): Macroscopically (1), yellowish to whitish wall thickening in the fundus of the GB was seen. Microscopic examination (2,3) showed poorly differentiated adenocarcinoma and the depth of invasion was to subserosal space. (T2)

References

1. Feldman, M., Brandt, J. L.: Choleserolosis of the Gallbladder. Sleisenger and Fordtran's Gastrointestinal and Liver Disease 2005;8th edition.
2. Katoh, T., Nakai, T., Hayashi, S., Satake, T.: Noninvasive carcinoma of the gallbladder arising in localized type adenomyomatosis. Am J Gastroenterol 1988;83:670–674.
3. Paraf, F., Potet, F.: Gallbladder carcinoma arising in adenomyomatosis. Am J Gastroenterol 1988;83:1439.
4. Ootani, T., Shirai, Y., Tsukada, K., Muto, T.: Relationship between gallbladder carcinoma and the segmental type of adenomyomatosis of the gallbladder. Cancer 1992; 69:2647–2652.
5. Ishizuka, D., Shirai, Y., Tsukada, K., Hatakeyama, K.: Gallbladder cancer with intratumoral anechoic foci: a mimic of adenomyomatosis. Hepatogastroenterology 1998;45:927–929.
6. Yoshimitsu, K., Irie, H., Aibe, H., Tajima, T., Nishie, A., Asayama, Y., Matake, K., Yamaguchi, K., Matsuura, S., Honda, H.: Well-differentiated adenocarcinoma of the gallbladder with intratumoral cystic components due to abundant mucin production: a mimicker of adenomyomatosis. Eur Radiol 2005;15:229–233.
7. Mizuguchi, M., Kudo, S., Fukahori, T., Matsuo, Y., Miyazaki, K., Tokunaga, O., Koyama, T., Fujimoto, K.: Endoscopic ultrasonography for demonstrating loss of multiple-layer pattern of the thickened gallbladder wall in the preoperative diagnosis of gallbladder cancer. Eur Radiol 1997;7:1323–1327.
8. Muguruma, N., Okamura, S., Okahisa, T., Shibata, H., Ito, S., Yagi, K.: Endoscopic sonography in the diagnosis of xanthogranulomatous cholecystitis. J Clin Ultrasound 1999;27:347–350.
9. Maeyama, R., Yamaguchi, K., Noshiro, H., Takashima, M., Chijiiwa, K., Tanaka, M.: A large inflammatory polyp of the gallbladder masquerading as gallbladder carcinoma. J Gastroenterol 1998;33:770–774.
10. Mekeel, K. L., Hemming, A. W.: Surgical management of gallbladder carcinoma: a review. J Gastrointest Surg 2007;11:1188–1193.
11. Fujita, N., Noda, Y., Kobayashi, G., Kimura, K., Yago, A.: Diagnosis of the depth of invasion of gallbladder carcinoma by EUS. Gastrointest Endosc 1999;50:659–663.

CHAPTER 25

Ampullary Lesions

Dr. Maria Chiara Petrone
Dr. Silvia Carrara
Dr. Paolo Giorgio Arcidiacono

Introduction

The ampulla is an extensive anatomic and functional region that includes not only the choledochopancreatic junction but also the sphincter of Oddi, traversing the duodenal wall to open at a small mucosal elevation: the papilla of Vater. The ampulla of Vater corresponds to the dilated junction of the common bile duct and main pancreatic duct. In the text we will use interchangeably the terms *papilla of Vater* and *ampulla of Vater*.

The minor papilla, also called the accessory pancreatic duct of Santorini, is 2 cm long, proximal and slightly anterior to the major papilla. Endoscopic ultrasonography (EUS) is effective and accurate in the preoperative evaluation of most ampullary pathologies. Available EUS devices include standard echoendoscopes, such as radial scanning and linear array echoendoscopes, and catheter ultrasound probes. Several reports suggest that EUS is superior to other conventional radiological modalities, including CT scan, in the staging of periampullary malignancies.[1-4] They demonstrate a significantly higher sensitivity and specificity in identifying periampullary lesions, assessing major vascular involvement, and determining lymph-node metastases with EUS compared with CT. Midwinter et al evaluated the findings from spiral computed tomography and EUS in 34 patients with suspected pancreatic and ampullary tumors.[5] EUS missed a 15 mm ductal adenocarcinoma, identifying it as biliary stricture, while CT missed eight lesions, six of which were resectable. In another study by Chen et al, of 74 patients with periampullary tumors, EUS was more sensitive than CT for tumor detection (EUS 97%; CT 39%) and T-staging (EUS 72%; CT 22%).[6]

EUS Exploration

The endosonographic exploration of the main and minor papilla is technically challenging due to the size of these two anatomic areas and their position in the superior genus and descending duodenum. For these reasons, sometimes the endosonographer needs some tricks in order to be sure to completely visualize these areas.

The choice of the best instrument to study the papilla is debated, but there are no published data showing a significant difference of accuracy among standard echoendoscopes. Catheter probes are reported to have a better efficacy in the staging of superficial lesions.[7] In periampullary lesions, the role of EUS role could not be not limited to diagnosing and staging. It is also used to help endoscopic treatment or to do an EUS guided treatment as well. Our policy is to perform all EUS ampullary procedures with a therapeutic linear probe.

The kind of sedation to be used has not been definitively established. In a recent randomized controlled study, our group showed a similar efficacy of conscious sedation and deep sedation during diagnostic and operative pancreatic endosonography.[8] This is usually a lengthy procedure, lasting for 45 minutes or more if a second therapeutic step is needed due to EUS results. For this reason, we think that in this setting a deep sedation with anaesthesiologist supervision is advocated.

As for all the other EUS procedures in the upper GI tract, the exam is performed with the patient laying on the left lateral side. The instrument is introduced under endoscopic view until it reaches the ssecond and third parts of the duodenum and then straightened in the same way as for the ERCP procedures. Then, the balloon on the probe is filled with water and, once the mesenteric vessels are targeted, the examination of the ampulla and periampullary region can start by slowly withdrawing the instrument, slightly releasing the little wheel that has been locked in the full right position since the beginning. Reaching the main papilla, the probe should be gently move away from the duodenal wall in order not to compress the papilla structure, risking false results. Sometimes, in cases of small and superficial lesions, it is better to retract the tip in the superior genus, with the probe looking down in the lumen of the second part of the duodenum right above the main papilla, and to fill the lumen with water after i.v. administration of spasmolytic drugs or glucagon to stop the motility; in this way, the main papilla and the onset of the ducts can be clearly seen on the same picture. The papilla of Vater is identified as a small hypoechoic structure, from which the two ducts, the upper common bile duct and the lower main pancreatic duct, can be traced and followed into the pancreatic head. The normal size of the major duodenal papilla is 10 × 5 mm (Figures 25–1 and 25–2).

Once the main pailla is targeted, the surrounding pancreatic parenchyma and both the pancreatic and common bile duct must be evaluated to clearly establish the presence and extent of tumor invasion. At each step, rotation of the instrument is necessary to scan through the entire pancreatic head.

The minor papilla is not generally visible during diagnostic EUS procedures because of its size and of its undefined structure, but if it is affected by a

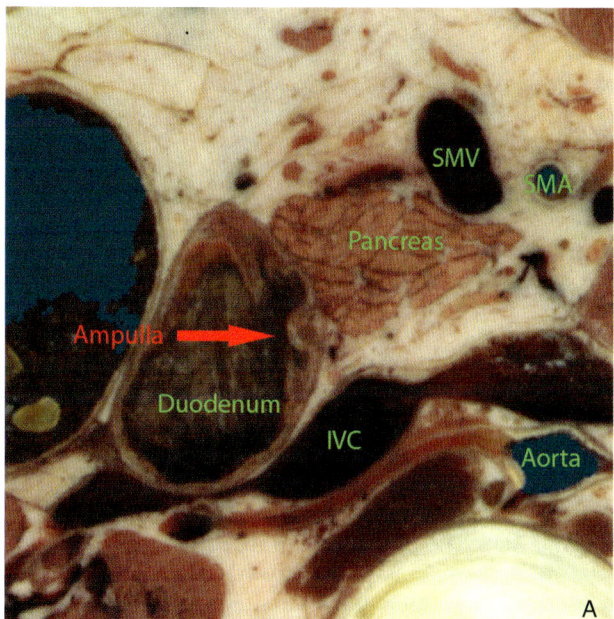
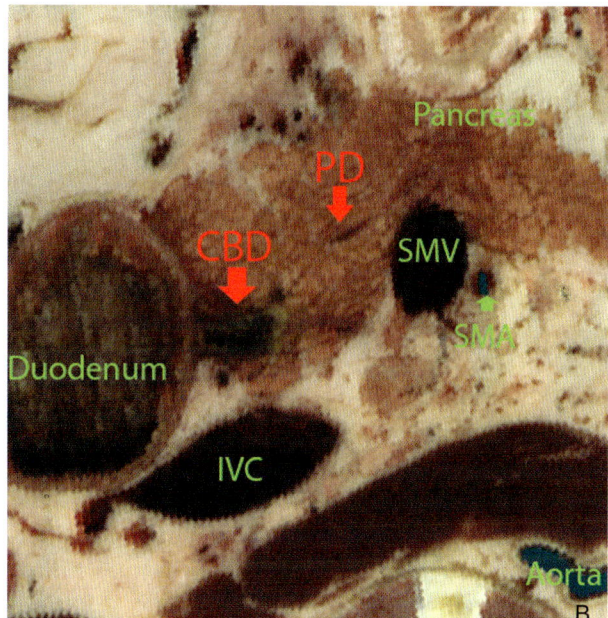
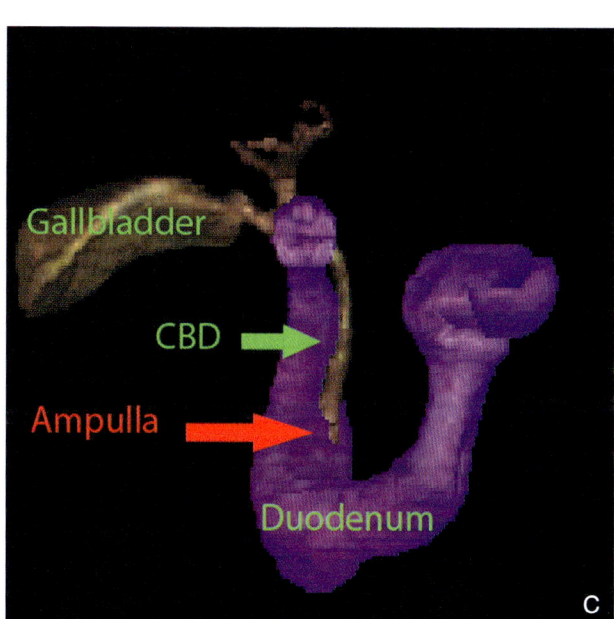
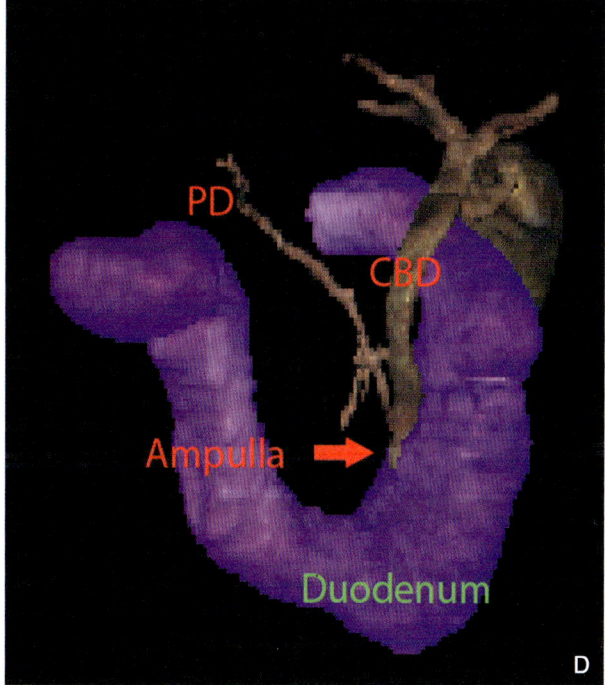

FIGURES 25–1. *A to D* (A and B) Visible Human axial cross-sections and models, (C) left anterior oblique view, (D) is left posterior oblique view from the region of the ampulla. CBD=common bile duct, PD=pancreatic duct, IVC=inferior vena cava, SMA=superior mesenteric artery, SMV=superior mesenteric vein.

disease, it can be better studied introducing the instrument in the duodenal bulb with the long maneuvre without balloon inflation and filling the lumen with water. Most of papillary lesions involve the main papilla, and these are distinguished as inflammatory and neoplastic.

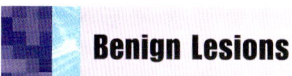 **Benign Lesions**

Among the inflammatory lesions, a well-known condition is the "fibrosis and stenosing papillitis," a

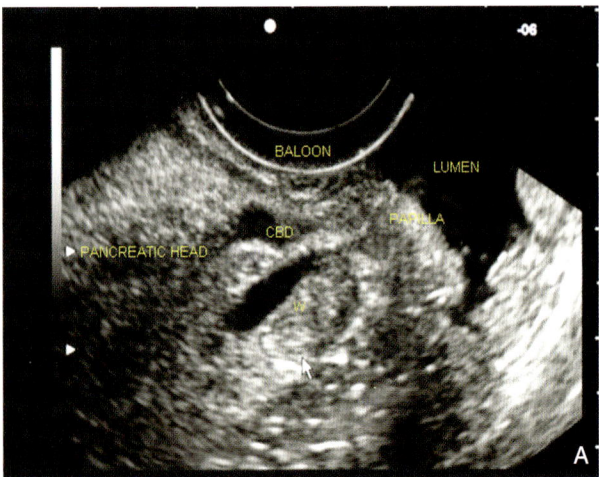 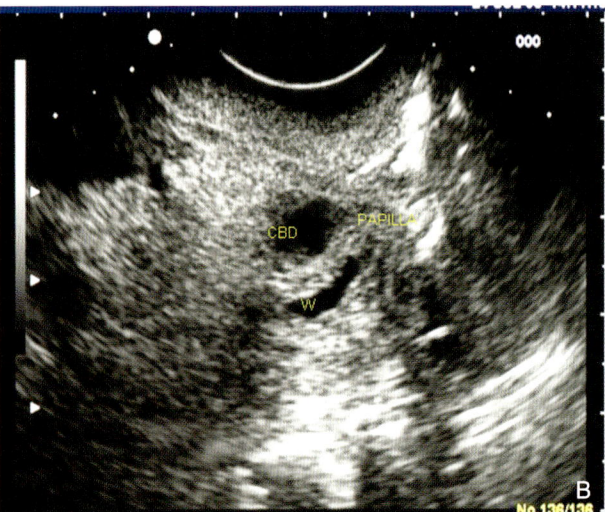

FIGURES 25–2. *A and B* Two examples of normal ampulla during EUS. The probe is placed in the second portion of the duodenum with the balloon inflated, but not pressed too hard against the duodenal wall, to avoid compression artefacts. The ampulla (papilla) is seen as an hypoechoic, well-delineated structure from which the two ducts, the common bile duct (CBD) and the Wirsung (W) can be traced and followed into the pancreatic head.

descriptive term for an anatomic deformity of the papilla of Vater that is characterized by the narrowing of the lower end of the common bile duct and the main pancreatic duct (Figure 25–3). The defect is secondary to inflammation and fibrosis due to the chronic passage of gallstones, episodes of acute pancreatitis, chronic pancreatitis, sclerosing cholangitis, peptic ulcer disease, and cholesterolosis. Patients with papillary stenosis from gallstone migration may present with episodes of severe upper-abdominal pain several years after cholecystectomy.

Microlithiasis may lead to pancreatitis through several mechanisms: transient impaction of small stones at the papilla, obstructing the pancreatic duct, or the repeated passage of stones (which may lead to papillary stenosis or SOD, both of which are associated with pancreatitis).[9] With the US probe positioned in the genu superior, the common bile duct (CBD) can be examined in longitudinal sections as far proximally as the hepatic duct and distally to the ampulla (Figure. 25–4). Withdrawal from the bulb under traction allows examination of the gallbladder

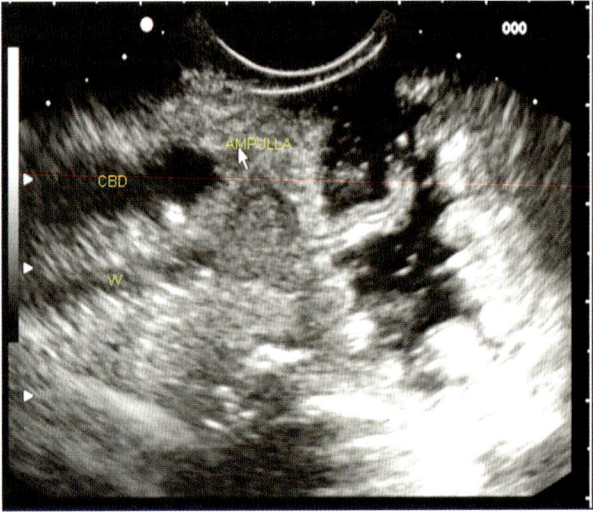

FIGURE 25–3. Sclerosis of the ampulla (papillitis): the inflammatory alteration of the ampulla is seen as hyperechoic, sign of fibrosis, that causes obstruction and dilation of the common bile duct. It's more frequent in elderly women with history of cholecystectomy or microlithiasis (See figure 25–4).

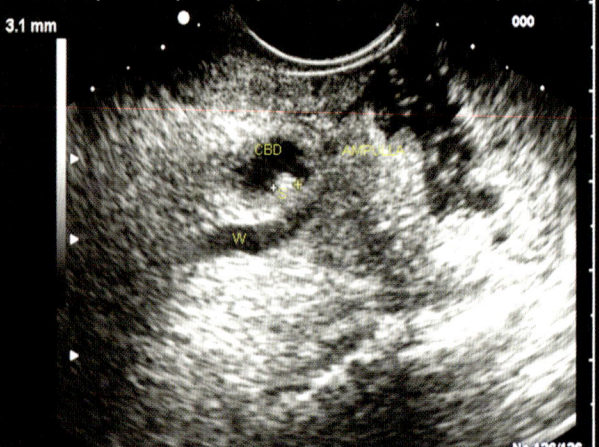

FIGURE 25–4. A 3.1 mm stone in the retro-ampullary tract of the CBD. EUS has an accuracy of 97% and a negative predictive value of 98% in the diagnosis of choledocholithiasis (Buscarini Gatrointestinal Endoscopy 2003).

and CBD, from its origin in the hilum to the convergence of the cystic and hepatic ducts and the proximal portion of the CBD.

In a prospective and competitive blind study in patients with CBD obstruction, EUS showed 100% accuracy for the diagnosis of choledocholithiasis. It was also significantly more sensitive than transabdominal ultrasonography or CT.[10]

In a recent study, Elek et al have described an inflammatory alteration of the papilla as the cause of biliary obstruction in 36% of their patients[11] (Figure 25–5). Adenomatous hyperplasia and adenomyomatosis were observed in 5% and 7% of examinations respectively. The clinical symptoms of these conditions are reflected in the Milwaukee classification of sphincter of Oddi dysfunction. At endosonographic exploration, concentric thickening of the papillary region is often present, with preserved layers of the duodenal wall; as the most important criterion, a funnel-shaped narrowing and filiform discharge of the CBD into the papilla.

Malignant Lesions

Tumors of the ampulla of Vater include neoplasia arising inside the ampulla (intra-ampullary type), tumors arising on the ampulla (peri-ampullary type), and tumors arising at the junction of the mucosa of the ampulla with that of the papilla or involving both the intra-ampullary and peri-ampullary region of the duodenum (mixed type). The periampullary region represents the junction of three different epithelia—pancreatic ducts, bile ducts, and duodenal mucosa. Carcinomas originating from the ampulla of Vater by gross inspection can arise from one of four epithelial types, terminal common bile duct, duodenal mucosa, pancreatic duct, or ampulla of Vater. Benign tumors of the ampulla of Vater are rare overall and include adenomas, gastrointestinal stromal tumor (GIST), lipomas, and neuroendocrine tumors.

Although classified as benign, ampullary adenomas are truly premalignant neoplasms arising from the mucosal epithelium of the papilla (Figures 25–6A, 25–6B). When present, symptoms of ampullary

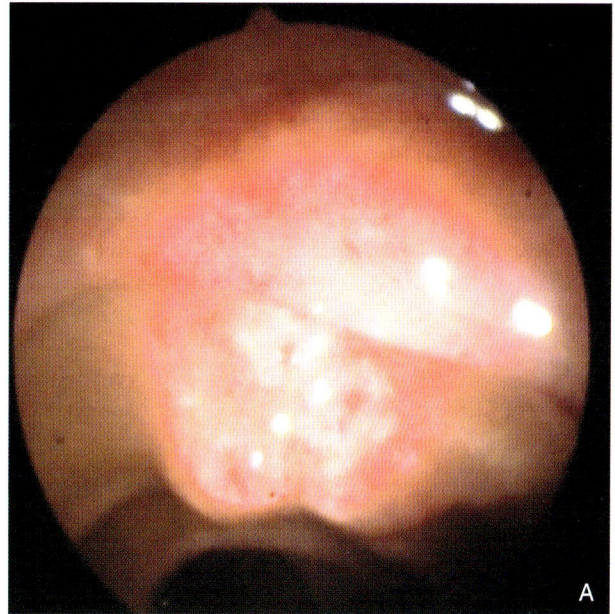

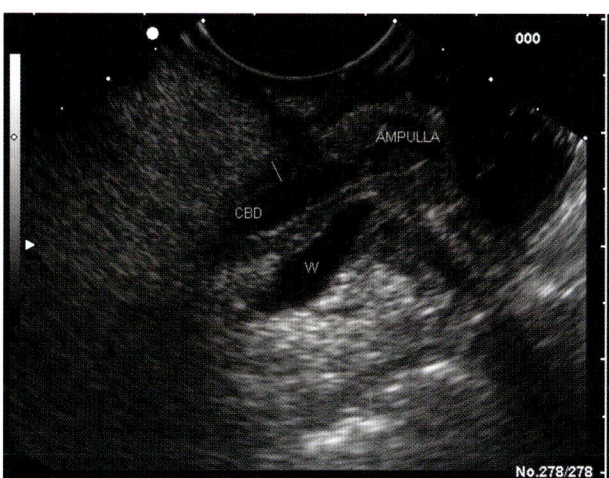

FIGURE 25–5. Oedema of the ampulla: the region is enlarged, hypoechoic and smooth. Cholangitis is seen as uniform, hypoechoic thickening of the CBD wall. There is also a mild dilation of the pancreatic duct (W).

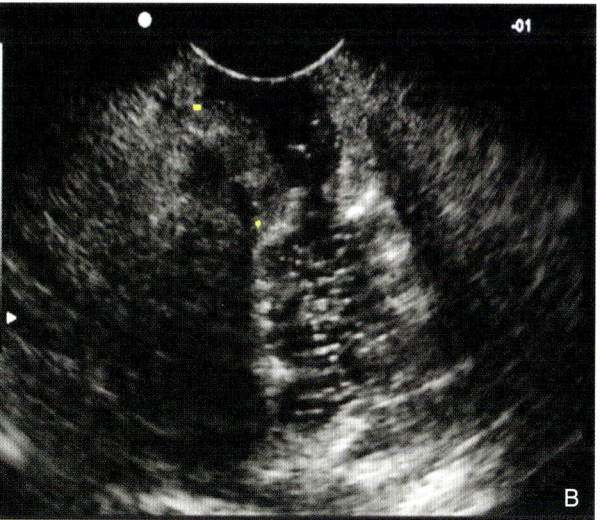

FIGURES 25–6. *A and B* (A) Endoscopic view of the ampulla with areas of dysplasia. (B) The same case of figure 25–7A at EUS: a mild thickening of the first layer (mucosa) without evidence of a clear focal lesion. The extension is marked by yellow points.

adenomas are usually nonspecific, reflecting ampullary (biliary or pancreatic) obstruction resulting from the mass effect of the adenoma compressing and impending biliary or pancreatic outflow. The most common of these symtoms is jaundice, which is usually painless. Common bile duct microstone secondary to cholestasis is associated in 15 to 30% of patients.[12-13] In biliary obstruction attributable to an ampullary neoplasm, EUS tipically demonstrates dilation of the common bile duct, consistent with obstruction at the level of the ampulla.

On the basis of autopsy investigations, the rate of neoplastic lesions of the ampulla was found to range between 0.063% and 0.21%.[14] Ninety percent of ampullary tumors are adenocarcinomas. They may occur as sporadic lesions or in patients with familial adenomatous polyposis (FAP). Histologically, most of these lesions are adenomas and, as in other adenomas of the gastrointestinal tract, malignant degeneration may develop through the adenoma-carcinoma sequence.[15-16]

Adenocarcinoma of the ampulla accounts for 5% of all gastrointestinal (GI) carcinomas, and must be differentiated from the carcinoma of the head of the pancreas (Figures 25–7A and 25–7B) and the common bile duct, because the prognosis and treatment are different. Klempnauer demonstrated five-year survival rates after resection of ampullary cancer and pancreatic head ductal cancer of 38% and 16% respectively.[17]

At endosonographic exploration, villous adenomas often correspond to a thickening of the first layer, the superficial mucosa (Figures 25–8A, 22–8B, 22–8C). A tumor of the ampulla is imaged as a hypoechoic focal mass. The bigger the lesion, the more heterogenous the echotexture. Invasion of the duodenal wall is seen as a disruption of the normal architecture of the layers. The staging is very important and may be affected by endoscopic procedures on the papilla, performed before diagnostic EUS, like papillosfinterotomy (PST) or biliary stenting, which is frequently performed in these patients.[18] In the same way as carcinomas of the pancreas, tumors of the papilla are classified using the TNM staging system. T1 tumors are confined to the papilla, without infiltration of the duodenal wall. T2 tumors are characterized by invasion of the duodenal wall no deeper than the muscularis propria (Figures 25–9A, 22–9B, 22–9C). T3 means that invasion of the pancreas is less than 2 cm (Figure 25–10). T4 includes tumors invading the pancreas by more than 2 cm or invading neighbouring vessels or organs.[19] Combined data from two centers reported the accuracy of ampullary tumor staging with multiple imaging modalities in patients with and without endobiliary stents.[20] EUS was shown to be more accurate than CT and MRI in the overall

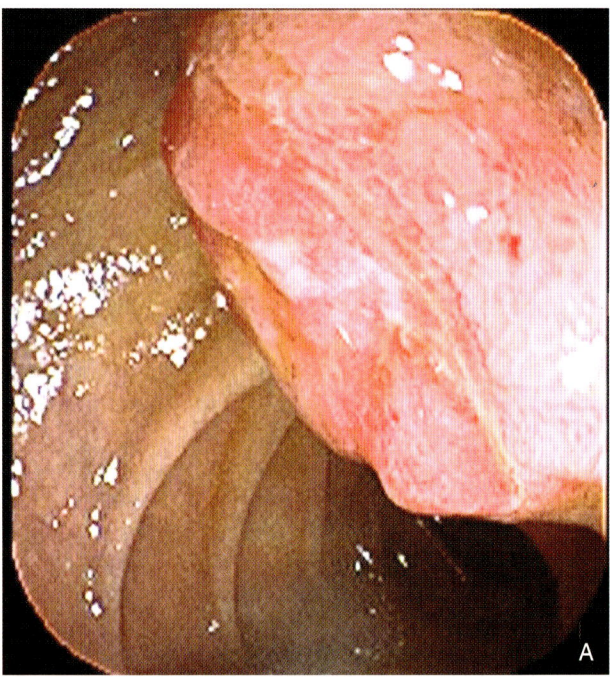

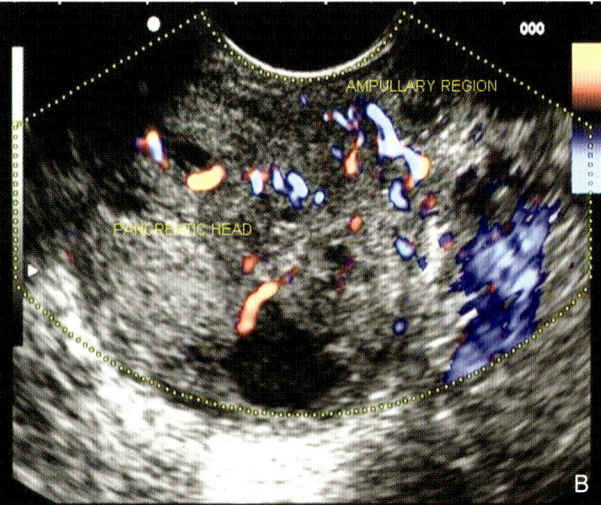

FIGURES 25–7. *A and B* (A) The ampulla is deformed and pressed by a mass growing beyond in the head of the pancreas in a patient with jaundice and abdominal pain. (B) At EUS scan, a mass into the pancreatic head was seen just beyond the ampulla, involving the ampulla and the two ducts; its echotexture was inhomogeneous with anechoic spaces and a rich vascularization. Fine needle aspiration biopsy revealed a mucinous tumor of the pancreas.

assessment of the T-stage of ampullary neoplasm (EUS 78%, CT 24%, MRI 46%). EUS T-stage accuracy was reduced from 84% to 72% in the presence of a transpapillary endobiliary stent. This is most prominent in the understaging of T2/T3 carcinomas.

The importance of EUS in defining vascular invasion by major duodenal papilla malignancies is based

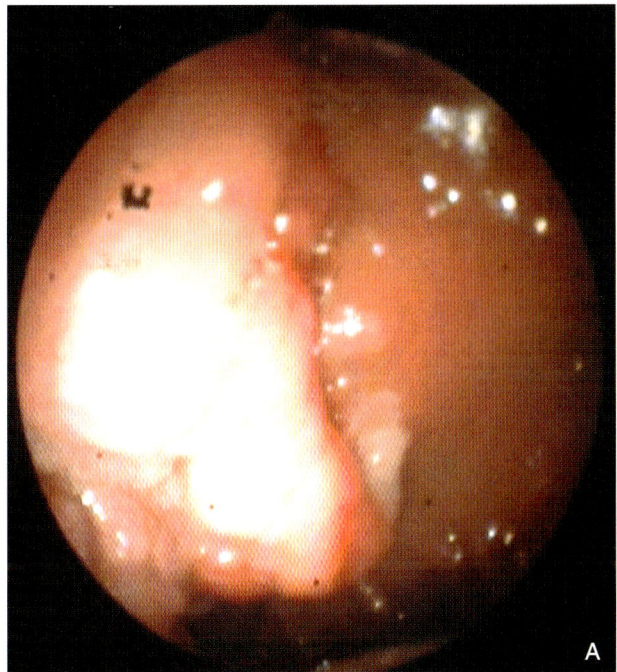
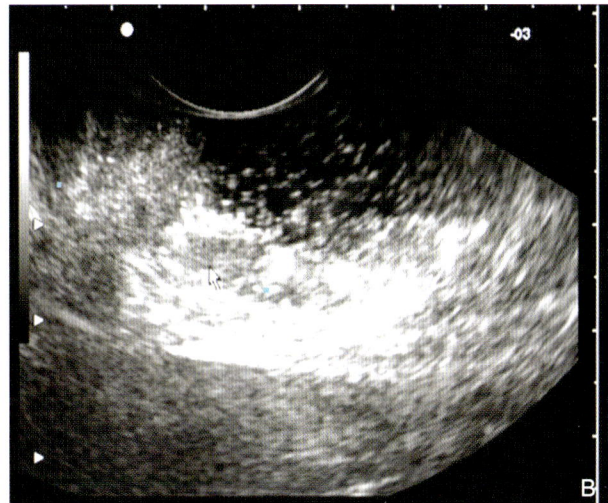
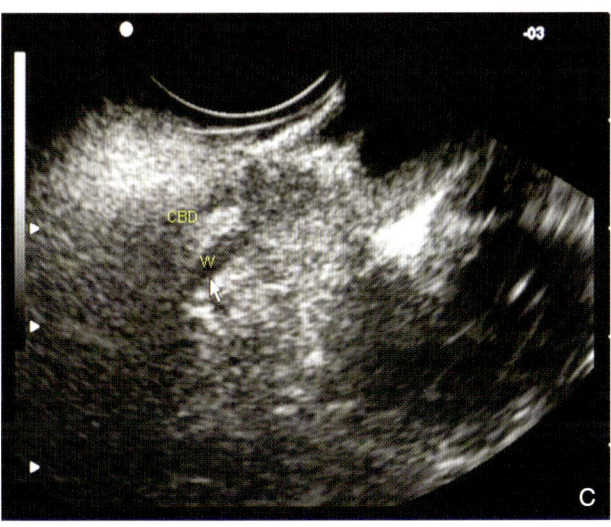

FIGURES 25–8. *A to C* (A) Ampullary adenoma (B) Endosonographic scan of the case from Figure 25–8A: the lesion is superficial, involving the mucosa. It is not possible to distinguish between a T1 papillary carcinoma and an adenoma using EUS alone, histological assessment is required. (C) The superficiality of the lesion, without involvement of the deeper muscular layer, is confirmed by the normal diameter of the two ducts, the pancreatic (W) and the biliary duct (CBD).

on the principal of surgical resectability. Patients with vascular invasion of peripancreatic vessels are not candidates for curative resection. The N classification categorizes the presence (N1) or absence (N0) of pathological lymphnodes. Tio et al evaluated the clinical tumor node metastasis (TNM) staging of ampullary and pancreatic carcinomas by EUS before surgery as compared with histology and/or surgery.[21] EUS was accurate in staging the depth of tumor invasion and diagnosing regional lymph-node metastasis. Nonresectabily was accurately assessed on the basis of vascular involvement. The overall accuracy in tumor staging for ampullary carcinomas was 84.4%.[21] Intraductal ultrasonography (IDUS) is preferable to EUS for small tumors. IDUS has a high resolution and can clearly demonstrate the duodenal papillary region and the Oddi's muscle layer, visualized as a single layer.[7]

Itoh et al. evaluated the usefulness of IDUS in diagnosing tumor extension of cancer of the papilla and compared preoperative diagnosis with that of histopathology. The accuracy rate of EUS was 87.5%. In assessing lymphnode metastases, sensitivity was 66% and specificity was 91%.[22]

Endoscopic biopsies, even when obtained after sphincterotomy, have proven unreliable in the diagnosis of papillary tumor-containing invasive carcinoma. Endoscopic brushings do not always yield

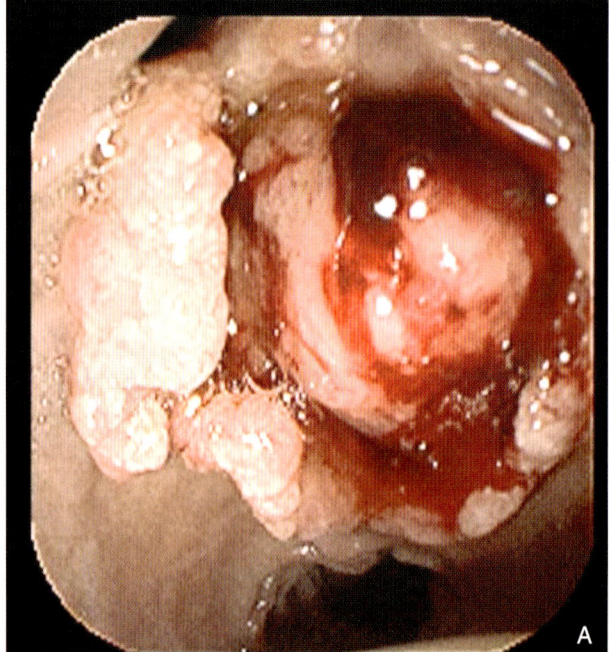

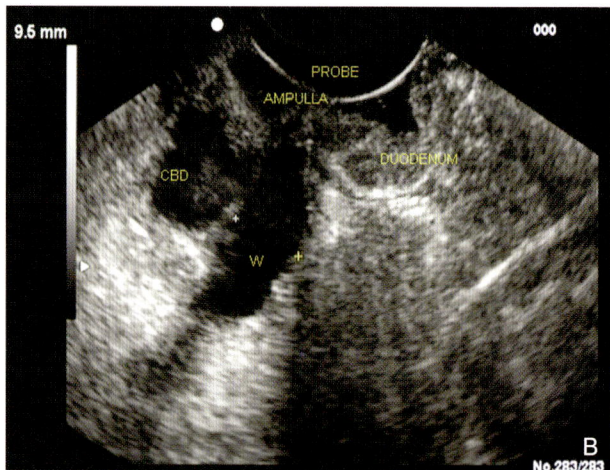

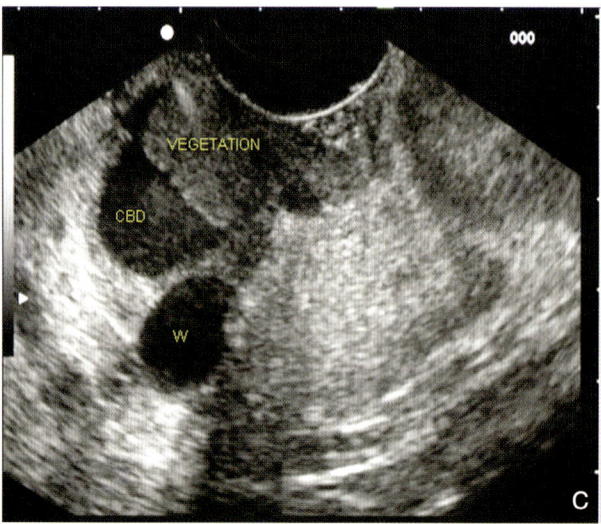

FIGURES 25–9. *A to C* Adenocarcinoma of the ampulla (B) EUS view of the case from Figure 25–9A: the regular architectural pattern of the ampullary region is destroyed by hypoechoic tissue; the biliary and pancreatic ducts are obstructed and dilated. Penetration of hypoechoic tissue into the muscolaris propria is defined as a T2 ampullary tumor. (C) A vegetation growing from the ampullary tumor involves the CBD. The probe is placed in front of the ampulla, in the straight position, with the balloon mildly filled with water without pressing too much in order to avoid artefacts.

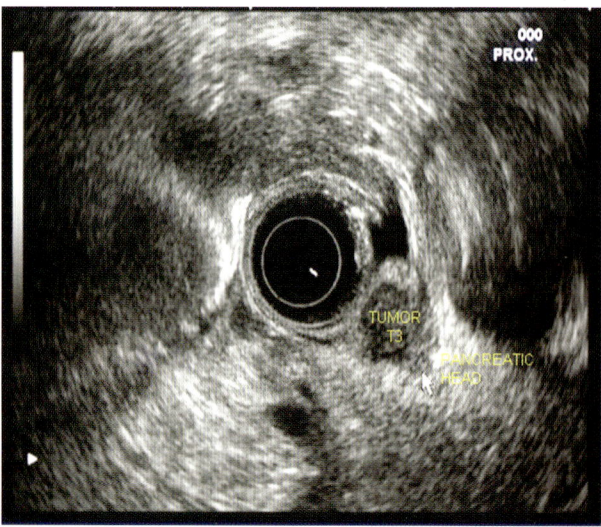

FIGURE 25–10. Radial scan of a T3 ampullary tumor. T3 is defined as a tumor invading 2 cm or less into the pancreas.

diagnostic material for an accurate assessment of the lesions.[23-24] With the increasing popularity of EUS-guided fine needle aspiration biopsy (FNAB) in the clinical evaluation and cytologic diagnosis of various neoplasms of the GI tract, pancreas, liver, lymph-node, and non-GI organs,[25-28] primary ampullary tumors are being sampled more frequently. In a recent paper, DeFrain et al evaluated EUS-FNAB accuracy, sensitivity, specificity and the cytomorphologic features of primary ampullary tumors showing that EUS is accurate in the evaluation of suspected ampullary malignancies. EUS-guided FNAB is effective in obtaining adequate diagnostic material.[29] The sensitivity and the specificity of cytologic evaluation of suspected ampullary lesions were 82.4% and 100%, respectively.

In contrast to pancreatic carcinoma, tumors of the papilla of Vater can usually be resected and therefore have a better prognosis. The choice of the resection method depends on the presence of intraductal growth. (Figures 25–11A, 25–11B, 22–11C) Intraductal extension of the tumor requires pylorus preserving pancreatoduodenectomy, while extraductal adenoma can be resected endoscopically. EUS allows visualization of the papilla of Vater and detects neoplastic intraductal growth or infiltration of the sorrounding structures. (Figures 25–12A, 25–12B, 25–12C, 25–12D)

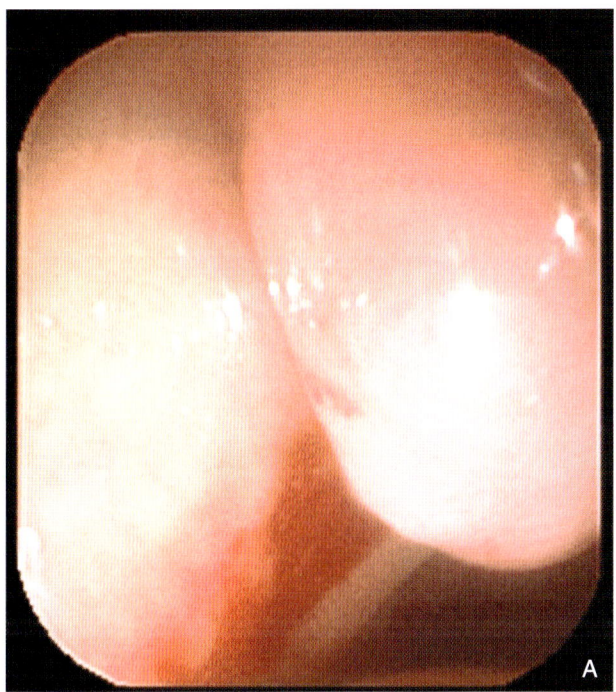

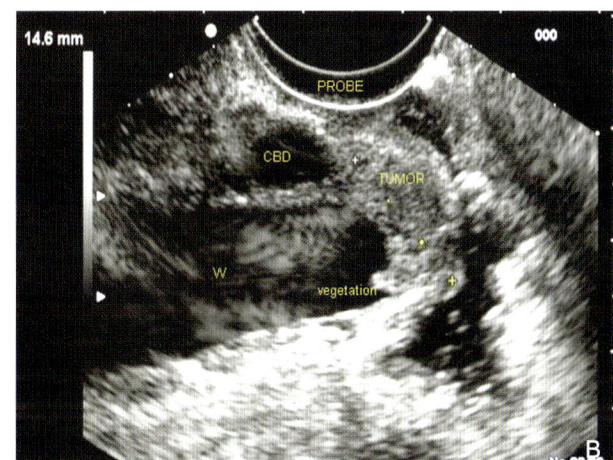

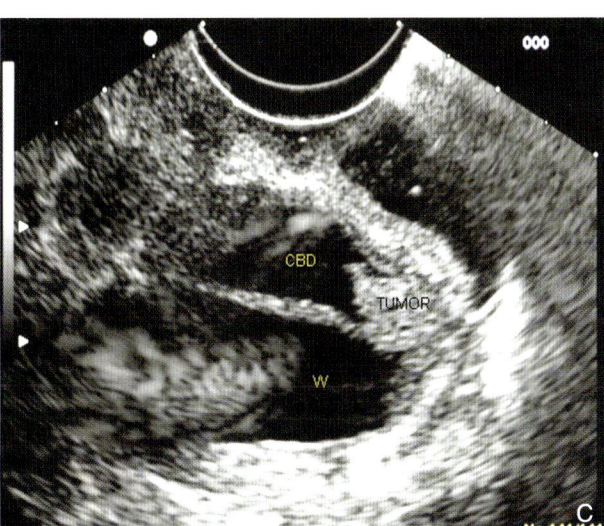

FIGURES 25–11. *A to C* (A) Tumor of the ampulla in a patient with jaundice (B) The tumor completely closes the pancreatic and biliary ducts with vegetation inside the Wirsung and the CBD (See Figure 25–11C). (C) A vegetation, growing from the ampullary tumor, invading the CBD

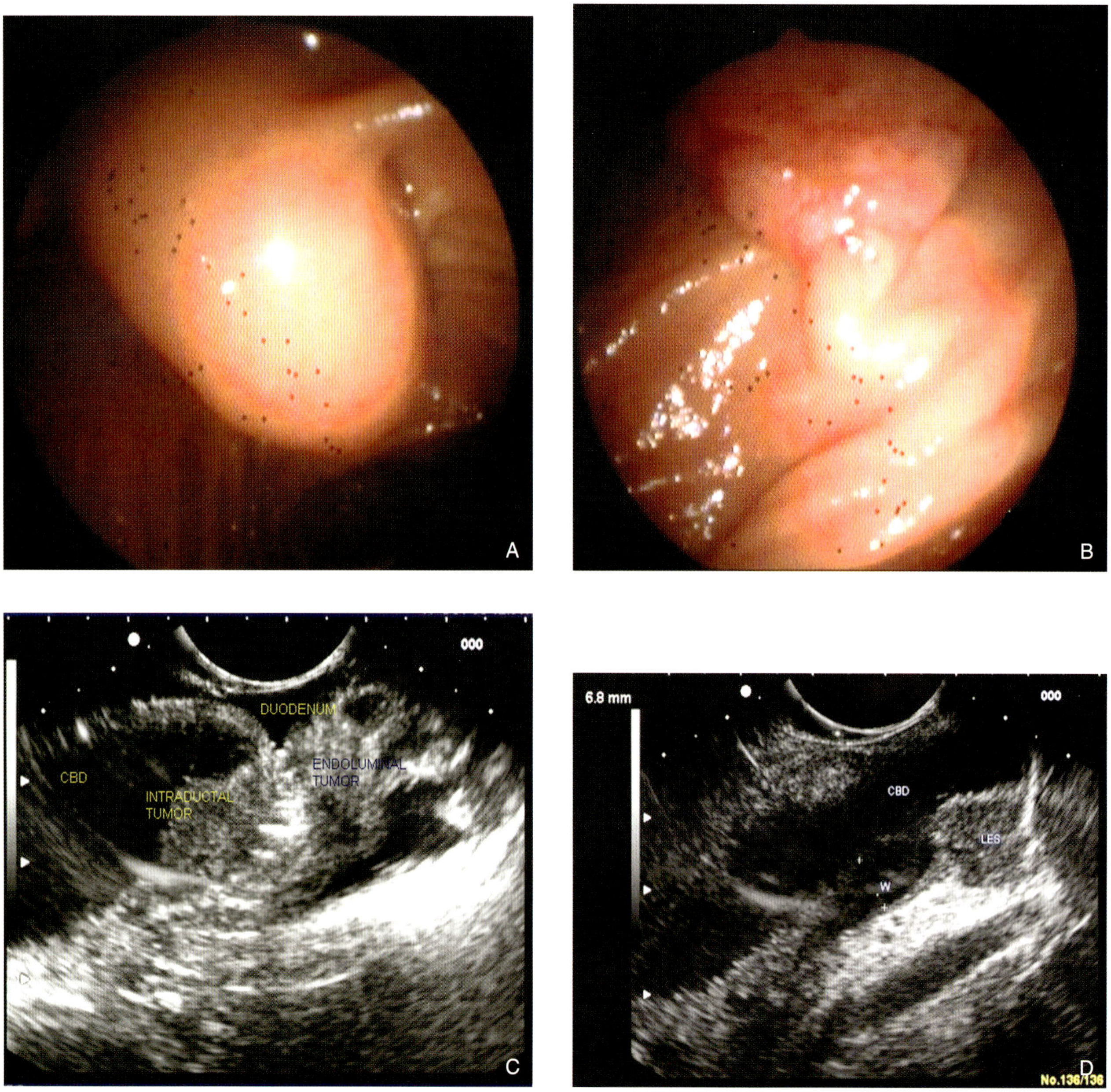

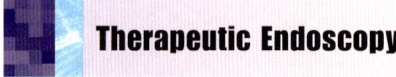

FIGURES 25–12. *A to D* (A) A prominent ampulla in a patient with jaundice (B) The biliary orifice is occluded by adenomatous tissue. (C) EUS view of the same case: the tumoral growth into the duodenal lumen and into the biliary duct (D) The lesion (LES) occluding the two ducts. The pancreatic duct is dilated (6.8 mm).

Therapeutic Endoscopy

Optimal management of neoplastic disease of the papilla of Vater is still not established. For a long time, radical surgery has been regarded as the only viable treatment modality for curative therapy.[30] In addition, the individual decision of the patient and general health status, comorbidity, and infiltration depth of the neoplastic lesion contribute to determine the therapeutic strategy. In cases of papillary invasive carcinoma, pancreaticoduodenectomy remain the type of resection of first choice.[31-32] Patients with a malignant neoplasm of the papilla, who are not fit for surgical resection due to severe comorbidity or who refuse any surgical procedure, can be taken into consideration for an endoscopic treatment or palliative endoscopic biliary drainage. Generally it depends on the ductal infilatration, whether the endoscopic excision of a papillary tumor is technically feasible or not.

Endoscopic snare resection is generally considered to be contraindicated if the tumor extends into the biliary or pancreatic duct,[33-35] but some authors have shown that less than 1 cm of extension into the common bile duct or pancreatic duct does not preclude endoscopic therapy because tissue invading to this level may be endoscopically exposed and ablated.[36-37]

The term *ampullectomy* refers to removal of the entire ampulla of Vater and is a surgical term for procedures that require surgical reimplantation of the distal common bile duct and pancreatic duct within the duodenal wall. Technically, when endoscopic resections of lesions at the major papilla are performed, only tissue from the papilla can be removed endoscopically, and thus the term *papillectomy* is more appropriate than the term *ampullectomy*, even if the two are often used interchangeably in the literature.[36]

There are no definitive guidelines as to the size or diameter beyond which endoscopic removal of ampullary adenomas should not be attempted. Most investigators recommend that, for endoscopic resction (ER), the size of the tumor should not exceed 4 cm in maximal diameter, even if there are reports of successful endoscopic resection of ampullary lesions of grater size. In a recent study, Eswaran et al have shown how removal of very large sessile lesions is possible with minimal increase in risk.[38] Due to their anatomically difficult location in the duodenum and at the biliary and pancreatic duct orifices, resection of papillary tumors is a much more complex procedure if compared to polypectomy in the colon. Techniques of endoscopic removal of ampullary adenomas remain unstandardized, likely because of the relatively small number of formal investigations into this practice.

Endoscopic snare papillectomy is being increasingly performed with curative intent for benign papillary tumors. There are some macroscopic criteria that suggest malignant transformation, such as the presence of spontaneous bleeding, ulceration, non-lifting sign at submucosal injection; friability and induration of the tissue—even if this last trait may also be caused by fibrosis.[39]

For endoscopic snare resection, a therapeutic duodenoscope with a large working channel should be preferred. Any polypectomy snare can be used; there is no evidence documenting the utility of one type of snare over another. Snare position during papillectomy is also not standardized, with investigators describing successful papillectomy with snares oriented in a cephalad to caudal orientation and vice versa; the majority of authors haven't specifically commented on the orientation of the snare during the procedures.[40-41] For resection, there is no consensus about which type of current should be used. Both pure cutting current and blended current have been used, and neither has been proven to be superior.[36] Submucosal injection prior to the resection is recommended by some authors, but not routinely required.[42] Endoscopic sphincterotomy of the biliary or pancreatic sphincter is frequently performed, assisting in pancreaticobiliary drainage after papillectomy, but there is no consensus about these maneuvers.[36]

Endoscopic papillectomy has an increased pancreatitis risk. Several studies have shown that placement of a prophylactic pancreatic duct stent reduces the risk of post-ERCP pancreatitis.[43]

The only prospective, randomized, controlled trial evaluating this method reports a statistically significant decrease in the rate of postprocedure pancreatitis in the stent group.[44] On the basis of these data, prophylactic pancreatic duct stenting during papillectomy is recommended to reduce the risk of postprocedural pancreatitis, but its use has yet to be evaluated in large randomized trials.[36]

If the adenoma cannot be resected completely, or if en-bloc resection is not technically feasible, additional treatment options are available. Ablative therapies such as argon plasma coagulation (APC), laser therapy, monopolar or bipolar electrocoagulation, are useful to destroy residual or recurrent adenomatous tissue not removed at primary snare resection. APC is the most frequently used modality given its widespread availability and superficial depth of tissue destruction, but in this way there is no spacimen for histological examination.

Successful papillectomy rates range from 46% to 92%; early complications after endoscopic papillectomy are similar to other complications of endoscopic procedures, overall ERCP including pancreatitis, perforation, bleeding, sedation complications, and cholangitis. Later complications may be the development of stenosis (pancreatic or biliary). It is recommended that all patients who have undergone endoscopic papillectomy undergo surveillance for the detection of recurrent neoplastic tissue.[36]

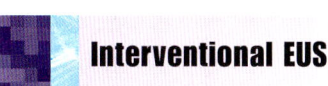

Interventional EUS

The detection of the pancreatic orifice and pancreatic stenting are still challenging procedures, with a failure rate around 5–10%. It can be difficult to visualize the pancreatic orifice after snare removal of the papilla because of edema and artifacts due to electro-cautery during ampullectomy. De Witt et al described the first use of EUS-guided methylene blue pancreatography (EUS-MBP) to identify the minor papilla after unsuccessful ERCP.[45] EUS-guided fine needle injection of

MB into the pancreatic duct provided excellent visualization of the minor papilla orifice.

Our group has recently described the EUS-guided MB injection into the pancreatic duct as a useful technique to assist the pancreatic stenting after ampullectomy in patients with ampullary tumors.[46-47-48-49] During EUS staging of ampullary lesions with a linear array echoendoscope, the pancreatic duct is punctured with a 22- or 25-gauge needle through the duodenal wall, as for EUS-FNA of the pancreatic head, and a few mL of MB are injected into the duct. After ampullectomy, a blue spot or flow identifies the pancreatic orifice, and a stent can be easily placed. (Figures 25–13A, 25–13B, 25–13C)

The same maneuvre can be used to perform a main pancreatic duct drainage with the insertion of a guidewire into the pancreatic duct under EUS guidance. This is mostly used as a second attempt in symptomatic patients with chronic pancreatitis, in whom endoscopic cannulation of pancreatic duct failed.[47]

A transduodenal approach is preferred to facilitate the puncture and to avoid intraperitoneal leakage of pancreatic fluid. The needle tip and the right placement of the guidewire can be followed under fluoroscopy, and contrast medium can be injected to contrast the pancreatic duct. The guidewire, inserted through the needle, is passed through the stricture and the major ampulla into the duodenum. The

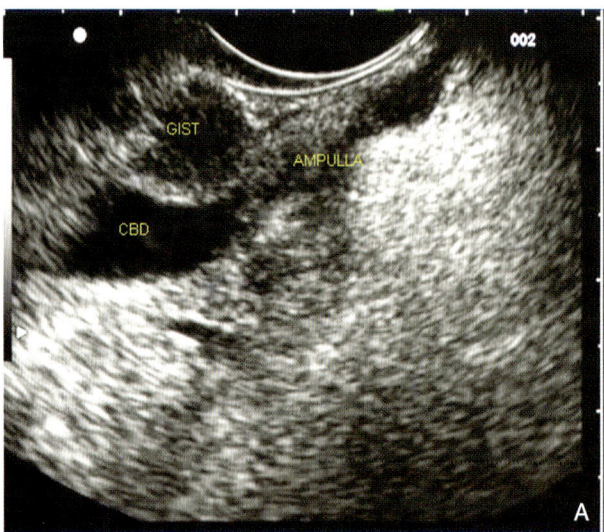

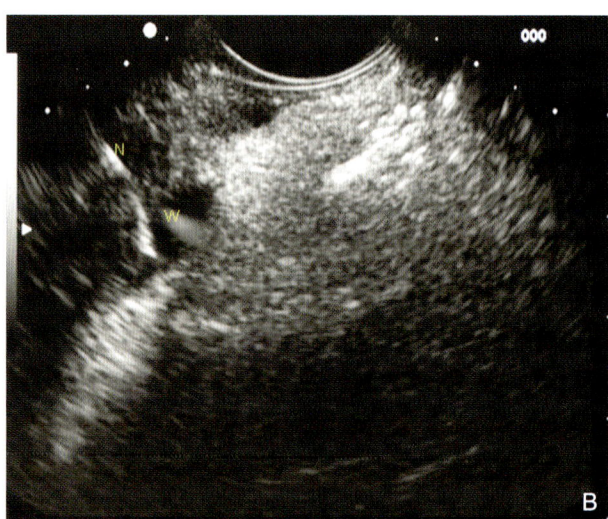

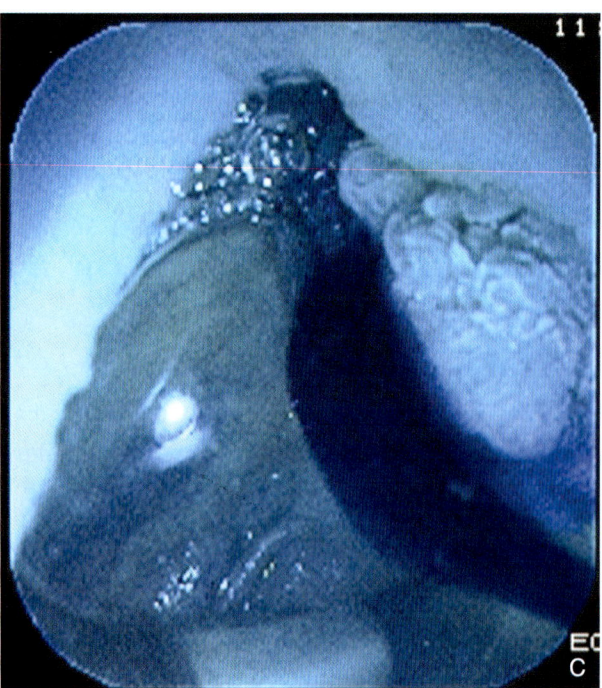

FIGURES 25–13. *A to C* (A) Ampullary region in an elderly patient with neurofibromatosis, who presented with abdominal pain, jaundice, and fever. The ampulla was prominent, and biopsies showed an adenoma. EUS confirmed a superficial lesion, without infiltration of the submucosa. The bile duct and the pancreatic duct, in the retro-ampullary region were dilated. Some hypoechoic solid focal lesions were found near the ampulla, growing from the muscolaris propria. One of these was located between the duodenal wall and the bile duct, giving a small compression to the duct. A fine needle aspiration biopsy showed mesenchimal stromal spindle cells positive to CD117 and actine, negative to S-100. (B) A 25-gauge needle was introduced into the Wirsung, and methylene blue (dilution 1.20000, 3 ml) was injected inside the duct. Its flow was observed from the ampullary orifice. A snare removal of the ampulla was performed with a duodenoscope in the same session. (C) The methylene blue flow from the pancreatic orifice was a helpful guide for the placement of a stent in the pancreatic duct to prevent postprocedural pancreatitis.

echoendoscope is then removed and the procedure is finished with a duodenoscope passed along the guidewire and placed in front of the papilla, near the distal tip of the guidewire that is grasped with a snare, withdrawn into the accessory channel of the duodenoscope, and a stent is inserted over the guidewire.

Hemorrhage, pancreatitis, and perforation are potential complications of interventional EUS of the biliary tract. This procedure should be attempted only by experienced endoscopists skilled in both EUS and ERCP. The risk of hemorrhage is decreased by the use of color Doppler for the visualization of interposing vessels. There are no guidelines about the use of prophylactic antibiotics administration.

Selective cannulation of the main pancreatic duct is more difficult in the presence of periampullary diverticula, and the rate of successful cannulation is lower in patients with intradiverticular papillae than in those with juxtapapillary diverticula.

We described a case of an older woman who presented with jaundice and abdominal pain and stones in the common bile duct, in which the ERCP failed because of the location of the papilla into a diverticulum. An EUS-guided rendezvous drainage of the obstructed biliary tract was performed with a linear array echoendoscope: the common bile duct was punctured from the bulb with a 22-gauge needle, and a 0.0018" guidewire was inserted through the needle and passed through the major ampulla into the duodenum. The procedure was finished with a duodenoscope, and the stones were removed from the biliary tract.

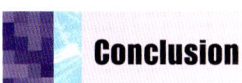

Conclusion

The detailed diagnosis of papillary lesions is an important area of application for endoscopic ultrasound before any diagnostic or therapeutic procedures such as sphincterotomy, ampullectomy, or surgical intervention. EUS is becoming more and more interventional with the improvement of echoendoscopes and accessories. In skilled hands, EUS will evolve as an important alternative technique to other more invasive drainage procedures with a minimal need of prescription drug assistance.

References

1. Rosch, T., Briag, C., Gain, T., et al.: Staging of pancreatic and ampullary carcinoma by endoscopic ultrasonography: comparison with conventional sonography, computed tomography, and angiography. Gastroenterology 1992;102:188–199.
2. Palazzo, L., Roseau, G., Gayet, B., et al.: Endoscopic ultrasonography in the diagnosis and staging of pancreatic adenocarcinoma: results of a prospective study, with comparison to ultrasonography and CT scan. Endoscopy 1993; 25:143–150.
3. Palazzo, L.: Staging of pancreatic carcinoma by endoscopic ultrasonography. Gastroenterology 1992;102: 188–199.
4. Mueller, M. F., Meyenberger, C., Bertschinger, P., et al.: Pancreatic tumors: evaluation with endoscopic US, CT, and MR imaging. Radiology 1994;190:745–751.
5. Midwinter, M. J., Beveridge, C. J., Wilsdon, J. B., et al.: Correlation between spiral computed tomography, endoscopic ultrasonography and findings at operations in pancreatic and ampullary tumors. Br F Surg 1999; 86:189–193.
6. Chen, C. H., Tseng, L. J., Yang, C. C., et al.: Preoperative evaluation of periampullary tumors by endoscopic sonography, transabdominal sonography, and computed tomography. J Clinical Ultrasound 2001; 29:313–321.
7. Yusuf, T. E., Bhutani, M. P.: Role of endoscopic ultrasonography in disease of the extrahepatic biliary system. J Gastroent Hepatol 2004;19:243–250.
8. Fanti, L., Agostoni, M., Arcidiacono, P. G., et al.: Target-controlled infusion during monitored anesthesia care in patients undergoing EUS: Propofol alone versus midazolam plus propofol. A prospective double-blind randomised controlled trial. Dig Liver Dis 2006 Oct 13.
9. Hernandez, C. A., Lerch, M. M.: Sphincter stenosis and gallstone migration through the biliary tract. Lancet 1993; 341:1371–1373.
10. Amouyal, P., Palazzo, L., Amouyal, G., et al.: Endosonography: promising method for diagnosis of extrahepatic cholestasis. Lancet 1989; 2: 1195–1198.
11. Elek, G., Gyori, S., Toth, B., Pap, A.: Histological evaluation of preoperative biopsies from Ampulla Vateri. Pathol Oncol Res 2003;9:32–41.
12. Binmoeller, K. F., Boaventura, S., Ramsperger, K., et al.: Endoscopic snare excision of benign adenomas of the papilla of Vater. Gastrointest Endosc 1993; 39:127–131.
13. Ponchon, T., Berger, F., Chavaillon, A., et al.: Contribution of endoscopy to diagnosis and treatment of tumors of the ampulla of Vater. Cancer 1989;64:161–167.
14. Perzin KH, Bridge MF. Adenomas of the small intestine: a clinicopathologic review of 51 cases and a study of their relationship to carcinoma. *Cancer*. 1981;48:799-819.
15. Hirota, W. K., Zuckerman, M. J., Adler, D. G., et al.: ASGE guideline: the role of endoscopy in the surveillance of premalignant conditions of the upper GI tract. Gastrointest Endosc 2006;63:570–580.
16. Stolte, M., Pscherer, C.: Adenoma-carcinoma sequence in the papilla of Vater. Scand J Gastroenterol 1996; 31:376–382.
17. Klempnauer, J., Ridder, G. J., Pichlmayr, R.: Prognostic factors after resection of ampullary carcinoma: multivariate survival analysis in comparison with ductal cancer of the papilla of Vater. Br. J. Surg. 1995; 82: 1686–91.
18. Chang, K. J.: State of the art lecture: Endoscopic ultrasound (EUS) and FNA in pancreatico-biliary tumors. Endoscopy 2006;38(S1):S56–S60.
19. Dietrich, C.F., Hocke, M., Seifert, H.: Endosonography of the hepatobiliary system. In: Christoph Frank Dietrich. Endoscopic Ultrasound. An introductory Manual and Atlas. Thieme Stuttgart, 2006 George Thieme Verlag Edition.

20. Cannon, M. E., Carpenter, S. L., Elta, G. H., et al.: EUS compared with CT, magnetic resonance imaging, and angiography and the influence of biliary stenting on staging accuracy of ampullary neoplasms. Gastrointest Endosc 1999;50(1):27–33.
21. Tio, T. L., Sie, L. H., Kallimanis, G. et al.: Staging of ampullary and pancreatic carcinoma: comparison between endosonography and surgery. Gatsrointest Endosc 1996;44:706–713.
22. Itoh, A., Goto, H., Naitoh, Y., et al.: Intraductal ultrasonography in diagnosing tumor extension of cancer of the papilla of Vater. Gastrointest Endosc 1997;45: 251–260.
23. Yamaguchi, K., Enjoji, M., Kitamura, K.: Endoscopic biopsy has limited accuracy in diagnosis of ampullary tumors. Gastrointest Endosc 1990;36:588–592.
24. Heidecke, C. D., Rosenberg, R., Bauer, M., et al.: Impact of grade of dysplasia in villous adenomas of Vater's papilla. World J Surg 2002;26:709–714.
25. Chang, K. J., Katz, K. D., Durbin, T. E., et al.: Edoscopic ultrasound guided fine needle aspiration. Gastrointest Endosc 1994;40:694–699.
26. Giovannini, M., Seitz, J. F., Monges, F., et al.: Fine needle aspiration cytology guided by endoscopic ultrasonography: results in 141 patients. Endoscopy 1995;27: 171–177.
27. Bhutani, M. S., Hawes, R. H., Baron, P. L., et al.: Endoscopic ultrasound guided fine needle aspiration of malignant pancreatic lesions. Endoscopy 1997;29: 854–858.
28. Shin, H. J., Lahoti, S., Sneige, N.: Endoscopic ultrasound-guided fine needle aspiration in 179 cases. The MD Anderson Cancer Experience. Cancer 2002;96: 174–180.
29. DeFrain, C., Chang, C., Srikureja, W., Nguyen, P. T., Gu, M.: Cytologic features and diagnostic pitfalls of primary ampullary tumors by endoscopic ultrasoun-guided fine-needle aspiration biopsy. Cancer 2005;105: 289–297.
30. Farouk, M., Niotis, M., Branum, G. D., et al.: Indications for and the technique of local resection of tumors of the papilla of Vater. Arch Surg 1991;126: 650–652.
31. Kim, M. H., Lee. S. K., Seo, D. W., et al.: Tumors of the maior duodenal papilla. Gastrointest Endosc 2001; 54: 609–620.
32. Beger, H. G., Treitschke, F., Gansauge, F., et al.: Tumor of the ampulla of Vater—experience with local or radical resection in 171 consecutively treated patients. Arch Surg 2001;247:526–532.
33. Norton, I. D., Gostout, C. J., Baron, T. H., et al.: Safety and outcome of endoscopic snare excision of the major duodenal papilla. Gastrointest Endosc 2002;56:239–243.
34. Catalano, M. F., Linder, J. D., Chak, A., et al.: Endoscopic management of adenoma of the major duodenal papilla. Gastrointest Endosc 2004;59:225–232.
35. Norton, I. D., Geller, A., Petersen, B. T., et al.: Endoscopic surveillance and ablative therapy for peri-ampullary adenomas. Am J Gastroenterol 2001;96: 101–106.
36. Adler, D. G., Qureshi, W., Davila, R., et al: Standards of Practice Committee. ASGE Guidelines. Gastrointest Endosc 2006;64:849–854.
37. Bohnacker, S., Seitz, U., Nguyen, D., et al.: Endoscopic resection of benign tumors of the duodenal papilla without and with intraductal growth. Gastrointest Endosc 2005;62:551–60.
38. Eswaran, S. L., Sanders, M., Bernardino, K. P., et al.: Success and complications of endoscopic removal of giant duodenal and ampullary polyps: a comparative series. Gastrointest Endosc 2006;64:925–932.
39. Cheng, C. L., Sherman, S., Fogel, E. L., et al.: Endoscopic snare papillectomy for tumors of the duodenal papillae. Gastrointest Endosc 2004;60:757–764.
40. Baille, J.: Endoscopic ampullectomy. Am J Gastroenterol 2005 ;100:2379–2381.
41. Kahaleh, M., Shami, V. M., Brock, A., et al.: Factors predictive of malignancy and endoscopic resectability in ampullary neoplasia. Am J Gastroenterol 2004;99: 2335–2339.
42. Bohnacker, S., Soehendra, N., Maguchi, H., et al.: Endoscopic resection of benign tumors ot the papilla of Vater. Endoscopy 2006;38:521–525.
43. Singh, P., Das, A., Isenberg, G., et al.: Does prophylactic pancreatic stent placement reduce the risk of post-ERCP acute pancreatitis? A meta-analysis of controlled trials. Gastrointest Endosc 2004;60:544–550.
44. Harewood, G. C., Pochron, N. L., Gostout, C. J.: Prospective, randomized, controlled trial of prophylacic stent placement for endoscopic excision of the duodenal ampulla. Gastrointest Endosc 2005;62:367–370.
45. De Witt, J., McHenry, L., Fogel, E., et al.: EUS-guided methylene blue pancreatography for minor papilla localization after unsuccessful ERCP. Gastrointest Endosc 2004;59:133–136.
46. Carrara, S., Arcidiacono, P. G., Diellou, M. G., et al.: EUS-guided methylene blue injected into the pancreatic duct as a guide for pancreatic stenting after ampullectomy. Endoscopy 2007 Feb;39 Suppl 1:E151-2. Epub 2007 Jul 4.
47. Will, U., Meyer, F., Manger, T., Wanzar, T.: Endoscopic ultrasound-assisted rendezvous maneuver to achieve pancreatic duct drainage in obstructive chronic pancreatitis. Endoscopy 2005; 37(2):171–173.
48. L. Bataille and P. Deprez.: A new application for therapeutic EUS: main pancreatic duct drainage with a "pancreatic rendezvous technique". Gastrointest Endosc 2002; 6: 740-743.
49. S. Mallery, J. Matlock, M. L. Freeman.: EUS-guided rendezvous drainage of obstructed biliary and pancreatic ducts: reports of 6 cases. Gastrointest Endosc 2004; 59(1): 100–107.

CHAPTER 26

Liver Lesions

Dr. Michael B. Wallace
Dr. Murli Krishna

The liver is commonly involved by lesions that originate in the liver, or have spread there from other sources. As shown in Figure 26–1, the left lobe of the liver and part of the right lobe are directly adjacent to the stomach and duodenum, and accessible to EUS imaging and biopsy.[1,2] Much of the right lobe, however, is better accessed by extracorporeal imaging and biopsy. This chapter illustrates lesions found in the liver with selected EUS pictures.

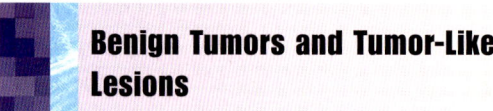

Benign Tumors and Tumor-Like Lesions

Cavernous Hemangioma

Cavernous hemangiomas are the most common benign tumors of the liver, often occurring in women. The size of these tumors may vary from less than a centimeter to large lesions replacing most of the liver ("giant hemangiomas").

Grossly, hemangiomas are circumscribed hemorrhagic lesions characterized by vascular spaces of variable size that are filled with blood. More solid areas in a hemangioma may represent thrombosis or scarring. Foci of calcification may also be present. Histologically, these tumors are characterized by vascular spaces that are lined by endothelium and contain blood. The spaces are separated by fibrous septae. The diagnosis is usually well established by imaging techniques, and fine needle aspiration is rarely performed for diagnosis. The aspirate specimen usually shows abundant fresh blood with scant benign endothelial and stromal cells.[3] (Figures 26–2, 26–3, 26–4)

Focal Nodular Hyperplasia

Focal nodular hyperplasia (FNH) is a localized nodular lesion in the liver consisting of nodules of hepatocytes separated by fibrous septae. It is not a true neoplasm, and may represent either a hamartoma or a proliferative response to vascular injury, the latter being currently favored. These lesions have a female sex predilection. They can occur at any age, but are most common in the third to fifth decades of life.

Grossly, FNH is a well-circumscribed, unencapsulated nodular mass with a characteristic central stellate scar. In 10–20% of patients, they may occur as multiple lesions. The background liver is usually normal. Histologically, FNH shows hyperplastic nodules of hepatocytes surrounded by fibrous septae that radiate from a central scar. Bile ductular proliferation is usually present, and the central scar often contains thick-walled arteries. The FNA specimen contains all normal liver cell types, with predominantly hepatocytes and smaller numbers of ductular cells and Kupffer cells.[4,5] (Figures 26-5, 26–6).

Liver Cell Adenoma

Liver cell adenoma is a benign neoplasm of hepatocytes. These tumors have an association with contraceptive or anabolic steroid use and are far more common in females. Like focal nodular hyperplasia, adenomas are most common in the third to fifth decades of life. Patients may present with pain, mass, or abdominal bleeding secondary to rupture. In 20–30% of patients, adenomas are multiple.

Grossly, liver cell adenomas are circumscribed fleshy masses. A capsule is usually absent in smaller adenomas, but larger lesions may be partially or completely encapsulated. Areas of hemorrhage, necrosis, and scarring may be present. Histologically, adenomas are characterized by proliferation of benign hepatocytes that are arranged in cords one to two cells thick. Vessels of variable size are present, but bile ducts are absent. In FNA biopsy specimens, a large tissue core is usually needed to suggest a diagnosis of adenoma. Smears are usually cellular, with bland hepatocytes that lack the typical widened trabecular arrangement seen in hepatocellular carcinomas. Nuclear-cytoplasmic ratio is low, and nucleoli are not prominent. These findings are helpful in distinguishing adenoma from hepatocellular carcinoma. However, in some cases, distinguishing an adenoma from a well-differentiated hepatocellular carcinoma may be difficult, especially if a tissue section is not available.[4,5] (Figures 26–7, 26–8, 26–9)

Bile Duct Adenomas and Hamartomas

Bile duct adenomas are small solitary well demarcated lesions that are usually located under the capsule. Histologically they are characterized by a benign proliferation of bile ducts within a fibrous stroma. Bile duct hamartomas (also known as von Meyenburg complexes) are developmental remnants of bile ducts. They are also usually subcapsular, but in contrast to adenomas they are centered in portal tracts and consist of dilated ducts that may contain bile. They are also found in association with fibropolycystic liver diseases. Bile duct adenomas and hamartomas are most commonly found incidentally at surgery or autopsy. FNA smears from both lesions are similar and may be hypocellular due to fibrosis. They show cohesive groups of benign duct epithelium with or without stroma.[6,7,8,9]

Liver Lesions 289

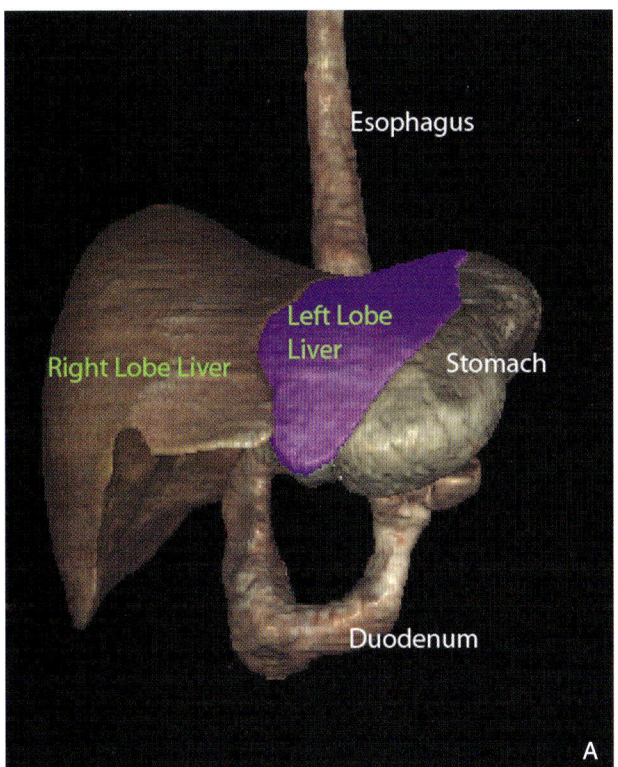
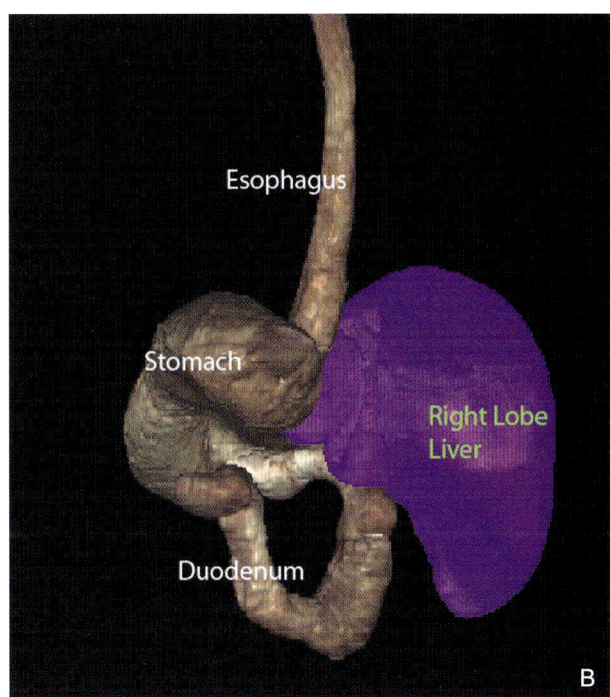
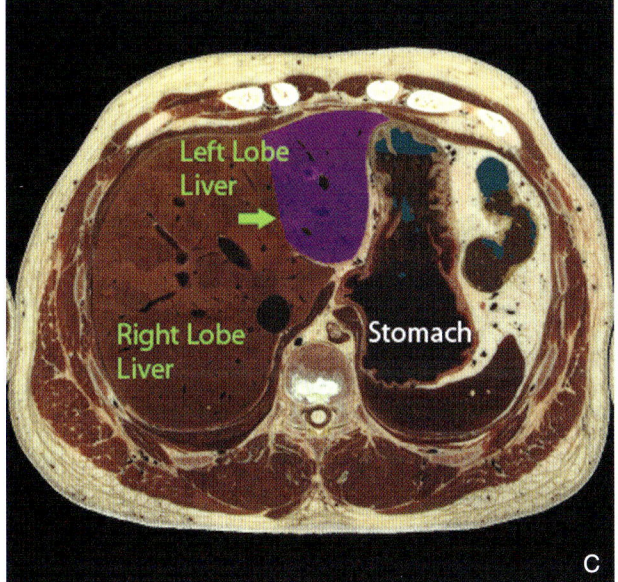
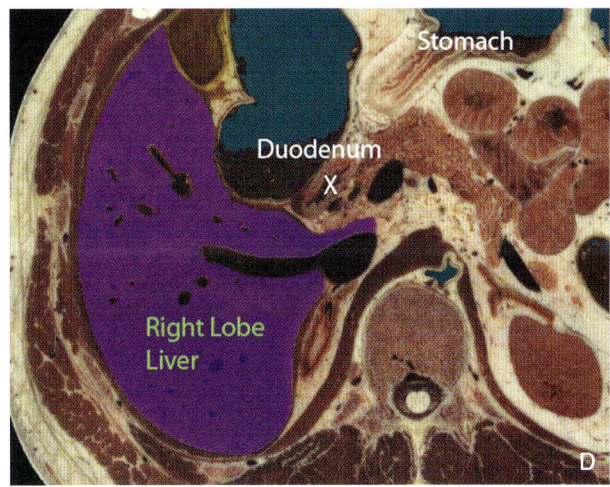
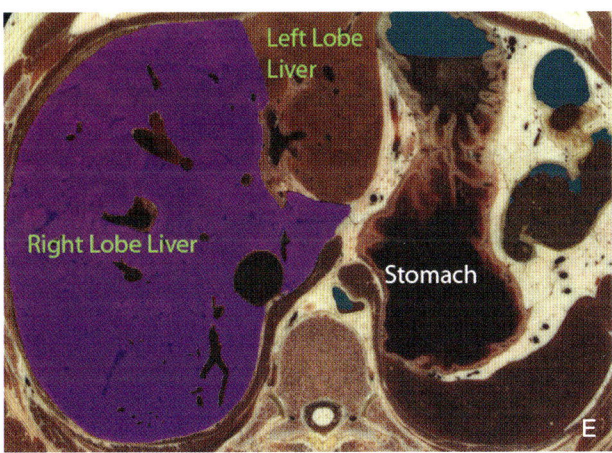

FIGURE 26–1. *A to E* (A) Model showing an anterior view with the left lobe of liver highlighted (B) Model of a posterior view showing right lobe of liver highlighted (C) Transaxial cross-section showing stomach as it relates to left lobe of liver (D) Transaxial cross-section showing stomach as it relates to right lobe of liver. (E) Transaxial cross-section showing duodenum as it relates to left lobe of liver.

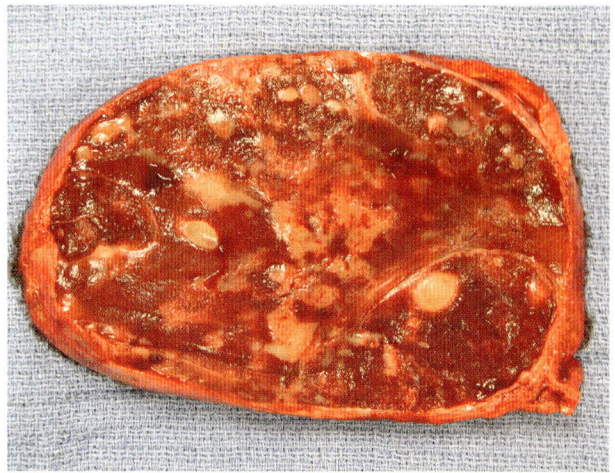

FIGURE 26–2. Hemangioma. The cut surface is hemorrhagic with grey-white areas of fibrosis and thrombosis.

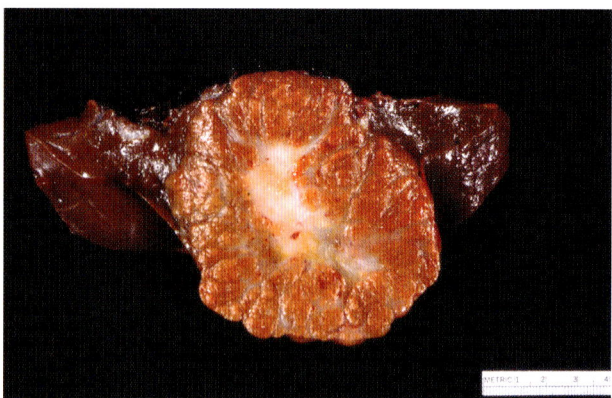

FIGURE 26–5. Focal nodular hyperplasia. A nodular, fleshy mass with a central stellate scar.

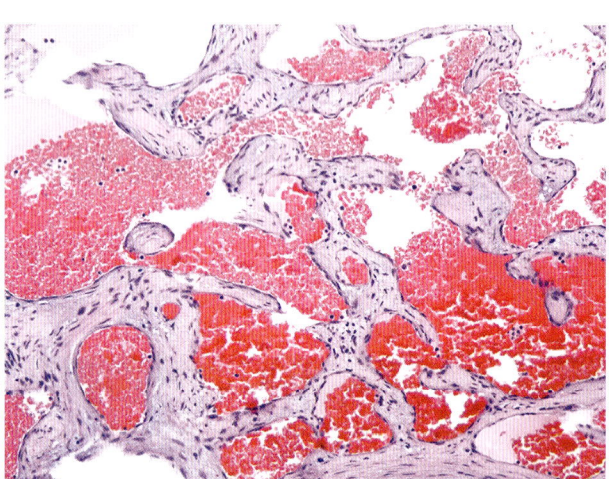

FIGURE 26–3. Hemangioma. Anastomosing vascular spaces filled with blood and lined by endothelium.

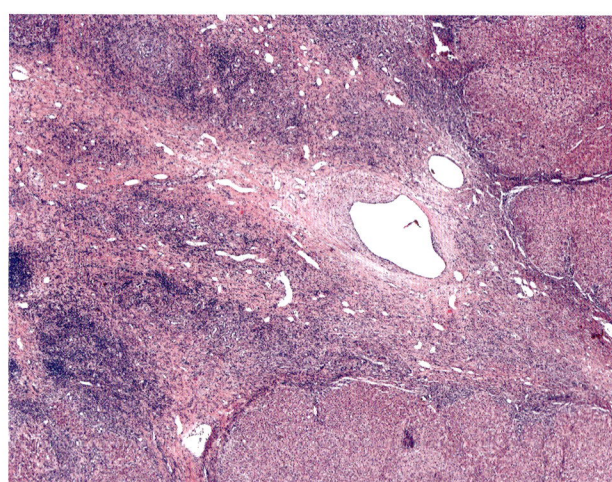

FIGURE 26–6. Focal nodular hyperplasia. A central scar is present with a thick-walled artery, radiating fibrous septae, and surrounding hyperplastic nodules.

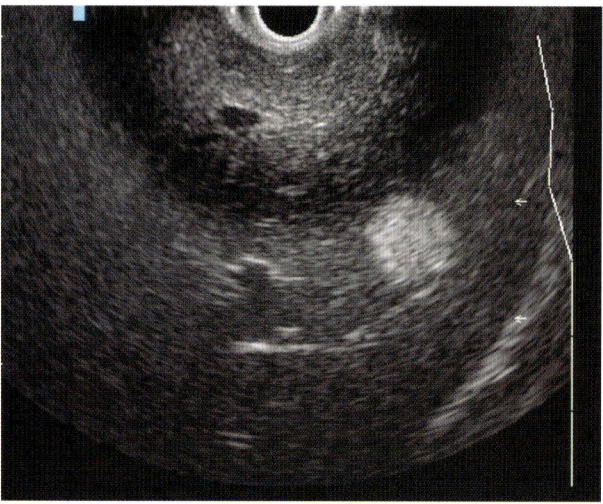

FIGURE 26–4. The image shows a classic, well-circumscribed hyperechoic (bright) round structure in the liver parenchyma consistent with a hemangioma.

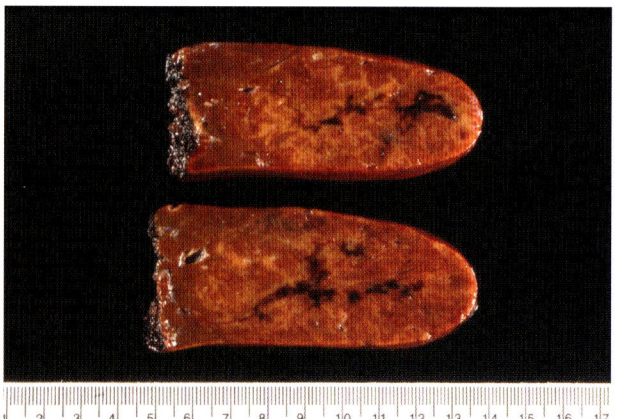

FIGURE 26–7. Liver cell adenoma. A fleshy, unencapsulated mass with patchy hemorrhage.

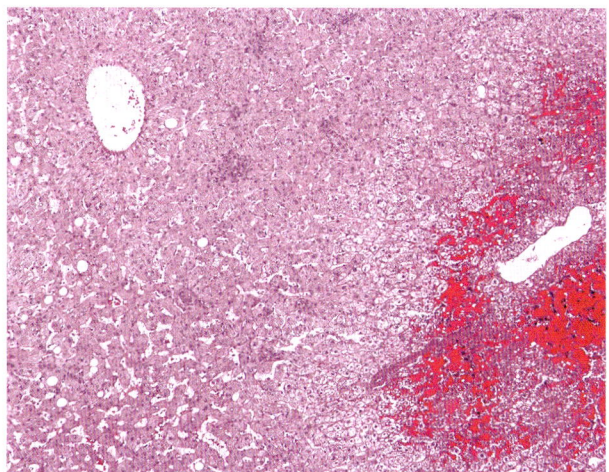

FIGURE 26–8. Liver cell adenoma: Benign hepatocytes arranged in thin cords, with interspersed thin-walled vessels and focal hemorrhage.

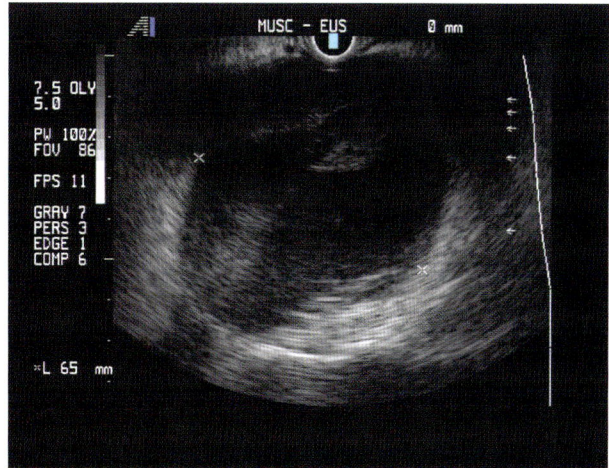

FIGURE 26–10. The EUS image reveals a large, 6 cm lesion, which is primarily anechoic (black) with some internal echos likely due to debris within the cyst.

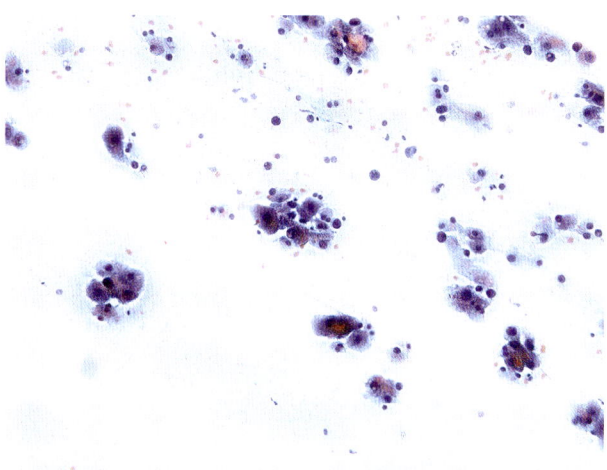

FIGURE 26–9. Liver cell adenoma. Smear shows scattered benign hepatocytes.

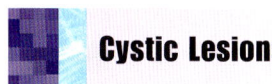

Cystic Lesions

Cystic lesions of the liver may be congenital or acquired. Congenital cysts include solitary bile duct cysts, polycystic disease, Caroli's disease, and ciliated foregut cysts. Aspirate smears from these cysts usually contain clear fluid with few benign cuboidal-to-columnar epithelial cells. Presence of ciliated cells is characteristic of ciliated foregut cysts.[8,9,10]

Acquired cystic lesions include abscesses, hematomas, hydatid cysts, and neoplastic cysts—including cystadenomas and cystic metastases. FNA specimen from an abscess contains acute inflammatory cells and necrotic debris. Specimen from a hepatobiliary cystadenoma shows extracellular mucin and benign mucinous epithelium. Clinical suspicion of a hydatid (echinococcal) cyst is usually a contraindication for FNA due to the risk of an anaphylactic reaction. When aspirated the diagnostic finding is the presence of scolices and hooklets.[8] (Figure 26–10).

Presence of cytologic atypia in a cystic lesion suggests a neoplastic cyst, and raises the possibility of high-grade dysplasia or malignancy. Cystic metastases reveal malignant cells, the appearance of which depends on the type of primary tumor.[10,11]

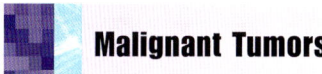

Malignant Tumors

Hepatocellular Carcinoma

Hepatocellular carcinoma (HCC) is a malignant tumor arising from hepatocytes. Overall it constitutes 70–80% of all primary hepatic malignancies, the remaining being mostly cholangiocarcinomas. The incidence of HCC varies significantly in geographic distribution, with most cases occurring in developing regions of the world, such as Asia and Africa. This variation is ascribed to the differences in incidence of risk factors, including hepatitis B virus infection and exposure to aflotoxin in developing countries, and alcohol and hepatitis C infection in developed countries. It is more common in males. Most (70–90%) HCCs arise in a background of cirrhosis, and a minority (10%) of cirrhotic livers develop HCC.[11,12]

Histologically, HCCs show malignant hepatocytes that are most commonly arranged in trabeculae. The trabeculae are usually more than two cells thick and lined by endothelial cells. Morphologic variations

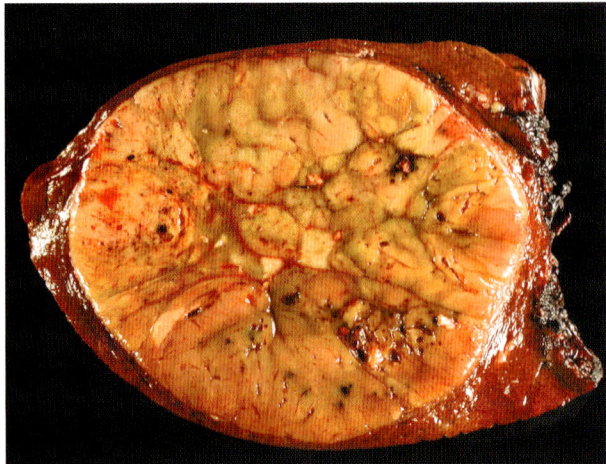

FIGURE 26–11. Hepatocellular carcinoma, forming a fleshy lobulated mass.

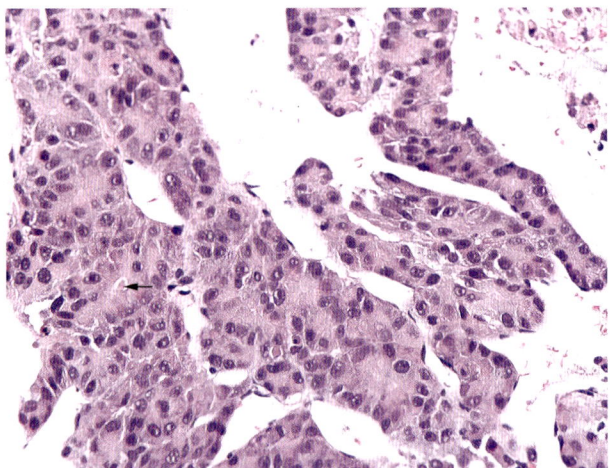

FIGURE 26–12. Hepatocellular carcinoma. Section of FNA cell block showing a trabecular pattern and prominent nucleoli. Focal canalicular bile is present (arrow).

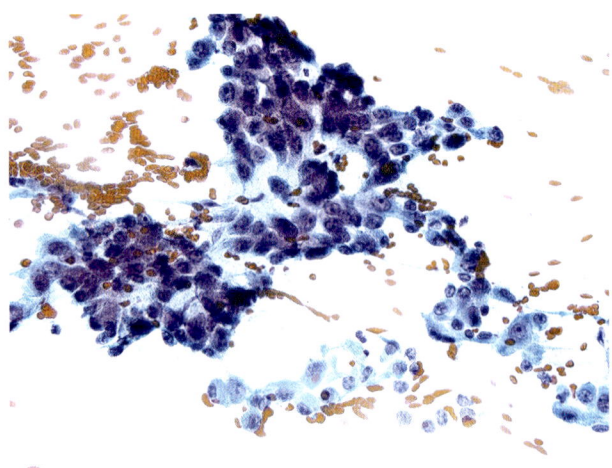

FIGURE 26–13. Hepatocellular carcinoma. Smear shows polygonal-to-round malignant cells with prominent nucleoli.

include pseudoacinar (pseudoglandular), clear cell, sarcomatoid, and small cell types. These variations may be seen within the same tumor. Cellular alterations seen in benign hepatocytes can also be seen in HCCs, including fatty change, cytoplasmic globules, Mallory's hyaline, and ground glass-type change (HBsAg negative). Iron and lipofuscin pigments are largely absent in HCCs. Bile production by the malignant cells may occur, and this feature is diagnostic of HCC.

A narrow-gauge FNA biopsy usually provides sufficient material for diagnosis of HCC. However, in patients clinically suspected to have HCC and who are candidates for resection or transplantation, FNA is not recommended to avoid tumor spread prior to surgery. FNA smears of well-to-moderately-differentiated HCC's are cellular and contain polygonal cells with increased nuclear-cytoplasmic ratio and prominent nucleoli. A trabecular arrangement may be evident when groups or sheets of cells are present. Other cytologic features described earlier may also be seen on smears. Typical cytologic appearance may not be seen in poorly differentiated tumors or those with variant morphology.[8,11,12,13] (Figures 26–11, 26–12, 26–13)

Fibrolamellar Hepatocellular Carcinoma

Fibrolamellar HCC is a rare variant of HCC that usually arises in noncirrhotic livers of adolescents or young adults. Women are more commonly affected, and there is no association with underlying liver disease. Similar to focal nodular hyperplasia, a central scar may be present. The tumor is histologically and cytologically characterized by large polygonal cells with abundant granular eosinophilic cytoplasm and prominent nucleoli. Intracytoplasmic globules and ground glass type inclusions ("pale bodies") may be present. The cells are arranged in trabeculae, and the intervening stroma shows lamellar fibrosis in which collagen is laid down in parallel strands.[11,14]

Intrahepatic Cholangiocarcinoma

Intrahepatic cholangiocarcinoma (ICC) is a malignant tumor composed of cells resembling those of the bile ducts, arising from any portion of intrahepatic bile ducts. ICC is the second-most common primary hepatic malignancy (15–20%), after HCC. These tumors arise in elderly patients, without a gender predilection. Etiologic associations include inflammatory bowel disease, parasites (*Opisthorchis viverrini* and *Clonorchis sinensis*), recurrent pyogenic cholangitis with hepatolithiasis, fibropolycystic

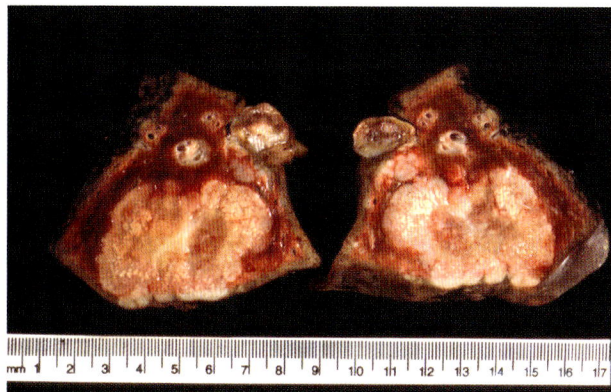

FIGURE 26–14. Intrahepatic cholangiocarcinoma, forming a fleshy nodular mass.

liver diseases, and exposure to Thorotrast.[11] (Figure 26-14)

Histologically, most cholangiocarcinomas are adenocarcinomas with tubular and/or papillary appearance. The neoplastic cells are cuboidal, columnar, or pleomorphic, and may contain mucin. Abundant fibrous stroma may also be present. Uncommon variants of ICC include adenosquamous or squamous carcinoma, mucinous carcinoma with abundant extracellular mucin, signet ring cell carcinoma, and sarcomatoid carcinoma.[11,12,15]

FNA smears are variably cellular depending on the degree of sclerosis in the tumor. The cytologic features are those of adenocarcinoma, with disorderly groups or sheets of cells. There is crowding, loss of nuclear polarity, irregular nuclei, and prominent nucleoli. The cytoplasm is delicate, and intracellular mucin may be evident. Findings corresponding to the variant phenotypes may be present.[8]

The morphologic features of ICC are similar to adenocarcinomas arising at other sites, with closest resemblance to those arising in the extrahepatic biliary tract and pancreas. Thus metastatic adenocarcinoma cannot be excluded on the basis of histologic or cytologic appearance alone, and diagnosis of ICC is made in the appropriate clinical setting.[10,13]

Combined Hepatocellular and Cholangiocarcinoma

Combined hepatocellular and cholangiocarcinoma is defined as a tumor containing unequivocal elements of both hepatocellular and cholangiocarcinoma that are intimately mixed. These tumors do not include those in which the two tumors are separate, even if close to each other ("collision tumors"). These tumors are rare, and the histologic and cytologic findings of the combined tumors are those of HCC and ICC[16].

Lymphoma

Primary lymphoma of the liver is defined as an extranodal lymphoma arising in the liver, with the bulk of the disease localized to this site. Primary lymphomas are rare; most are B-cell phenotype and usually occur in middle-aged white males. Primary hepatosplenic T-cell lymphomas almost always occur in young males.

Most primary hepatic lymphomas are diffuse, large B-cell type, expressing pan B-cell markers CD20 and CD79a (Figures 26–15, 26–16). Other uncommon primary lymphomas include Burkitt lymphoma and low grade B-cell lymphoma of mucosa-associated lymphoid tissue (MALT). Histologically, large-cell lymphoma is composed of sheets of large cells with large nuclei and prominent nucleoli. FNA smears are cellular, with loosely dispersed, large lymphoid cells.

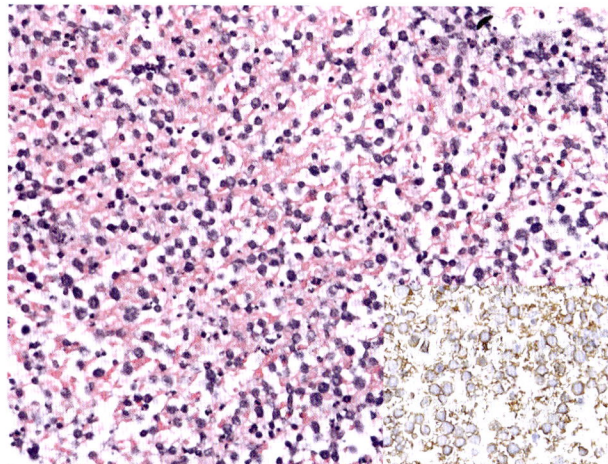

FIGURE 26–15. Large B-cell lymphoma. Section of FNA cell block with large atypical lymphoid cells. Tumor cells are positive for CD20 (inset).

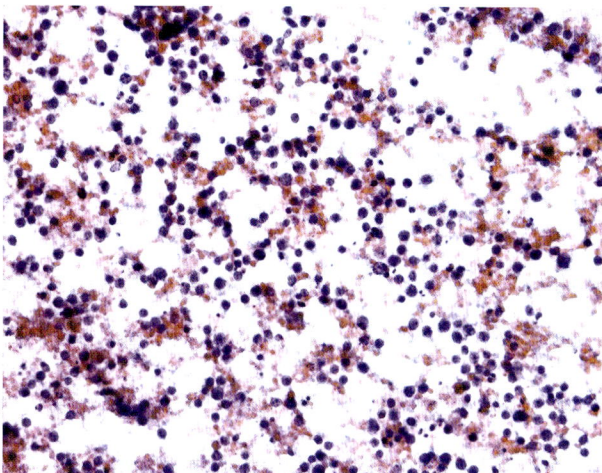

FIGURE 26–16. Large-cell lymphoma. Smear shows loosely dispersed large, atypical cells.

In contrast to primary lymphomas, secondary involvement of the liver is frequent, occurring in up to 20% of Hodgkin and non-Hodgkin lymphomas at presentation, and 55% at autopsy. The liver is also involved in 80–90% patients with chronic leukemia, and approximately 30% patients with myeloma.[11,17,18]

Epithelioid Hemangioendothelioma

Epithelioid hemangioendothelioma is a malignant vascular tumor of variable clinical course, ranging from indolent to aggressive. The tumor is more common in females (60%), with a mean age of 47 years. It is usually ill-defined and multifocal, with scattered grey-white lesions ranging from small to large with extensive involvement of the liver. It is characterized by epithelioid or spindle cells that form vascular spaces or grow along preexisting vascular spaces. The tumor typically contains prominent myxoid stroma that undergoes sclerosis as the lesions evolve.

FNA smears are usually hypocellular. Scattered atypical cells are present with epithelioid or spindle cell appearance. Intracytoplasmic vacuoles may be present, representing vascular spaces. Tissue sections are usually necessary to appreciate the characteristic morphology, and special stains may be performed to confirm the endothelial nature of the neoplastic cells.[8,11,19]

Angiosarcoma

Angiosarcoma is a high-grade, malignant vascular neoplasm that has an aggressive clinical course. It is more common in males, with a peak incidence in the fifth to sixth decades of life. The tumor is typically large, often involving almost the entire liver. Grossly, the tumor shows fleshy grey-white to hemorrhagic areas, including cavitating areas filled with blood. The cells of angiosarcoma can vary from spindle-shaped to round, and epithelioid to multinucleated. Mitoses are frequently seen. In addition to forming a dominant mass, the tumor cells also grow along preexisting vascular spaces. Like epithelioid hemangioendotheliomas, tissue sections and special stains are usually necessary to confirm the diagnosis.[8,11,20]

Metastatic (Secondary) Liver Tumors

In Europe and North America, metastatic tumors in a noncirrhotic liver are 30–40 times more common than primary tumors. However, in cirrhotic livers, primary tumors (mostly HCC) are approximately three times more common. Similarly, in some parts of Asia and Africa, primary tumors are more common due to the high incidence of hepatocellular carcinoma, shorter lifespan, and lower incidence of certain extrahepatic tumors. Although EUS is not typically used as the primary modality for detection of liver metastates, any patient undergoing EUS staging of upper GU and pancreatobiliary tumors should also undergo careful examination of the liver during EUS. Suspicious lesions can be safely sampled with EUS guided FNA. The typical apperance of liver metastates on EUS is shown in Figure 26–18.

The majority of metastatic tumors are carcinomas, followed by lymphomas. For carcinomas, the order of frequency in the Western population is: upper gastrointestinal tract and pancreas (44–78%), colon (56–58%), lung (42–43%), breast (52–53%), esophagus (30–32%), and genitourinary tract (24–38%). Metastases are often multiple and may appear long after the primary tumor has been removed. Histologic and cytologic features are those of the primary tumor, the most common being adenocarcinoma or non-small-cell cancer (Figures 26–17 - 26–24). Comparison with the original tumor and immunohistochemical stains may be helpful in determining the origin of the tumor. The most common metastatic sarcoma is a gastrointestinal stromal tumor (Figures 26–25 - 26–27), which can be identified by positive staining for KIT (CD117) in the appropriate clinical setting. Metastatic melanoma (Figures 26–28, 26–29) may contain melanin pigment; however, amelanotic melanomas can mimic other tumor types, such as carcinoma or sarcoma.[10,11] Other tumors include small-cell carcinoma (Figures 26–30, 26–31) and low-grade neuroendocrine tumors (Figures 26–32 - 26–34).

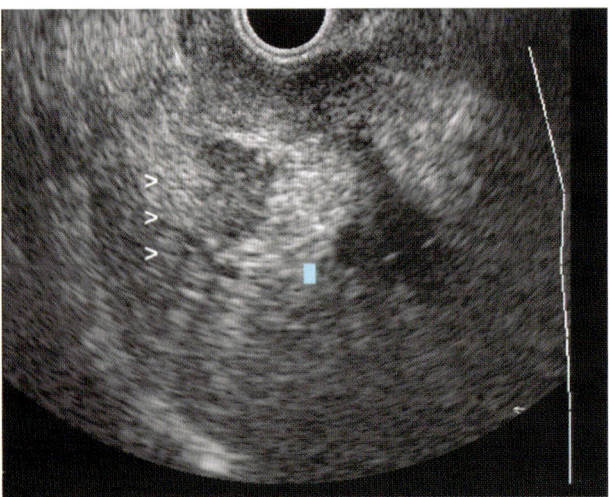

FIGURE 26–17. EUS image shows a complex lesion with mixed (hypo, hyper, and iso) echoic features, and irregular border within the liver parenchyma in a patient with a history of colon cancer. Fine needle aspiration confirmed adenocarcinoma.

Liver Lesions 295

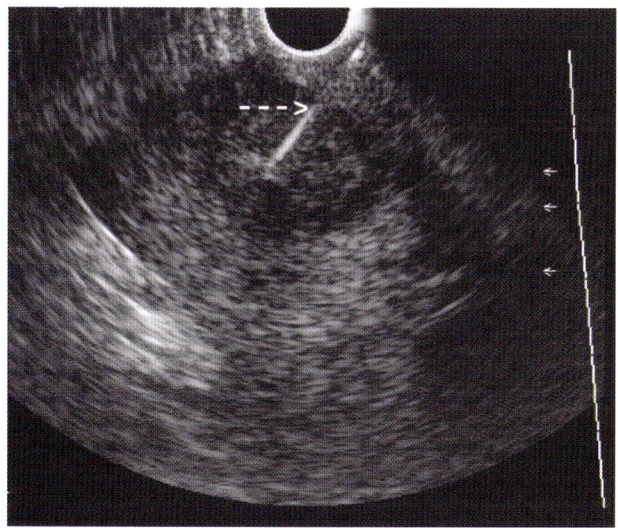

FIGURE 26–18. EUS showing a hypoechoic, irregular tumor within the liver parenchyma, biopsied in Figure 26–18.

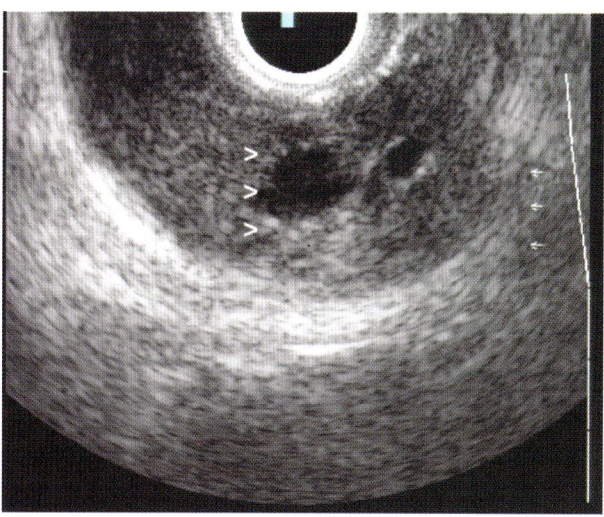

FIGURE 26–20. EUS showing hypoechoic lesion with FNA revealing non-small-cell carcinoma consistent with a lung primary.

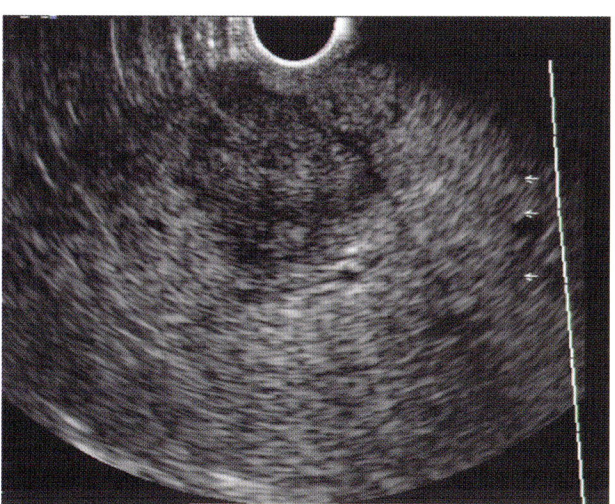

FIGURE 26–19. EUS-guided fine needle passing into the tumor (arrows). FNA confirmed metastastic pancreas cancer.

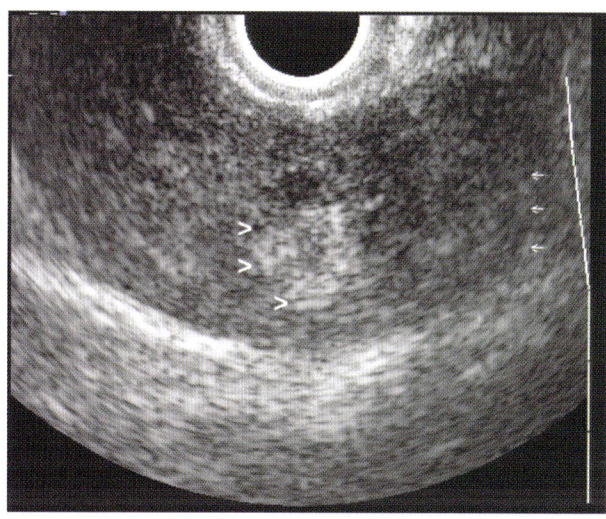

FIGURE 26–21. EUS showing mixed echotexture. Fine needle aspiration confirmed non-small-cell carcinoma consistent with a lung primary.

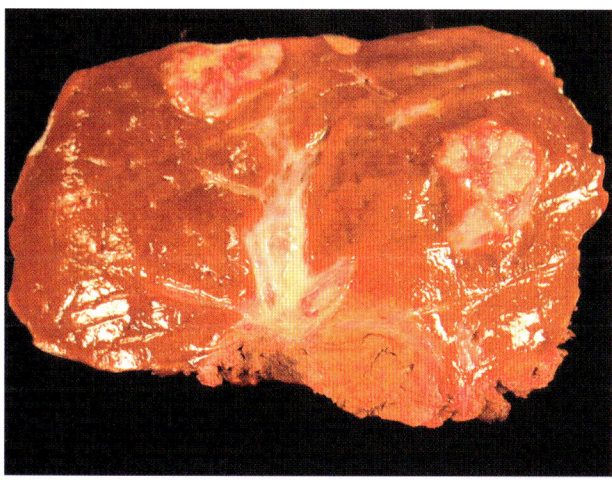

FIGURE 26–22. Metastatic colonic adenocarcinoma. Multiple tumor nodules are present, with central necrosis.

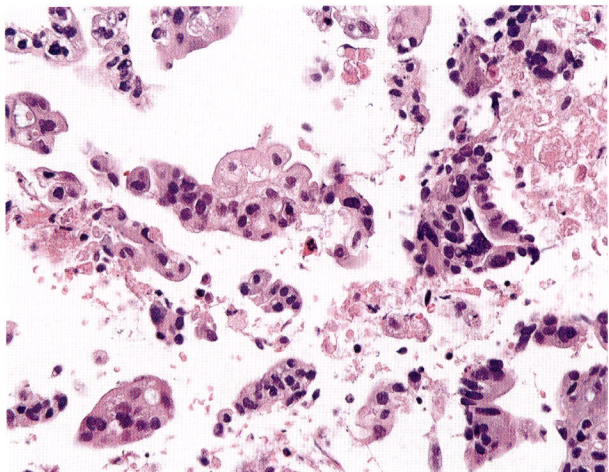

FIGURE 26–23. Adenocarcinoma. FNA cell block with malignant glandular epithelium.

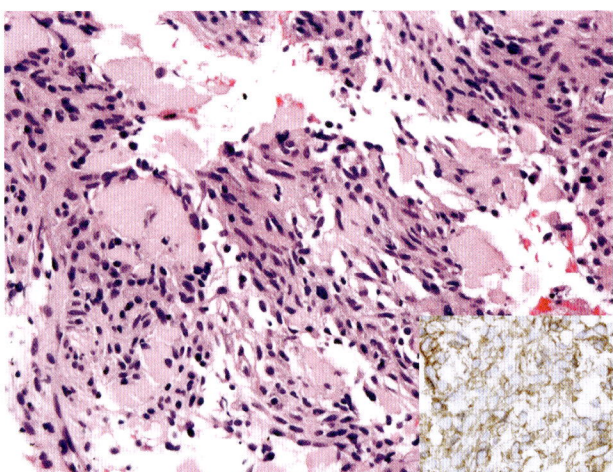

FIGURE 26–26. Metastatic gastrointestinal stromal tumor. Section of FNA cell block showing the typical spindle cell morphology. Tumor cells are positive for KIT (inset).

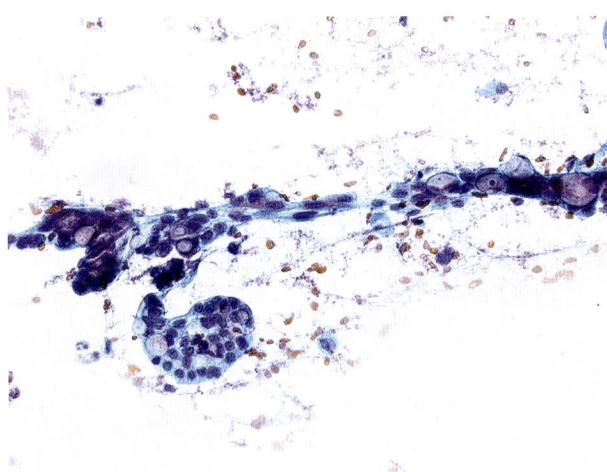

FIGURE 26–24. Adenocarcinoma. Smear shows malignant glandular epithelium with staining to highlight cytoplasmic mucin.

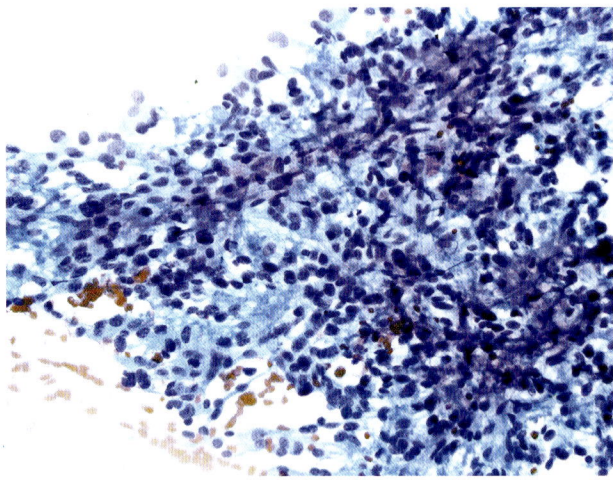

FIGURE 26–27. Metastatic gastrointestinal stromal tumor. FNA smear showing round-to-elongated tumor cells.

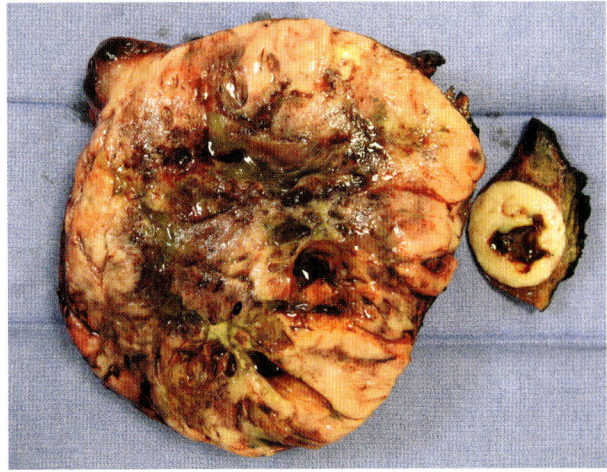

FIGURE 26–25. Metastatic gastrointestinal stromal tumor. A fleshy mass with areas of necrosis.

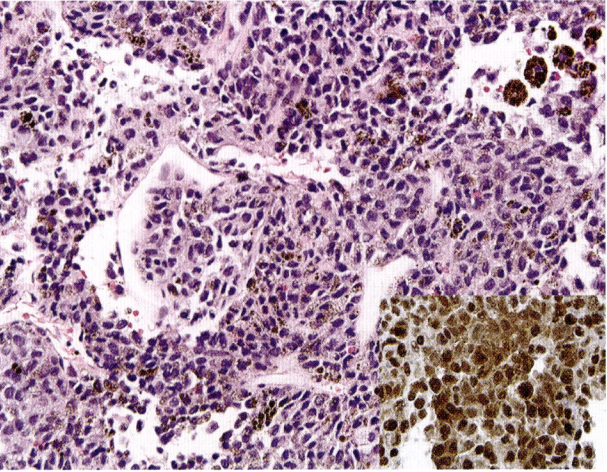

FIGURE 26–28. Metastatic melanoma. Section of FNA biopsy showing abundant melanin pigment within the tumor. Tumor cells are positive for S-100 protein (inset).

Liver Lesions 297

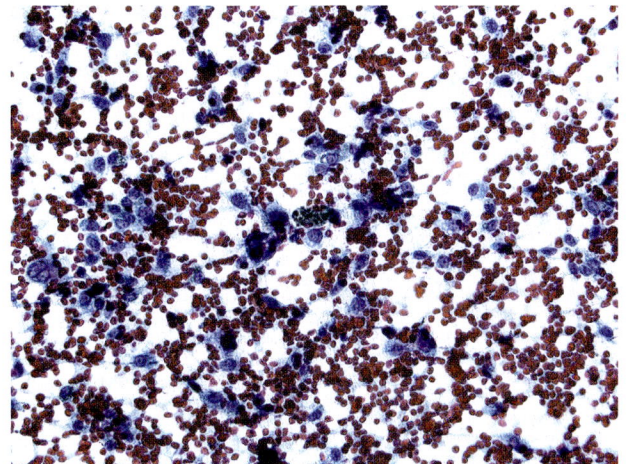

FIGURE 26–29. Metastatic melanoma. FNA smear with tumor cells containing melanin pigment.

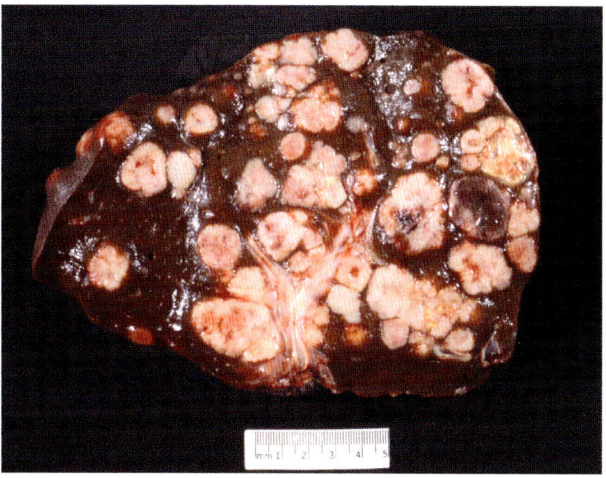

FIGURE 26–32. Metastatic carcinoid tumor, forming multiple nodules.

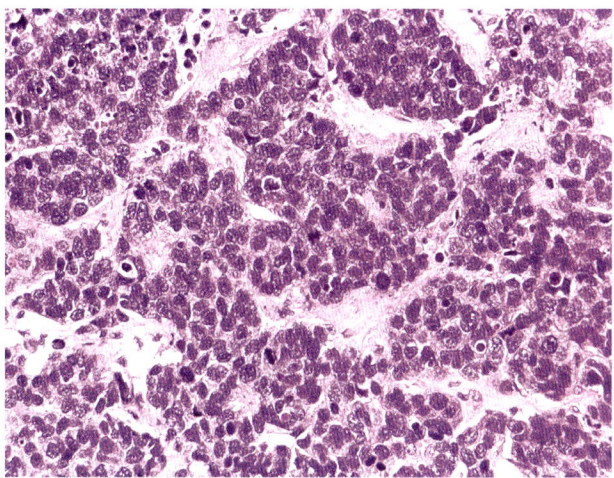

FIGURE 26–30. Small-cell carcinoma. Compact nests and cords of cells with scant cytoplasm. Mitoses are easily seen.

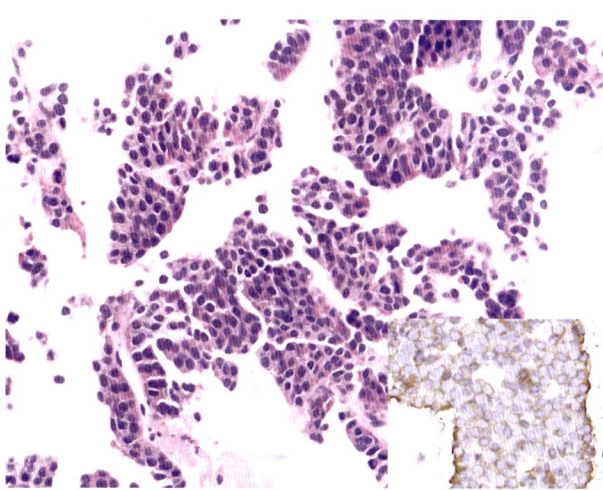

FIGURE 26–33. Metastatic carcinoid tumor. Section of FNA cell block showing cells with a trabecular arrangement and mild atypia. Tumor cells are positive for chromogranin (inset).

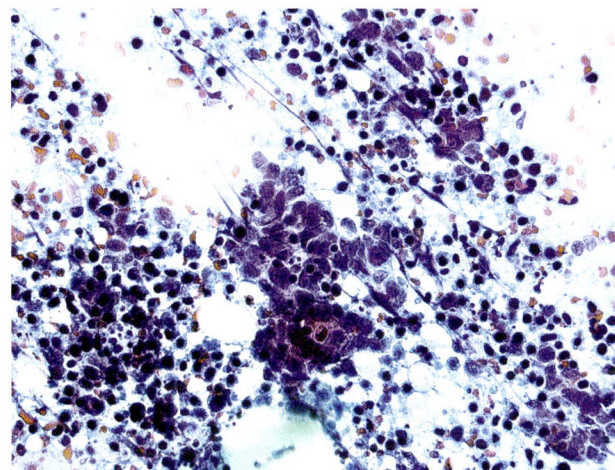

FIGURE 26–31. Small-cell carcinoma. FNA smear showing tumor cells with characteristic nuclear molding and background necrosis.

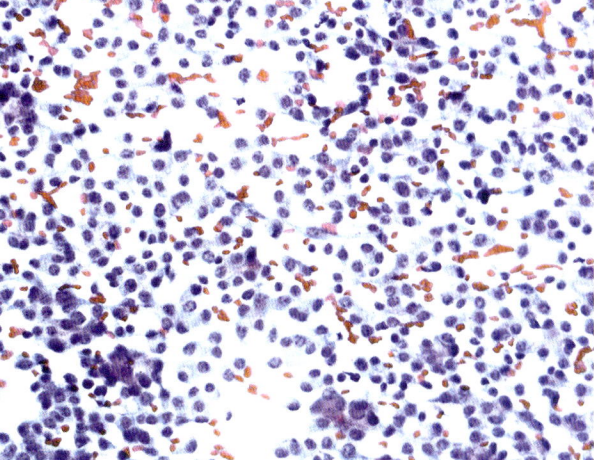

FIGURE 26–34. Metastatic carcinoid tumor. FNA smear showing a uniform population of cells with mild atypia. The nuclei are round with finely stippled chromatin.

References

1. DeWitt, J., LeBlanc, J., McHenry, L. et al.: Endoscopic Ultrasound-Guided Fine Needle Aspiration Cytology of Solid Liver Lesions: A Large Single-Center Experience. Am J Gastroenterol 2003; 98:1976–1981.
2. Hollerbach, S., Willert, J., Topalidis, T., et al.: Endoscopic Ultrasound-Guided Fine-Needle Aspiration Biopsy of Liver Lesions: Histological and Cytological Assessment. Endoscopy 2003; 35:743–749.
3. Caturelli, E., Rapaccini, G. L., De Simone, F. et al.: UIltrasound-guided fine-needle biopsy in the diagnosis of hepatic hemangioma. Liver 1986; 6(6):326–330.
4. Bioulac-Sage, P., Balabaud, C., Bedossa, P., et al.: Pathological diagnosis of liver cell adenoma and focal nodular hyperplasia: Bordeaux update. J of Hepatol 2007; 46: 521–527.
5. Lizardi-Cervera, J., Cuellar-Gamboa, L., Motola-Kuba, D.: Focal nodular hyperplasia and hepatic adenoma: A Review. Annals of Hepatol 2006; 5(3): 206–211.
6. Shiraki, K., Makino, Y., Sugimoto, K.: Multiple microhamartomas of the biliary tract system: von Meyenberg complexes. Clin Gastroenterol Hepatol 2006; 4(5):xxxii
7. Zheng, R. Q., Kudo, M., Onda, H., Inoue, T.: Imaging findings of biliary hamartomas. World J Gastroenterol 2005; 11(40):6354–6359.
8. DeMay, R. M.: The Art and Science of Cytopathology. Vol 2. Chicago: ASCP Press, 1996: 1017–1052.
9. Kanel, G. C., Korula, J.: Atlas of Liver Pathology 2nd ed. Philadelphia: Elsevier Saunders, 2005.
10. Ishak, K. G., Goodman, Z. D., Stocker, J. T.: In Rosai, J., Sobin, L. H. eds.: Atlas of Tumor Pathology: Tumors of the Liver the Liver and Intrahepatic Bile ducts. Third Series. Washington, D.C.: Armed Forces Institute of Pathology, 2001.
11. Hamilton, S. R., Aaltonen, L. A., eds.: World Health Organization Classification of Tumors. Pathology and Genetics of Tumors of the Digestive System. Lyon, France: IARC Press, 2000;157–202.
12. Goodman, Z.: Neoplasms of the liver. Modern Pathology 2007; 20: S49–60.
13. Das, D. K.: Cytodiagnosis of Hepatocellular Carcinoma in Fine-Needle Aspirates of the Liver: Its Differentiation From Reactive Hepatocytes and Metastatic Adenocarcinoma.. Diagn Cytopathol 1999; 21:370–377.
14. Jain, M., Niveditha, S. R., Bharadwaj, M., et al.: Cytological features of fibrolamellar variant of hepatocellular carcinoma with review of literature. Cytopathology 2002; 13:179–182.
15. Nakajima, T., Kondo, Y., Miyazaki, M., et al.: A histopathologic study of 102 cases of intrahepatic cholangiocarcinoma. Hum Pathol 1988; 19: 1228–1234.
16. Goodman, Z. D., Ishaq, K.G., Langloss, J. M. et al.: Combined hepatocellular-cholangiocarcinoma. A histologic and immunohistochemical study. Cancer 1985; 55: 124–135.
17. Sans, M., Andreu, V., Bordas, J. M., et al.: Usefulness of laparoscopy with liver biopsy in the assessment of liver involvement at diagnosis of Hodgkin's and non-Hodgkin's lymphoma. Gastrointest Endosc 1998; 47: 391–395.
18. Chim, C. S., Choy, C., Ooi, C. G., et al.: Hodgkin's disease with primary manifestation in the liver. Leuk Lymphoma 2000; 7:629–632.
19. Uchimura, K., Nakamuta, M., Osoegawa, M., et al.: Hepatic epithelioid hemangioendothelioma. J. Clin Gastroenterol 2001; 32:431–434.
20. Saleh, H. A., Tao, L. C.: Hepatic angiosarcoma: aspiration biopsy cytology and immunohistochemical contributions. Diagn Cytopathol 1998; 18: 208–211.

CHAPTER 27

Splenic Lesions

Dr. Annette Fritscher-Ravens
Dr. Theodoros Topalidis

The spleen is not a target generally attempted by endoscopic ultrasound (EUS). Mass lesions and focal abnormalities affecting the spleen are also relatively infrequent.[1,2] If a lesion is detected by computed tomography (CT) or transabdominal ultrasound (US), the possible benign and malignant diseases causing the abnormality are numerous. Therefore, the differential diagnosis of splenic lesions may even be of greater consequence in relation to disease management than the diagnosis of tumors in other locations within the abdomen.[3] However, although it is generally possible to image splenic lesions with CT and US, it should be noted that abnormalities with densities similar to the normal splenic parenchyma can occur and may then not be easily visible.[4,5,6] This is also true for visualization with EUS. Even if lesions are identified with any of the imaging modalities described previously, neither the echomorphology nor the density can determine the cause of the abnormality—the underlying disease.[2,4,6] This makes tissue sampling for diagnosis critically necessary. Figure 27–1A shows a Visible Human Model of the stomach, spleen, splenic artery, and splenic vein. A coronal cross-section is shown in Figure 27-1B. The proximity of the spleen to the stomach is evident, as well as the large blood vessels that comprise the splenic vasculature.

CT- or US-guided fine needle aspiration (FNA) or biopsy are safe in general. But biopsies of smaller lesions (Figures 27–2, 27–8), those adjacent to the splenic hilum, (Figure 27–4) or those without sufficient surrounding splenic tissue to protect the puncture site (Figures 27–5, 27–10) can be very difficult and sometimes even dangerous[7,8] (Figure 27–12). These and other issues such as possible clotting disorders, general fear of bleeding, and injury of possible interfering organs such as the colon have resulted in caution and antipathy to tissue sampling techniques of the spleen in some countries. Occasionally, diagnostic splenectomy is performed to achieve a necessary tissue diagnosis.[9-11]

EUS provides easy access to the spleen and can avoid some of the possible problems involved when percutaneous tissue sampling techniques are used. Real-time, guided EUS-FNA enables visualization of possible interfering vessels or detection of any structure within the pathway of the biopsy needle. It also allows sampling of lesions as small as 3 mm in size (Figure 27–2A). Although lesions found in the distal part of the spleen can be quite far away from the echoendoscope, resulting in a long needle pathway with a difficult target to aim, if small (Figures 27–2F, 27–8F), the actual organ is in close proximity to the echo-endoscope, and interfering structures are rare.

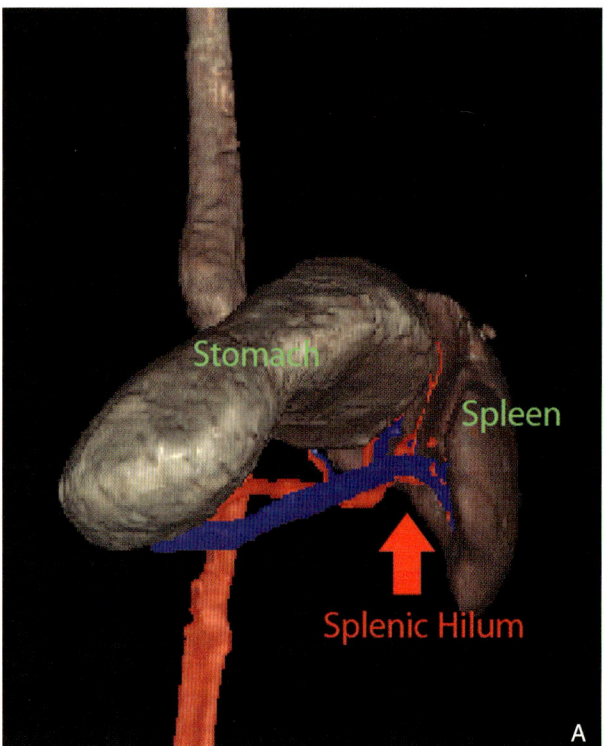

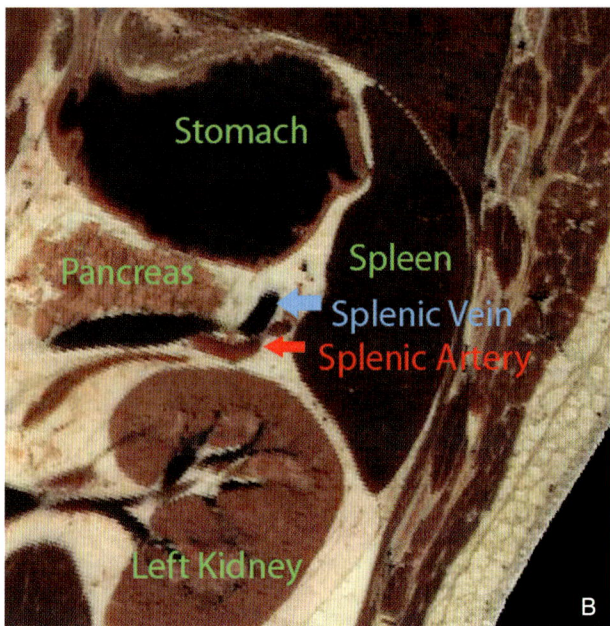

FIGURES 27–1. *A and B* (A) Visible Human Model showing the relation of the stomach to the spleen, splenic hilum, and major splenic vascularity (B) Coronal cross-section of the Visible Human Data showing the relation of the stomach to the spleen and major splenic vessels.

EUS-FNA allows cell sampling for cytology. Although the literature of this technique involving the puncture of the spleen is scarce, it enables characterization of solid focal splenic lesions for more efficient and effective management.[12,13]

This following overview of lesions and associated pathologies available to date may help endosonographers in their attempt to diagnose solid splenic lesions. Advantages and limitations of EUS-FNA will be discussed, including potential pitfalls in diagnosis.

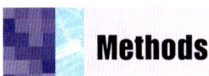
Methods

All of our previously published[12] and unpublished EUS-FNA procedures of the spleen were performed with 22-gauge needles, and only cytology obtained. Tru-cut or larger than 22-gauge needles for histological sampling were not used.

If bacterial infection could not be excluded, which was the case in most of the lesions detected, an additional puncture was performed for microbiological examination and culture.

Prophylactic antibiotics were only given if the patient had potential abscess formation suspected by pus within the needle aspirate, congenital cardiac defect, or cardiac valve replacement.

Smears of the aspirated material were air dried and sent for independent cytological review. All samples were stained using the May Gruenwald Giemsa staining method. A modified Papanicolaou classification was used for cytological differentiation of benign and malignant diseases.[14] Differentiation of

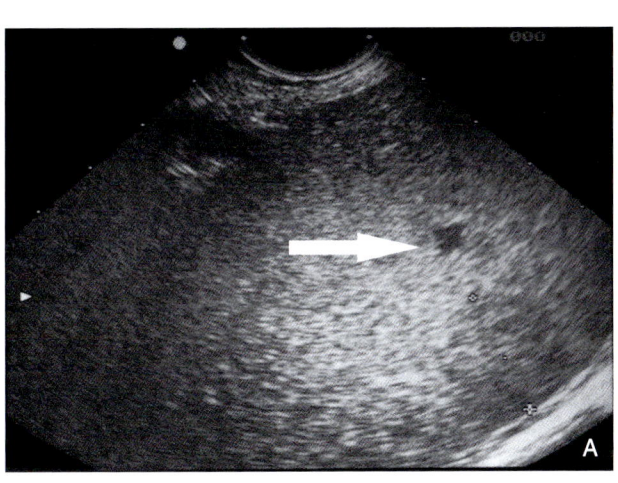
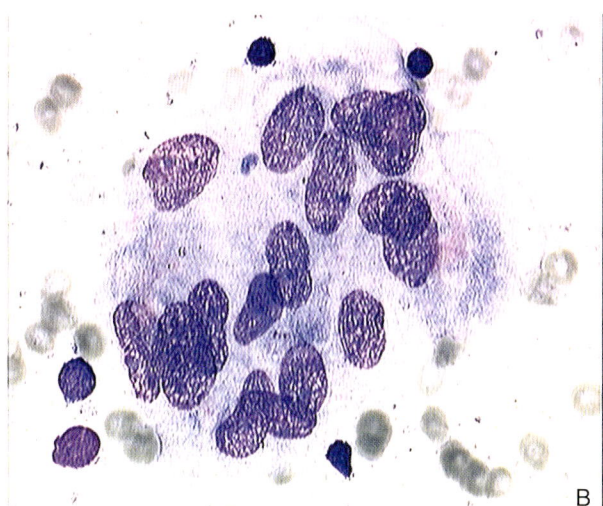
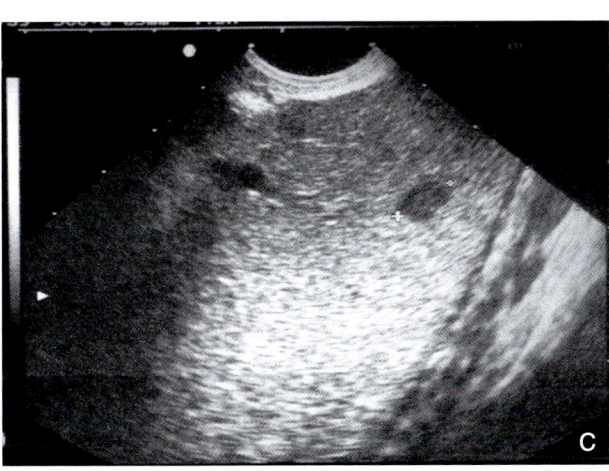
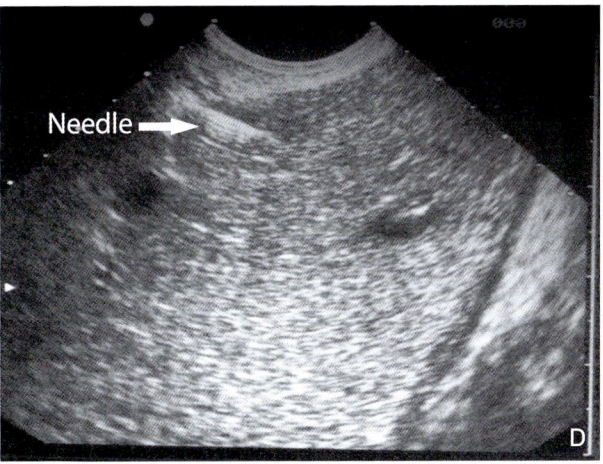

FIGURES 27–2. *A to D* (A) Tiny 2–3 mm echo-poor lesion in the spleen, which might be mistaken as a vascular structure (B) Cytology of FNA of Figure 27–1A shows epitheloid cell granuloma on a dirty background, suggestive of tuberculosis (C) 8 mm, well-defined, echo-poor lesion in the spleen (D) Fine needle aspiration of lesion from Figure 27–2C. The needle has to overcome a long path of about 7cm. This can be difficult if a small lesion of less than 1 cm has to be targeted.

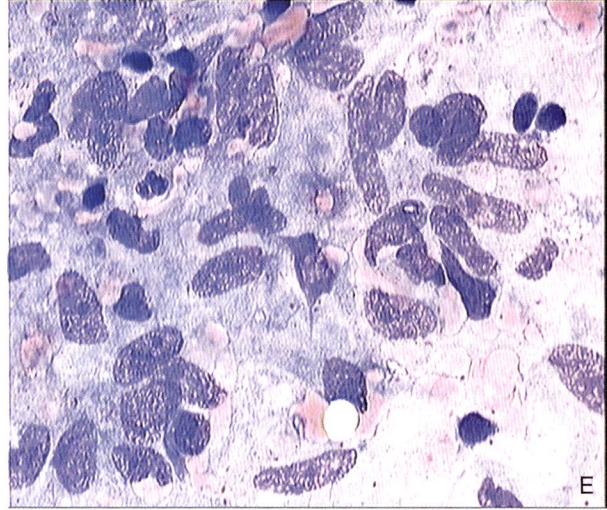

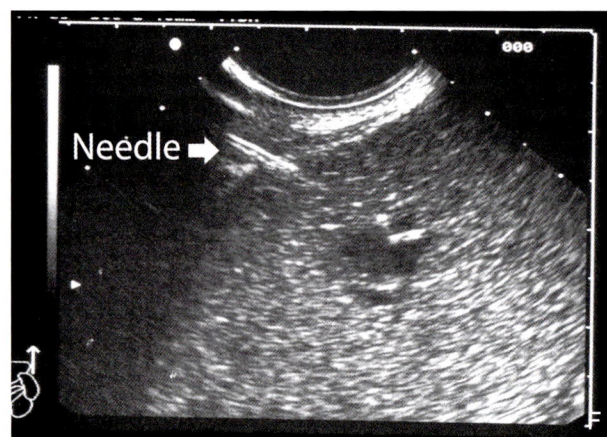

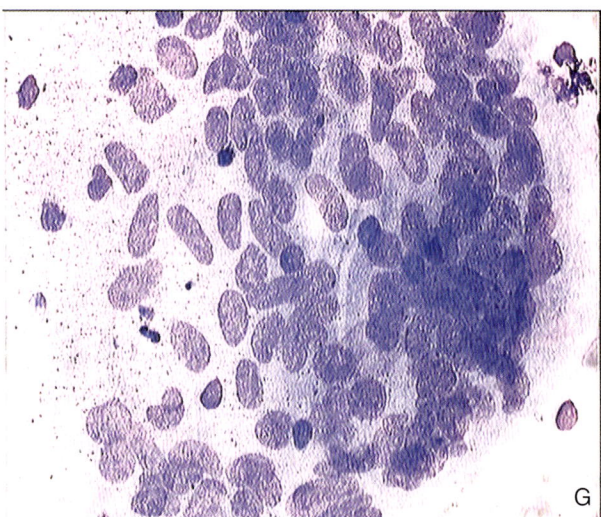

FIGURES 27–2. *E to G* (E) Fine needle aspirate of Figures 27–2C, 27–2D shows epitheloid cells on a dirty background, which represents cell detritus and protein precipitate. No intact granuloma seen. This cytology was suggestive of TB despite missing granulomata. Additional culture of aspirate proved tuberculosis. (F) Fine-needle aspiration of a 1 cm, well-demarcated lesion in the spleen. The location is less far from the gastric wall, enabling a shorter needle path. (G) Cytology shows one large epitheloid cell granuloma on a dirty background, in keeping with tuberculosis.

adenocarcinomas of different origins, such as gastric or colonic cancer, was possible using a combination of staining, evaluation of tumor markers in the cells, and immunocytochemical tests. Bacteriology tests included microscopy, culture, and sensitivity of the aspirated material.

Endoscopic ultrasound imaging of the spleen can be obtained after the echo-endoscope is placed into the subcardial area by turning the instrument anticlockwise, when the diaphragm and liver is in view. Its upper pole can be found in close proximity to the gastric wall. Color Doppler ultrasonography should be used to exclude the presence of any vessel lying in the path of the needle. It is especially useful when a lesion in the area of the splenic hilum is targeted. In this case it is necessary to rotate the endoscope into a position, where the hilum is out of the direct needle pathway.

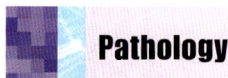 **Pathology**

With endoscopic ultrasound, appearances of the lesions of different diseases can look very much alike, which makes it impossible to even predict the underlying disease with any degree of certainty. In general, however, it can be said that any echo-poor lesion can represent benign as well as malignant pathology, and it is less probable that an echorich, well-defined lesion is of malignant etiology.

In this chapter the EUS images of the benign and malignant splenic foci will be shown next to the cytology results obtained by the EUS-guided fine-needle aspiration. In many cases, the images provided in this chapter may not meet the quality expected of published figures, as they were not specifically taken to be published and several have suffered damage.

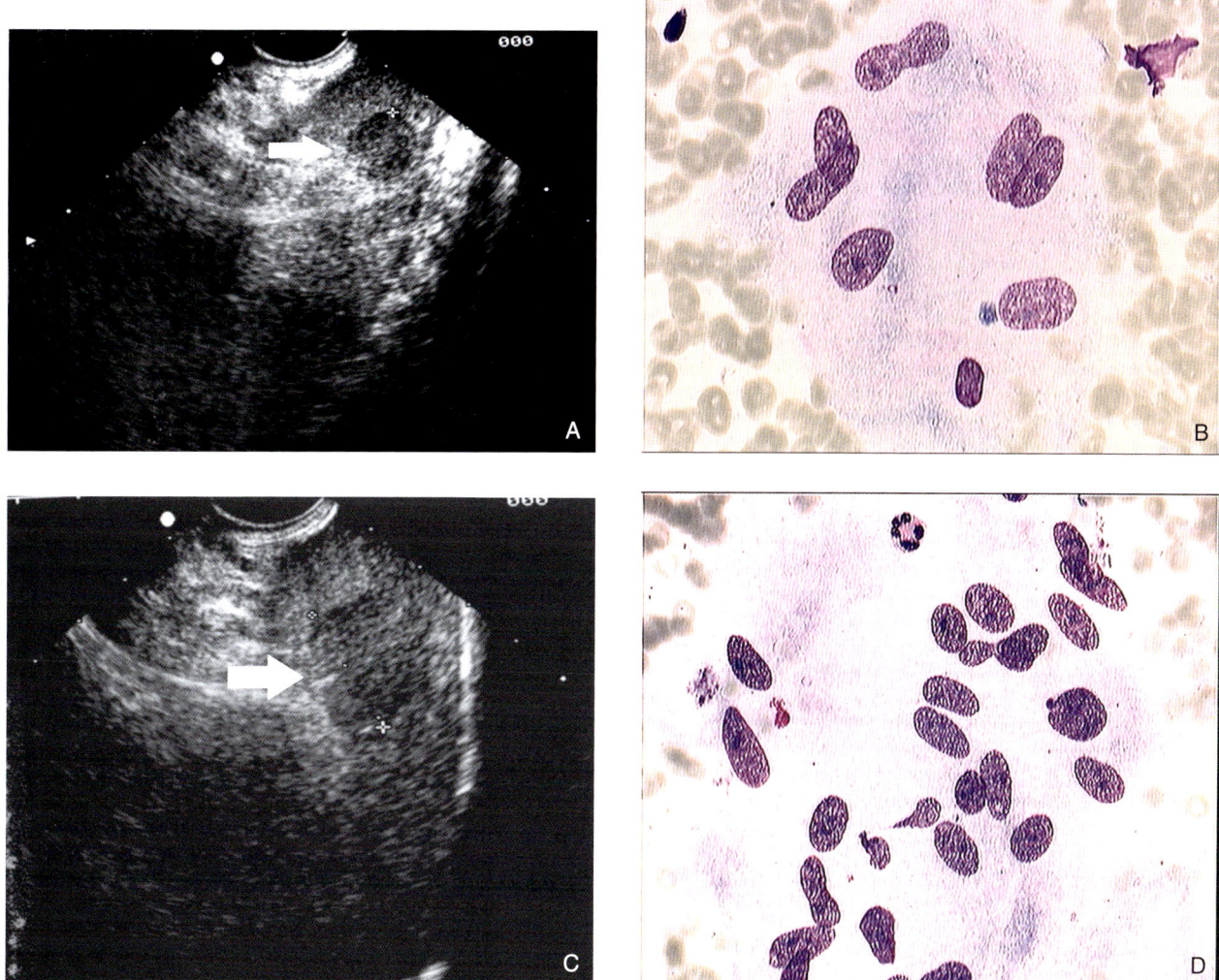

FIGURES 27–3. A to D (A) Echo-poor, round and well-demarcated 1.4 cm lesion in the spleen. Other such lesions can be imagined below this one, focused upon. (B) Fine-needle aspiration shows epitheloid cell granuloma on a clean background. Additional culture was negative. This kind of setting is in keeping with sarcoidosis. (C) 2 cm echo-poor lesion (D) Cytology of FNA from Figure 27–3C showing an epitheloid cell granuloma with clear background. Additional cultures were negative. Diagnosis: sarcoidosis.

Benign Splenic Lesions

Benign abnormalities of the spleen seen on EUS include tuberculosis (TB) (Figure 27–2) and sarcoidosis. (Figure 27–3). Both diseases are represented by single but mostly multiple echopoor well-defined, round foci. The size may vary from very tiny, of 2–3 mm shown in Figure 27–2A, to much larger, prominent echo-poor and well-defined configurations. The appearance of both diseases in echomorphology as well as in cytology is very similar. Some cytological criteria may make tuberculosis rather than sarcoidosis more likely. Such criteria for differential diagnosis include the presence of a "dirty" versus "clean" background. The "dirty" background represents cell detritus and protein precipitate. They can be found, when bacteria break up and are pathognomonic for tuberculosis. Further details for cytological differential diagnosis of both diseases are described elsewhere.[15] Whenever one of these diseases is suspected, additional FNA for bacteriology is strongly advisable. In all cases presented in this chapter, in addition to cytology, the tuberculosis was proven by positive results of mycobacterial cultures from the FNA material. In our experience from mediastinal FNA, it seems, however, not possible to obtain positive mycobacterial cultures with FNA in more than 50–70% of cases.

Possible abscess formation (Figures 27–4A, 27–4B), which can be similar in endoscopic ultrasound appearance to TB and sarcoidosis, might also need additional FNA for bacteriology, not only for proof of

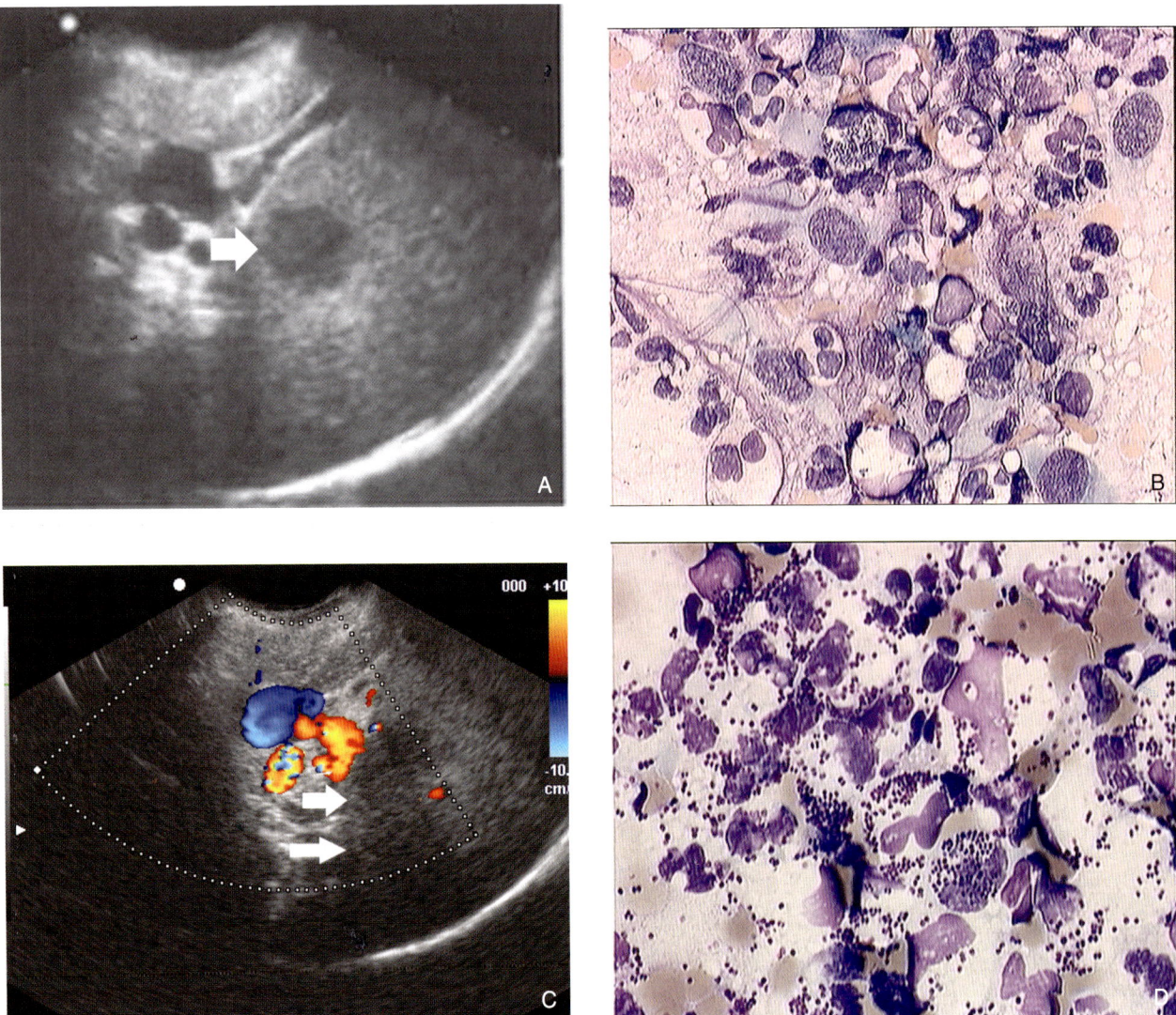

FIGURES 27-4. *A to D* (A) 1.4 cm vague, echo-poor lesion near the splenic hilum (Figure 27–2, reference 12). (B) Multiple, intracellular bacilli within a granulocyte (arrow), also some extracellular bacilli in the background (C) 2 cm echo-poor, ill-defined lesion in close proximity to the splenic hilum (arrows). For FNA the angle of view has to be changed to get the hilar vessels out of the needle pathway (D) Aspirate from lesion in Figure 27–4C shows massive amount of gram-positive cocci. Diagnosis: abscess

infective etiology, which can be achieved by cytology alone, but also for identification of the exact species and sensitivities for treatment. As can be seen in the figures provided, all of the lesions representing tuberculosis, sarcoidosis, and abscess formation are rather echo-poor and can be mistaken for malignant lesions.

Solitary abscesses in the spleen are rather uncommon in the Western world and may be seen more frequently in other geographic areas. In general they appear to present as an echo-poor area, but other than with TB or sarcoidosis and depending on the stage of disease, they may have irregular margins, as can be seen in Figure 27–4C.

Vascular-based abnormalities, such as an infarction, can show a broad variety of appearances, depending on the stage of the disease and how long ago the actual infarction took place. Directly and for a short period after the incident, it is characterized by an echo-poor mass.[6] Later stages of the disease appear as an echo-rich, well-demarcated mass lesions, as can be seen in Figure 27–5.

Vascular lesions, like splenic hemangiomas, (Figure 27–6A) are also rather infrequent and are represented by an echo-rich and well-demarcated focus, which is quite prominent and difficult to overlook. A cavernous haemangioma has been described elsewhere and can be seen to be of more heterogeneous appearance than the lesions shown in the chapter.[6] When fine-needle aspiration is carried out, it is pathognomonic, meaning a large amount of blood is aspirated (Figures 27–6B, 27–6D). Due to the risk of bleeding, it is strongly recommended to avoid biopsy

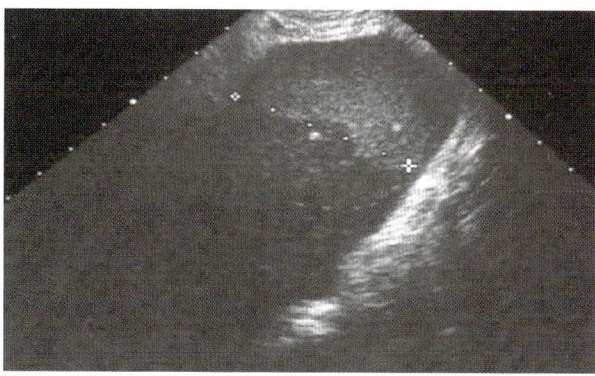

FIGURE 27-5. 2 cm hyperechoic lesion representing an infarction on EUS-FNA and on surgical histology (Reprinted from Fritscher-Ravens A, et al. Am J Gastroenterol 2003;98:1022–1027 with permission from Wiley-Blackwell)

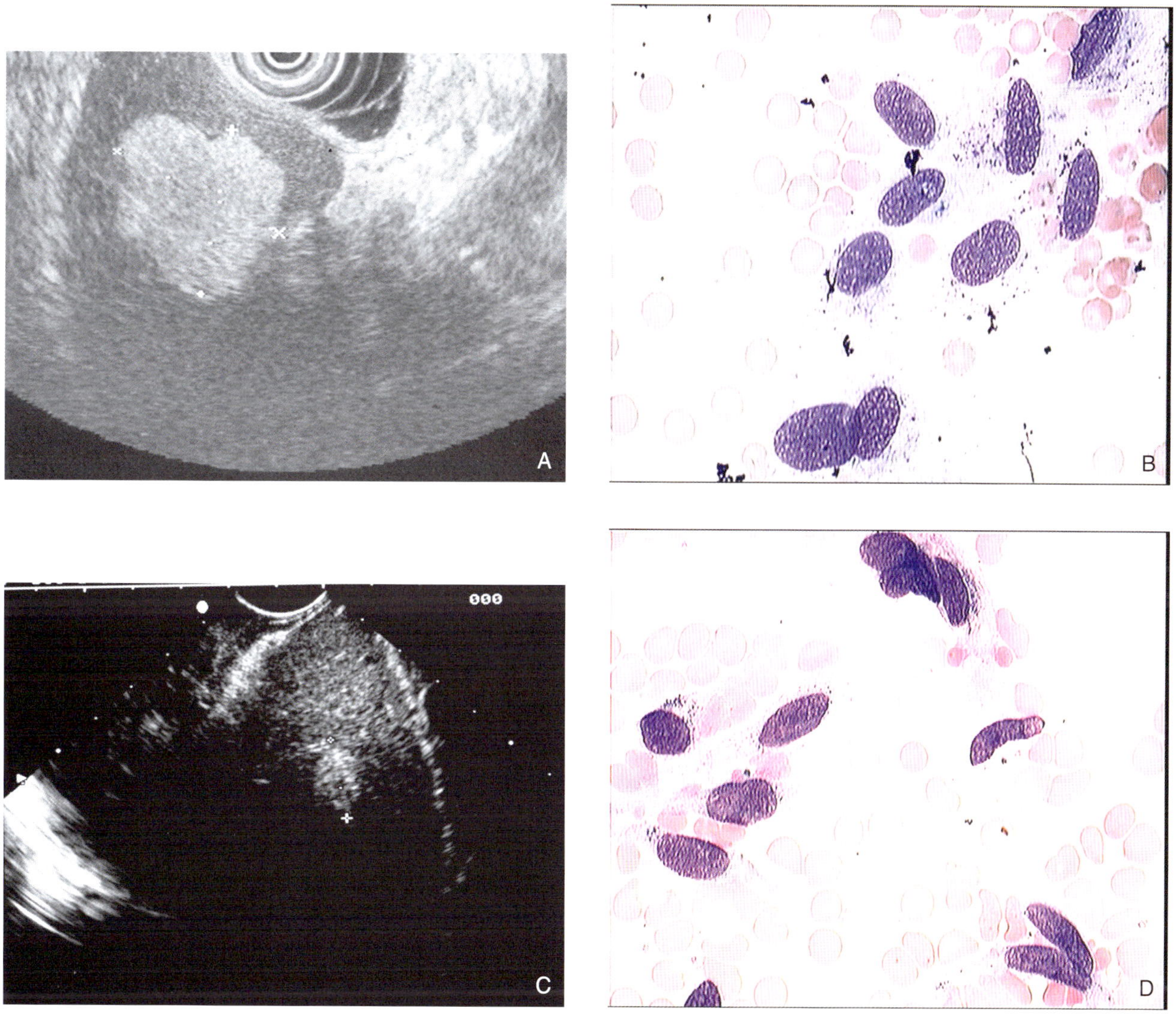

FIGURES 27-6. *A to D* (A) Large, irregular echorich area within the spleen vizualised with radial echoendoscopy. FNA was performed at a prior occasion with linear echoendoscopy. (B) Large amount of erythrocytes and endothelial cells with intracellular pigmantation (siderin), representing a haemangioma (C) Small 1 cm echorich and well-defined area within the spleen. This appearance represents the most frequently found image of a haemangioma. (D) FNA of lesion in Figure 27–6C with many erythrocytes and several endothelial cells with intracellular pigmantation, representing a haemangioma.

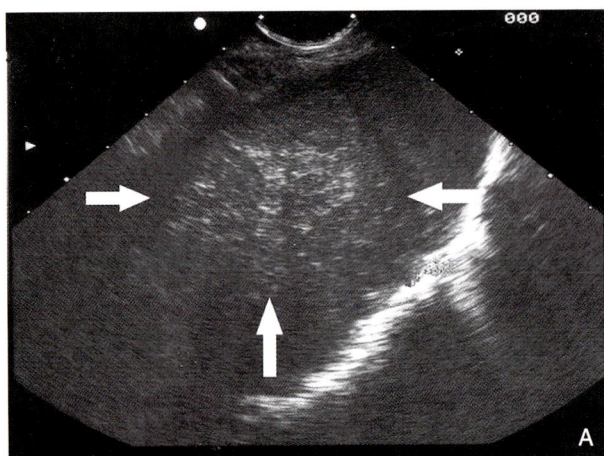
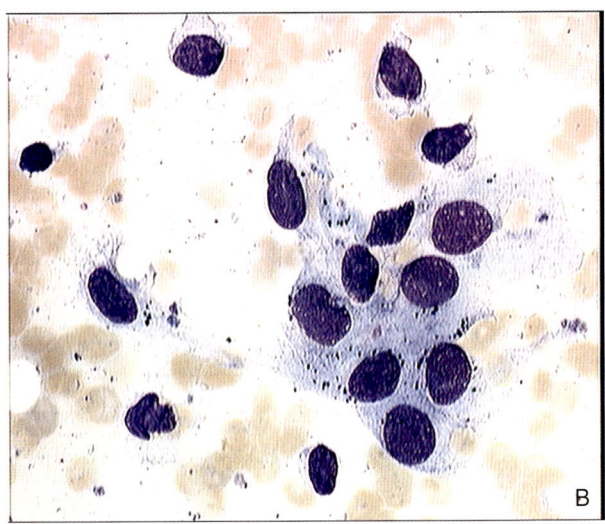

FIGURES 27–7. A and B (A) 3.5 cm inhomogeneous and mainly echo-rich area within the spleen. The lesion itself is well demarcated (arrows) but the echo-rich areas within appear branched out. The general appearance is similar to the haemangioma. (B) Aspirate of lesion in Figure 27–7A shows sinus endothelial cells with tailed cytoplasm and intracellular pigmentation representing a littoral cell angioma.

without splenic tissue to cover the needle path above the lesion in the area of the puncture site.

The rare littoral cell angioma in the red pulp of the spleen is a benign vascular tumor with an unknown natural history. It might be caused by different stimuli such as chronic infection or tumors. It has characteristic cytologic features shown in Figure 27–7B, including sinus endothelial cells with tailed cytoplasm and intracellular pigmentation. In the only case seen by the author, the lesion appeared as a roundish but not well-defined, heterogeneous area within the spleen with varying (echo-rich: isoechoic: echo-poor) but mainly echo-rich echomorphology when compared to the surrounding splenic tissue (Figure 27–7A). Other authors have described multiple such lesions within the spleen similar to this. The presumptive diagnosis might include hemangioma, lymphoma, or even abscess formation.

Malignant Diseases

Malignant diseases of the spleen may include lymphopoetic abnormalities as well as metastasis of various solid tumors. Non-Hodgkin lymphomas are heterogeneous and have a larger variation in appearance than other entities. In general they are represented by single or multiple, sharply demarcated, echo-poor lesions distributed throughout the spleen (Figure 27–8A). Some high-grade aggressive NHL lesions can also appear with rather ill-defined margins. In some cases, a single, small focus can be seen (Figure 27–8C). If this is small and located in a more distant area of the spleen in relation to the echo-endoscope, targeting for FNA can be quite challenging. It can at times also be very challenging to detect the lesions. It was especially difficult to visualize some of the few low-grade NHLs found within the spleen, as their echomorphology appeared to be very similar to the surrounding splenic tissue and the foci were of pale and weak appearance (Figures 27–8E, 27–8G). Some lesions, however, may not differ from the echomorphology of high-grade lymphomas and may present as echopoor foci with well-defined margins.

The EUS images obtained of Hodgkin's disease are similar to most of the NHLs. Imaging with echomorphology alone is not helpful for differential diagnosis, which again makes FNA necessary to obtain a tissue based diagnosis. Multiple echo-poor, mostly well-defined lesions, which are spread throughout and also across the organ, have been diagnosed to be of Hodgkin's disease. Their size can vary; each focus can measure from a few millimetres to about 3-4 cms (Figures 27–9A, 27–9B, 27–9C, 27–9D).

Splenic metastases are infrequent, but can originate from any primary tumor imaginable. Some metastases are easily visible on the EUS image, such as those of small-cell lung cancer (Figure 27–10A) with multiple echo-poor lesions throughout the spleen or that of a gastric primary appearing as a single echo-poor mass in Figure 27–10B. Others, such as the metastases of a colon cancer presented in Figure 27–10C may be hard to visualize, as their appearance can be of similar echogenicity as the surrounding splenic tissue. Some of the filiae have an echo-poor

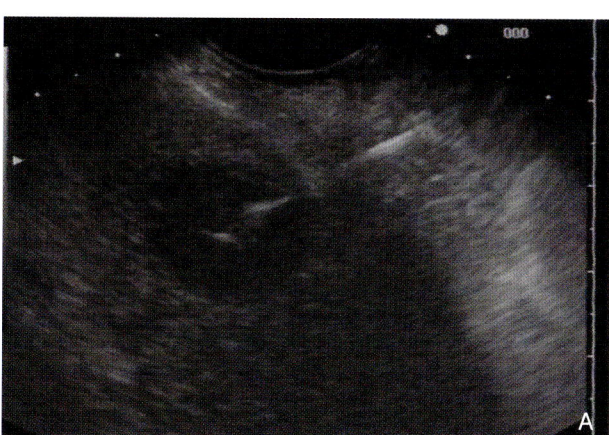
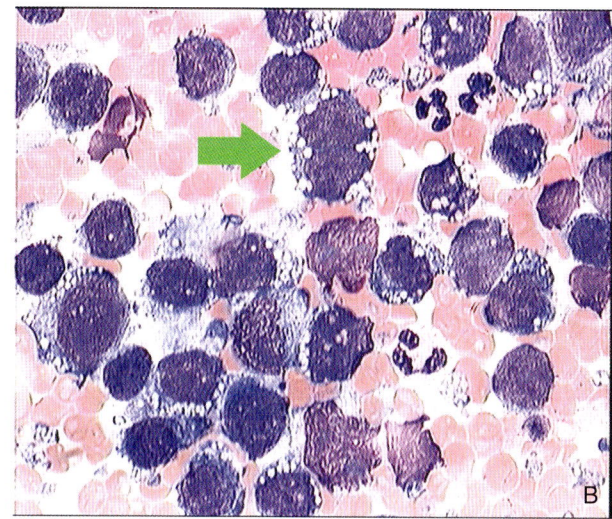
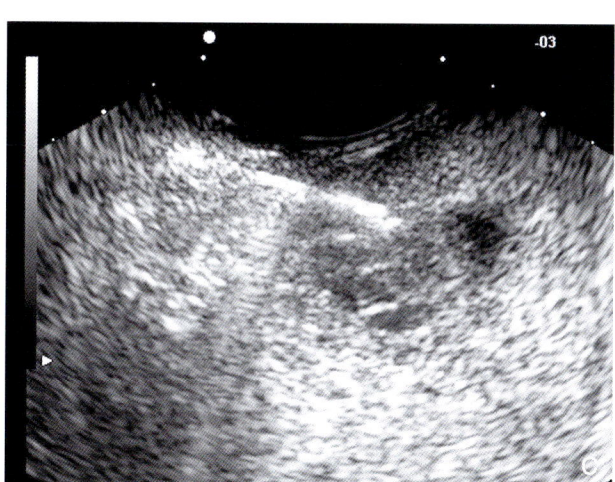
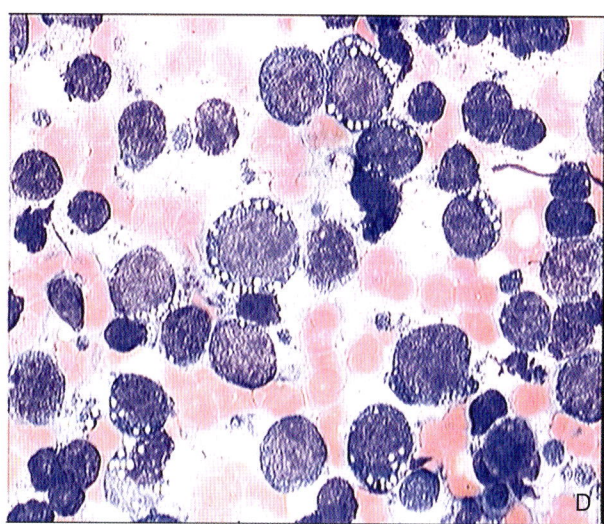
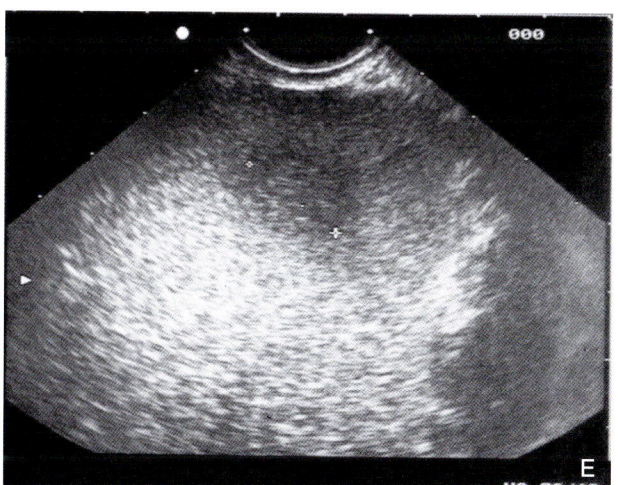

FIGURES 27–8. A to E (A) 1.5 cm echo-poor lesion in the spleen, aspiration revealed large-cell non-Hodgkins lymphoma (Courtesy John Deutsch). (B) Cytology: Diffuse large B-call lymphoma, variant: immunoblastic. Arrow: multinucleated immunoblast with abundant cytoplasm. (C) EUS-FNA of a 2 cm echo-poor, well-defined lesion in the spleen in close proximity to the gastric wall, making the puncture easier than the average long distance FNA of the spleen. Several such lesions were found within the organ. (D) FNA cytology shows diffuse, large B-call lymphoma variant: centroblastic. (E) 1.4 cm rather well-defined echo-poor lesion in the spleen. The appearance is rather pale and weak rather than prominent.

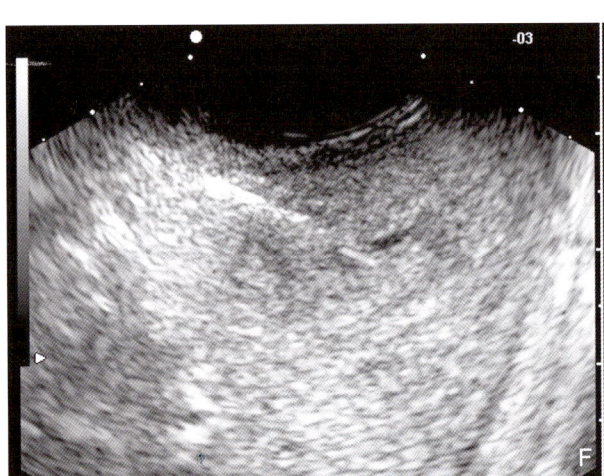
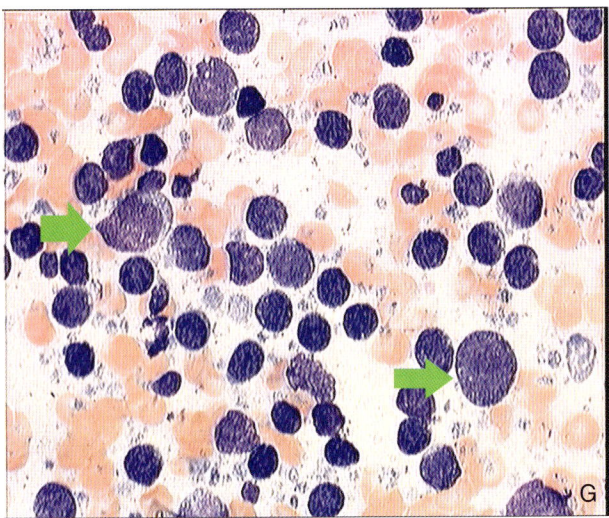

FIGURES 27–8. *F and G* (F) EUS-FNA of the lesion from Figure 27–8E (G) Cytology shows follicular lymphoma (centroctic-centroblastic) represented by multiple centrocytes with a few centroblasts (arrow).

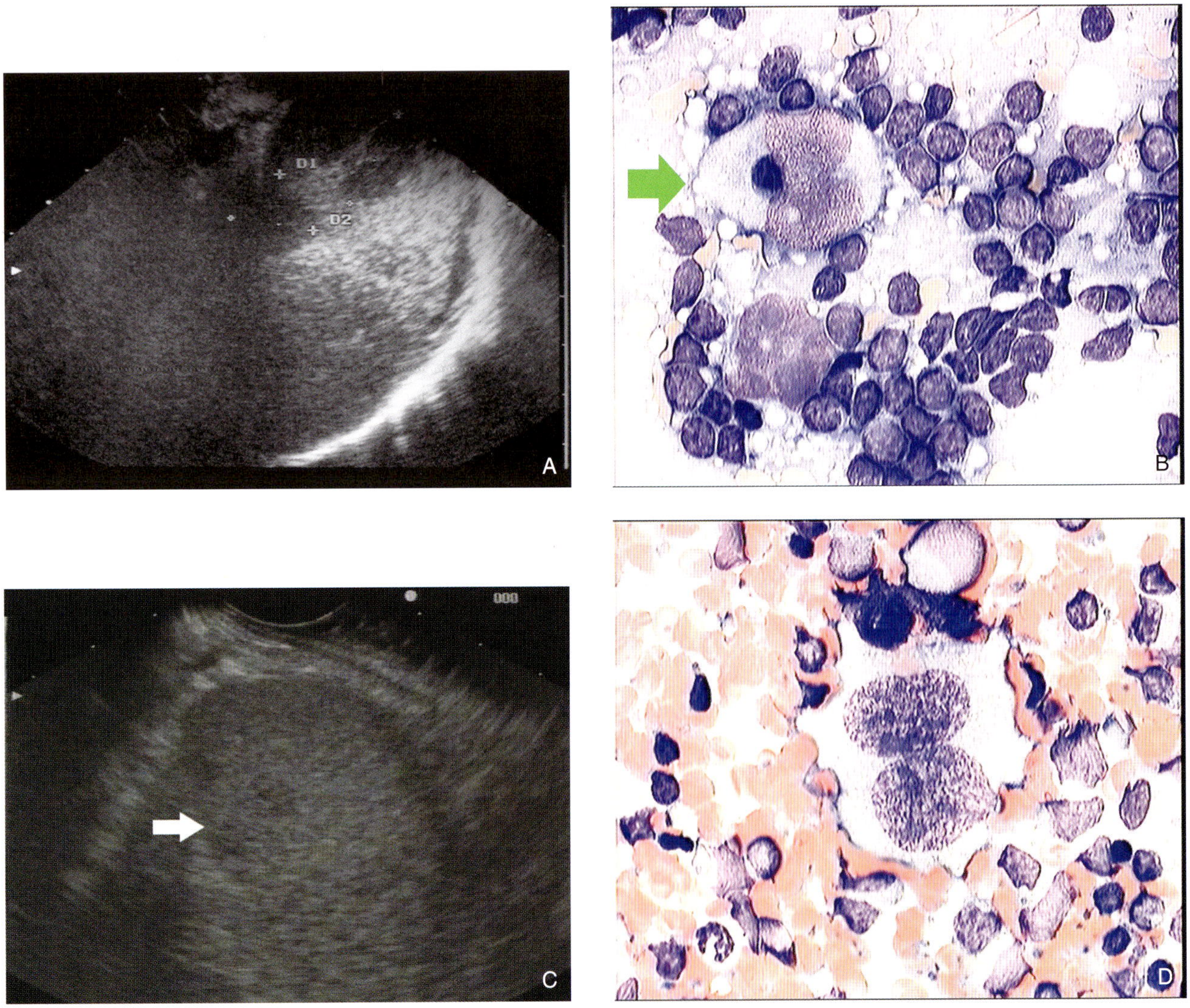

FIGURES 27–9. *A to D* (A) Multiple echo-poor lesions within the spleen of varying sizes. Some foci appear well demarcated, others have rather irregular borders. (B) Cytology of FNA of Figure 27–9A shows a typical Hodgkin's cell (arrow) with Reed Sternberg cell with multiple or multi-lobed nuclei below. (C) Another EUS image of a echo-poor splenic Hodgkin's lymphoma (Courtesy John Deutsch). (D) Hodgkin's cell within larger and smaller lymphocytes and pulp cells representing the spleen.

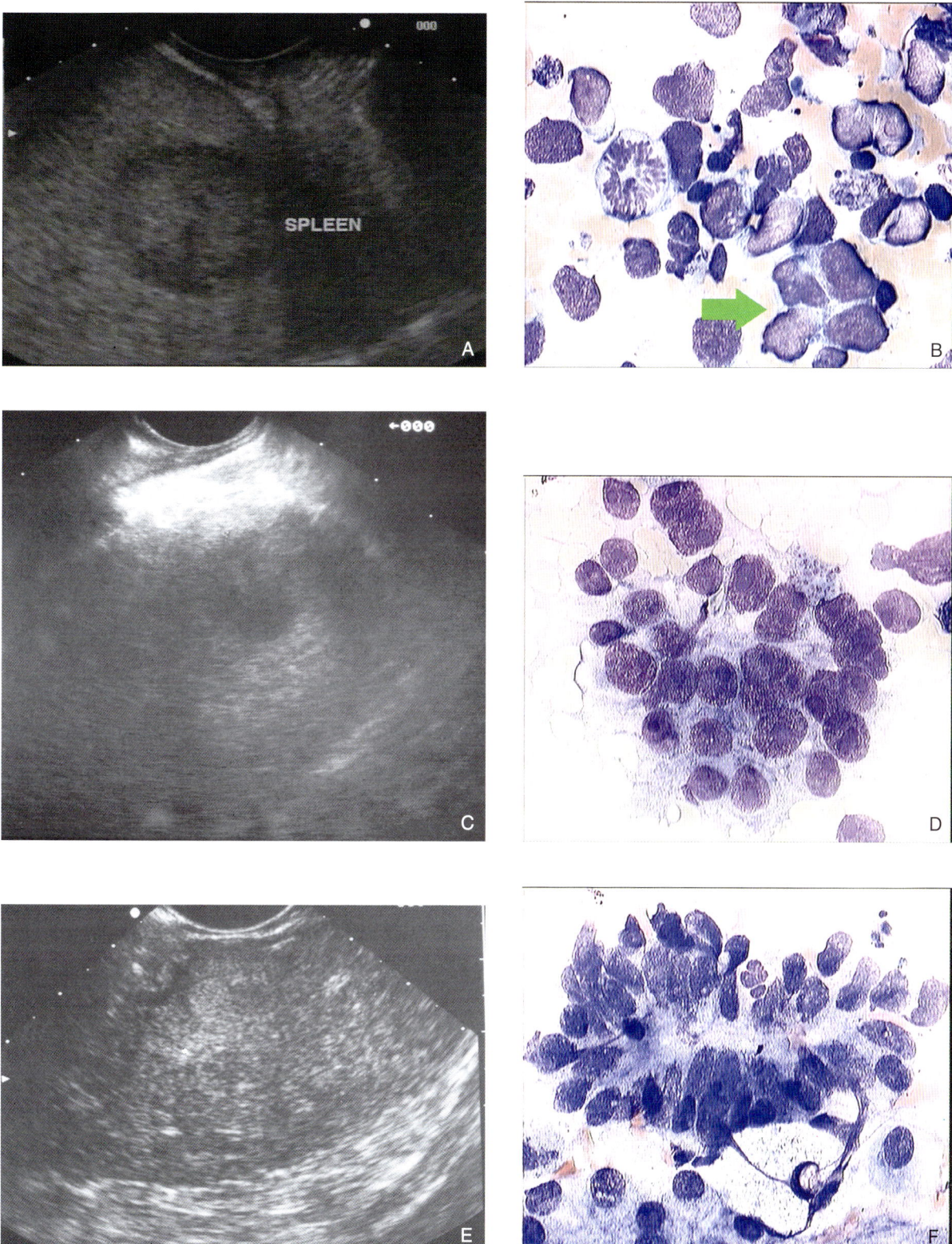

FIGURES 27–10. *A to F* (A) The spleen shows a prominent echo-poor lesion (Courtesy John Deutsch). (B) Cytology proves metastasis of small-cell lung cancer (oat cell type). Typical arrangement of moulding cells (white arrow) and mitotic figure at 9° (black arrow). (C) Single 1 cm echo-poor lesion within otherwise normal-appearing spleen (D) Group of adeno carcinoma cells. According to additional tests (immuno-cytochemistry), this was classified a metastasis of a gastric cancer. (E) The spleen is nearly replaced by multiple, large lesions, which even grow across its margins. The lesions are hard to see as their echomorphology is so similar to the surrounding splenic tissue. Some have a typical echo-poor rim around them. (F) Cytology of Figure 27–10E showing adenocarninoma. The typical morphology with papillary groups and pallisarde arrangement of cells classifies this as a metastasis of colon cancer.

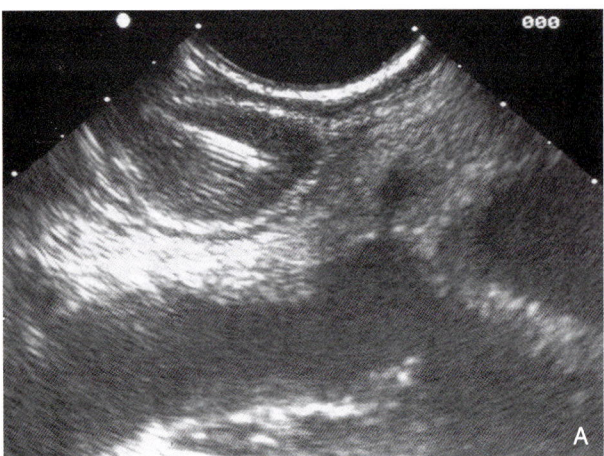 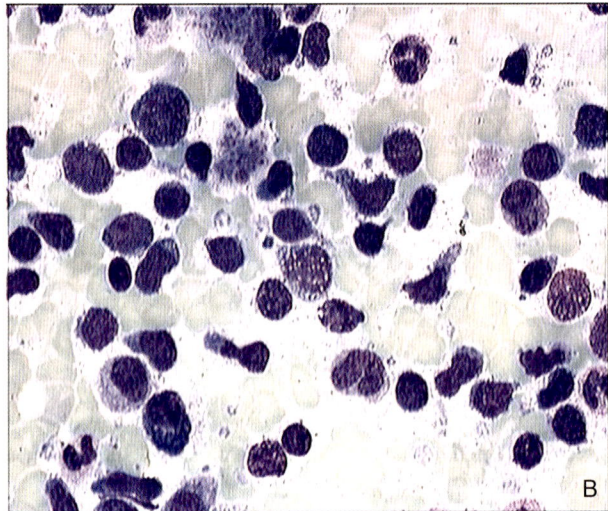

FIGURES 27–11. A and B (A) FNA of echo-poor lesion adjacent to stomach and spleen (B) Histology from the aspiration in Figure 27–10A shows splenic tissue.

rim around them, which can be seen in Figure 27–10F and may hint toward such a disease. This may be of some help for detection and selection of masses suitable for fine-needle aspiration.

Other malignant diseases, which can involve the spleen, may include plasmocytoma and vascular lesions such as hemangiosarcoma. Images, however, are not available to the author.

Accessory Spleen

The possibility of an accessory spleen to be found in various locations of the abdominal cavity should in general not be neglected. Figure 27–11A shows an echo-poor, well-demarcated lesion in close proximity to the gastric wall. It has an echo-poor rim or wall around it and may be mistaken for a GIST tumor, if detected in such a close proximity to the gastric wall as in this case. However, EUS-FNA showed splenic tissue (Figure 27–11B). If not biopsied and/or pulp cells are not found, some such lesions might be mistaken for malignant lesions or GIST tumors.

Conclusion

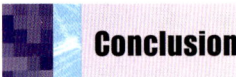

In recent years there has been an increasing use of FNA to establish a diagnosis when focal splenic lesions are identified at US or CT.[3-7,16-19] But only a few reports are available of results using endoscopic ultrasound for fine needle aspiration.[12,13] There have been occasional reports of the use of FNA to obtain a diagnosis of splenomegaly without focal abnormalities.[20]

Percutaneous biopsy has been reported to be safe for obtaining a tissue diagnosis of splenic lesions in more than 1000 patients as early as the 1970s,[21] FNA has never been completely accepted as a routine diagnostic method by the general medical community despite reports of high sensitivity and specificity. In relation to EUS, the reluctance cannot be due to difficulties in assessing the organ or damaging others with the needle. Some may feel that the procedure carries a substantial risk of complications, particularly haemorrhage or rupture, which are thought to be higher when compared to biopsy of other abdominal organs.[18] In published series of percutaneous puncture, the most serious complication include bleeding or rupture and are reported to occur in 0–2.5% of cases.[5,7,19,21] Using EUS, some possible complications can be avoided, as the needle path between the echoendoscope within the stomach and the spleen itself is generally short and does not interfere with other organs. The two publications reporting EUS-FNA in small series of 12 and 6 patients respectively, did not report any complications at all. In our overall experience, very few patients reported some pain for a few hours after the procedure, and one patient had a small intra-splenic haematoma, but no relevant complication occurred.

Limitations with EUS-FNA may include clotting disorders, which make prior and subsequent treatment necessary. Diagnosis of low-grade non-Hodgkin's lymphoma via cytology may not always be reliable or possible. In such cases larger needles should be considered to provide histology, but may result in a higher complication rate. In our limited experience, cytology was valid in about 90% of cases, making EUS-FNA a valuable diagnostic tool for focal splenic lesions.

References

1. Wolf, B. C., Neimann, R. S.: Disorders of the spleen. In: Bennington JL. (ed.). Major problems in pathology. Philadelphia: Saunders, 1989: 5-204.
2. Wan, Y. L., Cheung, Y. C., Lui, K. W., et al.: Ultrasonographic findings and differentiation of benign and malignant focal splenic lesions. Postgrad Med J 2000; 76:488–493.
3. Douglas, B. R., Charboneau, W., Reading, C. C.: Ultrasound guided intervention. Radiol Clin N Am 2001;39:415–428.
4. Morita, K., Numata, K., Tanaka, K., et al.: Sonographically guided core-needle biopsy of focal splenic lesions: report of four cases. J Clin Ultrasound 2000;28:417–423.
5. Civardi, G., Vallisa, D., Berte, R., et al.: Ultrasound guided fine-needle aspiration biopsy of the spleen: high clinical efficacy and low risk in a multicerter Italian study. Am J Haematol 2001;67:93–99.
6. Solbiati, L., Bossi, M. C., Bellotti, E., et al.: Focal lesions in the spleen: Sonographic patterns and guided biopsy. AJR 1983;140:59–65.
7. O'Malley, M., Wood, B. J., Boland, W., et al.: Interventional Radiology Case Conference. Percutaneous Imaging guided biopsy of the spleen. AJR 1999;172: 661–665.
8. Smith, E. H.: Complications of percutaneous abdominal fine-needle biopsy. Radiology 1991;178:253–258.
9. Kraus, M. D., Fleming, M. D., Vonderheide, R. H.: The spleen as a diagnostic specimen. Cancer 2001;91:2001–2009.
10. Wiernik, P. H., Rader, M., Becker, N. H.: Inflammatory pseudotumor of the spleen. Cancer 1990; 66: 597–600.
11. Westra, W. H., Anderson, B. O., Klimstra, D. S.: Carcinosarcoma of the spleen. An extragenital malignant mixed muellerian tumor? Am J Surg Pathol 1994;18:309.
12. Fritscher-Ravens, A., Mylonaki, M., Pates, A., et al.: Endoscopic ultrasound-guided biopsy for the diagnosis of focal lesions of the spleen. Am J Gastroenterol 2003;98:1022–1027.
13. Eloubeidi, M.A., Varadarajulu, S., Eltoum, I., et al.: Transgastric endoscopic ultrasound-guided fine-needle aspiration biopsy and flow cytometry of suspected lymphoma of the spleen. Endoscopy 2006; 38:617–620.
14. Atay, Z.: The reliability of cytodiagnosis in determining malignancy histogenetic tumor type. In: Nakhosteen, J. A. and Maassen. W., eds.: Bronchology: Research, Diagnostic and therapeutic aspects. Boston: Martinus Nijhoff Publishers 1981:37–42.
15. Fritscher-Ravens, A., SriRam, P. V. J., Meyer, A., et al.: Diagnosis of sarcoidosis by endosonography-guided fine-needle aspiration. Chest. 2000; 118:928–935.
16. Zeppa, P., Vetrani, A., Luciano, L., et al.: Fine needle aspiration biopsy of the spleen. Acta cytologica 1994; 38:299–309.
17. Keogan, M. T., Freed, K. S., Paulson, E. K., et al.: Imaging guided biopsy of focal splenic lesions: Update on safety and effectiveness. AJR 1999; 172: 933–937.
18. Caraway, N. P., Fanning, C. V.. Use of fine needle aspiration biopsy in the evaluation of splenic lesions in a cancer centre. Diagn Cytopathol 1997; 16:312–316.
19. Venkataramu, N. K., Gupta, S., Sood, B. P., et al.: Ultrasound-guided fine needle aspiration biopsy of splenic lesions. Brit J Radiol 1999; 72:953–956.
20. Lishner, M., Lang, R., Hamlet, Y., et al.: Fine-needle aspiration biopsy in patients with diffusely enlarged spleens. Acta cytological 1996; 40:196–198.
21. Sodestrom, N.: How to use cytodiagnostic spleen puncture. Acta Med Scand 1976; 199:1–5.

CHAPTER 28

Adrenal Lesions

Dr. Shyam Varadarajulu
Dr. Mohamad A. Eloubeidi

The adrenal gland is a common site for metastasis of lung and other tumors. As morphological characteristics on imaging studies *per se* are inadequate for establishing definitive diagnosis, safe procurement of tissue is of paramount importance. Although this can be achieved via the percutaneous route under computed tomogram (CT) or ultrasound-guidance, inadequate tissue sampling and procedural risks make endoscopic ultrasound (EUS) a better alternative. This chapter provides an outline on the evaluation of patients with adrenal lesions utilizing EUS.

Identification of the Left Adrenal Gland

As shown in the Visible Human Models of Figures 28–1A amd 28–1B, the adrenal glands are situated adjacent to the kidneys and in close proximity to the posterior stomach on the left, and the duodenum on the right. Coronal cross-sectional anatomy (Figure 28–1C) of the stomach shows the close proximity of the stomach to the left adrenal gland. As can be appreciated from the transaxial cross-section in Figure 28–1D, the right adrenal gland can sometimes be hard to reach from the duodenum due to other intervening structures, such as the inferior vena cava.

The left adrenal gland can be identified in greater than 95% of EUS examinations, using either of the two techniques described in the text that follows.[1]

Technique 1: The descending aorta is first traced up to the celiac trunk (usually located about 40–45 cm from the incisor teeth). At that level, gentle clockwise torque of the echoendoscope rapidly identifies the left adrenal gland.[2]

Technique 2: The echoendoscope is advanced into the proximal stomach and the abdominal aorta is identified just below the gastroesophageal junction.[1] The splenic vein is then isolated by advancing the transducer forward with a clockwise rotation. The splenic hilum is found by following the splenic vein laterally (further clockwise rotation and slight withdrawal). The left kidney is then imaged by advancing the scope from the splenic hilum. The left kidney is seen in cross-section with a central pelvis, with the caliceal system appearing echogenic with the surrounding hypoechoic cortex. The left adrenal gland is found just below the splenic vein between the left kidney and the abdominal aorta.

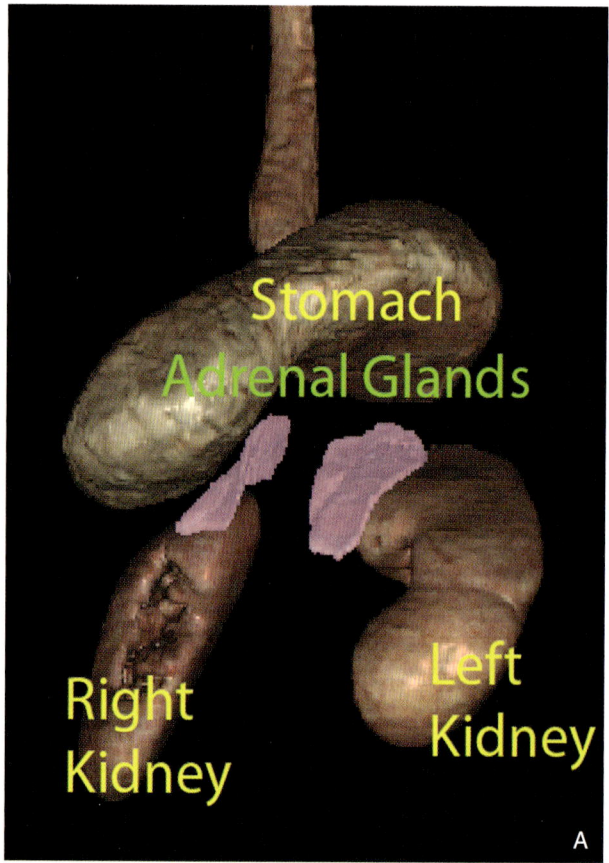
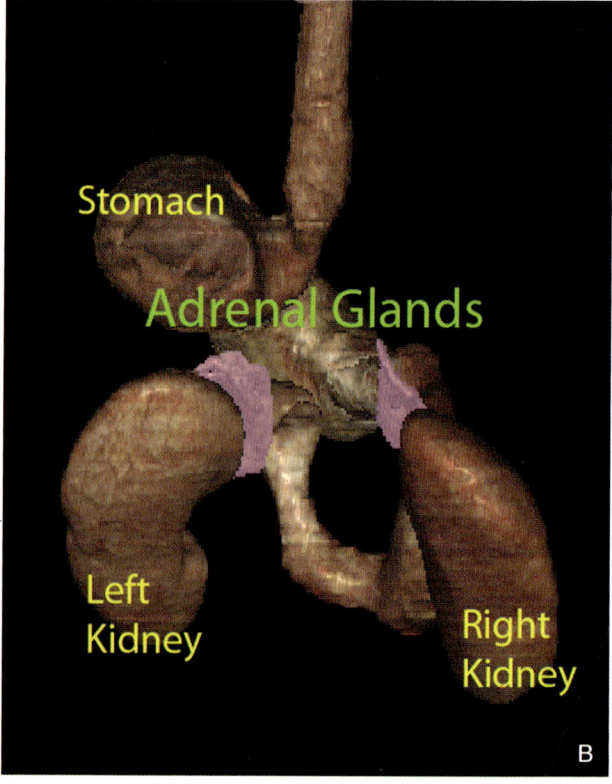

FIGURES 28–1. *A and B* (A) anterior and (B) posterior views of models created from Visible Human Anatomy. The adrenal glands are in pink.

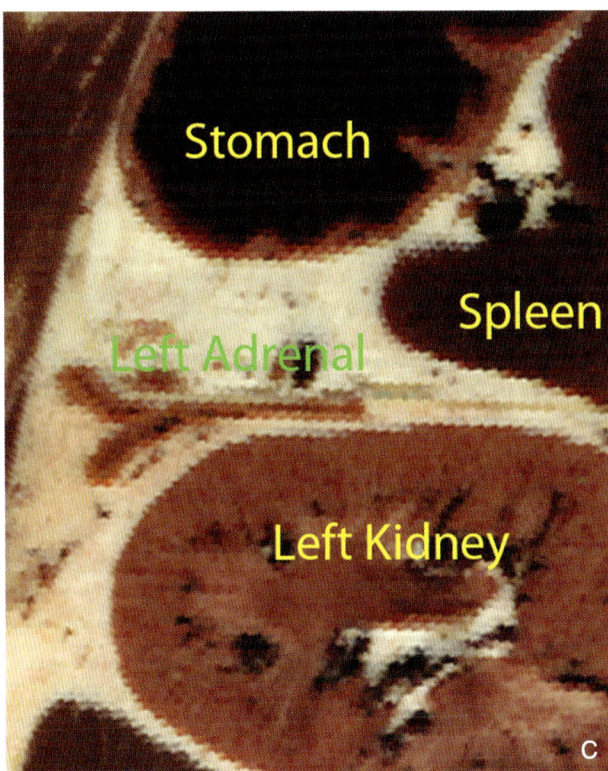
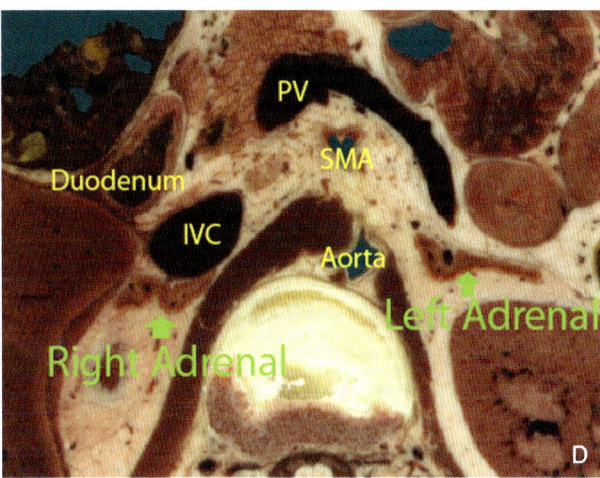

FIGURES 28–1. *C and D* (C) A coronal cross-section of the region of the posterior stomach. (D) a transaxial cross-section of the adrenal glands. IVC = inferior vena cava, PV = portal vein confluence, SMA = superior mesenteric artery.

The right adrenal gland generally cannot be well visualized at EUS because it is located farther away from the stomach and is superior to the duodenal sweep. In 20% of cases it can be seen with the transducer deep into the duodenal lumen beyond the ampulla with morphological characteristics similar to the left adrenal gland. Even when detected by EUS, the right adrenal gland usually is located deep or adjacent to the inferior vena cava, thereby making EUS-guided FNA difficult but not impossible. Radiologists familiar with EUS-guided FNA can predict the ability to sample the right adrenal from cross sectional imaging. Typically, there is a small window through the duodenum.

Glandular Morphology

The normal adrenal gland on EUS appears homogeneous and hypoechoic with a characteristic "seagull" or "elliptical" shape (Figures 28–2A, 28–2B). The adrenal gland can appear as both shapes with a slight change in the orientation of the EUS probe tip. This variation in shape represents different ultrasound cuts of the gland. The adrenal gland exhibits a hypoechoic rim that corresponds histologically to the adrenal cortex. The hyperechoic central region represents the adrenal medulla.[1] This distinction can be best appreciated at a frequency of 12 MHz or higher (Figure 28–2A). The length of the gland is measured from the end of one wing to the other, and the width is measured at the widest mid portion or body of the gland. The average long-axis dimension of the adrenal gland is 2.5 cm and the short-axis dimension is 0.8 cm.[1]

The most common malignant pathology involving the adrenal gland is metastasis from lung cancer.[1-7] Others include metastasis from the GI tract, pancreas, melanoma, renal cell cancer, primary pheochromocytoma, paraganglioma, adrenal cortical cancer, multiple endocrine neoplasia, and adrenal adenoma.[1-10]

When pathologically involved, as in case of malignancy, the adrenal glad tends to loose its "seagull" morphology and appears at EUS to have a mass-like appearance (Figure 28–3) or one of its wings may appear enlarged (Figure 28–4).[1,2] When the size of the adrenal gland exceeds 3 cm, the lesion is more likely to be malignant.[2] The configuration of the adrenal gland appears to be well preserved when enlargement is caused by benign processes.[2] However, as with CT and magnetic resonance imaging, the diagnostic accuracy for EUS based on morphology alone is poor and leads to misclassification (benign versus malignant) in 20% of cases.[2,11,12] Only an EUS-guided FNA can provide definitive diagnosis in a majority of patients who present with adrenal masses.

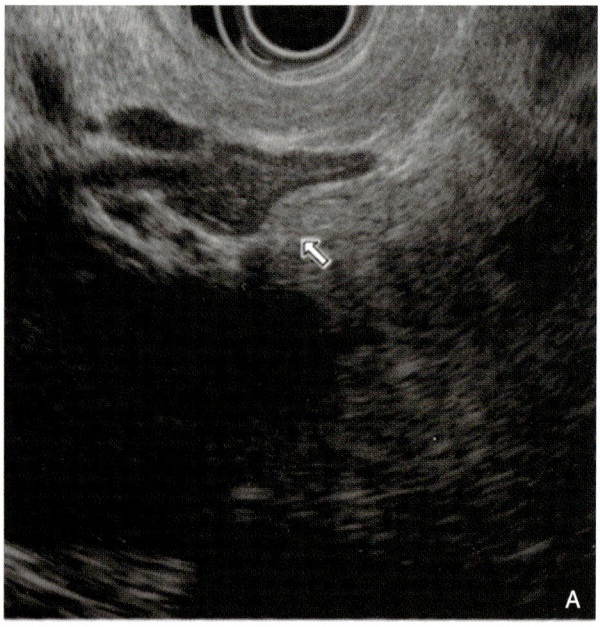
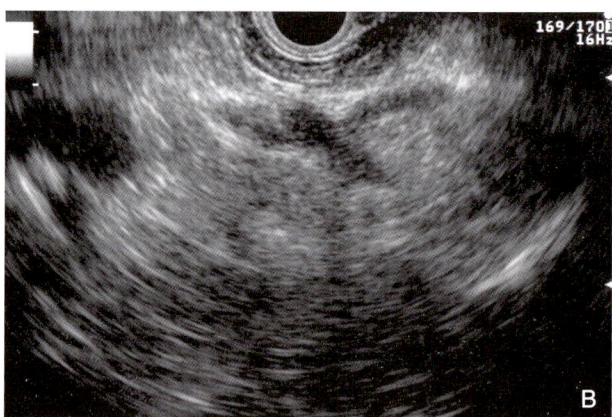

FIGURES 28–2. A and B (A) EUS performed using a radial echoendoscope at 12 Mhz reveals adrenal gland with a hypoechoic cortex and hyperechoic inner medulla. (B) Normal-appearing adrenal gland imaged with the curvilinear echoendoscope (7.5 Mhz).

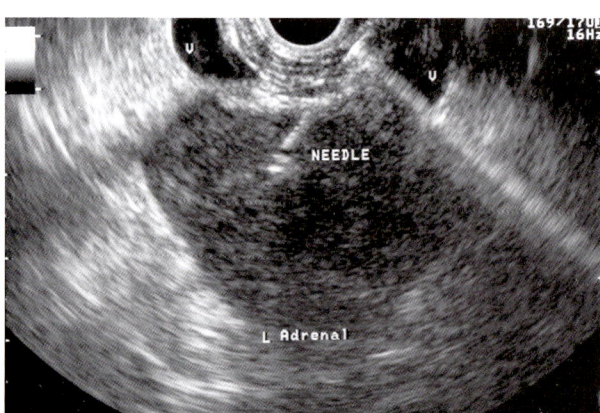

FIGURE 28–3. EUS performed using a linear echoendoscope reveals an adrenal mass. The normal configuration of the gland is lost in this patient with metastatic cancer.

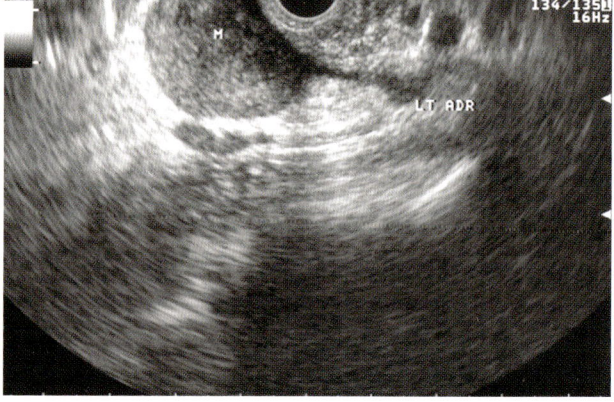

FIGURE 28–4. EUS performed using a linear echoendoscope reveals an enlarged left wing of the adrenal gland due to metastasis from non-small-cell lung cancer. The architecture of the right wing appears intact.

EUS-Guided FNA

After excluding the presence of vessels along the path of the needle using color-flow and Doppler ultrasound, the adrenal gland is punctured using a 22-gauge needle (Figure 28–5). When the tip of the needle catheter sheath is visualized endosonographically, the needle is advanced from the sheath, through the wall of the stomach, and into the target lesion under US guidance (Video 28–1). Once in the target lesion, the stylet is removed, and the needle is moved back and forth for 15 to 30 seconds and then withdrawn. Suction is not required unless the first pass yields no cellular material.

As the stomach is the only organ that needs to be traversed, EUS-guided FNA of the adrenal gland appears to be very safe when compared to techniques such as CT or ultrasound that pursue the percutaneous route.[13-15] Diagnostic material can be procured in most instances within a median of five passes with an accuracy that exceeds 75% (Table 28–1).

Recently, Tru-cut biopsy (TCB) has been advocated by some investigators when the yield at EUS-FNA is low or when histopathological analysis of the adrenal

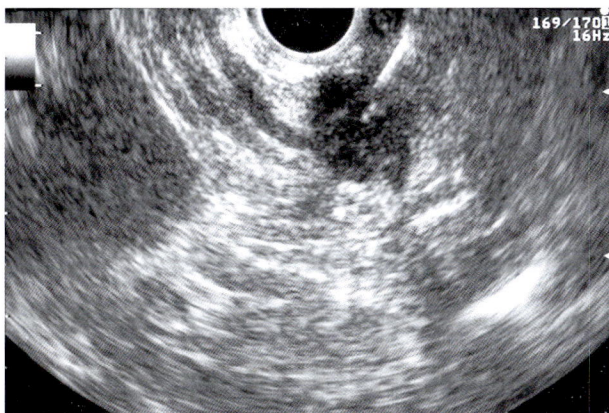

FIGURE 28–5. A 11 mm nodule in one wing of a normal appearing adrenal gland. PET scan showed avid uptake (SUV greater than 5). EUS-FNA confirmed malignant involvement.

mass is desired.[16] Although experience with EUS-guided TCB of the adrenal gland is limited, the technique appears safe when clinically indicated and in the appropriate clinical setting.

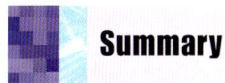 **Summary**

EUS and EUS-guided fine-needle aspiration are minimally invasive and safe techniques for evaluating the adrenal gland. These techniques have high diagnostic accuracy and provide definitive diagnosis in most patients, thereby optimizing clinical care.

Video: Available at www.pmph-usa.com/bhutani
Video 28–1: EUS-guided FNA of a patient with left adrenal mass secondary to metastatic lung cancer.

Table 28–1	Major Studies Evaluating the Role of EUS-Guided FNA in Patients with Adrenal Masses		
Author Accuracy (%) (reference)	No. of patients	passes	No. of FNA
Eloubeidi (2)	31	4.5 (median)	81
DeWitt (3)	38	3.6 (mean)	76
Stelow (7)	22	Not reported	88

References

1. Chang, K. J., Erickson, R. A., Nguyen, P.: Endoscopic ultrasound (EUS) and EUS-guided fine-needle aspiration of the left adrenal gland. Gastrointest Endosc 1996; 44: 568–572.
2. Eloubeidi, M. A., Seewald, S., Tamhane, A., et al.: EUS-guided FNA of the left adrenal gland in patients with thoracic or GI malignancies. Gastrointest Endosc. 2004; 59:627–633.
3. DeWitt, J., Alsatie, M., LeBlanc, J., et al. : Endoscopic ultrasound-guided fine-needle aspiration of left adrenal gland masses. Endoscopy 2007; 39:65–71.
4. Jhala, N. C., Jhala, D., Eloubeidi, M. A., et al.: Endoscopic ultrasound-guided fine-needle aspiration biopsy of the adrenal glands: analysis of 24 patients. Cancer 2004; 102: 308–314.
5. Mercier, O., Fadel, E., de Perrot, M., et al.: Surgical treatment of solitary adrenal metastasis from non-small cell lung cancer. J Thorac Cardiovasc Surg. 2005; 130:136–140.
6. Lucchi, M., Dini, P., Ambrogi, M. C., et al.: Metachronous adrenal masses in resected non-small cell lung cancer patients: therapeutic implications of laparoscopic adrenalectomy. Eur J Cardiothorac Surg. 2005; 27: 753–756.
7. Stelow, E. B., Stanley, M. W., Mallery, S.: Synchronous primary pancreatic endocrine neoplasm and adrenal pheochromocytoma diagnosed by EUS-guided FNA. Gastrointest Endosc. 2004; 59: 136–139.
8. Bovio, S., Cataldi, A., Reimondo, G., et al.: Prevalence of adrenal incidentaloma in a contemporary computerized tomography series. J Endocrinol Invest. 2006;29: 298–302.
9. Kim, H. Y., Kim, S. G., Lee, K. W., et al.: Clinical study of adrenal incidentaloma in Korea. Korean J Intern Med. 2005;20:303–309.
10. Ettinghausen, S. E., Burt, M. E.: Prospective evaluation of unilateral adrenal masses in patients with operable non-small-cell lung cancer. J Clin Oncol 1991; 9:1462–1466.
11. Oliver, T. W., Bernardino, M. E., Miller, J. I., Mansour, K., Green, D., Davis, W.A.: Isolated adrenal masses in non-small-cell bronchogenic carcinoma. Radiology 1984;153:217–218.
12. Burt, M., Heelan, R. T., Coit, D., et al.: Prospective evaluation of unilateral adrenal masses in patients with operable non-small-cell lung cancer. J Thorac Cardiovasc Surg 1994;107:584–589.
13. Silverman, S. G., Mueller, P. R., Pinkney, L. P., Koenker, R. M., Seltzer, S. E.: Predictive value of image-guided adrenal biopsy: analysis of results of 101 biopsies. Radiology 1993; 187:715–718.
14. Bernardino, M. E., Walther, M. M., Phillips, V. M., Graham, S. D. J., Sewell, C. W., Gedgaudas-McClees, K., et al.: CT-guided adrenal biopsy: accuracy, safety, and indications. AJR Am J Roentgenol 1985;144: 67–69.
15. Mody, M. K., Kazerooni, E. A., Korobkin, M.: Percutaneous CT-guided biopsy of adrenal masses: immediate and delayed complications. J Comput Assist Tomogr 1995;19:434–439.
16. Gerke, H., Robinson, R. A., Luo, P.: Diagnosis of focal metastasis to the adrenal gland by EUS-guided core biopsy. Gastrointest Endosc. 2005 Sep; 62:469–471.

CHAPTER 29

Portal Vein Thrombosis

Dr. William R. Brugge
Dr. Kunal Jajoo

Portal Vein Thrombosis

Thrombosis of the portal vein, a pre-hepatic cause of portal hypertension, results in a broad range of clinical manifestations. Acute thrombosis can be can present incidentally, discovered on cross-sectional imaging done for other clinical reasons, or with acute abdominal pain and ascites, particularly if the mesenteric veins are involved.[1] Chronic thrombosis of the portal vein results in portal hypertension and its complications: variceal hemorrhage, splenomegaly, ascites, and thrombocytopenia.[2] Portal vein thrombosis (PVT) occurs equally in children and adults,[3] though the etiologies in these groups differ greatly. In children, the most common cause of PVT is infection, largely umbilical vein sepsis. In adults, the causes range from hypercoagulable states, to inflammatory diseases, to cirrhosis with or without hepatocellular carcinoma (HCC).[4] In up to one-third of patients with PVT, no etiology is found.

The diagnosis of PVT classically required invasive contrast angiography. Techniques in imaging using ultrasound with color Doppler and cross-sectional imaging by computed tomography (CT) with tri-phase contrast or magnetic resonance angiography (MRA) often obviate the need for more invasive testing. However, if PVT is highly suspected and noninvasive imaging is inconclusive, venous angiography remains the gold standard.

Endoscopic ultrasound (EUS) provides an additional modality for the detection of PVT. EUS offers the advantage of minimizing the distance between the ultrasound transducer and the portal venous system, thereby decreasing the chance of interference by bowel gas, contrast, or adipose tissue. In an early study of EUS for the detection of PVT, 9 of 11 patients with a clinical presentation of PVT and negative CT scan were found to have thrombus by EUS.[5] A more recent study by our group demonstrated that linear array EUS is very sensitive (81%) and highly specific (93%) for the detection of thrombus among a group of patients with PVT confirmed by CT scan and/or surgery.[6] Figure 29–1A shows typical Visible Human Anatomy in the region of the pancreatic head and portal confluence. In practice, the finding of PVT by EUS often occurs in patients referred for tumor staging of pancreatic or biliary malignancy. (Figures 29–1B - 29–1D)

The portal vein is typically identified by EUS at its confluence with the splenic vein and with the transducer in the duodenal bulb. The tip of the endoscope is then rotated and slowly withdrawn in order to follow the portal vein toward the porta hepatis. Thrombus may be visible as hyperechoic material within the otherwise hypoechoic vein. Confirmation with color flow Doppler can demonstrate retained venous flow (Figure 29–2) or cavernous transformation. The complications of PVT can also be identified by EUS (Figure 29–3A - 29–3D). EUS is highly sensitive for the detection of ascites, even when other imaging is negative.[7] Para-gastric and para-esophageal varices not visible by endoscopy can also be detected by EUS. Though the role of EUS in the detection and management of portal hypertension is evolving, it has demonstrated value in detecting PVT, especially in the setting of malignant disease.

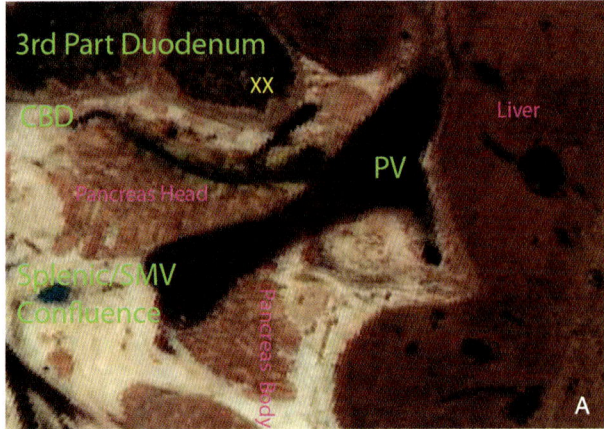
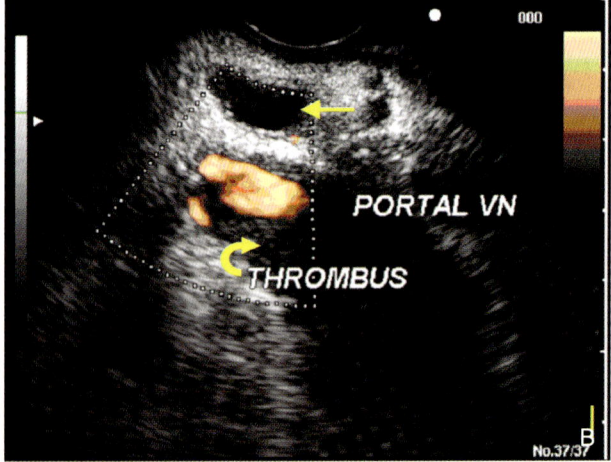

FIGURES 29–1. A and B (A) Visible Human Anatomy, which approximates the position of EUS images shown below. The image is made from the left lateral decubitis position. This image shows the portal vein from the liver hilum to the confluence. The third part of the duodenum is in the superior aspect of the image, and the yellow XX is in the vicinity of where the EUS probe would be located with the endoscope coming out of the plane of the image. CBD=common bile duct, PV=portal vein, SMV =superior mesenteric vein. (B) Partially occlusive thrombus (bent arrow) seen in the portal vein as it courses beneath a dilated distal common bile duct (straight arrow)

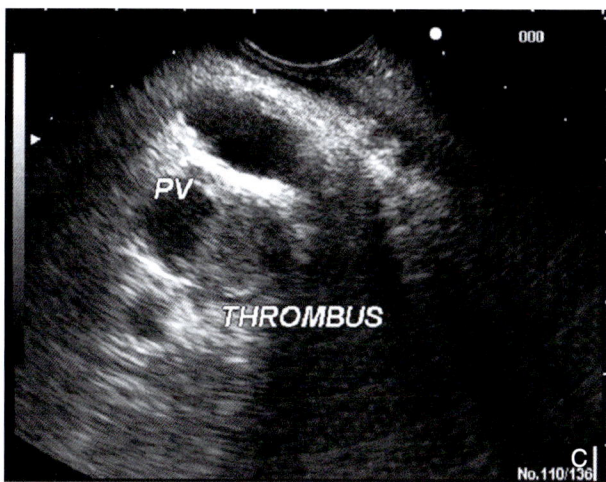 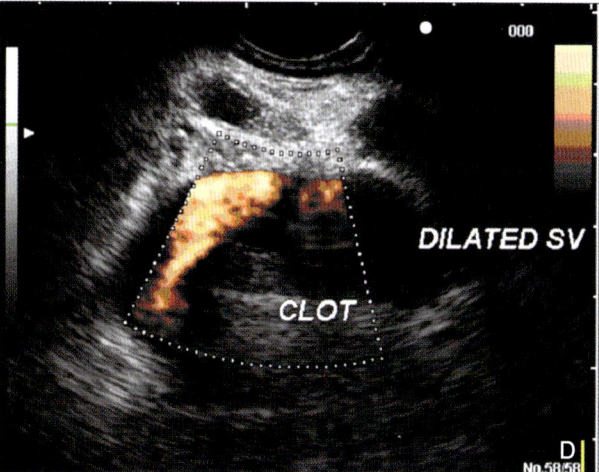

FIGURES 29–1. *C and D* (C) Further toward the porta hepatis, the thrombus occupies a greater proportion of the vessel lumen. (D) The thrombus extends toward the confluence, causing dilation of the splenic vein.

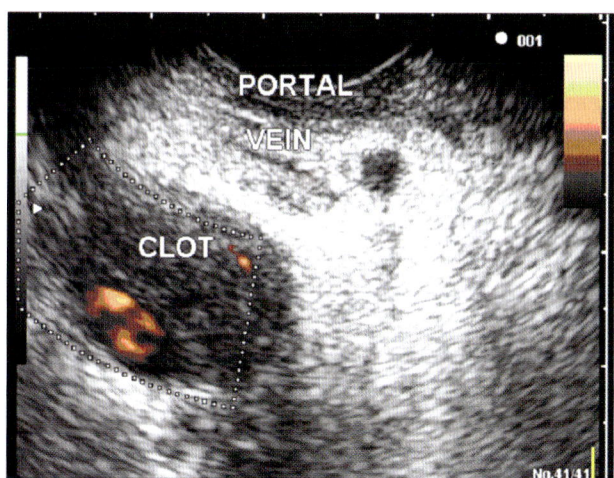

FIGURE 29–2. Linear EUS image with color flow Doppler demonstrates a thrombus (clot) in the portal vein. A minimal amount of retained venous flow is seen in red-orange.

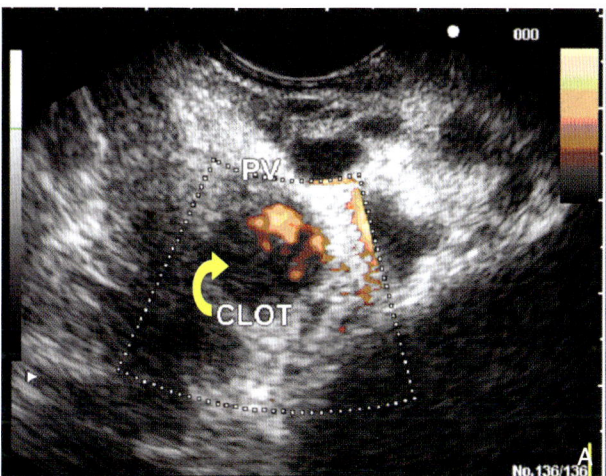 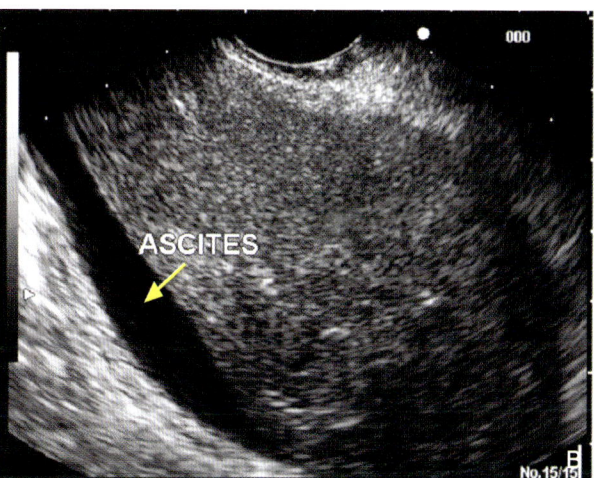

FIGURES 29–3. *A and B* Linear EUS image with color flow Doppler demonstrates a thrombus (curved arrow) in the portal vein. A moderate amount of retained venous flow is seen in red-orange. (B) Perihepatic ascites (arrow) are seen as anechoic fluid at the liver edge in the same patient.

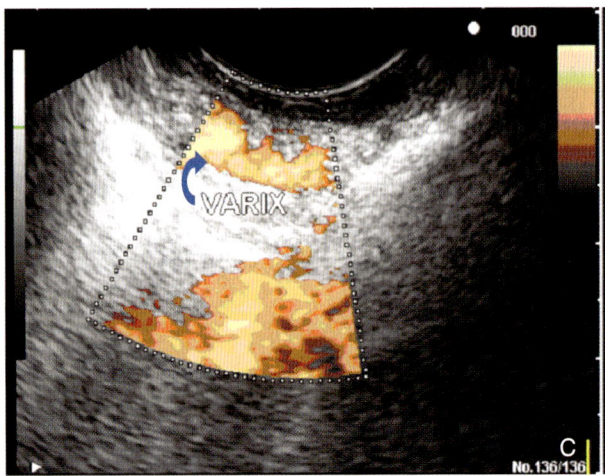 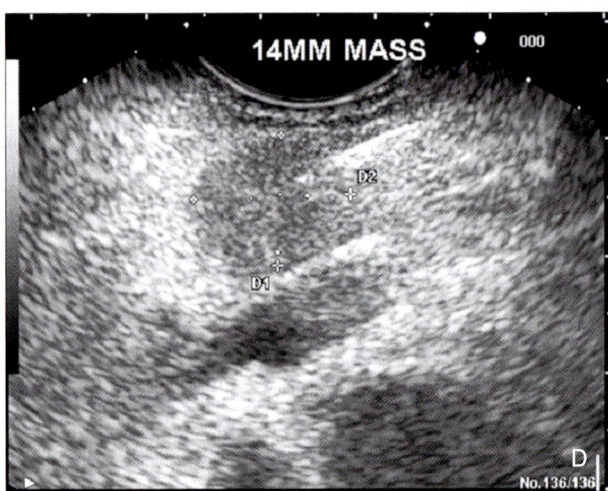

FIGURES 29–3. *C and D* (C) Peri-gastric varix (curved arrow), as a result of PVT, seen with color flow Doppler (D) PVT in this patient was caused by metastatic cholangiocarcinoma.

PVT in the setting of hepatocellular carcinoma may result from tumor thrombus or may be due to underlying cirrhosis. The differentiation of these two processes is important because the presence of tumor thrombus is a contraindication to liver transplantation and portends a poor prognosis. Transabdominal ultrasound with FNA has been demonstrated to be safe and effective for the diagnosis of portal vein tumor thrombus by HCC.[8,9,10] EUS-guided FNA of the portal vein has been described in this setting and offers the advantage of a short needle track. It also circumvents a transhepatic approach, thereby minimizing the probability of false-positive results.[11] Further study of this EUS staging modality is required.

with SVT and incidentally detected varices will experience bleeding.[13]

EUS is highly specific and fairly sensitive for the detection of SVT (Figure 29–4).[5] The majority of studies of EUS and SVT have involved its utility in the staging of pancreatic cancer. In this setting, EUS is effective in detecting invasion of the porto-splenic vessels by pancreatic cancer.[14] However, the sensitivity of EUS for the detection of invasion of the superior mesenteric vein and other adjacent vessels is limited.[15,16] Overall, EUS with FNA is highly accurate in the staging of pancreatic cancer, particularly for small tumors.[17]

Splenic Vein Thrombosis

Splenic vein thrombosis (SVT) is most commonly seen in association with chronic pancreatitis. Other etiologies of SVT include acute pancreatitis, malignancy, and the causes of PVT. Thrombosis of the splenic vein can result in splenomegaly as well as sinistral (left-sided) portal hypertension and gastroesophageal varices. Variceal hemorrhage in this setting, particularly when isolated gastric varices are present, is difficult to control and may necessitate urgent splenectomy.[12] Previous studies suggested that SVT frequently lead to variceal hemorrhage and had prompted the recommendation of prophylactic splenectomy for such patients. In contrast, recent studies have demonstrated that a minority of patients

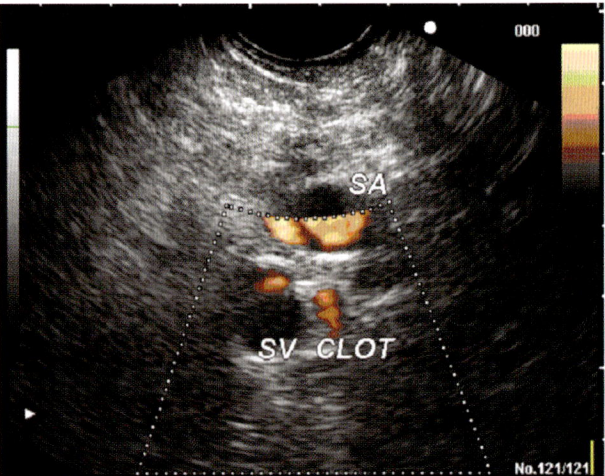

FIGURE 29–4. Linear EUS image demonstrating the splenic artery (SA) and splenic vein (SV). The SV contains a hyperechoic thrombus, which obstructs flow as demonstrated by color flow Doppler.

References

1. Webster, G. J., Burroughs, A. K., Riordan, S. M.: Portal vein thrombosis — new insights into aetiology and management. Aliment Pharmacol Ther 2005;21:1–9.
2. Sarin, S. K., Agarwal, S. R.: Extrahepatic portal vein obstruction. Semin Liver Dis 2002;22:43–58.
3. Webb, L. J., Sherlock, S.: The aetiology, presentation and natural history of extrahepatic portal venous obstruction. Q J Med 1979;192:627–639.
4. Sobhonslidsuk, A., Reddy, K. R.: Portal vein thrombosis: a concise review. Am J Gastroenterol 2002;97:5335–5341.
5. Wiersema, M. J., Chak, A., Kopecky, K. K., Wiersema, L. M.: Duplex Doppler endosonography in the diagnosis of splenic vein, portal vein, and portosystemic shunt thrombosis. Gastrointest Endosc 1995;42:19–26.
6. Lai, L., Brugge, W. R.: Endoscopic ultrasound is a sensitive and specific test to diagnose portal venous system thrombosis (PVST). Am J Gastroenterol 2004;99:40–44.
7. Nguyen, P. T., Chang, K. J.: EUS in the detection of ascites and EUS-guided paracentesis. Gastrointest Endosc 2001;54:336–339.
8. Vilana, R., Bru, C., Bruix, J., et al.: Fine needle aspiration biopsy of portal vein thrombus: value in detecting malignant thrombosis. AJR Am J Roentgenol 1993;160:1285–1287.
9. Dusenbery, D., Dodd, G. D., 3rd, Carr, B. I.: Percutaneous fine needle aspiration of portal vein thrombi as a staging technique for hepatocellular carcinoma. Cytologic findings of 46 patients. Cancer 1995;75:2057–2062.
10. De Sio, I., Castellano, L., Calandra, M., et al.: Ultrasound-guided fine needle aspiration biopsy of portal vein thrombosis in liver cirrhosis: results in 15 patients. J Gastroenterol Hepatol 1995;10:662–665.
11. Lai, R., Stephens, V., Bardales, R.: Diagnosis and staging of hepatocellular carcinoma by EUS-FNA of a portal vein thrombus. Gastrointest Endosc 2004;59:574–577.
12. Weber, S. M., Rikkers, L. F.: Splenic vein thrombosis and gastrointestinal bleeding in chronic pancreatitis. World J Surg 2003;27:1271–1274.
13. Heider, T. R., Azeem, S., Galanko, J. A., Behrns, K. E.: The natural history of pancreatitis-induced splenic vein thrombosis. Ann Surg 2004;239:876-80; discussion 880–882.
14. Brugge, W. R., Lee, M. J., Kelsey, P. B., et al.: The use of EUS to diagnose malignant portal venous invasion by pancreatic cancer. Gastrointest Endosc 1996;43:561–567.
15. Aslanian, H., Salem, R., Lee, J., et al.: EUS diagnosis of vascular inasion in pancreatic cancer: surgical and histologic correlates. Am J Gastroenterol 2005;100:1381–1385.
16. Rosch, T., Dittler, H. J., Strobel, K., et al.: Endoscopic ultrasound criteria for vascular invasion in the staging of cancer of the head of the pancreas: a blind reevaluation of videotapes. Gastrointest Endosc 2000;52:469–477.
17. Varadarajulu, S., Eloubeidi, M. A.: The role of endoscopic ultrasonography in the evaluation of pancreaticobiliary cancer. Gastrointest Endosc Clin N Am 2005;15:497–511.
18. Adapted from Schafer, D. F., Sorrell, M. F.: Vascular diseases of the liver. In Feldman, M., Friedman, L. S., Sleisenger, M. H., eds. Sleisenger and Fordtran's gastrointestinal and liver disease: pathophysiology, diagnosis, management. Vol2. 7th ed. Philadelphia: Saunders, 2002:1369.

CHAPTER 30

Peritoneal and Pleural Fluid

Dr. Nundhini Thukkani
Dr. Douglas O. Faigel

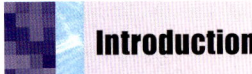

Introduction

In staging of known or suspected malignancy, endoscopic ultrasound has become an invaluable tool. While primarily used in the locoregional staging of cancers, EUS may be useful in identifying and sampling sites of distant metastases such as the liver.[1]

Certain malignancies may spread to the pleura or peritoneum and result in pleural effusions or ascites. For the endosonographer, these most commonly include cancers of the stomach, pancreas, or lung, but can be seen with a variety of other malignancies as well. Breast and lung cancers are most often associated with pleural seeding and the development of malignant effusions. Peritoneal seeding and malignant ascites are often seen in the setting of advanced gastrointestinal, hepatic, and genitourinary malignancy. The finding of malignant ascites or pleural effusions represents metastatic, unresectable disease (M1) and is a poor prognostic indicator with approximate one-year survival often less than 10%.[2]

Common benign conditions, however, are also associated with fluid accumulation, such as congestive heart failure, nephrotic syndromes, cirrhosis, pancreatitis, tuberculous disease, constrictive pericarditis, severe malnutrition, and protein-losing enteropathy.

Several approaches have been used to image pleural and peritoneal fluid. Standard imaging for pleural effusions includes ultrasonography, chest x-rays, and computerized tomography. Pleural effusions can also be seen on magnetic resonance imaging and echocardiography. Peritoneal fluid is commonly identified by ultrasonography or computerized tomography. Several studies have shown greater sensitivity of EUS at detection of peritoneal fluid. In a prospective study by Lee et al in 250 patients with gastric adenocarcinoma, the sensitivity of EUS (87.1%) for the detection of ascites was greater than that of ultrasound and CT combined (16.1%). On multivariate analysis, detection of ascites by EUS was found to be the only significant predictor for peritoneal metastases, with an OR of 4.7 (95% CI 2-11.2).[3]

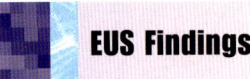

EUS Findings

The detection of pleural and peritoneal fluid by EUS is often in the context of staging known malignancy, most often of the stomach, pancreas, and lung. Malignant ascites or pleural fluid are most common in tumors of higher T- and N-stage.[3]

Pleural Effusions

EUS is most sensitive at detecting right-sided pleural effusions. This is due to positioning the patient in the left lateral decubitus position, which allows fluid to layer adjacent to the esophagus. The relation of the pleura to the esophagus is illustrated by the Visible Human axial image shown in Figure 30–1A. The collection is most commonly visualized as an anechoic triangular-shaped structure adjacent and lateral to the azygous vein and is Doppler negative (Figure 30–1B). These characteristics make the effusion amenable to fine-needle aspiration (Figure 30–1C).

Pericardial Effusions

Small pericardial effusions are commonly seen on the posterior wall of the left atrium adjacent to the anterior wall of the esophagus. The axial cross-section Visible Human Anatomy is shown in Figure 30–2A. These small effusions, however, are typically not physiologically or clinically relevant (Figure 30–2B). Larger pathologic effusions are rarely encountered. EUS-guided FNA of pericardial effusions has not been described. The risk of infection with FNA is a major concern.

Ascites

Ascites on EUS appear as anechoic structures with an irregular, triangular, Doppler-negative shape extrinsic to the viscus (Figure 30–3A). The Visible Human Anatomy of this region is shown in Figure 30–3B.

Transgastric EUS can detect ascites adjacent to the left lobe of the liver or layering dependently next to the greater gastric curve or spleen. Fingers of omentum or loops of bowel may be seen floating in the ascites. Bowel contractions may cause the shape of these collections to change during real-time imaging. In patients with massive ascites, the stomach will be completely surrounded by anechoic fluid.

Transduodenal ascites may appear as triangular pockets of fluid or larger collections adjacent to the duodenal bulb, liver, or gallbladder (Figure 30–4A). Pericholecystic fluid may be an indication of cholecystitis or ascites. The differentiation may be made by the presence of gallbladder pathology such as stones or wall thickening.

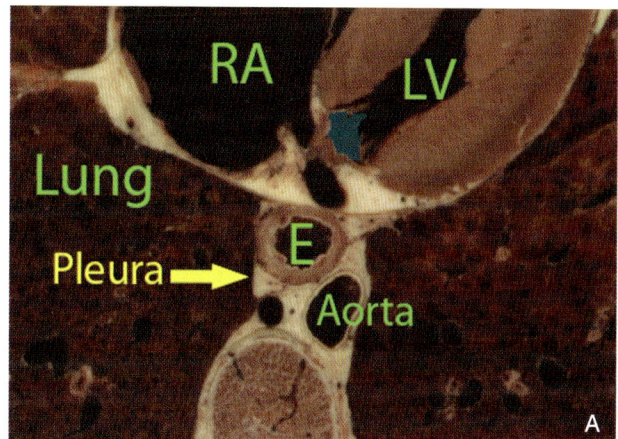
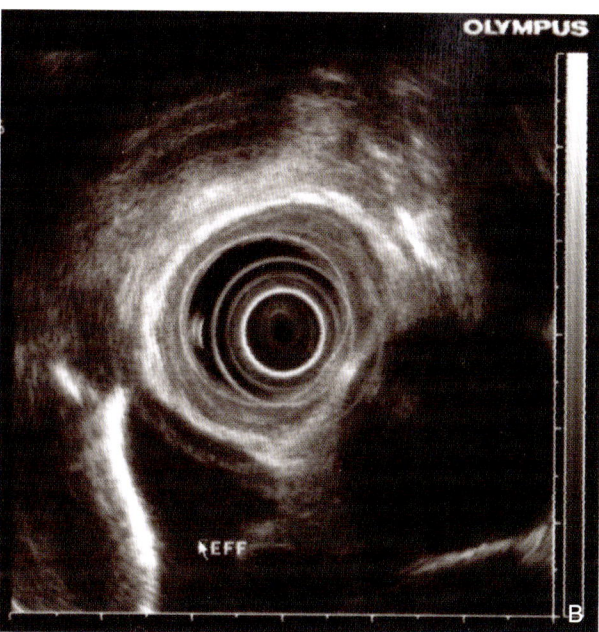
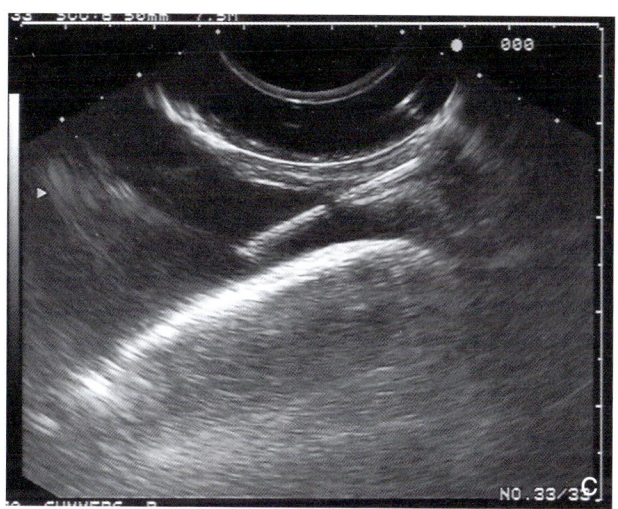

FIGURES 30–1. *A to C* (A) Axial cross-section anatomy of the thorax. E=esophagus, LV=left ventricle, RA=right atrium (B) Pleural Effusion. Large pleural effusion in a patient with T1 N0 adenocarcinoma of the esophagus. (EFF = effusion) (C) Transesophageal EUS-guided fine-needle aspiration of the effusion in 1A. Cytology was negative for malignancy. Subsequent surgical resection confirmed a T1 N0 M0 esophageal carcinoma.

Distinguishing ascites from fluid within adjacent loops of bowel is important. Ascites will be directly adjacent to the stomach or duodenum with a single five-layer wall between the transducer and the fluid. Fluid within adjacent loops will have two walls between the transducer and the fluid.

 EUS-Guided Fine-Needle Aspiration

Using curved, linear array echoendoscopes, EUS-guided FNA of pleural effusions (Figure 30–1B) and ascites (Figure 30–4B) may be performed. Doppler ultrasonography ensures that fluid within the target fluid collection is not blood within a flowing vessel. This also ensures avoidance of intervening blood vessels, such as gastric varices, in patients with portal hypertension or splenic vein thrombosis. Ascites and effusions will be Doppler negative. Small effusions near the heart or large vessels (including the azygous vein) may have weak Doppler signal due to transmitted pulses from adjacent vasculature. Doppler should be routinely performed before fine-needle aspiration.

A tumor should be avoided in attempts to aspirate adjacent fluid. The piercing of a tumor may give false-positive cytology and risk seeding into the fluid collection.[4,5] Typically a 22-gauge needle may be used; the fluid is nonviscous and aspirates easily. A 19-gauge needle is rarely needed.

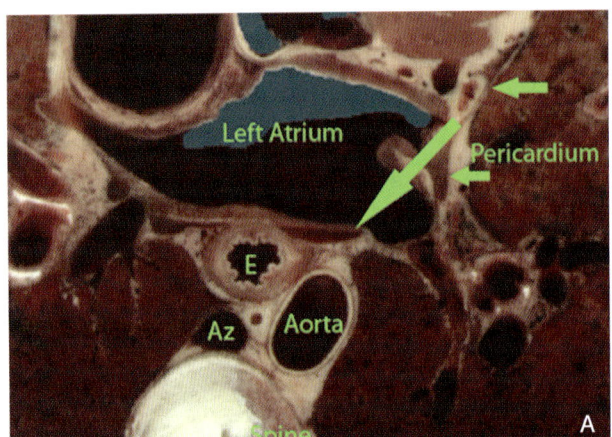
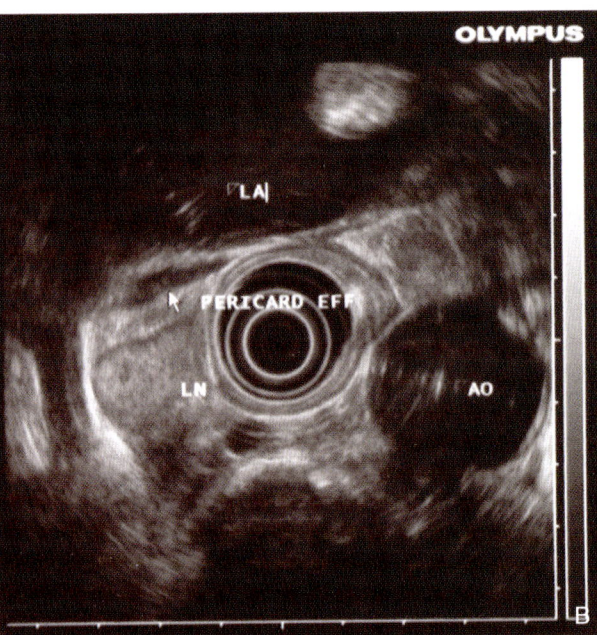

FIGURES 30–2. A and B (A) Axial cross-section anatomy at the level of the left atrium. E=esophagus, Az=azygous vein. (B) Pericardial effusion. A small pericardial effusion is seen adjacent to the left atrium (LA) in a patient with interstitial lung disease. An enlarged lymph node (LN) is also seen. (AO = Aorta).

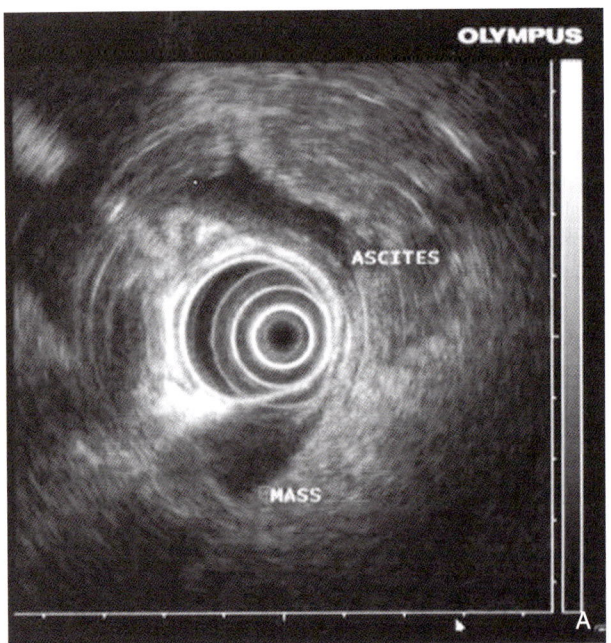
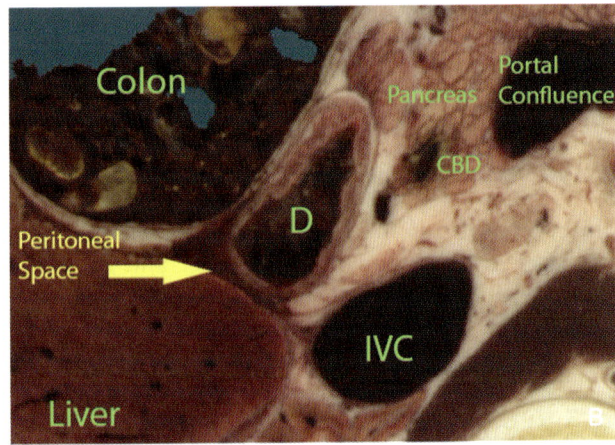

FIGURES 30–3. A and B (A) Ascites. A small pocket of ascites is visualized adjacent to the gastric wall in a patient with gastric cancer. (B) Cross-sectional anatomy near the second portion of the duodenum. D=duodenum, CBD=common bile duct, IVC=inferior vena cava.

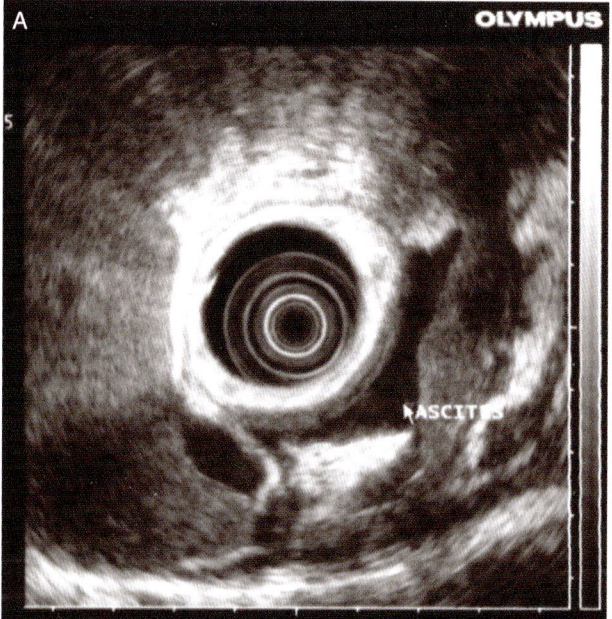 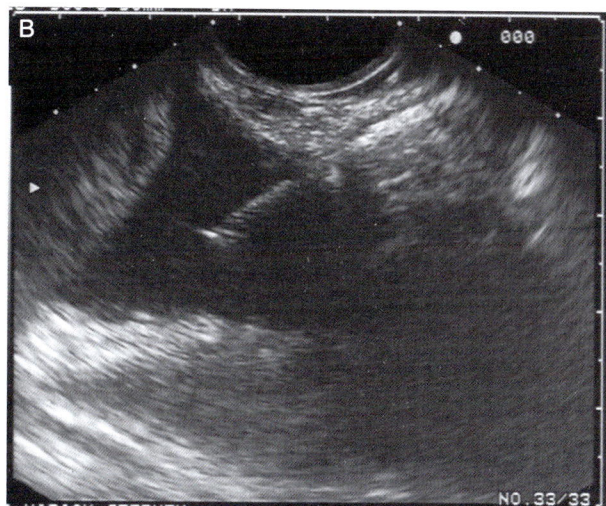

FIGURES 30–4. *A and B* (A) Periduodenal ascites. Ascites seen surrounding the duodenal bulb in a patient with adenocarcinoma of the pancreatic head. Extensive lymphadenopathy and a liver mass were also identified. (B) Ascites FNA. EUS-guided fine-needle aspiration of the ascites seen in Figure 30–4A is performed via a transgastric puncture. Cytology showed atypical cells suspicious for malignancy. Ascitic fluid CEA was elevated at 43.7 ng/ml. Ascitic fluid albumin was 2.3 g/dl and the serum albumin was 2.1 g/dl. Taken together, these findings indicate peritoneal metastasis.

Technique

In performing the fine-needle aspiration, the fluid pocket is first identified with the linear array echoendoscope, confirming also that the tumor will not be traversed. Doppler is then used to ensure that the target fluid is not blood and that intervening vessels are excluded. If the needle has a dull-tipped stylet, the stylet must be pulled back to 'sharpen' the needle. The gastrointestinal tract can then be pierced with a swift, stabbing motion. If desired, a restraining knob on the needle can be set to prevent inserting the needle too far. The needle can then be cleared of cells from the GI tract wall by advancing the stylet fully into the needle. The stylet is then removed and suction applied to collect fluid.

Fluid Analysis

In aspirating fluid, as much as possible should be collected. The quality of the fluid should be noted (color, viscosity, clarity). Fluid should be sent for cytology and other clinically relevant studies. Most commonly, cell count with differential (1-2cc in purple-topped sodium citrate containing tube) is sent. Albumin (1-2cc in red-topped tube) may also be sent, and the serum albumin concentration should also be measured in order to calculate the serum-ascites albumin gradient (serum albumin minus the ascites albumin). High gradients (more than 1.1 g/dL) are associated with ascites due to portal hypertension, while low gradients are associated with malignancies and infections.[6] Bacterial culture should not be routinely performed as the sample will be contaminated and will grow polymicrobial oral flora. An acid fast bacilli culture and stain should be considered if clinically indicated.

Carcinoembryonic antigen (CEA) and other tumor markers have been studied for their use in malignant effusions. Passebosc-Faure et al evaluated the use of molecular markers in serous effusions, 104 pleural and 10 ascitic, and found that the combination of cytology with reverse-transcriptase PCR CEA and epithelial cell adhesion molecule (Ep-CAM) improved the detection of malignancy in cytology negative effusions. There was a sensitivity of 90.1% and specificity and positive-predictive value of 100% and 86%, respectively[7]. A CEA level more than 11 ng/ml has been reported to significantly increase the diagnostic yield over cytology alone to over 85%.[8] An ascites CEA level greater than 5 ng/ml has a sensitivity for malignancy that is in excess of 95%.[9]

Pleural fluid should be sent for lactate dehydrogenase (LDH), total protein, cell count and differential, and glucose, pH, and amylase if clinically indicated. Transudative effusions are characterized by fluid protein less than 3 g/dL, LDH less than 200 IU/L, and white blood cell count less than 1000/mm.[3] Transudates are typically benign and prone to fluid overload states, especially congestive heart failure. Exudates may be due to malignancies or infections, underlining the importance of distinguishing them from transudates.

Tumor marker measurement within the pleural fluid is also useful. While CEA has been the most commonly used marker, a variety of others have been reported. Porcel et al conducted a blind comparison of tumor markers in malignant and benign pleural fluid in 416 patients. They found that the combined use of CEA, cancer antigen 125 (CA-125), carbohydrate antigen 15-3 (CA 15-3), and cytokeratin 19 fragments (CYFRA 21-1) had 100% specificity. The combined sensitivity was 54%; High cutoff points were established to exclude benign effusions (CEA greater than 40ng/ml, CA-125 greater than 1000ng/ml, CA 15-3 greater than 53 U/ml, and CYFRA 21-1 greater than 150U/L). When used with cytology, the diagnostic yield was increased by 18%.[10] CEA remains the single-most clinically useful marker having an accuracy of 85%, while CA 15-3 and CYFRA 21-1 are considered to be alternative options.[11]

Complications and Their Avoidance

General complications of EUS (bleeding and perforation) should be considered in addition to those of fine-needle aspiration. FNA is an inherently nonsterile procedure, thus infection is always a concern. In one study of EUS-FNA of ascites, one of 25 patients who underwent EUS-FNA of ascites developed bacterial peritonitis despite the use of prophylactic antibiotics.[14] Prophylactic antibiotics have been administered in most studies. A recommended course includes a 400 mg intravenous dose of ciprofloxacin at the time of the procedure followed by 500 mg oral ciprofloxacin twice a day for five to seven days (adjust dose for renal insufficiency, if needed).[12,13]

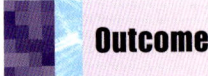

Outcome

The detection of malignant ascites or pleural fluid has prognostic and therapeutic implications as it indicates advanced, nonresectable disease (M1). The prevalence of ascites on EUS done for locoregional staging in known or suspected malignancy varies between 5.3-15%.[14,15,16,17] In a prospective study of 629 patients by Kaushik et al, 25 patients underwent EUS-FNA of ascites of either periduodenal or perigastric fluid collections. Of these, 64% (16/25) had cytology positive for malignancy.[14] The sensitivity of EUS-guided paracentesis for diagnosing malignant ascites was 94% in this study, with a positive predictive value of 100% and a negative predictive value of 89%. In a retrospective study by the authors, 47 of 231 (20.3%) patients noted to have ascites on EUS underwent FNA.[17] Of these, 17 patients (36.2%) had malignant cells noted on cytology. Ten of these patients had no known nodal metastases and six would have been offered aggressive management if not for the malignant ascites found on EUS. (The other four patients had T4 unresectable pancreatic masses). No complications were noted. Thus, the impact of these findings has prognostic implications on the course of management, helping to direct towards palliation rather than aggressive, curative approaches.

There is less experience with EUS and pleural effusions, and the precise role remains undefined. EUS-guided thoracentesis has been described and may reveal malignant cells on cytology.[18] In our experience, small right-sided pleural effusions are commonly identified and almost always benign. EUS-guided FNA should be reserved for those with a high index of suspicion in patients with effusions too small to undergo standard percutaneous thoracentesis.

Conclusions

Ascites and effusions are frequent findings during EUS examinations. When identified in patients with known or suspected cancer, they may indicate pleural or peritoneal metastasis. For this reason, the endosonographer should be alert to the presence of these fluid collections, and their presence or absence noted. Pleural effusions and ascites are amenable to EUS-guided FNA, and cytological examination may reveal malignant cells. The presence of cancer cells in the fluid carries an M1 designation and portends a poor prognosis. The major risk of EUS guided FNA is infection, and prophylactic antibiotics are indicated.

References

1. Ten Berge, J.: EUS guided Fine Needle Aspiration of the Liver. Indications, Yield, and Safety based on an

International Survey of 167 Cases. Gastrointestinal Endoscopy, 55(7):859–862, 2002.
2. Abeloff, Martin D., et al.: Clinical Oncology. 3rd edition: Philadelphia, PA: Churchill Livingstone, 2004.
3. Lee, Y. T., Ng, E., Hung, L., Chung, S., Ching, J., Chan, W., Chu, W., Sung, J.: Accuracy of endoscopic ultrasonography in diagnosing ascites and predicting peritoneal metastases in gastric cancer patients. Gut, 54:1541–1545, 2005.
4. Paquin, S. C., Gariepy, G., Lepanto, L., Bourdages, R., Raymond, G., Sahai, A.: A first report of tumor seeding because of EUS-guided FNA of a pancreatic adenocarcinoma. Gastrointestinal Endoscopy, 61(4):610–611, 2005.
5. Shah, J. N., Fraker, D., Guerry, D., Feldman, M., Kochman, M. L.: Melanoma seeding of an EUS-guided FNA needle track. Gastrointestinal Endoscopy, 59(7): 923–924, 2004.
6. McHutchison, J. G.: Differential diagnosis of ascites. Semin Liver Dis 1997;17:191–202.
7. Passebosc-Faure, K., Li, G., Lambert, C., Cottier, M., Gntil-Perret, A., Fournel, P., Perol, M., Genin, C.: Evaluation of a panel of molecular markers for the diagnosis of malignant serous effusions. Clinical Cancer Research, 11:6862–6867, 2005.
8. Torresini, R. J., Prolla, J. C., Diehl, A. R., Morais, E. K., Jobim, L. F.: Combined carcinoembryonic antigen and cytopathologic examination in ascites. Acta Cytol. 2000 Sep-Oct;44(5):778–782.
9. Pinto, M. M., Bernstein, L. H., Brogan, D. A., Criscuolo, E. M.: Carcinoembryonic antigen in effusions. A diagnostic adjunct to cytology. Acta Cytol. 1987 Mar-Apr;31(2):113–118.
10. Porcel, J. M., Vives, M., Esquerda, A., Salud, A., Pere, B., Rodrigue-Panandero, F.: Use of a panel of tumor markers (carcinoembryonic antigen, cancer antigen 125, carbohydrate antigen 15-3, and cytokeratin 19 fragments) in pleural fluid and differential diagnosis of benign and malignant effusions. Chest, 126: 1757–1763, 2004.
11. Shitrit, D., Zingerman, B., Shitrit, A. B., Shlomi, D., Kramer, M. R.: Diagnostic value of CYFRA 21-1, CEA, CA 19-9, CA 15-3, and CA 125 assays in pleural effusions: analysis of 116 cases and review of the literature. Oncologist. 2005 Aug;10(7):501–507.
12. Jacobsen, B. C., Adler, D. G., Davila, R. E., Hirota, W. K., Leighton, J. A., Oureshi, W. A., Rajan, E., Zuckerman, M. J., Fanelli, R. D., Baron, T. H., Faigel, D. O.: ASGE Guideline: Complications of EUS. Gastrointestinal Endoscopy 61 (1): 8–12, 2005.
13. Hirota, W. K., Peterson, K., Baron, T. H., Goldstein, J. L., Jacobson, B. C., Leighton, J. A., Mallery, J. S., Waring, J. P., Fanelli, R. D., Wheeler-Harbough, J., Faigel, D. O.: ASGE Guideline: Guidelines for Antibiotic Prophylaxis for GI Endoscopy. Gastrointestinal Endoscopy 58(4): 475–482, 2003.
14. Kaushik, N., Khalid, A., Brody, D., McGrath, K.: EUS-guided paracentesis for the diagnosis of malignant ascites. Gastrointestinal Endoscopy, 64(6): 908-13, 2006.
15. Chu, K. M., Kwok, K. F., Law, S., Wong, K. H.: A prospective evaluation of catheter probe EUS for the detection of ascites in patients with gastric carcinoma. Gastrointestinal Endoscopy, 59(4): 471–475, 2004.
16. Nguyen, P. T., Chang, K. J.: EUS in the detection of ascites and EUS-guided paracentesis. Gastrointestinal Endoscopy, 54(3): 336–339, 2001.
17. Thukkani, N., Davila, R. E., Faigel, D. O.: Diagnostic yield of EUS-FNA of ascites. Gastrointestinal Endoscopy, 63(5): AB275, 2006.
18. Chang, K. J., Albers, C. G., Nguyen, P.: Endoscopic ultrasound-guided fine needle aspiration of pleural and ascetic fluid. Am J Gastro 1995;90:148–150.

SECTION III

Colorectal

CHAPTER 31

Rectal Cancer

Dr. Marc Giovannini

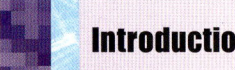
Introduction

Colorectal cancer is among the most common cancer affecting adult men and women. There are nearly 38,000 new rectal cancers diagnosed each year in the United States. While part of a functional continuum, rectal cancers are distinguished from colon cancers based on some very real anatomic, prognostic, and practical differences. These differences command staging and therapies unique to rectal lesions. Stage-based therapy for rectal cancer has achieved broad acceptance and is considered the standard of care. This submission reviews the role of endoscopic ultrasound (EUS) for the evaluation and management of rectal cancers.

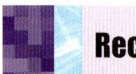
Rectal Anatomy

The rectum originates beneath the peritoneal reflection, extending 15–20 cm from the anal verge. The rectum is contained within the narrow pelvis, confined by the pubic bones anteriorly and the lumbosacral spine and coccyx posteriorly. A relevant Visible Human Model is shown in Figure 31–1A. The rectum is surrounded by structures vital to urinary and sexual function. Using transrectal EUS, the urinary bladder, seminal vesicles, prostate, and urethra are well seen in the male. The urinary bladder, uterus, and vagina are less well-appreciated in women. Transaxial Visible Human images are shown in Figures 31–1B, 31–1C. The anatomy of the anorectum is specifically designed for storage and controlled evacuation of the fecal bolus. Defecation and continence require the coordinated interaction of several muscular structures in and surrounding the anorectum. The circular muscle of the anus forms a prominent internal anal sphincter, which provides tonic closure of the anus. Specialized skeletal muscles descending from the levator ani apparatus provide a muscular sling and terminate to form the external anal sphincter. When viewed with a radial scanning echoendoscope at the level of the anal verge, the internal and external anal sphincters can be viewed as two distinct rings.[1] The lymphatic drainage of the rectum follows the route of its venous drainage along the inferior, middle, and superior hemorrhoidal veins to the inferior mesenteric veins and along the iliac veins and onto the portal vein.

Rectal Cancer

The prognosis for rectal cancer correlates with the pathologic stage at the time of diagnosis. So too,

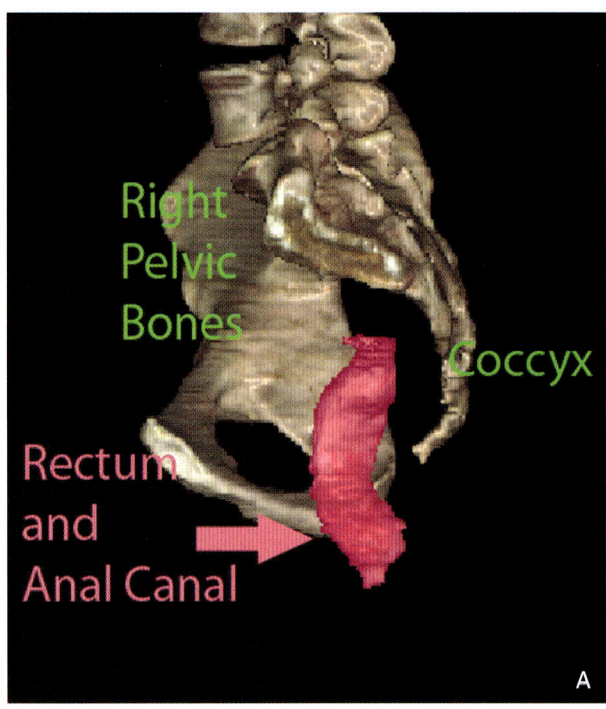
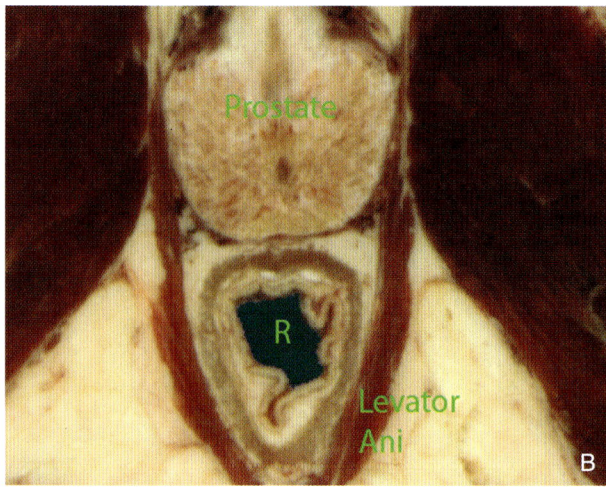

FIGURES 31–1. *A and B* (A) A Visible Human Model showing the right pelvic bones, coccyx and rectum. (B) A Visible Human transaxial cross-section of the male at the level of the prostate.

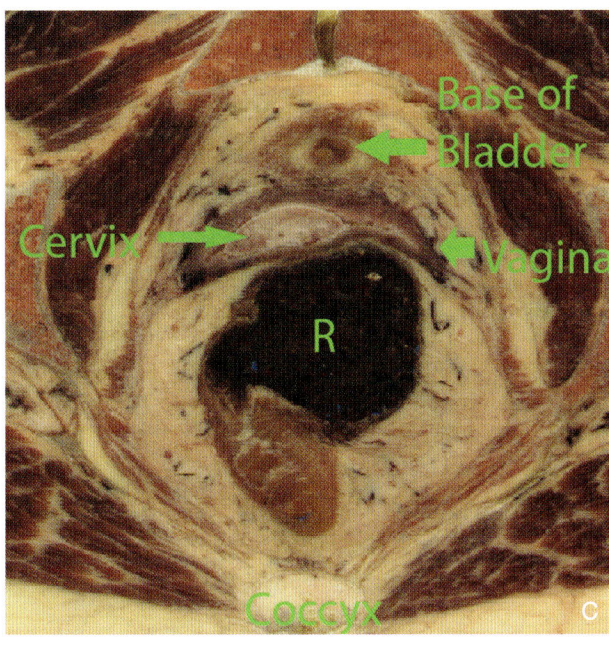

FIGURE 31–1. *C* (C) A Visible Human transaxial cross-section of the female at the level of the cervix. R=rectum

management is predicated based upon tumor stage at diagnosis and response to induction therapy. A wide variety of surgical techniques have been developed for rectal neoplasms in consideration of the anatomic constraints, preservation of function, and intent to achieve cure.[2] These are associated with disparate rates of postoperative morbidity. Cancer-containing superficial villous adenomas can be cured with endoscopic mucosal resection (EMR). Lesions confined to the wall may be resected by transanal excision or low anterior resection. Lesions involving, or in close proximity to, the anus may warrant abdominoperineal resection preserving anal sphincter function. Patients with locoregionally-advanced lesions (extension onto the perirectal fat and/or perirectal or pelvic adenopathy) should be considered for neoadjuvant chemoradiotherapy. Neoadjuvant therapy has been demonstrated to reduce local recurrence and permit increased likelihood of a sphincter-sparing operation with less toxicity when compared to postoperative regimes.[3] Thus, unlike more proximal colon cancer, the optimal method of management for rectal carcinoma is critically dependent on the accurate preoperative staging of the disease, as shown in Table 31–1.[4]

Table 31–1 Tumor Staging

Tumor Stage/Location	Treatment Option
Polypoid T1m cancer	Snare polypectomy
Sessile T1m cancer	EMR
	TAEX
T1sm, N0	EMR OR TAEX
	LAR
T2, N0/High	LAR
T2, N0/Low	TAEX or APR
T2 T3, N1/High	LAR
T2,T3, N1/Low	RT followed by APR
T4, any N	RT-CT followed by APR

EUS tumor stage and lesion location determines treatment options for rectal cancers.

High = <u>more than</u> 2 cm from dentate line; Low = <u>less than</u> 2 cm from dentate line; EMR = endoscopic mucosal resection; TAEX = transanal excision; LAR = low anterior resection; APR = abdominoperineal resection; RT = neoadjuvant radiotherapy, RT-CT: neoadjuvant radiochemotherapy.

Equipment and Technique

Endorectal Ultrasound (ERUS) can be performed either with blind, rigid probes (Figure 31–2) or with flexible echoendoscopes. ERUS is an ambulatory procedure. Patients prepare the rectum with two Fleet® enemas in advance. Intravenous sedation is optional. With the patient in the left-lateral-decubitus position, digital rectal exam (DRE) should be

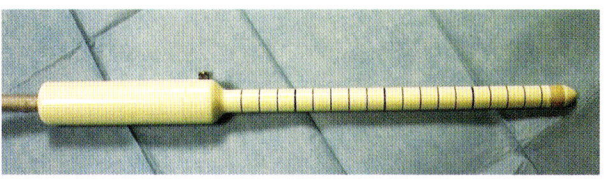

FIGURE 31–2. Rectal rigid probe from Hitachi (R54)

performed. DRE should allow assessment of sphincter tone and palpation of the lesion. If palpable, the lesion should be described in terms of location, distance from the anal verge, and fixation or mobility. Forward viewing sigmoidoscopy should be performed to image the lesion both in the forward and retroflexed scope positions. This allows familiarity with the anatomic configuration of the patient's rectum and the location and distribution of the tumor.

The echoendoscope is inserted and advanced beyond the lesion, under direct vision, to the rectosigmoid junction. ERUS imaging should begin at 5-7.5 MHz during withdrawal of the scope. The lumen is deflated of air and the water-fill balloon adjusted for acoustic coupling. Tip deflection should be passive allowing the transducer to find the right axis to the lumen. During this phase of the exam, surrounding adenopathy is the quarry. Any lymph nodes seen should be interrogated for size, shape, and echoqualities. The scope is withdrawn to the level of the anal verge. Next, the tumor itself should be targeted to determine depth of penetration into or through the rectal wall. The choice of frequency is dependent on the lesion size, but 5 and 7.5 frequencies are most commonly employed for T-staging. The degree of tip deflection and water-balloon fill should be adjusted to avoid false-findings owing to tumor compression, tangential imaging, and air artifact. Water-filling the lumen through the accessory channel is often necessary to achieve optimal imaging. The echoendoscope is advanced and withdrawn over the lesion to achieve satisfactory imaging over the length of the lesion. Lastly, the scope is withdrawn to the anal verge to interrogate anal sphincters for tumor invasion. Sphincter interrogation is an active process and should incorporate voluntary squeezing and relaxation of the muscles during imaging.

ERUS Staging of Rectal Cancer

The American Joint Committee on Cancer has identified the TNM classification as the preferred staging system.[5] This system is based on the determination of depth of tumor invasion (T-classification), the presence of regional lymph node metastases (N-classification), and the presence of distant metastases (M-classification). The individual classifications are combined to provide an overall stage.

EUS Tumor Stage

Endosonographically, the rectal wall is seen as five alternating hyper- and hypoechoic layers (Figure 31–3). The histologic correlation of the echolayers is as follows:

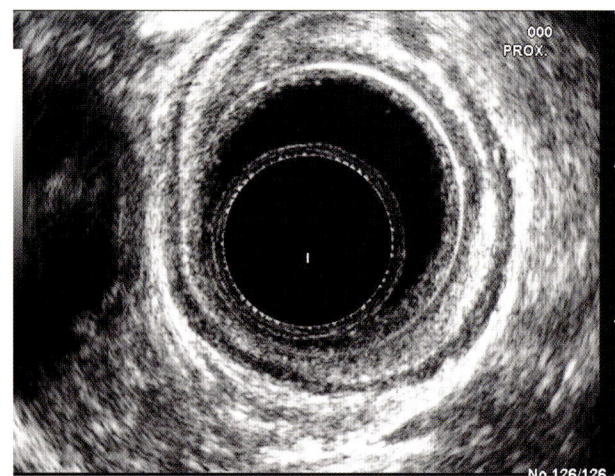

FIGURE 31–3. Normal rectal wall

First layer (hyperechoic): interface between water or water-filled balloon and the superficial mucosa.
Second layer (hypoechoic): represents the deep mucosa and the muscularis mucosa.
Third layer (hyperechoic): represents the submucosa and its interfaces.
Fourth layer (hypoechoic): represents the muscularis propria.
Fifth layer (hyperechoic): interface between the serosa and perirectal fat.

Rectal cancer appears as homogeneous hypoechoic soft tissue. Invasion appears as disruption of the normal wall echolayer pattern. A tumor that by EUS appears to be limited to the mucosa or the submucosa (first three echo layers) is classified as a T1 lesion (Figure 31–4). A tumor that invades into the muscularis propria (the hypoechoic fourth EUS layer) is a T2 lesion (Figure 31–5). A T3 lesion penetrates

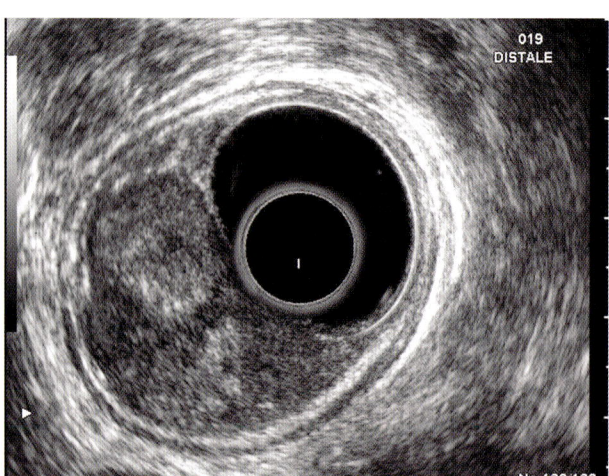

FIGURE 31–4. US T1 rectal cancer

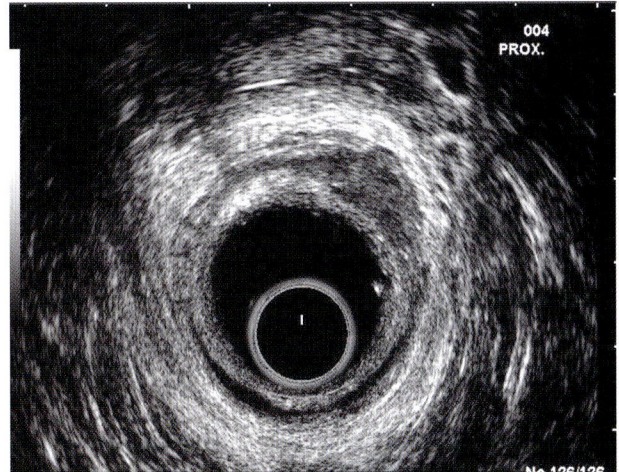

FIGURE 31–5. US T2 rectal cancer

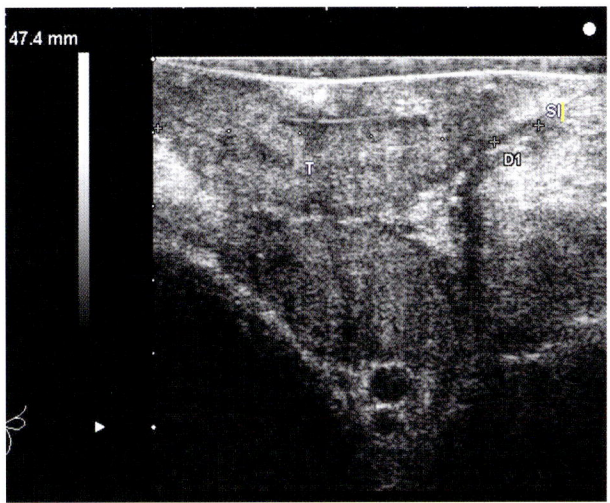

FIGURE 31–7. US T4 rectal cancer (prostate involvement)

through the rectal wall, extending beyond the five echo layers and into the surrounding perirectal fat (Figure 31–6). A T4 lesion displays direct invasion into an adjacent organ, such as the prostate gland, sacrum, vagina, and bladder (Figure 31–7).

EUS Lymph Node Staging

Endosonographically, lymph nodes appear as round or oval structures (Figure 31–8), which are hypoechoic compared to the surrounding perirectal fat. Endosonographic criteria applied to perilesional adenopathy in other regions of the digestive tract for the determination of malignancy versus benignity may not be so well applied in rectal cancer. Data obtained primarily in patients with esophageal carcinoma have identified four sonographic criteria predictive of malignancy: large size (greater than 1cm), hypoechoic echodensity, sharply demarcated borders, and round (rather than ovoid or flat) shape.[6] These criteria may not apply so well to rectal carcinoma, however. Up to 50% of metastatic lymph nodes associated with rectal cancers are smaller than 5 mm.[7] While EUS-guided fine-needle aspiration (FNA) of an individual lymph node might confirm accuracy, it is only rarely called upon for this purpose in initial staging.

Accuracy of EUS in Staging Rectal Cancer

Accuracy of tumor and nodal staging is dependent on the experience and expertise of the endosonographer.[8] The overall accuracy of T-staging for rectal cancer varies between 70% to 90%.[9-17] When EUS is

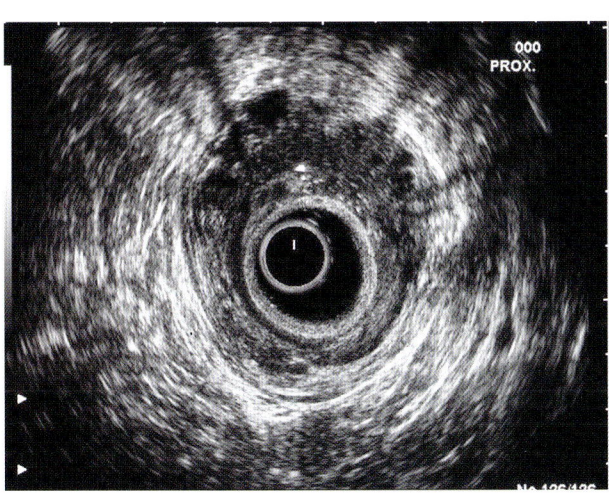

FIGURE 31–6. US T3 rectal cancer

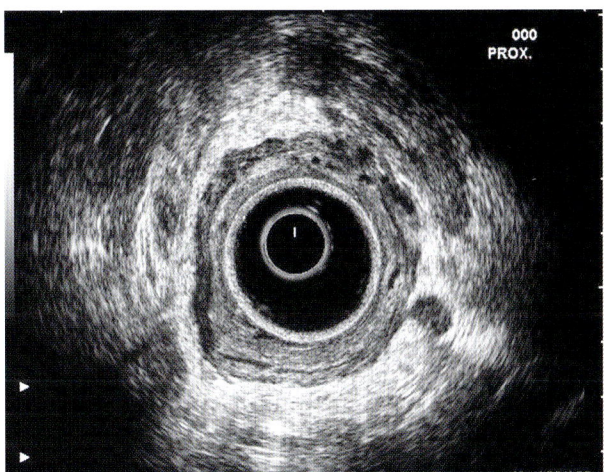

FIGURE 31–8. US T3N1 rectal cancer

incorrect for T-stage, it is typically due to overstaging rather than understaging. EUS tends to overstage cancers because high-resolution ultrasound can detect, but not separate inflammation adjacent to the malignancy from the tumor itself. Understaging is attributed to undetected microscopic invasion of cancer cells beyond that observed by EUS Accuracy is generally lowest for lesions classified as T2 by EUS, which may be overstaged as T3 lesions. Overstaging is apt to occur when imaging tumors located on a haustral fold, due to artifact induced by tangential imaging. Water-filling the rectal vault will improve technical results and likely enhances T-stage accuracy.

The overall accuracy of N-staging by EUS is 73% to 83%.[9-16] Lower nodal staging accuracy is attributed to the observation that up to 50% of malignant nodes are less than 5 mm in diameter, and EUS detection rates of these nodes may be as low as 20%.[7]

Nonetheless, ERUS has been reported to be equal to or superior to computed tomography (CT) for T- and N-staging. Among several comparative studies, ERUS has a greater accuracy than CT scan for staging of rectal cancer: 67% to 93% versus 53% to 86% for T-stage, and 80%- 87% versus 57% to 72% for N-stage.[19-21] Magnetic resonance imaging (MRI) with endorectal surface coils has compares similarly but not better that ERUS in accuracy.[22-26] MR imaging is more expensive than transanal ultrasound and endorectal MRI is not widely available.

While there is little published experience for EUS-FNA for rectal cancer, experience extrapolated from other malignancies has suggested that the performance of fine- needle aspiration cytology can markedly increase the accuracy and specificity of EUS nodal classification. Management may be altered when nodal metastasis is identified in a patient in whom T-classification would otherwise suggest the possibility of local endoscopic or transanal resection as a curative option. This applies to the 10% of patients with T1 lesions that have positive lymph nodes.

Restaging After Neoadjuvant Therapy

Preoperative neoadjuvant chemoradiotherapy is commonly used to down-stage rectal cancers. In addition to improving long-term survival and local recurrence, this approach allows sphincter-preserving low-anterior resection (LAR) in many patients who would require abdominoperineal resection (APR) based on findings at initial presentation. Neoadjuvant therapy of rectal cancer results in tumor regression/necrosis and inflammatory and fibrotic changes in the rectal wall. These changes may be sonographically indistinguishable from viable tumor. As such, accuracy of T- and N-staging after chemoradiation therapy is considerably compromised.[27] Therefore, we do not apply TNM staging when inspecting lesions for response to preoperative chemoradiatherapy. Rather we assess evidence for tumor regression from surrounding organs, in particular the anal sphincters, vagina, and prostate. In this way, EUS can direct therapy in patients who have undergone neoadjuvant therapy as a prelude to possible sphincter-sparing surgery.[28]

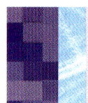

EUS for Local Recurrence of Colorectal Carcinoma

Local recurrence of rectal cancer after presumed curative resection occurs in 10–15% of cases, usually within the first two years after surgery. It is hypothesized that early detection of recurrent local tumor prompting early retreatment would improve survival. While this notion may be logical, it remains unproved. EUS may be useful in the detection of suspected local recurrence when no mucosal lesions are seen during surveillance sigmoidoscopy. Preliminary data obtained using blind/rigid ultrasound probes suggested that transrectal ultrasound was highly sensitive for the detection of anastamotic recurrence.[29,30] A more recent study using a radial scanning echoendoscope reported EUS as highly sensitive (greater than 90%) in the detection of local rectal tumor recurrence.[31] However, the sonographic changes of local tumor recurrence are not specific. Postoperative and postradiation inflammatory/fibrotic changes have similar appearances.[32] EUS should be used to complement sigmoidoscopy when local recurrence is suspected (Figure 31–9). In these instances, extraluminal local recurrence suspected by EUS can be confirmed by EUS-guided fine-needle aspiration.

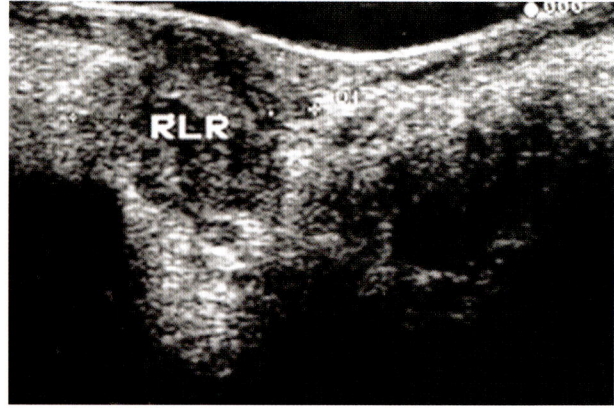

FIGURE 31–9. Deep pelvic recurrence of rectal cancer

Three-Dimentional EUS

Several studies in the field of endoscopic ultrasound (EUS) technology have reported advantages for three-dimensional (3-D) EUS.[33-45] However, most of 3-D EUS studies have been performed using catheter-type miniature probe system.[35,38,41] Some studies have previously reported benefits of a prototype 3-D EUS using a linear-array echoendoscope for 3-D guidance of interventional procedures, but the applicable scanning method of this system was systemically limited and, because the US probe was not positioned at the tip of the endoscope, it was difficult to obtain clinically sufficient images without geometrical distortion in the stomach.[45,47,48] A recent study tried to resolve this problem and maximize the performance of the 3-D EUS using a linear echoendoscope with a miniature electromagnetic position sensor attached to the tip of the scope, which can be used in freehand scanning in any position.[49] But the problem of this technique is that this electromagnetic sensor increase the size of the probe. We report our experience of a totally new software of 3-D EUS working without any electromagnetic sensor, which can be used even with electronic radial or linear rectal probes. Two types of systems have been developed, making use of either a series of 2-D images produced by 1-D arrays, or 2-D arrays to produce 3-D images directly. Two criteria must be met to avoid inaccuracies: the relative position and angulation of the acquired 2-D images must be known accurately; and the images must be acquired rapidly and/or gated to avoid artefacts due to respiratory, cardiac, and involuntary motion.

Tracked Free-Hand Systems

The operator holds an assembly composed of the transducer and an attachment, and manipulates it over the anatomy. 2-D images are digitized as the transducer is moved while meeting two criteria: the exact relative angulation and position of the ultrasound transducer must be known for each digitized image; and the operator must ensure that no significant gaps are left when scanning the anatomy .

3-D Reconstruction

The 3-D reconstruction process refers to the generation of a 3-D image from a digitized set of 2-D images. The approach used was the voxel-based volume. The 2-D images are built into a 3-D voxel-based volume (3-D grid) by placing each digitized 2-D image into its correct location in the volume. The main advantage was that no information was lost during the 3-D reconstruction and a variety of rendering techniques were possible, but large data files are generated.

Visualization of 3-D Ultrasound Images

The ability to visualize information in the 3-D image depends critically on the rendering technique. Three basic types are being used :

Surface-Based Viewing Technique

An operator or algorithm identifies boundaries of structures to create a wire-frame representation. These are shaded and illuminated, so that surfaces or structures or organs are visualized.

Multiplane Viewing Techniques

Orthogonal views: Three perpendicular planes are displayed simultaneously and can be moved or rotated.

Polyhedron: The 3-D images is presented as a multi-sided volume (polyhedron). The appropriate ultrasound image is "painted" on each face of the polyhedron, which can be manipulated.

Volume-Based Rendering Techniques

The 3-D image is projected onto a 2-D plane by casting rays through the 3-D image. The voxel values intersected by each ray can be multiplied by factors and summed to produce different effects: multiplied by 1 and then added to form a radiographic-like image; multiplied by factors to produce translucency; or display only the voxel with the maximum intensity along each ray.

3-D EUS is a new technique still in development (Figure 31–10). Recently, Sumiyama et al have reported their experience using 3-D EUS and electronic linear probe. They concluded that 3-D EUS using linear-array echoendoscope was accurate and represented a consistent method. They claimed that 3-D EUS facilitated anatomical interpretation of sonographic images and reduced procedural difficulty of scanning. Previous experience using 3-D EUS using mechanical mini-probes was reported for cardiovascular procedure[50] and using rigid electronic probes for gynecologic tumor assessment.[51,52] More recently, 3-D EUS using mechanical miniprobes was published for pancreatico-biliary diseases (35,38,41) and anal diseases.[39] Our experience is a bit different; we use 3-D EUS with a new software allowing the use of linear-curved or radial electronic probe because the software is integrated in the computer of the US machine and

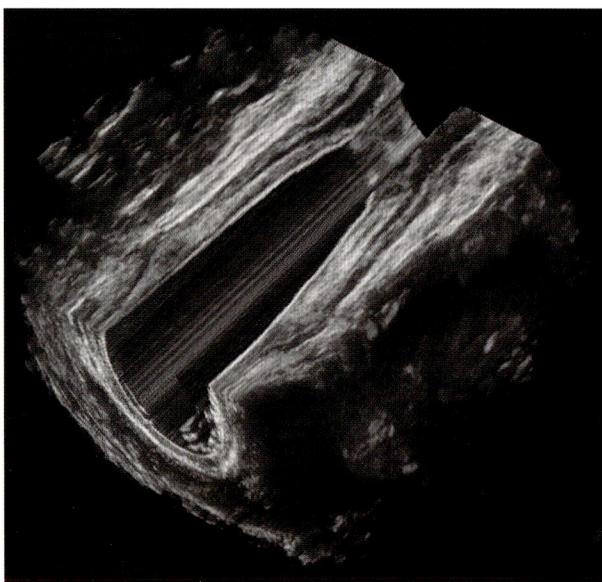

FIGURE 31–10. Normal 3-D reconstruction of the rectum

didn't need an external sensor attached at the tip of the EUS scope. However, the usefulness of 3-D EUS has not been clearly defined.[53,54] Regarding the locoregional staging of rectal cancer, several studies showed an important interest as better parietal staging[36,37] possibility of an accurate staging even in the case of stenotic lesion and also to perform more precisely an EUS-guided biopsy.[55] Our results showed that the mesorectum margins are better defined using 3-D EUS than using 2-D EUS—allowing a more accurate parietal staging. This precise definition of the mesorectum involvement has a direct impact on the therapeutic decision making because cancer reaching the margins of the mesorectum as considered as T4 lesion even without involvement of a pelvic organ.[56] (Figure 30–11) Such lesions must be treated by a preoperative radio-chemotherapy.

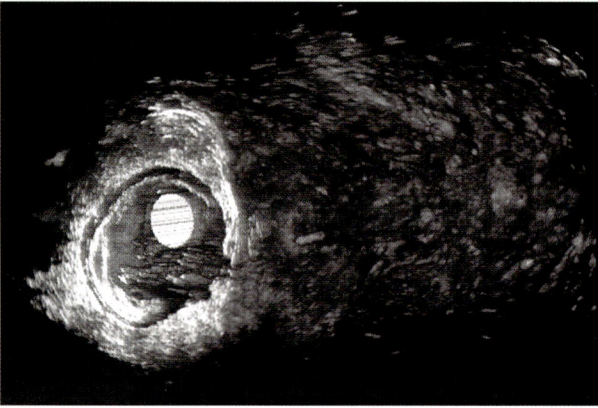

FIGURE 31–11. 3-D reconstruction of rectal cancer with complete involvement of the mesorectum

Conclusion

EUS is the most accurate tool for local staging of rectal carcinoma. In addition to providing accurate T- and N-stage, EUS allows assessment of the internal and external anal sphincters. Accurate endosonographic staging directs the optimal method of management of rectal carcinoma, type of resection, and candidacy for neoadjuvant therapy. Repeat sigmoidoscopic and endosonographic imaging may be considered in selected patients following neoadjuvant therapy. EUS-guided FNA can be used to detect suspected local recurrence.

References

1. Schwartz, D. A., Harewood, G. C., Wiersema, M.J.: EUS for rectal disease. Gastrointestinal Endoscopy 2002; 56:100–109.
2. Ramamoorthy, S. L., Fleshman, J. W.: Surgical treatment of rectal cancer. Hematol Onco Clin N Am 2002; 16(4):927–946.
3. Santiago, R. J., Metz, J. M., Hahn, S.: Chemoradiotherapy in the treatment of rectal cancer. Hematol Onco Clin N Am 2002;16(4):995–1014.
4. Ahmad, N. A., Kochman, M. L., Ginsberg, G. G.: Endoscopic ultrasound and endoscopic mucosal resection for rectal cancers and villous adenomas. Hematol Onco Clin N Am 2002;16(4):897–906.
5. American Joint Committee on Cancer. Colon and Rectum. Manual for staging of cancer, 4th Ed. Philadelphia: J. B. Lippincott, 1992:75–79.
6. Catalano, M. F., Sivak, M. V., Jr., Rice, T., et al.: Endosonographic features predictive of lymph node metastasis. Gastrointest Endosc 1994; 40:442–446.
7. Spinelli, P., Schiavo, M., Meroni, E., et al.: Results of EUS in detecting perirectal lymph node metastases of rectal cancer: The pathologist makes the difference. Gastrointest Endosc 1999;49: 754–758.
8. Boyce, G. A., Sivak, M. V., Jr., Lavery, I. C., Fazio, V. W., Church, J. M., Milsom, J., et al.: Endoscopic ultrasound in the preoperative staging of rectal carcinoma. Gastrointest Endosc 1992;38:468–471.
9. Marone, P., Petrulio, F., de Bellis, M., et al. : Role of endoscopic ultrasonography in the staging of rectal cancer: a retrospective study of 63 patients. J Clin Gastroenterol 2000; 30:420–424.
10. Gualdi, G. F., Casciani, E., Guadalaxara, A., et al.: Local staging of rectal cancer with transrectal ultrasound and endorectal magnetic resonance imaging: comparison with histologic findings. Dis Colon Rectum 2000; 43:338–345.
11. Glaser, F., Kuntz, C., Schlag, P., et al.: Endorectal ultrasound for control of preoperative radiotherapy of rectal cancer. Ann Surg 1993;217:64–71.
12. Herzog, U., von Flue, M., Tondelli, P., et al.: How accurate is endorectal ultrasound in the preoperative staging of rectal cancer? Dis Colon Rectum 1993; 36:127–134.
13. Cho, E., Nakajima, M., Yasuda, K., et al.: Endoscopic ultrasonography in the diagnosis of colorectal cancer invasion. Gastrointest Endosc 1993; 39:521–527.

14. Boyce, G. A., Sivak, M. V., Lavery, I. C., et al.: Endoscopic ultrasound in the preoperative staging of rectal cancer. Gastrointest Endosc 1992; 38:468–471.
15. Yamashita, Y., Machi, J., Shirouzu, K., et al.: Evaluation of endorectal ultrasound for the assessment of wall invasion of rectal cancer: Report of a case. Dis Colon Rectum 1988; 31:617–623.
16. Beynon, J.: An evaluation of the role of rectal endosonography in rectal cancer. Ann R Coll Surg Eng 1989;71: 131–139.
17. Feifel, G., Hildebrandt, U., Dhom, G.: Assessment of depth of invasion of rectal cancer by endosonography. Endoscopy 1987;19: 64–67.
18. Faigel, D. O., Ginsberg, G. G., Bentz, J. S., Gupta, P. K., Smith, D. B., Kochman, M. L.: Endoscopic ultrasound-guided real-time fine-needle aspiration biopsy of the pancreas in cancer patients with pancreatic lesions. Journal of Clinical Oncology 1997;15:1439–1443.
19. Herzog, U., von Flue, M., Tondelli, P., et al.: How accurate is endorectal ultrasound in the preoperative staging of rectal cancer? Dis Colon Rectum 1993; 36: 27–34.
20. Rifkin, M. D., Ehrlich, S. M., Marks, G.: Staging of rectal carcinomas: prospective comparison of endorectal ultrasound and CT. Radiology 1989;170: 319–322.
21. Pappalardo, G., Reggio, D., Frattaroli, F. M., et al.: The value of endoluminal ultrasonography and computed tomography in the staging of rectal cancer: A preliminary study. J Surg Oncol 1990; 43:219–222.
22. Waizer, A., Powsner, E., Russo, I., et al.: Prospective comparative study of MRI versus transrectal ultrasound for pre-operative staging and follow-up of rectal cancer. Dis Colon Rectum 1991; 34:1068–1072.
23. Thaler, W., Watzka, S., Martin, F., et al.: Preoperative staging of rectal cancer by endoluminal ultrasound vs. magnetic resonance imaging: Preliminary results of a prospective, comparative study. Dis Colon Rectum 1994; 37:1189–1193.
24. Schaefer, H., Gossmann, A., Heindel, W., et al.: Comparison of endorectal MR imaging and transrectal ultrasound with pathology in rectal tumors. Endoscopy 1996; 28:S9.
25. Hunerbein, M., Pegios, W., Rau, B., et al.: Prospective comparison of endorectal ultrasound, three-dimensional endorectal ultrasound, and endorectal MRI in the preoperative evaluation of rectal tumors. Preliminary results. Surg Endosc 2000;14: 1005–1009.
26. Meyenberger, C., Huch Boni, R. A., Bertschinger, P., et al.: Endoscopic ultrasound and endorectal magnetic resonance imaging: a prospective, comparative study for preoperative staging and follow-up of rectal cancer. Endoscopy 1995; 27:469–479.
27. Napoleon, B., Pujol, B., Berger, F., et al.: Accuracy of endosonography in staging of rectal cancer treated by radiotherapy. Br J Surg 1991;78:785–788.
28. Loren, D. E., Kochman, M. L., Forman, L. M., Ahmad, N. A., Goldsmith, J. D., Rosato, E. F., Ginsberg, G. G.: Endoscopic and EUS directed therapy for rectal cancer. Gastroenterology 2002;122(4):A-331.
29. Beynon, J., Mortensen, N. J. M. C, Foy, D. M. A., et al.: The detection and evaluation of locally recurrent rectal cancer with rectal endosonography. Dis Colon Rectum 1989; 32: 509–517.
30. Feifel, G., Hildebrandt, U.: Diagnostic imaging in rectal cancer: Endosonography and immunoscintigraphy. World J Surg 1992; 16: 841–847.
31. Muller, C., Kahler, G., Scheele, J.: Endosonographic examination of gastrointestinal anastamoses with suspected locoregional tumor recurrence. Surg Endosc 2000;14:45–50.
32. Hunerbein, M., Dohmoto, M., Haensch. Evaluation and biopsy of recurrent rectal cancer using three-dimensional endosonography. Dis Colon Rectum 1996; 39:1373–1378.
33. Kallimanis, G., Garra, B. S., Tio, T. L.: The feasibility of three-dimensional endoscopic ultrasonography: a preliminary report. Gastrointest Endosc 1995;41: 235–239.
34. Odegaard, S., Nesje, L. B., Molin, S, O., Gilja, O. H., Hausken, T.: 3-D intraluminal sonography in the evaluation of gastrointestinal diseases. Abdo Imaging, 1999, 24:449–451.
35. Kanemaki, N., Nakazawa, S., Inui, K., Yoshino, J., Yamao, J., Okushima, K.: 3-D intraductal ultrasonography: preliminary results of a technique for diagnosis of diseases of pancreatobiliary system. Endoscopy, 1997, 28:726–731.
36. Hünerbein, M., Schlag, P. M.: Three-dimensional endosonography for staging of rectal cancer. Ann Surg 1997;225:432–438.
37. Ivanov, K. D., Diavoc, C. D.: Three-dimensional endoluminal ultrasound: new staging technique in patients with rectal cancer. Dis Colon Rectum 1997;40:47–50.
38. Tokiyama, H., Yanai, H., Nakamura, H., Takeo, Y., Yoshida, T., Okita, K.: 3-D endoscopic ultrasonography of lesions of the upper gastrointestinal tract using a radial-linear switchable thin ultrasound probe. J Gastroenterol Hepatol. 1999,14:1212–1218.
39. Gold, D. M., Bartram, C. I., Halligan, S., Humphries, K. N., Kamm, M. A., Kmiot, W. A.: 3-D endoanal sonography in assessment anal canal injury. Br J surg, 1999, 86:365–370.
40. Calleja, J. L., Albillos, A.: 3-D endosonography for staging of rectal cancer. Gastrointest Endosc. 1998, 47: 317–318.
41. Marusch, F., Koch, A., Schmidt, U.: Routine use of transrectal ultrasound in rectal carcinoma: results of a prospective multicenter study. Endoscopy, 2002, 34(5):385–390.
42. Chung, C. Y., McCrary, W. H., Dhaliwal, S.: 3-D esophageal varix model quantification of variceal volume by high-resolution endoluminal US. Gastrointest Endosc, 2000,52:87–91.
43. Hünerbein, M., Ghadimi, B. M., Gretschel, S., Schlag, P. M.: 3-D endoluminal ultrasound: A new model for the evaluation of gastrointestinal tumors. Abdom Imaging, 1999, 24:445–448.
44. Hünerbein, M., Ghadimi, B. M., Gretschel, S., Schlag, P. M.: 3-D endoscopic ultrasound of the esophagus, preliminary experience. Surg Endosc, 1997, 11: 991–994.
45. Liu, Y. T., Miller, L. S., Chung, J. Y., McCrary, W. H., Dhaliwal, S. : Validation of volume measurements in esophageal pseudotumors using 3-D endoluminal ultrasound. Ultrasound Med Biol, 2000, 26: 735–741.
46. Tamura, S., Hirano, M., Chen, X., Sato, Y., Narumi, Y., Hori, M., Takahashi, S., Nakamura, H. : Intrabody 3-D position sensor for an ultrasound endoscope. IEEE Trans Biomed Eng, 2002, 49 : 1187–1194.
47. Sumiyama, K., Suzuki, N., Katutani, H., Hino, S., Tajiri, H. : A novel 3-D EUS technique for real-time visualization of the data reconstruction process. Gastrointest Endosc. 2002, 55:723–726.
48. Molin, S. O., Nesje, L. B., Gilja, O. H., Hausken, T., Martens, D., Odegaard, S. : 3-D endosonography in

gastroenterology: methodology and clinical implications. Eur J Ultrasound 1999, 10, 171–177.
49. Sumiyama, K., Suzuki, N., Tajiri, H.: A linear-array freehand 3-D endoscopic ultrasound. Ultrasound Med Biol, 2003, 29;1001–1006.
50. Klingensmith, J. D., Schoenhagen, P., Tajaddini, A., Halliburton, S. S., Tuzcu, E. M., Nissen, S. E., Vince, D. G.: Automated 3-D assessment of coronary artery anatomy with intravascular ultrasound scanning. Am Heart J, 2003,145:795–805.
51. Ayoubi, J. M., Franchin, R., Ferretti, G., Pons, J. C., Bricault, I.: 3-D ultrasonography reconstruction of the uterine cavity virtual hysteroscopy ? Eur Radiol. 2002, 12: 2030–2033.
52. Liu, J. B., Miller, J. S., Bagley, D. H., Goldberg, B. B.: Endoluminal sonography of the genitourinary and gastrointestinal tract. J Ultrasound Med. 2002, 21: 323–327.
53. Yoshimoto, K.: Clinical application of ultrasound 3D imaging system in lesions of the gastrointestinal tract. Endoscopy, 1998, 30, 145–148.
54. Yoshino, J., Nakazawa, S., Iniu, K.: Surface-rendering imaging of gastrointestinal lesions by 3-D EUS. Endoscopy, 1999, 31:541–545.
55. Hünerbein, M., Dohmoto, M., Haensch, W., Schlag, P. M.: Evaluation and biopsy of recurrent rectal cancer using three-dimensional endosonography. Dis Colon Rectum 1996; 39: 1373–1378.
56. Heald, R.J., Ryall, R. D. : Recurrence and survival after total mesorectal excision for rectal cancer. Lancet, 1986, 1479–1481.

CHAPTER 32

Perirectal Abscesses

Dr. Christa Meyenberger
Dr. Franc H. Hetzer

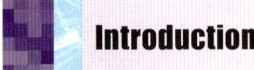

Introduction

The majority of anorectal abscesses occur through an infected proctodeal gland, which usually drains into anal crypts. A small number of abscesses may also appear perirectally. They have their origins in the visceral organs, especially the anorectal abscess with enteritis granulomatosa (Crohn's disease). These abscesses often form above the proctodeal glands with and without concurrent proctocolitis.

An abscess should preferably be opened near to its source, because this causes the fistula, which will definitely follow, to appear with a short tract. Therefore, correct localisation of the opening is mandatory. The endoanal ultrasound (EUS) is relatively simple, well tolerated, rapid diagnostic tool used to identify an abscess and to localise all purulent areas to ensure complete surgical drainage[1]. Additionally the EUS predicts the relationship between the abscess and the sphincter mechanism with a high accuracy. [2,3]

The anatomy of the perianal area is shown. Figure 32–1 provides Visible Human Models of the anal sphincters and levator ani as they relate to each other as well as the rectum and coccyx. Figure 32–2 shows sagittal, coronal, and axial cross-sections from the male, and a coronal cross-section from the female.

Anorectal abscess are classified, similarly to the perianal fistulas, into intersphincteric, ischorectal, supralevatoric or perianal.[4] See Figure 32–2F.

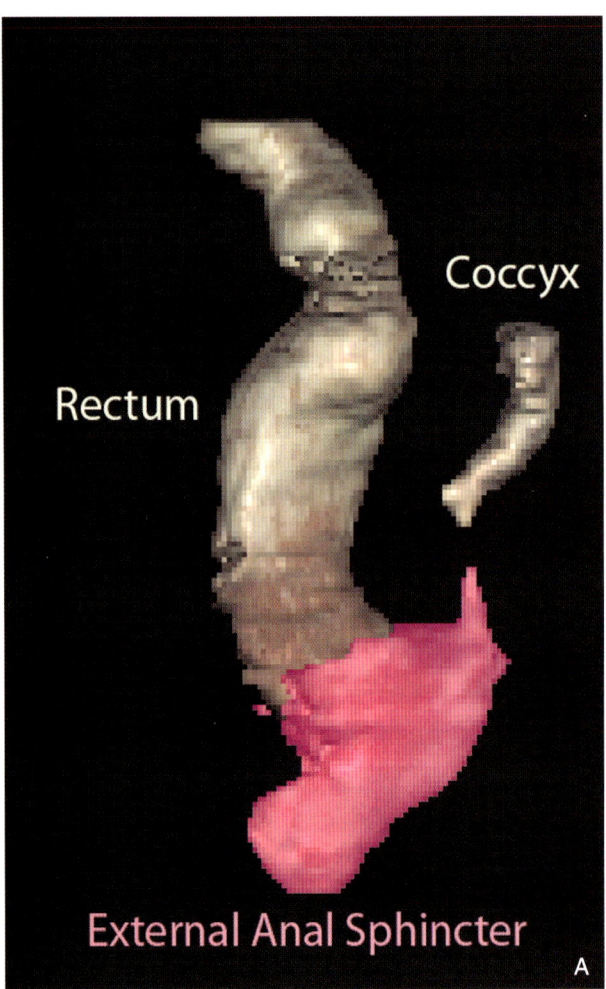
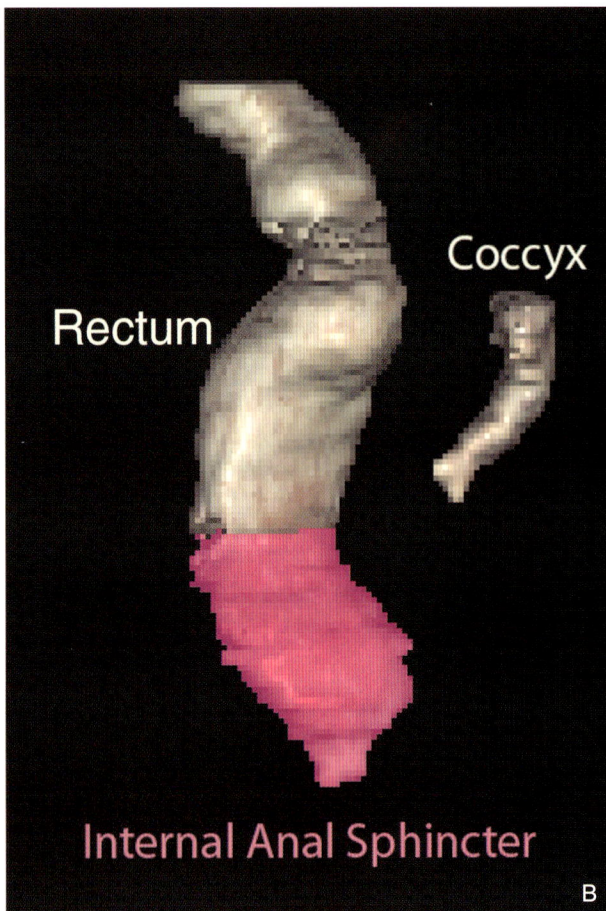

FIGURES 32–1. *A and H* (A) Visible Human Models of the rectum, coccyx levator ani and anal sphuincters. Left lateral view of rectum, coccyx and (A) external anal sphincter, (B) internal anal sphincter.

Perirectal Abscesses 347

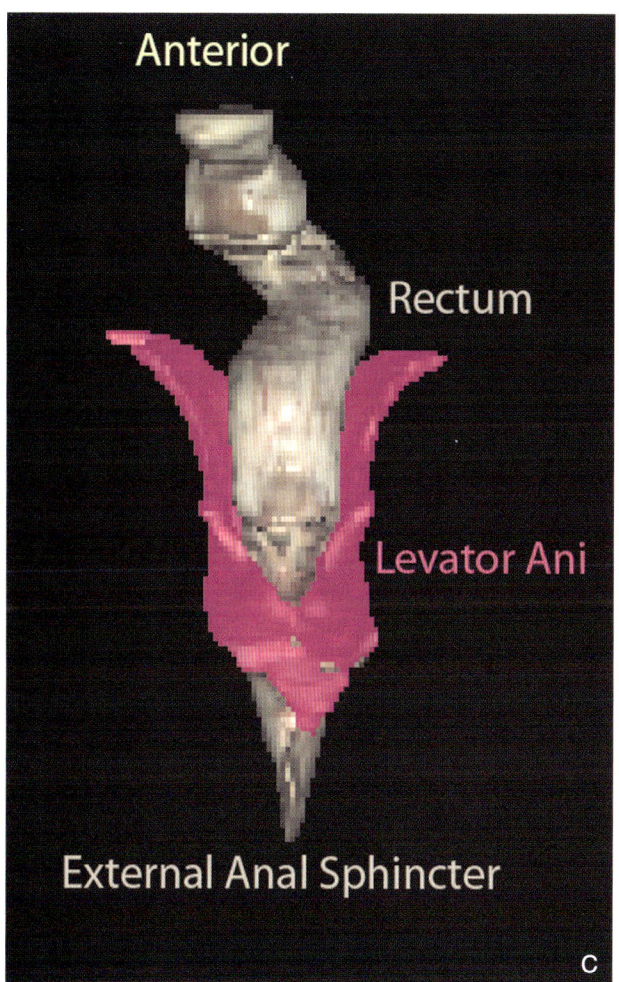

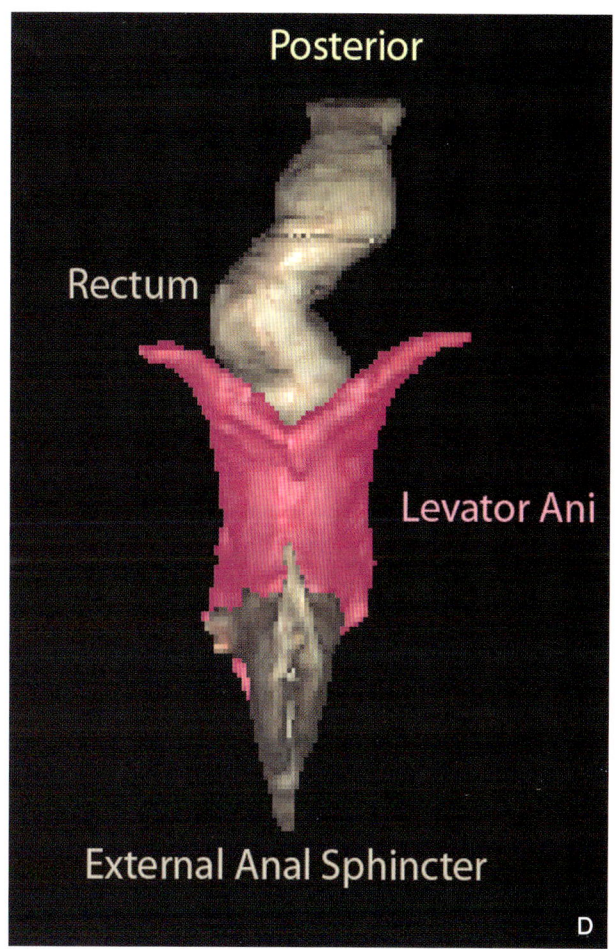

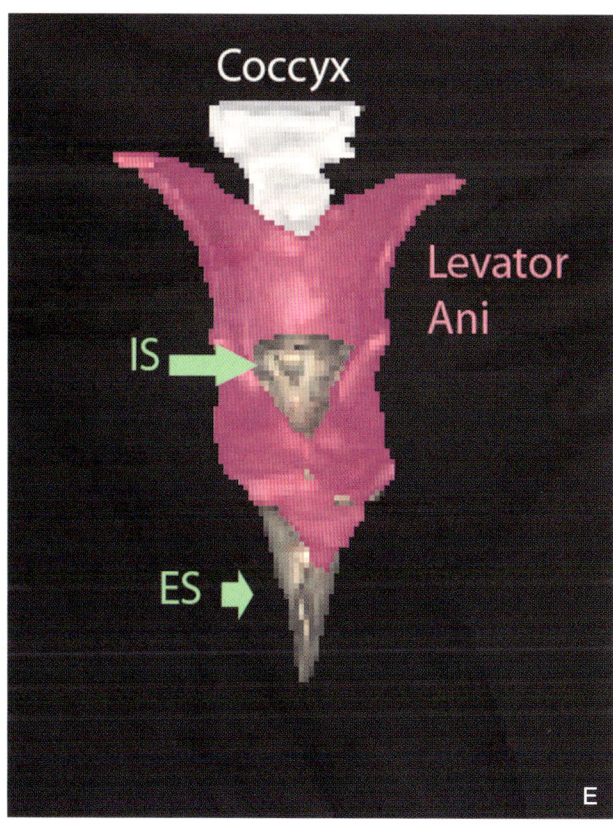

FIGURES 32–1. *C to E* (C) Levator ani from anterior and (D) posterior views. (E) Levator ani from anterior view without rectum, with internal anal sphincter (IS) and external anal sphincter (ES). Lateral views without the rectum, showing the coccyx.

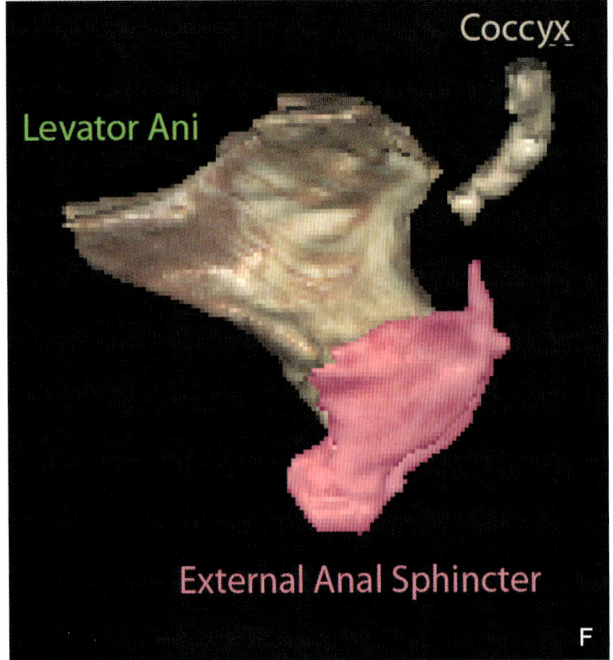
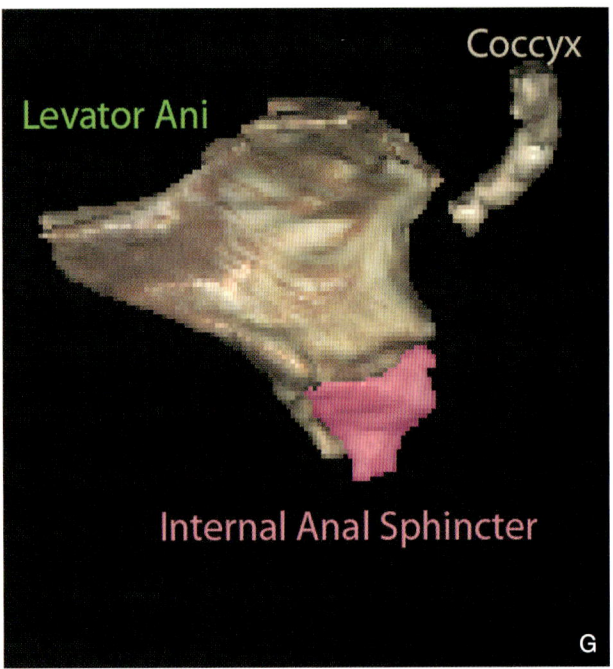
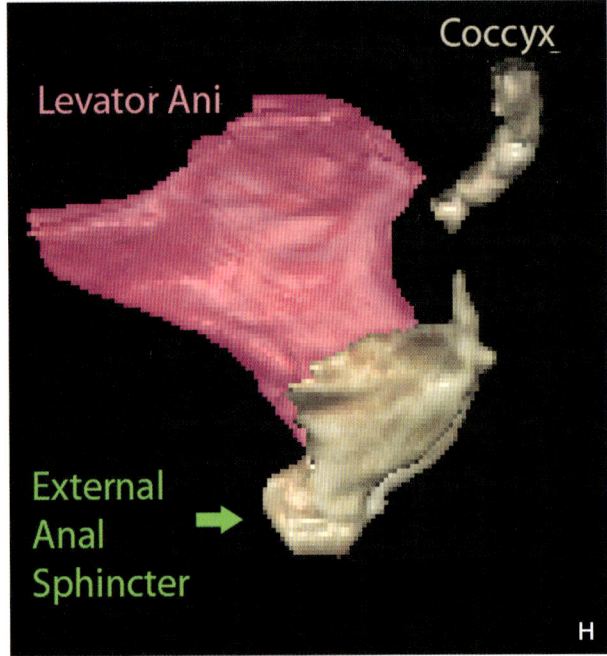

FIGURES 32-1. *F to H* (F) external anal sphincter, (G) Internal anal sphincter, and (H) Levator ani.

Perirectal Abscesses 349

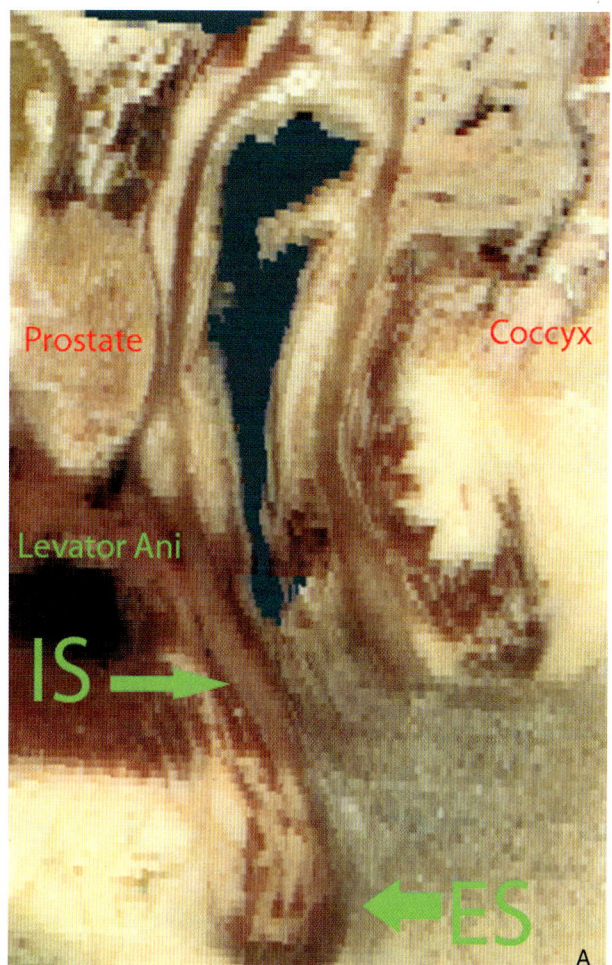

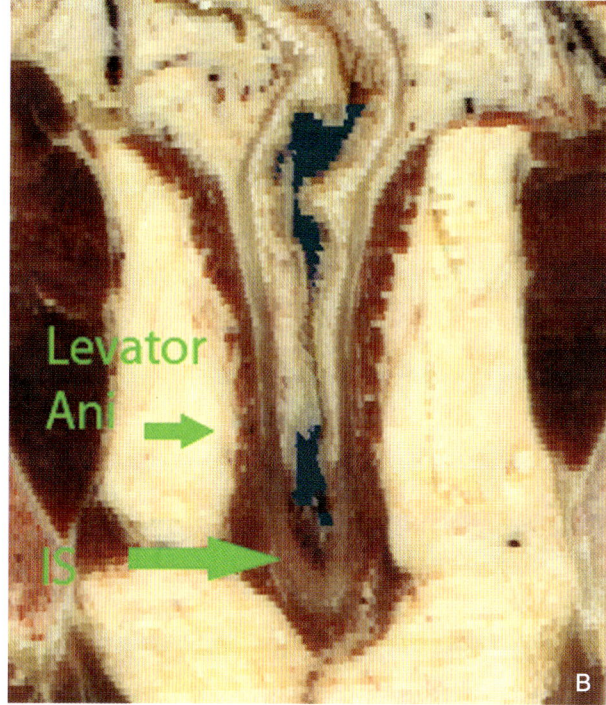

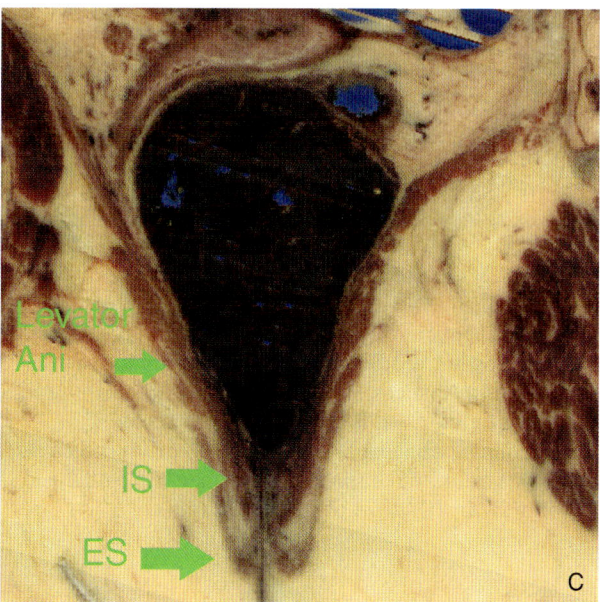

FIGURES 32–2. *A to C* Visible Human cross-section anatomy showing (A) sagittal view of anal canal (IS = internal anal sphincter, ES = external anal sphincter), (B) Coronal view of anal canal in male, (C) Coronal view of anal canal in female.

350 EUS Pathology with Digital Anatomy Correlation

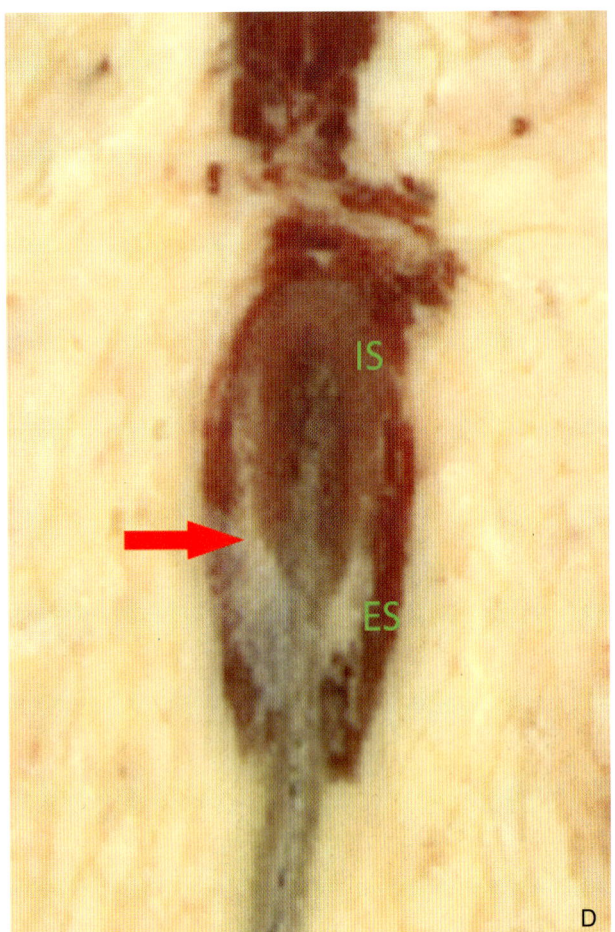

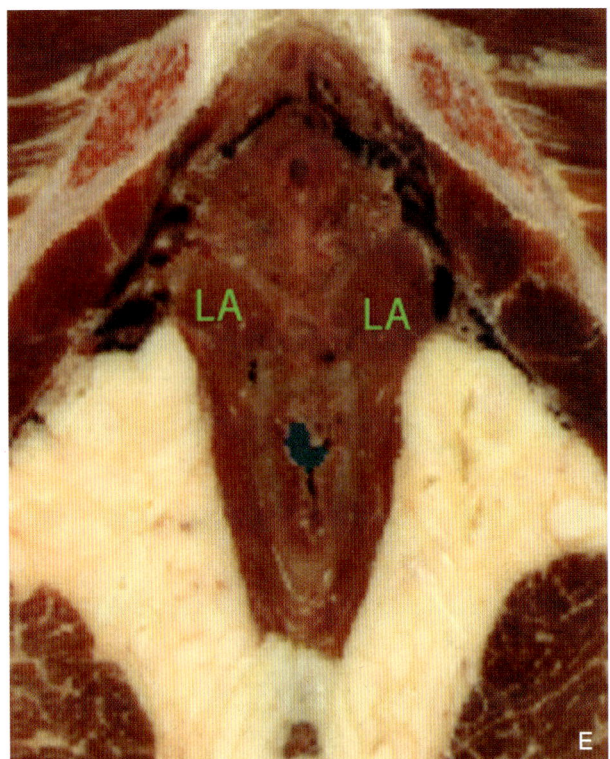

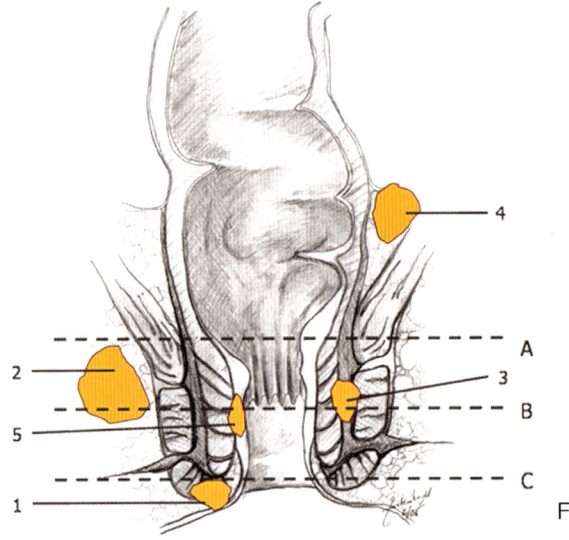

FIGURES 32–2. *D to F* (D) transaxial view of distal anal canal. The red arrow shows the intersphincteric space. (E) trans axial view of mid-anal canal. LA=levator ani. (F) Schema of the various types of perirectal Abscess: 1. Perianal 2. Ischorectal 3. Intersphincteric 4. Supralevatoric abscess, 5. Submcosal abscess. The coronal diagram indicates three different anal canal levels; upper (A), middle (B) and lower (C) level of the anal canal.

Endoanal Ultrasound in Perirectal Abscess

In the endoanal ultrasound (EUS) a perirectal abscess is presented as a hypoechoic cavity, seldom containing air. In the majority of cases, a coexisting fistula or a fistula that had developed the abscess will not be found, i.e. the source passage, because it will be swollen. The seeking of a fistula tract and even more the treatment of such a finding during deroofing of the abscess is controversial. Tang found in his study that only half of the patients will develop a fistula after abscess drainage and, even when a fistula has been found and treated, it will have no influence on the recurrence rate.[5] (Figures 32–3A, 32–3B, 32–4A, 32–4B).

On the one hand, EUS lacks the ability to image beyond the external sphincter, and therefore cannot reliably identify perianal, ischiorectal, or supralevator abscesses. Magnetic resonance imaging is indeed very effective for identifying the anatomical site of those complex cases. On the other hand, simple perirectal abscesses can certainly be identified and treated without the aid of any imaging. However, EUS can identify previously unsuspected purulent locations, define the relationship between abscess and sphincter mechanism, and help the surgeon to correctly drain the most frequent intersphincteric abscess. Figures 32–4AB, 32–5AB, 32–6, 32–7, 32–8.

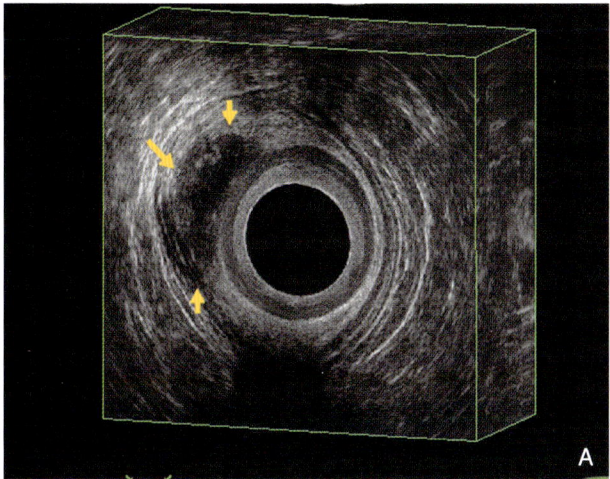
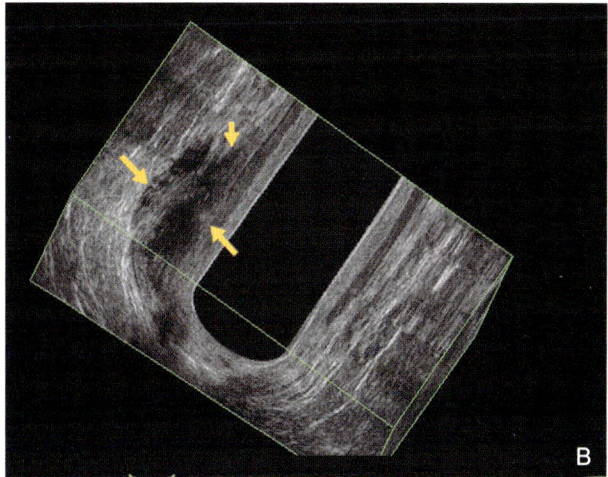

FIGURES 32–3. *A and B* A 23-year-old man with a intersphincteric abscess (Brüel&Kjaer, ProFocus, Naerum, Danemark, Transducer type 2050, 16MHz). (A) Axial, mid-anal canal imaging of a hypoechoic abscess from 8 to 11 o'clock in lithotripsy position (arrows). (B) Three-dimensional view with coronal plane is applied from 9 to 3 o'clock in lithotripsy position. Arrows indicate the abscess.

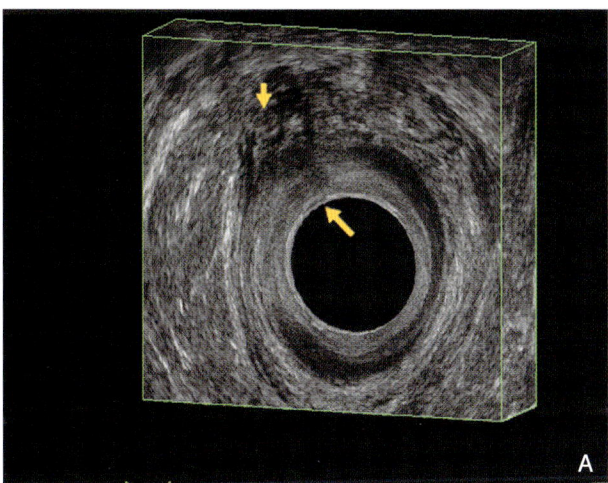
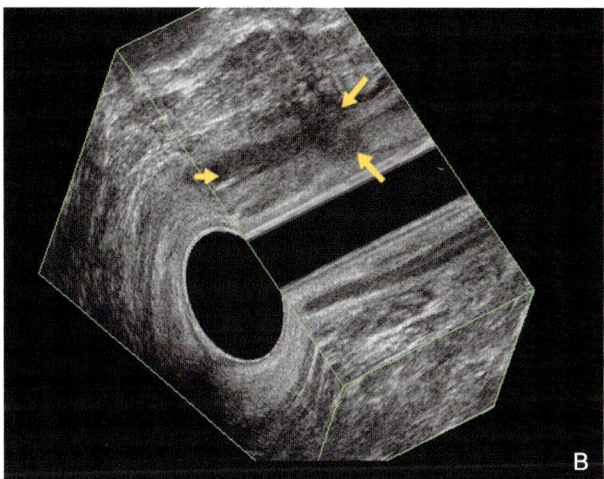

FIGURES 32–4. *A and B* A 37-year-old man with an intersphincteric abscess (Brüel&Kjaer, ProFocus, Naerum, Danemark, Transducer type 2050, 16MHz). (A) Axial, mid-anal canal imaging of a hypoechoic abscess between 9 to 12 o'clock in lithotripsy position (arrows) with a fistula and an internal opening at 11 o'clock (arrow). (B) Three-dimensional view with coronal plane is applied between 10 to 2 o'clock in lithotripsy position. Arrows indicate the abscess and fistula tract.

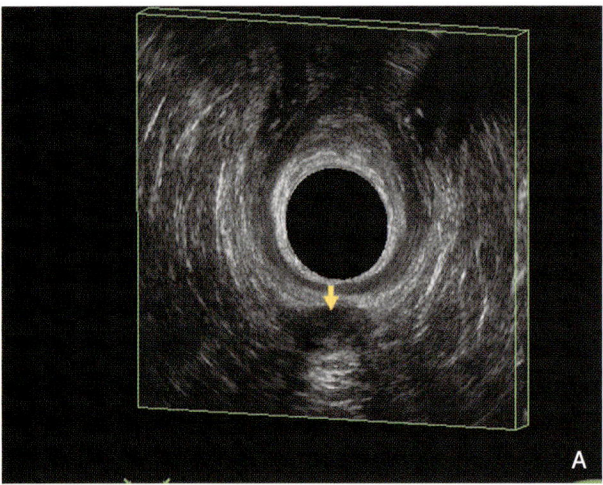
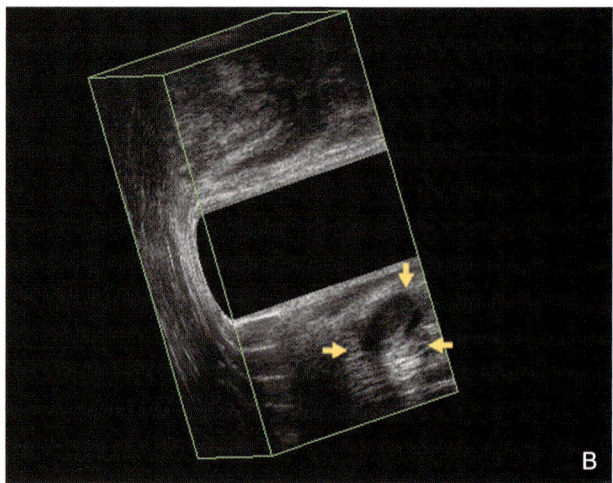

FIGURES 32–5. *A and B* A 53-year-old man with an ischorectal abscess (Brüel&Kjaer, ProFocus, Naerum, Danemark, Transducer type 2050, 16MHz) (A) Axial, upper-anal canal imaging of a hypoechoic abscess between 5 to 7 o'clock in lithotripsy position (arrows). (B) Three-dimensional view with coronal plane is applied between 12 to 6 o'clock in lithotripsy position. Arrows indicate the abscess.

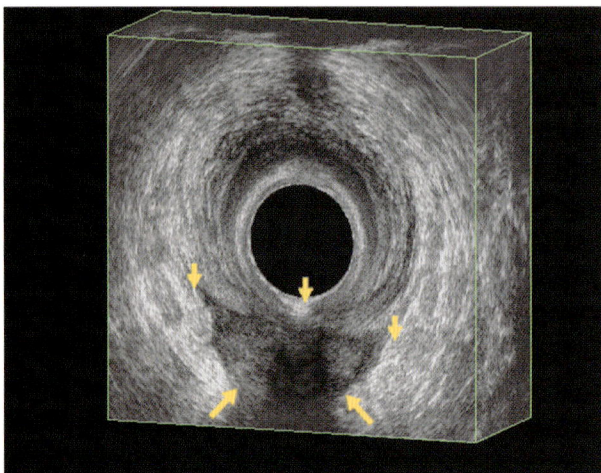

FIGURE 32–6. A 67-year-old male with a simple perianal abscess. Axial, middle anal canal imaging of a hypoechoic abscess between 5 to 7 o'clock in lithotripsy position (arrows). (B&K ProFocus, Transducer type 2050, 16MHz)

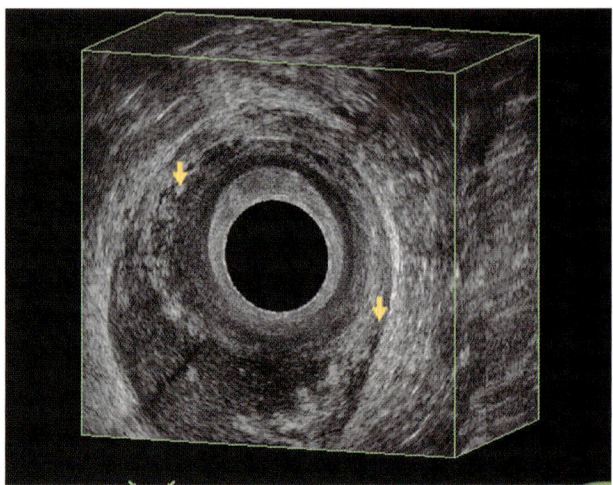

FIGURE 32–7. A 26-year-old female with a complex perianal, horseshoe abscess. Axial, middle anal canal imaging of a hypoechoic abscess between 4 to 10 o'clock in lithotripsy position (arrows). (B&K ProFocus, Transducer type 2050, 16MHz)

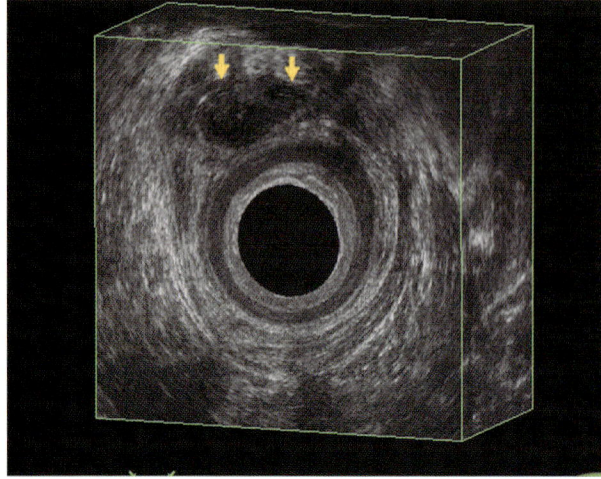

FIGURE 32–8. A 24-year-old female with Crohn's disease and supralevatoric abscess. Axial, upper-anal canal imaging of a hypoechoic abscess between 10 to 12 o'clock in lithotripsy position (arrows). (B&K ProFocus, Transducer type 2050, 16MHz)

References

1. Ratto, C., Grillo, E., Parello, A., Costamagna, G., Doglietto, G. B.: Endoanal ultrasound-guided surgery for anal fistula. Endoscopy 2005;37:722–728.
2. Cataldo, P. A., Senagore, A., Luchtefeld, M. A.: Intrarectal ultrasound in the evaluation of perirectal abscesses. Dis Colon Rectum 1993; 36:554–558.
3. Law, P. J., Talbott, R. W., Bartram, C. I., Northover, J. M.: Anal endosonography in the evaluation of perianal sepsis and fisula in ano. Br J Surg 1989;76:752–755.
4. Parks, A. G., Gordon, P. H., Hardcastle, J. D.: A classification of anal fistula. Br J Surg 1976;63:1–12.
5. Tang, C. L., Chew, S. P., Soew-Choen, F.: Prospective randomized trial of drainage alone vs. drainage and fistulotomy for acute perianal abscesses with proven internal opening. Dis Colon Rectum. 1996;39(12):1415–1417.

CHAPTER

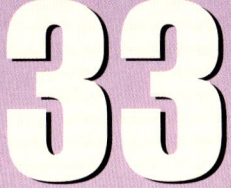

Anorectal Fistulae

Dr. Christa Meyenberger
Dr. Franc H. Hetzer

Introduction

Anorectal fistulas are abnormal tubular tracts communicating between the anus or the rectum and the perianal skin. The perianal abscess is an acute manifestation, and the fistula a chronic condition of the same disease. An inflamed proctodeal gland is the basis for the genesis of the nonspecific anal fistulas disease.[1] These eccrine glands, of rudimentary primordial origin, form a pathological anatomical unit together with the anal crypts. By comparison, other aetiology factors are rare e.g. Crohn's disease, tuberculosisi or rectovaginal fistula.

All nonspecific fistulae have their starting point in the intersphincteric space. Perianal fistulas are classified according to their primary path extension in inter-sphincteric, trans-sphincteric, suprasphincteric, or extrasphincteric,[2] see Diagram 33–1. Visible Human Anatomy has previously been shown in Figures 32–1 and 32–2 in Chapter 32, Perirectal Abscesses. In the previously described classification, about 95% of the fistulas are either inter- or transsphincteric.

Endoanal Ultrasound in Nonspecific Anorectal Fistula

The endoanal ultrasound (EUS) sign of a fistula is continuous hypoechoic linear structure with possible hyperechoic reflection (air). The assessment with ultrasound provides detailed information about the extent of the fistula track. The internal fistula opening can even be identified applying the appropriate technique.[3,4] Furthermore, the EUS can provide the capability to identify hidden sphincter muscle defects. Having both the information on the known fistula as well as any possible hidden fistulas, simplifies the planning of the surgical access point and the surgical repair of the fistula. In a series of operations, Lengyel et al, for instance, found in 82% of cases a coincidence with the preoperative EUS and the surgical findings. The authors consider the technique useful for the preoperative planning of fistula surgery.[5]

Figures 33–1 - 33–6 show different types of fistula tracts. Attention should be focused on integrity of the internal and external anal sphincters. Tears and defects may be associated with the fistula (focal infection) or a previous surgery.

Sometimes the classification by EUS of the perianal fistula can be difficult. Specifically, an active tract is often difficult to differentiate from scarring of healed fistulous tract. Injecting hydrogen peroxide into the fistula has been suggested to improve the diagnostic accuracy.[6-8] Figure 33–4 shows a transsphincteric fistula indicated by 3% hydrogen peroxide injection. However, the benefit of the peroxide-enhanced EUS is currently being discussed. A recently published literature review could not indicate significantly better accuracy for the additional use of hydrogen peroxide injection. It showed that unenhanced EUS had an accuracy of 64–94%, whereas peroxide-enhanced EUS, 60–95%.[9] Additionally the injection may cause some pain in acute inflamed tissue.

In general, anorectal fistulas do not heal spontaneously. Even though anal fistula disease is not life threatening, the treatment of complex fistula tracks constitutes one of the greatest problems facing anal surgery today. Adequate preoperative diagnosis is the key step to prevent failure in the surgical treatment of fistula. Missing secondary tracts or internal openings during surgical exploration may lead to recurrence. This is more likely when the fistula is complex. In these cases a three-dimensional (3-D) EUS with hydrogen peroxide injection alone[10] or combined with magnetic resonance (MR) assessment[11] may prove more accurate for detecting primary and secondary tracks and internal openings. The MR imaging seems to be superior to the EUS with a sensitivity of 87%, a specificity of 98%, and an accuracy to surgical findings up to 97 %.[9,12] However, the lack of widespread availability of MR imaging makes using the extended EUS for complex anal fistulae still attractive. Figure 33–5 presents a 3D-EUS in a patient with a complex transsphincteric fistula.

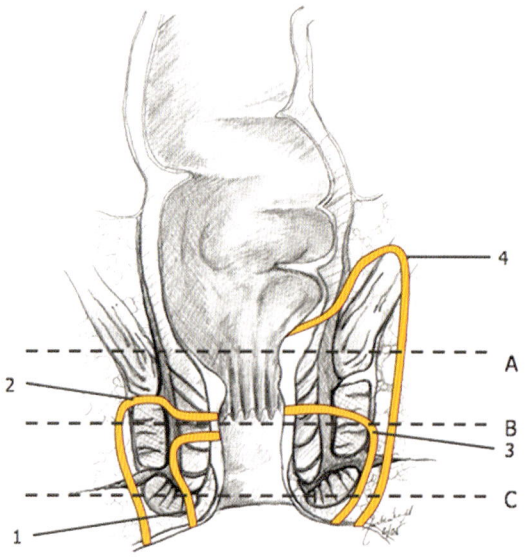

DIAGRAM 33–1. Schema of the various types of anal fistulas: 1. Intersphincteric, 2. Suprasphincteric, 3. Transsphincteric, 4. Extrasphincteric fistula tract. The coronal diagram indicates three different anal canal levels; upper (A), middle (B) and lower (C) level of the anal canal.

Anorectal Fistulae 357

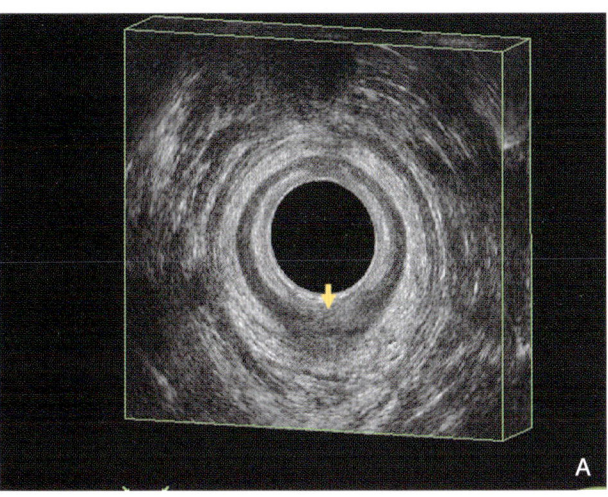
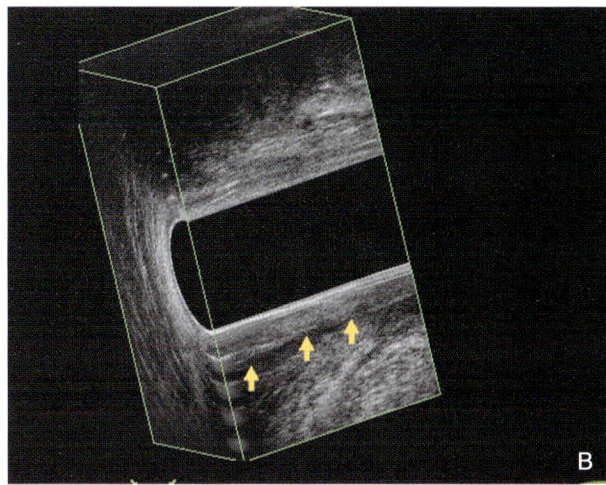

FIGURE 33–1. *A and B* (A) A 43-year-old man with an intersphincteric fistula (Brüel&Kjaer Naerum, Danemark, ProFocus, Transducer type 2050, 16MHz). 33–1A: Axial, mid-anal canal imaging of a hypoechoic fistula tract at 6 o'clock in lithotripsy position (arrow). (B) Three-dimensional view with coronal plane is applied from 12 to 6 o'clock in lithotripsy position.

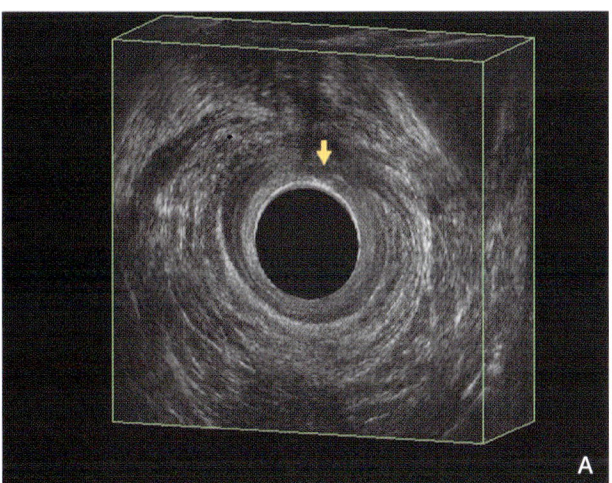
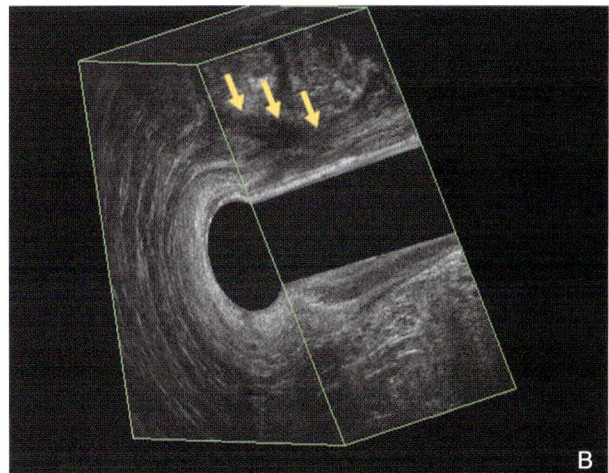

FIGURE 33–2. *A and B* A 43-year-old man with an extrasphincteric fistula (Brüel&Kjaer Naerum, Danemark, ProFocus, Transducer type 2050, 16MHz) (A) Axial, mid-anal canal imaging of a hypoechoic fistula tract at 12 o'clock in lithotripsy position, arrow indicates the internal opening. (B) Three-dimensional view with coronal plane is applied from 1 to 5 o'clock in lithotripsy position.

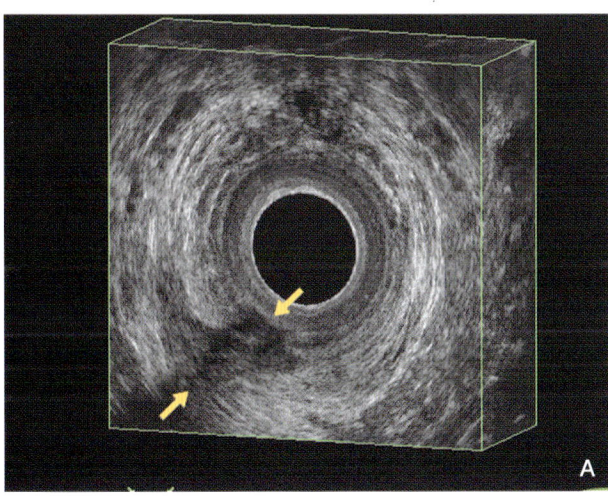

FIGURE 33–3. *A* A 37-year-old man with a transsphincteric fistula (Brüel&Kjaer Naerum, Danemark, ProFocus, Transducer type 2050, 16MHz) (A) Axial, mid-anal canal imaging of a hypoechoic fistula tract at 7 o'clock in lithotripsy position, arrow indicates the internal opening.

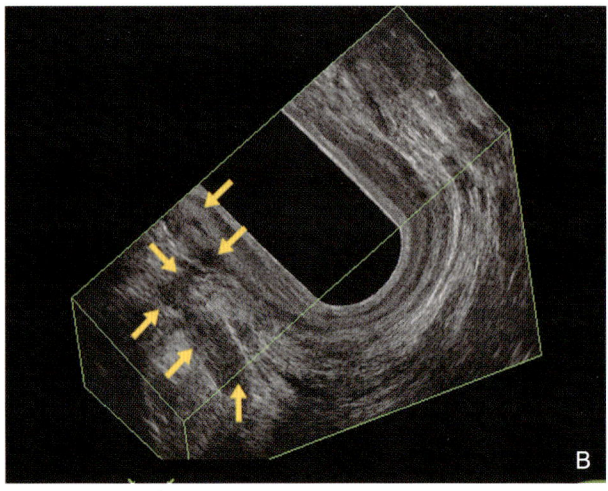

FIGURE 33–3. *B* (B) Three-dimensional view with coronal plane is applied from 4 to 7 o'clock in lithotripsy position. Arrows indicate the fistula tract.

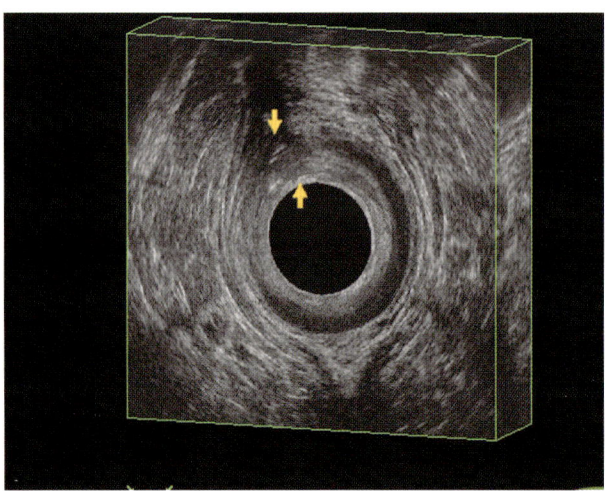

FIGURE 33–4. Axial, mid-anal canal, peroxide-enhanced endoanal ultrasound in a 63-year-old man with a transsphincteric fistula. The detection of the fistula tract becomes easier by the hyperechoic H_2O_2 injection. (Brüel&Kjaer Naerum, Danemark, ProFocus, Transducer type 2050, 16MHz)

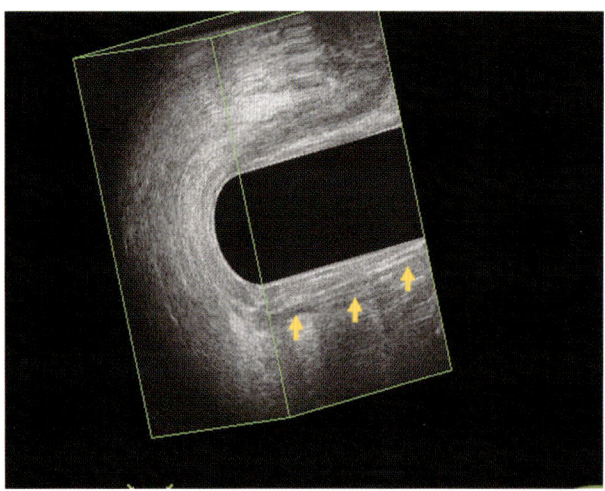

FIGURE 33–5. Peroxide-enhanced endoanal ultrasound in a 33-year-old female with an intersphincteric, thin fistula. (Brüel&Kjaer Naerum, Danemark, ProFocus, Transducer type 2050, 16MHz)

Promising results were found in this field with the new technique of transperianal ultrasound (TPUS). However, at present time, TUPS has not been subject to an outcome-based standard of success in fistula management and must, therefore, still be regarded as an experimental tool.[13-15]

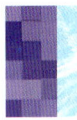

Endoanal Ultrasound in Specific Anorectal Fistula

Contrary to cryptoglandular fistulas the primary center of the inflammation is found in the cases of anal fistulas associated with M. Crohn and colitis ulcerosa in the mucosa and/or submucosa area of the rectal wall. From there the fistula tracks spread in different directions, irrespective of the existing anatomical structures.[16] For this reason, anal fistulas associated with M. Crohn and ulcerative colitis cannot be adequately classified according to the known classifications. Figure 33–6 presents a complex perianal inflammatory lesion in Crohn's disease imaged by EUS.

The diagnosis and treatment of perianal Crohn fistulas include conservative as well as surgical approach, however the treatment can be difficult and represent a challenge for physicians and surgeons. A comprehensive imaging is recommended. The combination of MR imaging and EUS is capable of detecting perianal fistulae with a sensitivity of up to 100%.[17,18]

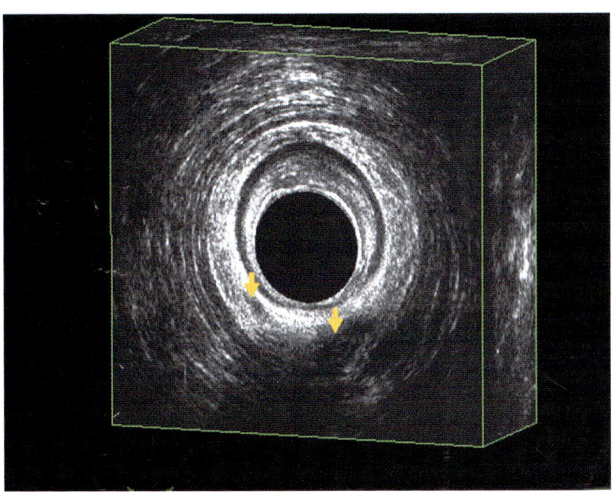

FIGURE 33–6. A 46-year-old man with a superficial fistula (Brüel&Kjaer Naerum, Danemark, ProFocus, Transducer type 2050, 16MHz). Axial, mid-anal canal imaging shows two fistula tracts indicated by arrows.

References

1. Parks, A. G., Morson, B. C.: The pathogenesis of fistula-in-ano. Proc R S Med 55: 551–554.
2. Parks, A. G., Gordon, P. H., Hardcastle, J. D.: A classification of anal fistula. Br J Surg 1976;63:1–12.
3. Law, P. J., Bartram, C. I.: Anal endography: Technique and normal anatomie. Gastrointest Radiol.1989;14:349.
4. Navarro, J. A., Garcia-Domingo, M. I., Rius Macias, J., Marco-Molina, C.: Ultrasound study of anal fistulas with hydrogen peroxyde enhancement. Dis Colon Rerctum 2004;47:108–114.
5. Lengyel, A. J., Hurst, N. G., Williams, J. G.: Pre-operative assessment of anal fistulas using endoanal ultrasound. Colorectal Dis 2002;4:436–440.
6. Cheong, D. M., Nogueras, J. J., Wexner, S. D., Jagelman, D.E.: Anal endosonography for recurrent anal fistulas: image enhancement with hydrogen peroxide. Dis Colon Rectum. 1993;36(12):1158–1160.
7. Poen, A. C., Felt-Bersma, R. J., Eijsbounts, Q. A., Cuesta, M. A., Meuwissen.: Hydrogen peroxide-enhanced transanal ultrasound in the assessment of fistula-in-ano. Dis Colon Rectum. 1998;41(9):1147–1150.
8. Ratto, C., Gentile, E., Merico, M., Spinazzola, C., Mangini, G., Sofo, L., Doglietto, G.: How can the assessment of fistula-in ano be improved? Dis Colon Rectum. 2000;43(10):1375–1382.
9. Zbar, A. P., Armitage, N. C.: Complex perirectal sepsis: clinical classification and imaging. Tech Coloproctol. 2006;10(2):83–93.
10. Buchanan, G. N., Bartram, C. I., Williams, A. B., Halligan, S., Cohen, C.R.: Value of hydrogen peroxide enhancement of three-dimensional endoanal ultrasound in fistula-in-ano. Dis Colon Rectum. 2005;48(1):141–147.
11. West, R. L., Zimmermann, D. D., Dwarkasing, S., Hussain, S. M., Hop, W. C., Schouten, W. R., Kuipers, E. J., Felt-Bersma, R. J.: Prospective comparison of hydrogen peroxide-enhanced three-dimensional endoanal ultrasonography and endoanal magnetic resonance imaging of perianal fistulas. Dis Colon Rectum. 2003;46(10):1407–1415.

12. Halligan, S., Stoker, J.: Imaging of fistula in ano. Radiology. 2006;239(1):18–33.
13. Rubens, D. J., Strang, J. G., Bogineni-Misra, S., Wexler, I. E.: Transperineal sonography of the rectum: anatomy and pathology revealed by sonography compared with CT and MR imaging. Am J Roentgenol 1998;170: 637–642.
14. Zbar, A. P., Oyetunji, R. O., Gill, R.: Transperineal versus hydrogen peroxide-enhanced endoanal ultrasonography in never operated and recurrent cryptogenic fistula-in-ano: a pilot study Tech Coloproctol. 2006 Nov 27.
15. Domkundwar, S. V., Shinagare, A. B.: Role of transcutaneous perianal ultrasonography in evaluation of fistulas in ano. J Ultrasound Med. 2007;26(1):29–36.
16. Singh, B., McMortensen, N. J., Jewell, D. P., George, B.: Perianal Crohn's disease. Br J Surg 2004;91:801–814.
17. Schwartz, D. A., Wiersema, M. J., Dudika, K. M., Fletcher, J. G., Clain, J. E., Tremaine, W. J., Zinsmeister, A. R., Norton, I. D., Boardman, L. A., Devine, R. M., Wolff, B. G., Young-Fadok, T. M., Diehl, N. N., Pemberton, J. H., Sandborn, W. J.: A comparison of endoscopic ultrasound, magnetic resonance imaging, and exam under anesthesia for evaluation of Crohn's perianal fistulas. Gastroenterology 2001;121(5):1064–1072.
18. Orsoni, P., Barthet, M., Portier, F., Panuel, M., Desjeux, A., Grimaud, J. C.: Prospective comparison of endosonography, magnetic resonance imaging and surgical findings in anorectal fistula and abscess complicating Crohn's disease. Br J Surg 1999;86(3):360–364.

CHAPTER 34

Anal Sphincter Defects

Dr. Christa Meyenberger
Dr. Franc H. Hetzer

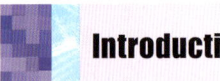

Introduction

Endoanal ultrasonography (EUS) is an accepted technique in the assessment of both acute perianal trauma and chronic sphincter defects. During the past ten years, its application has become more established, mainly because of improvements in the technology of endoscopes and ultrasound transducers. EUS has been validated both intraoperatively[1,2] and histologically.[3] Therefore, EUS is the accepted gold standard for anal sphincter anatomy.

However the technique has its limits. The interpretation of EUS images is still difficult causing inter- and intraobserver agreement to be only moderately reliable.[4,5] With the introduction of three-dimensional ultrasound imaging, the anatomic interpretation of the sphincters has significantly improved and allows for review of the acquired data at any time independently of the examiner.[6,7] Visible Human Anatomy has been previously illustrated in Figure 32–1 and Figure 32–2 of Chapter 32, Perirectal Abscesses. Figures 34–1A, 34–1B, and 34–1C present the normal ultrasound anatomy of the upper-anal canal level, middle canal level and lower canal level in a female. (Diagram 34-1) Figure 34–2 shows the corresponding normal ultrasound anatomy of the sphincter complex in three-dimensional section. Figures 34–3A, 34–3B, 34–3C and 34–4 present the same images in a healthy man. By using three-dimensional reconstructions, the relationship between the radial and linear extent of anal sphincters tears can be explored more accurately. Gender differences in anal canal and sphincter length can also be established.[8,9]

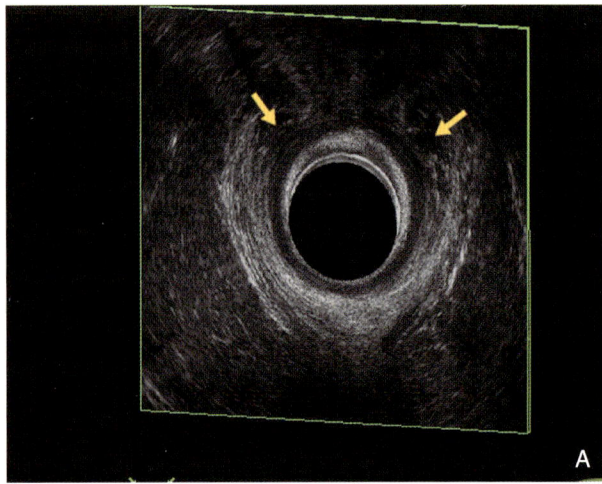

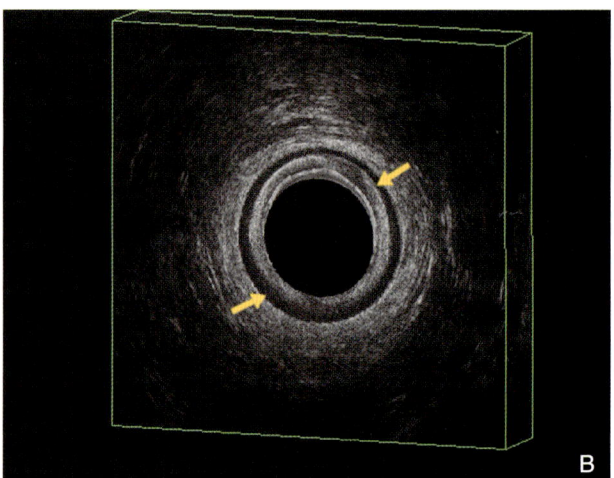

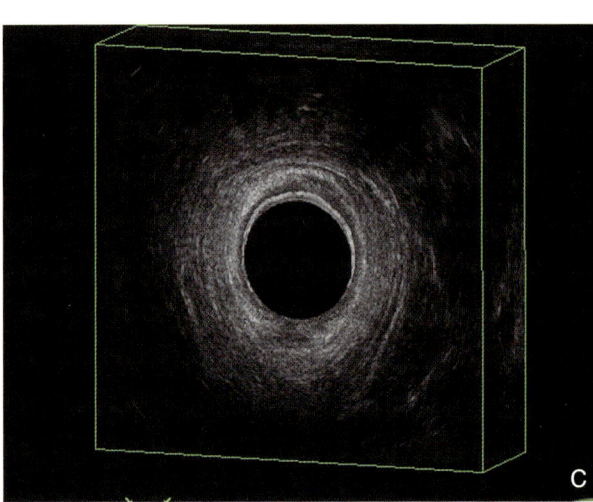

FIGURE 34–1. *A to C* Normal ultrasound anatomy of the upper (A), middle (B) and lower (C) level of the anal canal in a 47-year-old nulliparous female. (Brüel&Kjaer, ProFocus, Naerum, Danemark, Transducer type 2050, 16MHz). (A) Normal appearance of the anal canal at upper level in an axial image. At the cranial end of the anal canal, the external sphincter muscle becomes more hypoechoic and gives rise to the levator ani sling above this level (arrows).
(B) Normal appearance of the anal canal at middle level in an axial image. The internal sphincter is seen as a continous hypoechoic ring (arrows) that surrounds the submucosal space. The external anal sphincter appears as less well-defined hyperechoic band immediately outside the internal sphincter.
(C) At the anal verge, the lower level, the internal anal sphincter is typically seen as an incomplete ring or disappears completely. The external sphincter encircles the anal canal as a hyperechoic band.

Anal Sphincter Defects 363

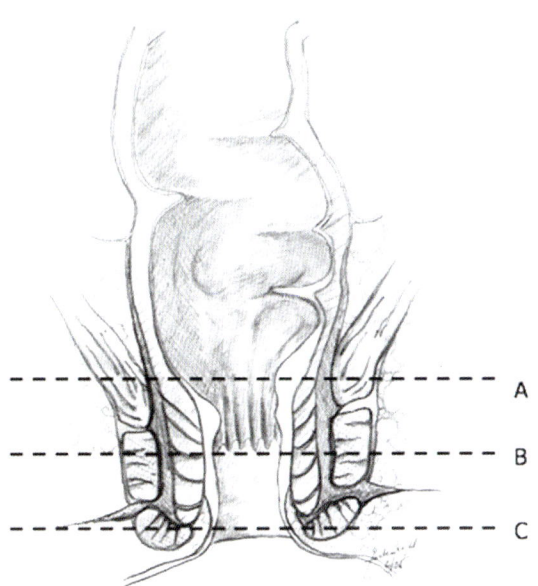

DIAGRAM 34–1. Coronal diagram of the three different anal canal levels; upper (A), middle (B) and lower (C) level of the anal canal.

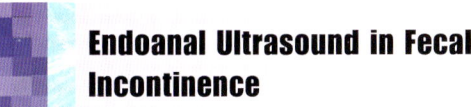

Endoanal Ultrasound in Fecal Incontinence

Although fecal incontinence may be the result of several causes, anal sphincter injury is often a consequence of obstrectic trauma, anorectal surgery, or accidental injury.[10] While there is no strong relationship between muscle injuries and the severity of clinical symptoms, about two-thirds of patients with faecal incontinence are diagnosed with a sphincter lesion using EUS.[11] This type of lesion can be identified through a discontinuity in the sphincter in the EUS image. Other diagnoses that can be made using EUS are scarring, which is characterized by a loss of the normal texture. Loss of normal texture is characterized by low reflectivity, and the localized internal anal sphincter defect is visible as an interruption of the hypoechoic centric structure. Figures 34–5A and 34–5B show a rupture of the internal anal sphincter caused by a direct trauma. The patient shown fell from a ten-meter diving board directly on his buttocks as a young man. Seven years later, he is now seeking medical advice because of passive fecal incontinence.

In Figure 34–6 complicated lesions of the internal anal sphincter after haemorrhoidectomy are presented. The remaining sphincter muscles show local thickening.

An external sphincter injury is the most common sphincter disruption because it is related to a complicated vaginal delivery.[12] The lesion is typically located anteriorly as shown in figure Figures 34–7A and 34–7B. The defect is seen indirectly as a change in echogenicity in this area.

At present, EUS is the first step in the evaluation of patients with fecal incontinence. EUS is performed to identify those patients with sphincter damage who may benefit from sphincter repair. For example, Figures 34–8A and 34–8B show a 45-year-old female with a combination of internal and external anal sphincter damage after three childbirths. The integration of EUS will permit planning the best treatment for this patient particularly if the colorectal surgeon himself is directly involved in the diagnostic process.

EUS is an important contribution to the correct imaging of the external anal sphincter particularly in

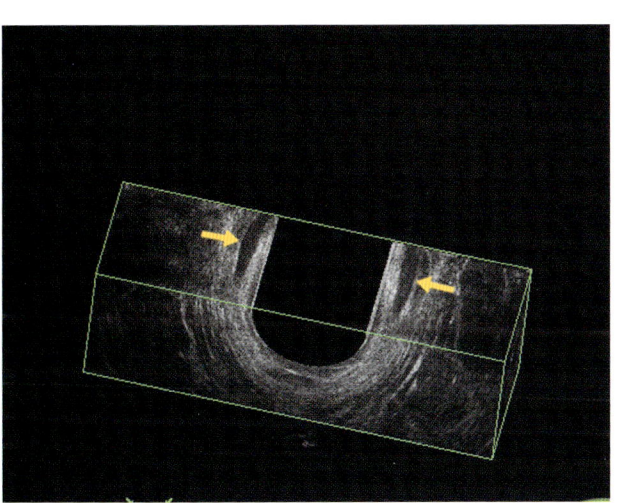

FIGURE 34–2. Normal ultrasound anatomy of the sphincter complex in 3-D in the same 47-year-old nulliparous female from Figure 34–1. (Brüel&Kjaer, ProFocus, Naerum, Danemark, Transducer type 2050, 16MHz). A coronal plane is applied from 3 to 9 o'clock in lithotripsy position. Internal anal sphincter appears as a hypoechoic ring in the middle an upper part of the anal canal (arrows).

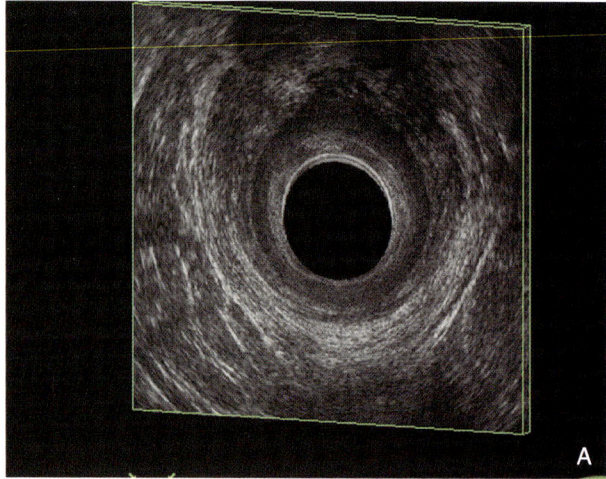
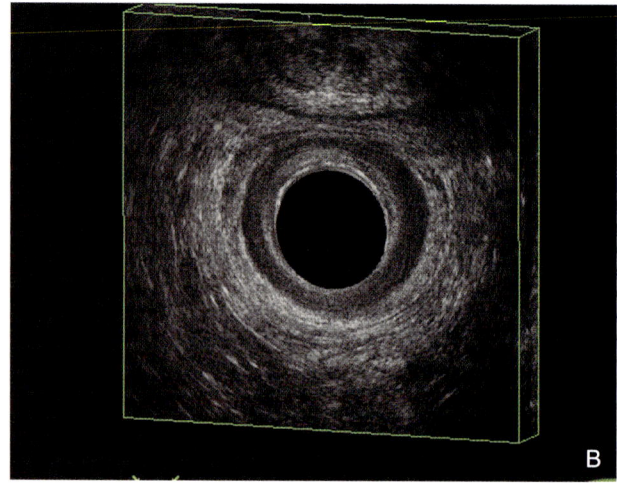
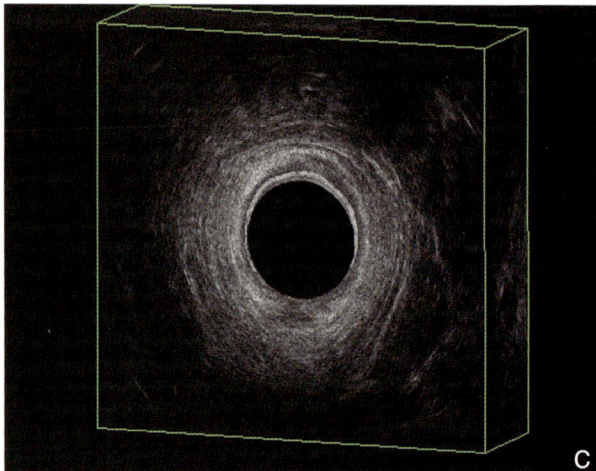

FIGURE 34–3. *A to C* Normal ultrasound anatomy of the upper (A), middle (B) and lower (C) level of the anal canal in a 42-year-old male. (Brüel&Kjaer, ProFocus, Naerum, Danemark, Transducer type 2050, 16MHz). (A) A shows normal appearance of the anal canal at upper level in an axial image. At the cranial end of the anal canal, the external sphincter muscle becomes more hypoechoic and gives rise to the levator ani sling above this level. The external ring, hyperechoic, is anteriorly more closed than in a female. (B) The sphincter rings in a male are better defined and thicker than in a female. A normal appearance of the anal canal at middle level in an axial image is shown. The internal sphincter is seen as a continous, strong hypoechoic ring that surrounds the submucosal space. The external anal sphincter appears as a less well-defined hyperechoic band immediately outside the internal sphincter. (C) At the anal verge, the lower level of the anal canal, the internal anal sphincter is typically seen as an incomplete ring or disappears completely. The external sphincter encircles the anal canal as a hyperechoic band.

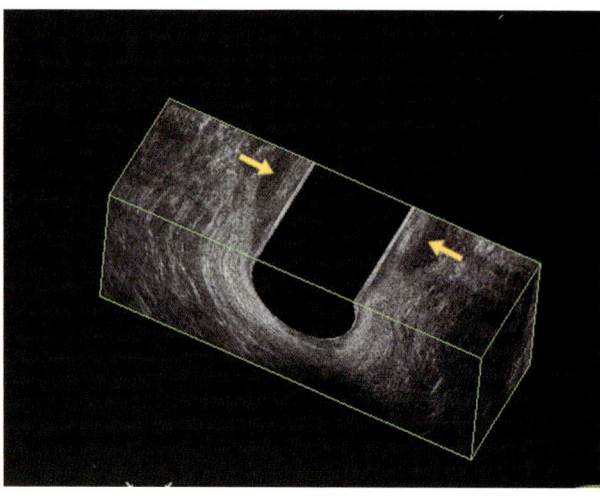

FIGURE 34–4. Normal ultrasound anatomy of the sphincter complex in 3-D in the same 42-year-old male from Figure 34–3. (Brüel&Kjaer, ProFocus, Naerum, Danemark, Transducer type 2050, 16MHz). A coronal plane is applied from 3 to 9 o'clock in lithotripsy position. Internal anal sphincter appears as a hypoechoic ring in the middle and upper part of the anal canal (arrows).

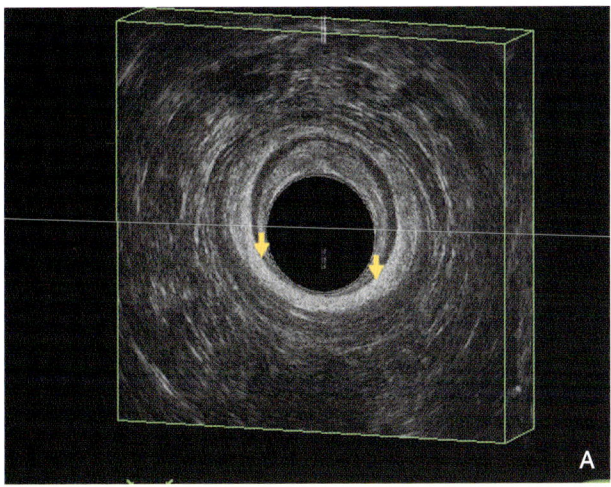 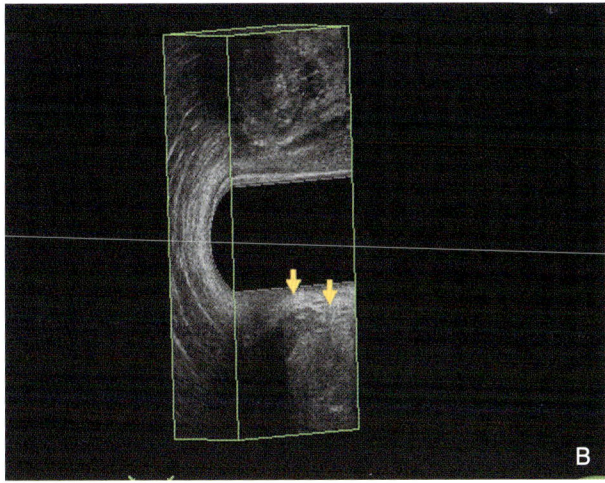

FIGURE 34–5. *A and B* Disruption of the internal anal sphincter in a 28-year-old man. (Brüel&Kjaer, ProFocus, Naerum, Danemark, Transducer type 2050, 16MHz) (A) Internus defect in an axial middle anal canal image. Large defect of the hypoechoic internal anal sphincter ring (arrows). (B) Three-dimensional view with coronal plane is applied from 12 to 6 o'clock in lithotripsy position. Hypoechoic scaring tissue posteroirly, indicated by arrows, where normally the internal anal sphincter appears.

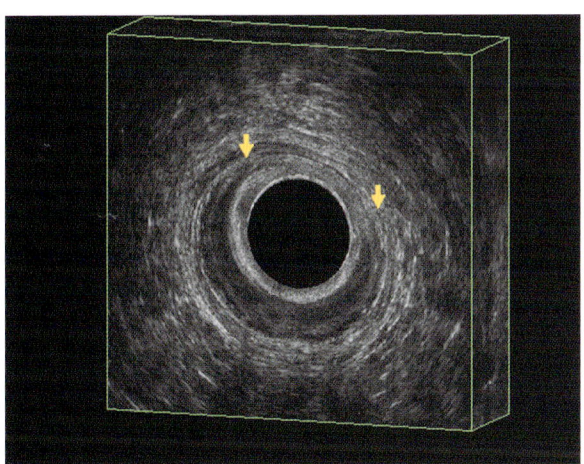

FIGURE 34–6. Lesions of the internal sphincter after haemorrhoidectomy in a 56-year-old man. Arrows indicate the remaining sphincter with local thickening in the axial middle-anal canal image. (Brüel&Kjaer, ProFocus, Naerum, Danemark, Transducer type 2050, 16MHz)

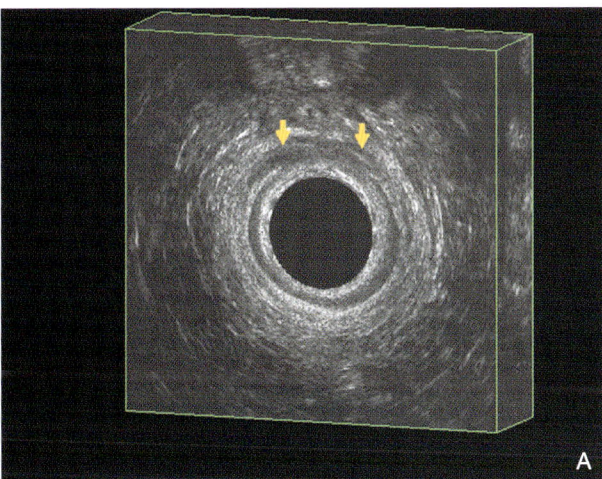 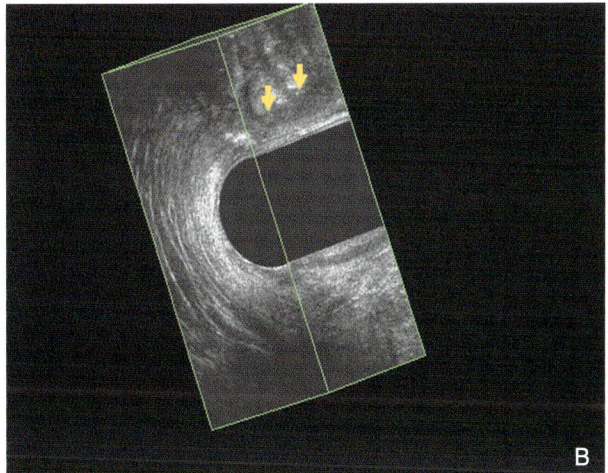

FIGURE 34–7. *A and B* Typically located anteriorly external anale sphincter defect in a 63-year-old female many years after a complicated vaginal delivery. (Brüel&Kjaer, ProFocus, Naerum, Danemark, Transducer type 2050, 16MHz. (A) Axial middle-anal canal image shows an anterior defect of the external anal sphincter (arrows) between 11 and 1 o'clock in lithotripsy position. (B) Three-dimensional view of the anterior sphincter lesion. A coronal plane is applied from 12 to 6 o'clock in lithotripsy position.

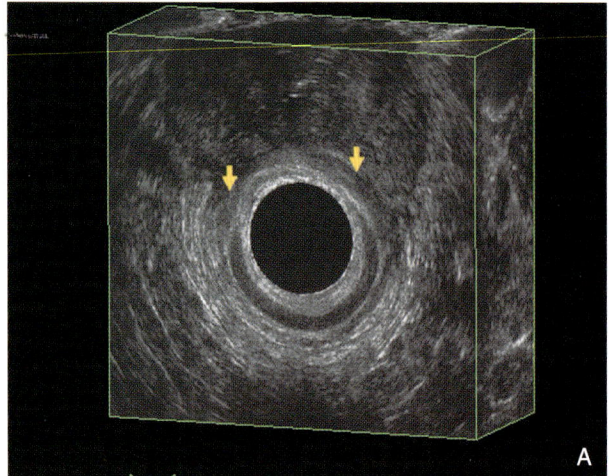 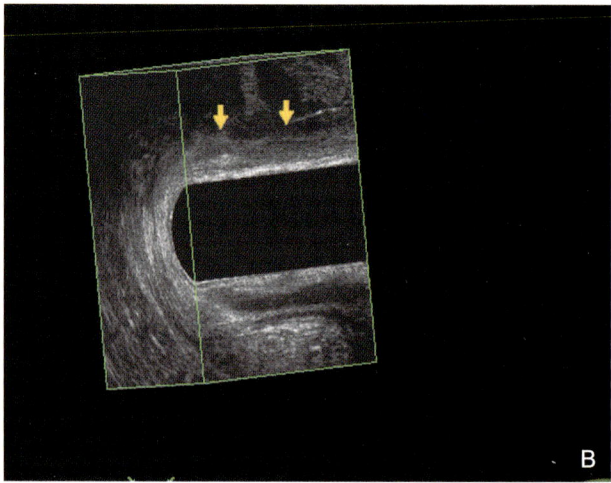

FIGURE 34–8. *A and B* Anteriorly localized combined defect of the internal and external anal sphincter in a 45-year-old female after three vaginal deliveries. (Brüel&Kjaer, ProFocus, Naerum, Danemark, Transducer type 2050, 16MHz). (A) Axial middle-anal canal image shows an anterior defect of both sphincters (arrows) between 9 and 1 o'clock in lithotripsy position. (B) Three-dimensional view of the anterior internal and external anal sphincter defect. A coronal plane is applied from 12 to 6 o'clock in lithotripsy position.

differentiating between females and males. In females it is well documented that a shorter external anal sphincter exists on the anterior side than on the posterior side.[13] It is not always easy to differentiate between the natural gaps, (hypoechoic areas with smooth, regular edges), shown in Figure 34–9, and the sphincter ruptures (mixed echogenicity, due to scarring, with irregular edges), in Figures 34–8A and 34–8B. The correct assessment of the external anal sphincter plays a key rule in the therapeutic option chosen in symptomatic patients. Symptomatic patients with a wide external sphincter rupture are potential candidates for sphincter repair or neosphincter procedures (dynamic gracilosplasty or artificial bowel sphincter), whereas patients without a discontinuity of muscle may benefit from less invasive treatments, such as sacral nerve stimulation.

Although it seems normal, without any lesion, sometimes the internal anal sphincter has differences in echogenicity and thickness. This degeneration of the internal sphincter has been regarded as a cause of passive faecal incontinence.[14] In Figure 34–10, the EUS reveals an intact but thinner than normal and hyperechoic internal sphincter. This 87-year old woman, examined due to sever passive incontinence, presented reduced resting pressure and normal squeeze pressure, rectal sensitivity and pudendal latency at anorectal manometry.

EUS is not only an ideal diagnostic tool in the hands of surgeons with special interest of restorative

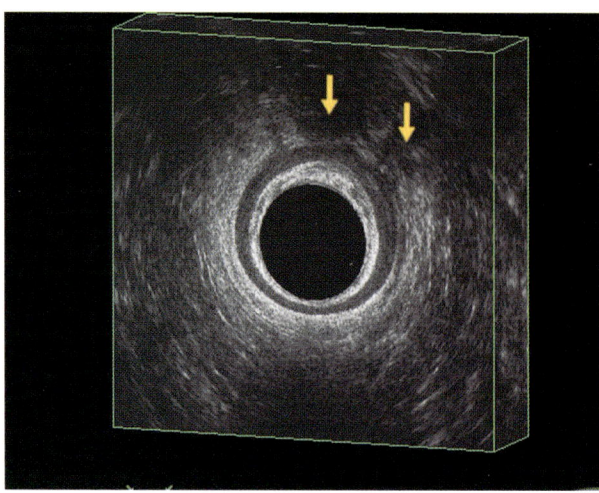

FIGURE 34–9. A 35-year-old nulliparous female with a natural gap anteriorly at the mid-anal canal level. (Brüel&Kjaer, ProFocus, Naerum, Danemark, Transducer type 2050, 16MHz). The natural gaps appear with hypoechoic areas with smooth, regular edges (arrows).

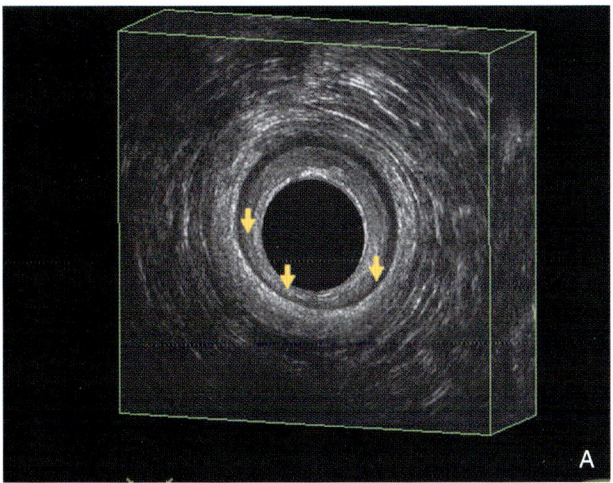
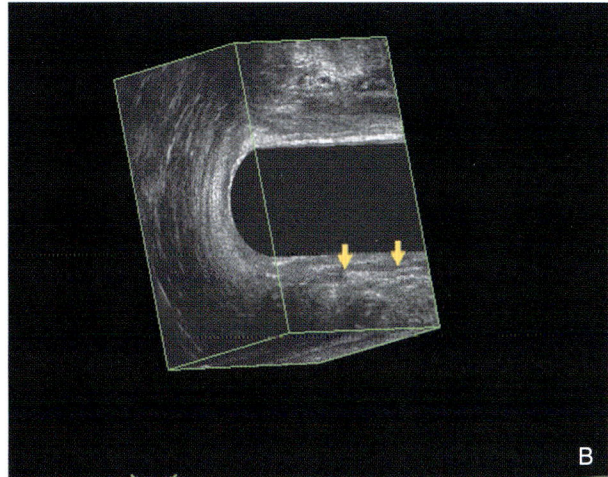

FIGURE 34–10. *A and B* Internal anal sphincter degeneration in an 87–year–old female with passive faecal incontinence. (Brüel&Kjaer, ProFocus, Naerum, Danemark, Transducer type 2050, 16MHz). (A) Mid anal canal axial imaging of posteriorly sphincter degeneration. The internal sphincter appears intact but thinner than normal and hyperechoic. (B) Three-dimensional view of the posteriorly internal anal sphincter degeneration. A coronar plane is applied from 12 to 6 o'clock in lithotripsy position.

procedure. The intraoperative EUS helps surgeons to perform procedures such as the sphincter augmentation with bulky injectable biomaterials. Guided by the EUS, the surgeon introduces the needle of the applicator in the intersphincteric space and injects under vision the material, e.g. silicone (Figures 34–11A and 34–11B).[15]

The EUS allows not only applying surgical interventions, it is also an excellent tool to control postoperatively the quality of surgery, for instance the anal sphincter repair, (Figures 34–12A and 34–12B).

The quality of magnetic resonance (MR) assessment in pelvic floor disorders has also improved however for detection of sphincter lesions, especially internal anal sphincter lesions, EUS is still superior.[16] The combination of MR and EUS in an overlay technique will increase the accuracy of the interpretation of sphincter damage in future.[17]

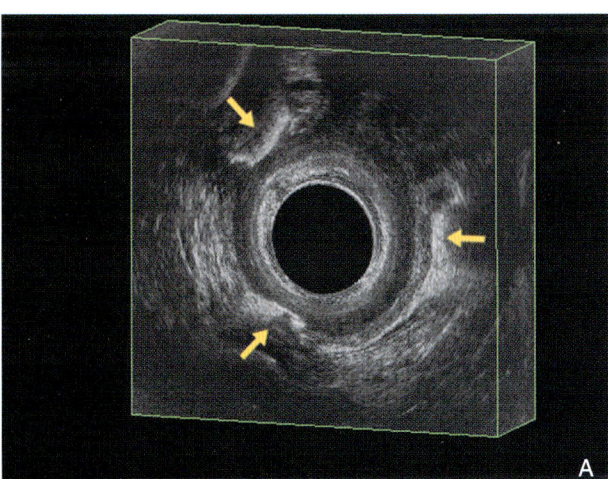
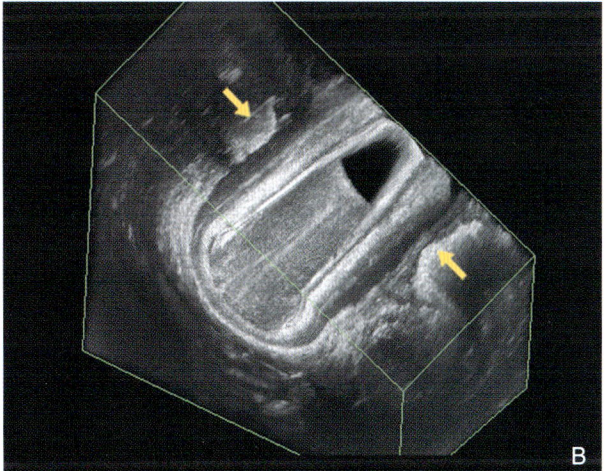

FIGURE 34–11. *A and B* Injection of bulking agents in a 76-year-old female with passive fecal incontinence. (Brüel&Kjaer, ProFocus, Naerum, Danemark, Transducer type 2050, 16MHz). (A) Silicone cushions in the mid anal canal level as a hyperechoic alterations at 3, 7, and 11 o'clock (arrows). (B) Three-dimensional view of the sphincter augmentation with Silicon. A coronal plane is applied from 10 to 5 o'clock in lithotripsy position and rander modus is activated for enhanced contrast.

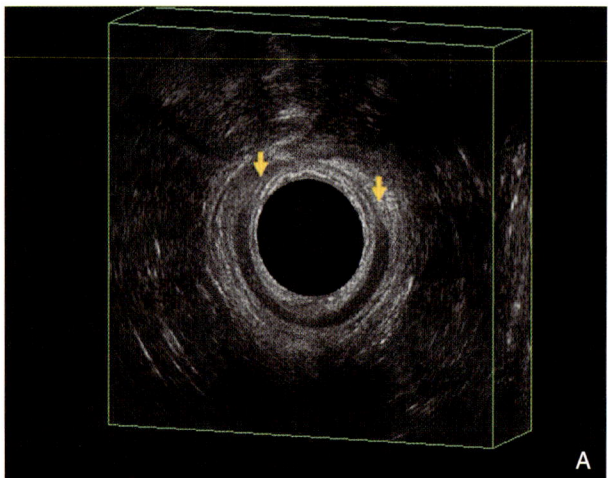 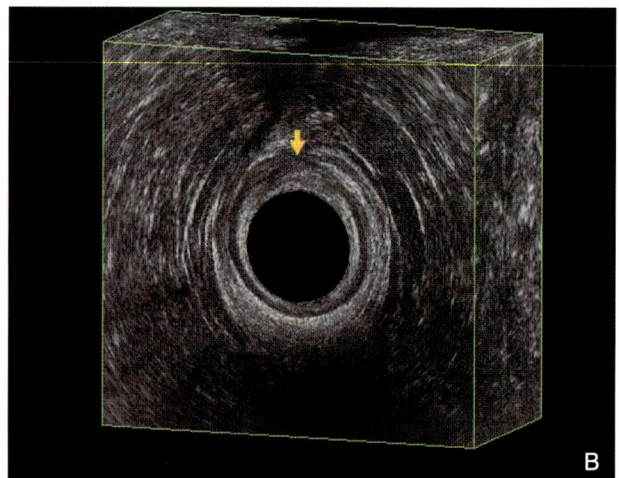

FIGURE 34–12. *A and B* Pre- and postoperative EUS in a 26-year-old female with anterior sphincter defect and overlapping sphincter repair. (Brüel&Kjaer, ProFocus, Naerum, Danemark, Transducer type 2050, 16MHz). (A) Preoperatively an internal and external sphincter defect five years after a complicated delivery. Arrows indicate the internal sphincter gap. (B) Six months after successful overlapping sphincter repair. The internal sphincter ring is nearly completely closed anteriorly (arrow).

References

1. Sultan, A. H., Nicolls, R. J., Kamm, M. A., Hudson, C. N., Beynon, J., Bartram, C. I.: Anal endosonography and correlation with in vitro and vivo anatomy. Br J Surg 1993;80:508–511.
2. Meyenberger, C., Bertschinger, P., Zala, G. F., Buchmann, P.: Anal sphincter defects in fecal incontinence: correlation between endosonography and surgery. Endoscopy. 1996;28(2):217–224.
3. Sultan, A. H., Kamm, M. A., Talbot, I. C., Nicholls, R. J., Bartram, C. I.: Anal Endosonography for identifying external sphincter defects conformed histological. Br J Surg 1994;81:463–446.
4. Faltin, D. L., Boulvain, M., Stan, C., Epiney, M., Weil, A., Irion, O.: Intraobserver and interobserver agreement in the diagnosis of anal sphincter tears by postpartum endosonography. Ultrasound Obstet Gynecol. 2003;21(4):375–377.
5. Gold, D. M., Halligan, S., Kmiot, W. A., Bartram, C. I.: Intraobserver and interobserver agreement in anal endosonography. Br J Surg. 1999;86(3):371–375.
6. Williams, A. B., Bartram, C. I., Halligan, S., Marshall, M. M., Nicholls, R. J., Kmiot, W. A.: Multiplanar anal endosonography-normal anal canal anatomy. Colorectal Dis. 2001;3(3):169–174.
7. Gregory, W. T., Boyles, S. H., Simmons, K., Corcoran, A., Clark, A. L.: External anal sphincter volume measurements using 3-dimensional endoanal ultrasound. Am J Obstet Gynecol. 2006;194(5):1243–1248.
8. Gold, D. M., Bartram, C. I., Halligan, S., Humphries, K. N., Kamm, M. A., Kmiot, W.A.: Three-dimensional endoanal sonography in assessing anal canal injury. Br J Surg. 1999;86(3):365–370.
9. West, R. L., Felt-Bersma, R. J., Hansen, B. E., Schouten, W. R., Kuipers, E. J.: Volume measurements of the anal sphincter complex in healthy controls and fecal-incontinent patients with a three-dimensional reconstruction of endoanal ultrasonography images. Dis Colon Rectum. 2005;48(3):540–548.
10. Lunniss, P. J., Gladman, M. A., Hetzer, F. H., Williams, N. S., Scott, S. M.: Risk factors in acquired fecal incontinence. J R Soc Med. 2004;97:111–116.
11. Voyvodic, F., Rieger, N. A., Skinner, S., Schloithe, A. C., Saccone, G. T., Sage, M. R., Wattchow, D. A.: Endosonographic imaging of anal sphincter injury: does the size of the tear correlate with the degree of dysfunction? Dis Colon Rectum. 2003;46(6):735–741.
12. Sultan, A. H., Kamm, M. A., Hudson, C. N., Thomas, J. M., Bartram, C. I.: Anal sphincter disruption during vaginal delivery. N Engl J Med 1993;329:1905–1911.
13. Oh, C. H., Kark, A.: Anatomy of the external anal sphincter. Br J Surg 1972;59:717.
14. Vaizey, C. J., Kamm, M. A., Bartram, C. I.: Primary degeneration of the internal anal sphincter as a cause of passive faecal incontinence. Lancet. 1997;349(9052):612–615.
15. Tjandra, J. J., Lim, J. F., Hiscock, R., Rajendra, P.: Injectable silicone biomaterial for fecal incontinence caused by internal anal sphincter dysfunction is effective. Dis Colon Rectum 2004;47(12):2138–2146.
16. Malouf, A. J., Williams, A. B., Halligan, S., Bartram, C. I., Dhillon, S., Kamm, M. A.: Prospective assessment of accuracy of endoanal MR imaging and endosonography in patients with fecal incontinence. AJR Am J Roentgenol. 2000;175(3):741–745.
17. Williams, A. B., Bartram, C. I., Halligan, S., Marshall, M. M., Nicholls, R. J., Kmiot, W. A.: Endosonographic anatomy of the normal anal canal compared with endocoil magnetic resonance imaging. Dis Colon Rectum. 2002;45(2):176–183.

CHAPTER 35

Ovarian and Gynecological Lesions

Dr. Brian R. Weston
Dr. Manoop S. Bhutani

The published literature to date on the use of endorectal ultrasonography (EUS) for the evaluation and diagnosis of primary or secondary gynecologic disorders is sparse. Most such problems are initially referred to a gynecologist where evaluation via transabdominal or transvaginal approach is conventional. Referral to a gastroenterologist for endosonography may occur when it is deemed necessary (either clinically or radiographically) to evaluate colorectal or perirectal involvement, or on occasion for diagnosis of a denovo or incidental process.

Rectal EUS has been effectively utilized for the diagnosis and evaluation of a variety of extra-rectal benign and malignant pelvic disorders. Multi-planar high-resolution sonographic imaging is not only possible of the rectal wall layers but also of adjacent perirectal, perineal, and pelvic structures and organs that are in close proximity to the ultrasound probe. (Visible Human Anatomy shown in Figures 35–1A - 35–1D) The diagnostic capacity for transrectal EUS is greatly enhanced by the capacity for fine-needle aspiration. Accurate real-time tissue sampling of lesions as small as 5-10 mm is possible using a linear echoendoscope.[1,2] Fine needle aspiration is relatively noninvasive and safe in comparison to laparoscopy and open surgery. Low complication rate, minimal patient preparation and need for sedation, and ability to be performed on an outpatient basis are all attractive features.

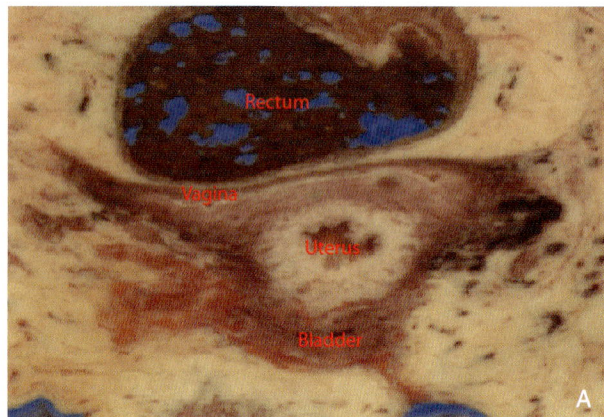
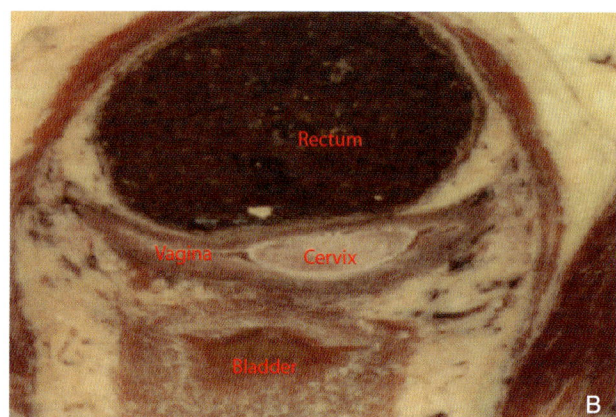
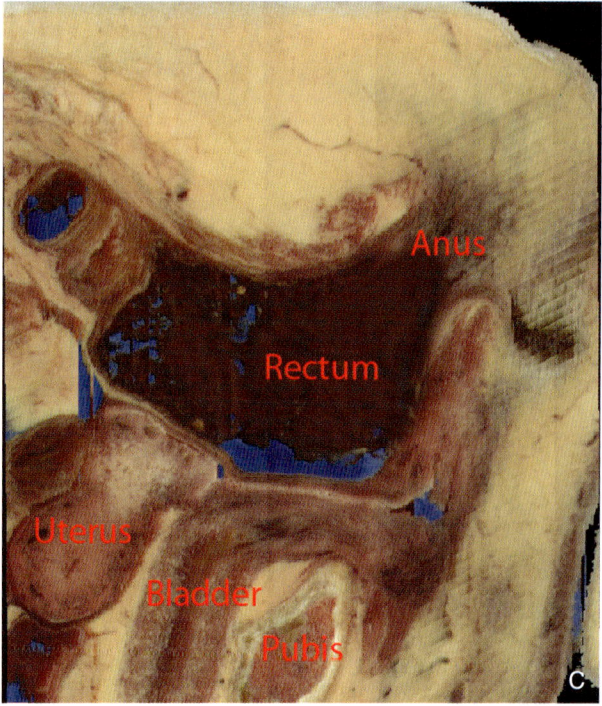
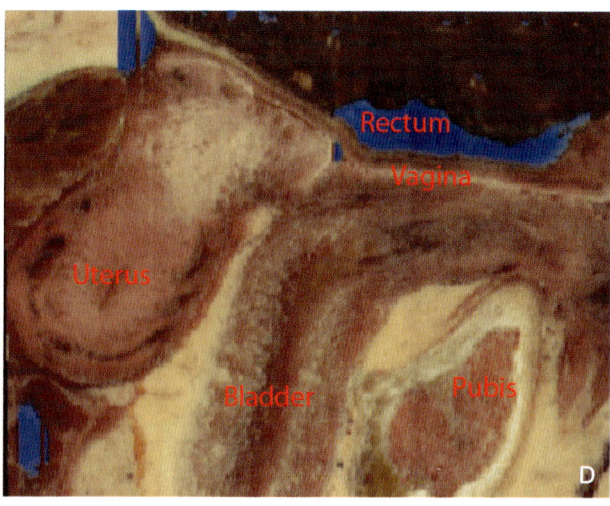

FIGURE 35–1. *A to D* (A) Transaxial Visible Human Anatomy of female pelvis through the uterus (B) Transaxial Visible Human Anatomy of female pelvis through the cervix (C) Sagittal Coronal Visible Human Anatomy of female pelvis (D) Magnified Sagittal Coronal Visible Human Anatomy of female pelvis

Evaluation and diagnosis of primary or recurrent pelvic tumors originating from the uterus, ovary, or vagina are all potentially feasible via rectal EUS (Figures 35–2A and 35–2B). Direct local invasion or extrinsic compression of the rectal wall or perirectal space may occur from either benign or malignant pelvic solid tumors or infiltrative inflammatory processes. Echofeatures of such processes are tumor specific and dependent on the presence of necrosis, hemorrhage, inflammatory change, or infection. Most of the current literature is limited to small case studies and reports.[1-3]

Metastatic disease and/or perirectal lymph node involvement related to either local or distant primary disease processes are not infrequently sought for staging or restaging (Figures 35–3, 35–4). FNA is readily

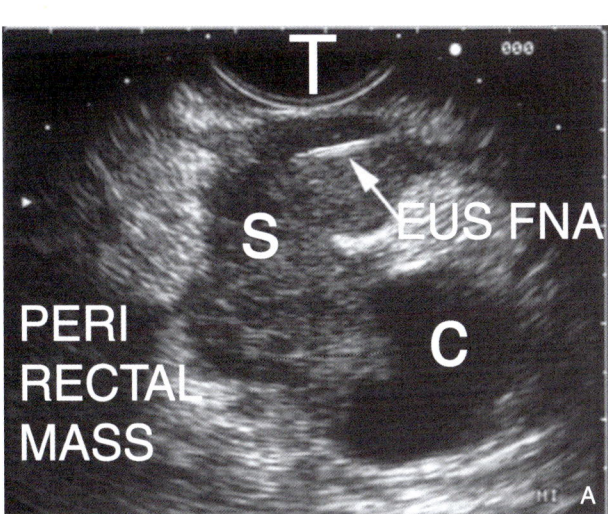
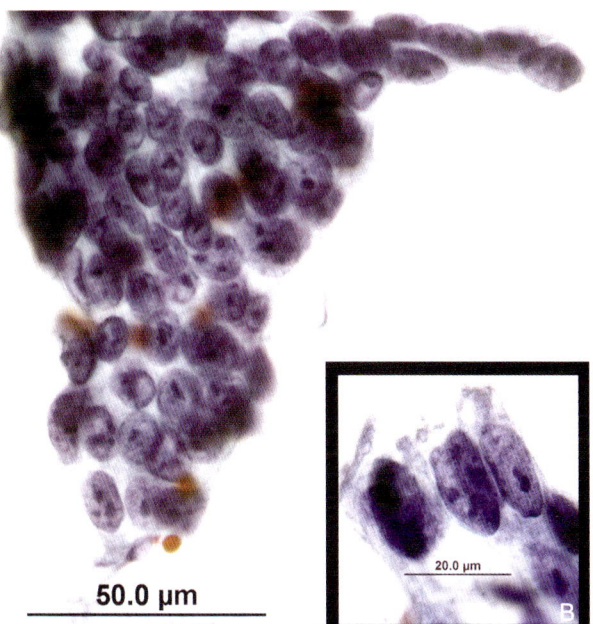

FIGURE 35–2. *A and B* (A) Linear transrectal EUS with FNA of a perirectal mass with solid (S) and cystic (C) components. T: transducer in the rectum. (B) Perirectal mass, EUS-guided fine-needle aspiration: A cluster of tall, columnar-shaped neoplastic cells are seen consistent with a carcinoma of ovarian origin. (Papanicolaou stain, medium and high power).

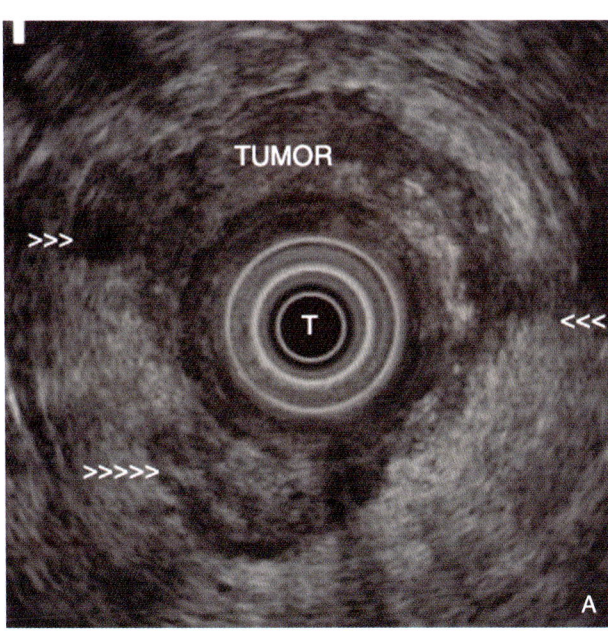
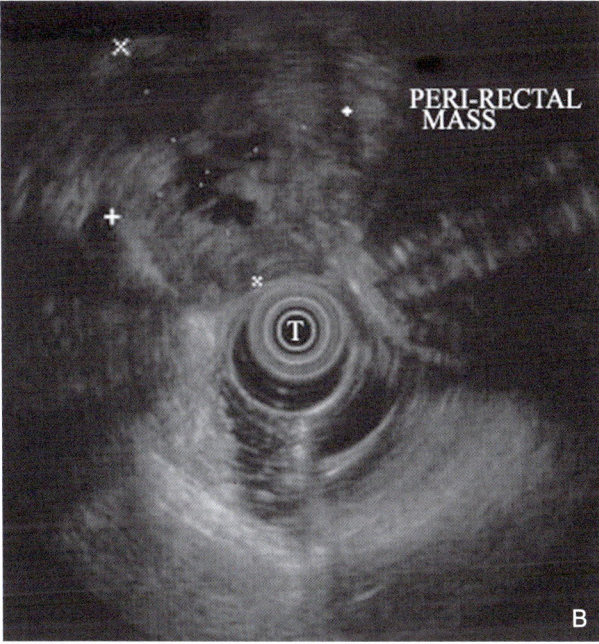

FIGURE 35–3. *A and B* (A) Rectosigmoid cancer staged as T3 (with penetration into perirectal fat shown with arrowheads) with a radial EUS transducer (T). (B) A 5 cm perirectosigmoid mass is seen by EUS distal to the rectal cancer by radial EUS in the patient shown in Figure 35–2A.

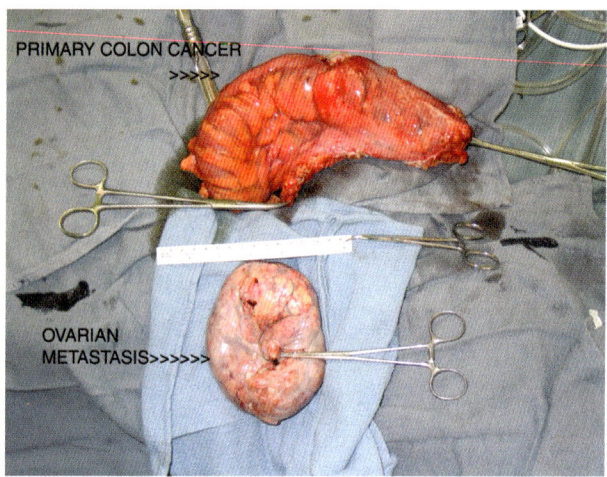

FIGURE 35–4. Surgical findings in the patient in figures 35–3A and 35–3B. A primary colorectal cancer is found along with a solitary 5 cm ovarian metastasis correlating with the EUS findings.

performed in such circumstances. Lymph node enlargement may be related to local inflammatory/infectious processes, surgery or post chemo-radiation treatment. Several infiltrative processes that may involve the perirectal or pelvic region such as lymphoma, sarcoma/leiomyosarcoma, stromal tumors, teratoma, chordoma, and melanoma have also been reported.

 ## Pelvic Inflammatory Disorders

EUS may be of benefit in evaluation of certain pelvic inflammatory disorders or potentially any condition associated with a perirectal fluid collection, pelvic abscess, or fistula. Endometriosis, a condition defined by the presence of extrauterine functioning endometrial tissue, has been the most extensively studied. This condition may affect 5–20% of menstruating woman, who often present with pelvic pain and infertility.[4.] Ectopic endometriotic implants are most commonly found in the pelvis. Deep pelvic endometriosis may include the uterosacral ligaments, the rectouterine pouch (pouch of Douglas), and rectovaginal lesions that may infiltrate the intestinal wall. The rectosigmoid colon is the most common site of extrapelvic involvement present in approximately 3–37% of patients.[5,6] Gastrointestinal involvement is found at surgery in 5–15% of women who undergo laparoscopy or laparotomy for endometriosis.[7,8] While many patients may be asymptomatic or have nonspecific symptoms, the disease can present as an obstructing colonic neoplasm, inflammatory process, or hematochezia. Preoperative imaging is often recommended to diagnose the extent of rectosigmoid infiltration when surgical management is indicated.

EUS has been shown to be useful in the evaluation of deeply infiltrating endometriosis (see Table, 35–1,

Table 35–1 Comparison Between Published Series in the EUS Diagnosis of Endometriosis

	Patients	RVS; s/s	UTS; s/s	Rectal Wall
Schroder 1997	16	8(100/100%)		100/91%
Fedele 1998	140	34 (97/96%)	- (80/97%)	100/98%
Chapron 1998	38			16(100/100%)
Dumontier 2000	48	6 (50/100%)	15 (60/80%)	6 (100/100%)
Roseau 2000	46			24 (100/100%)
Camagna 2002	32	17 (94/100%)	-	14 (100/75%)
Doniec 2003	65			97/97%
Bazot 2003	30			82/87.5%
Abrao 2004	32			100/67%
Chapron 2004	81			97/89%
Camagna 2004	31			100/71%
Thomassin 2004	27			89/100%
Delpy 2005	30	26 (96/100%)	22 (42/82%)	12 (92/66%)
Bahr 2006	37			8 (87.5/97%)

(Adapted in part from references 18,19) Abbreviation: n = number of patients, rvs = rectovaginal septum, utl = uterosacral ligament, s/s = sensitivity and specificity

References 9-16). Many studies have demonstrated a negative predictive value greater than 90 percent.[10,11,13-19] Endometriotic infiltration of the recto-sigmoid intestinal wall is well visualized by EUS. Other forms of imaging (transabdominal USS, transvaginal USS, endoscopy, CT, MRI, and even laparoscopy) may be suboptimal in the evaluation of the rectovaginal septum and rectal wall. Accurate determination of depth of infiltration and layers involved is often possible. Most intestinal involvement is seen within the serosa or adventitia (fifth layer) and muscularis propria (fourth layer) (Video 35–1); the lesions less frequently infiltrate deeper into the wall.[8,19] Involvement of the mucosa and submucosa occurs in less than 30 percent of cases.[19] Evaluation of perirectal structures and the subperitoneal space[4,18] is also possible. The sonographic appearance of endometriosis may be variable. Focal or diffuse irregular nodular thickening of endometriotic implants that vary in size (ranging from a few millimeters to several centimeters) and/or echotexture may be present (Figure 35–5, Video 35–1). Endometriotic nodules or implants are more often hypoechoic than hyperechoic.[19] and may be either homogenous or heterogenous in appearance depending on the absence or presence of hormone induced hemorrhage or necrosis within the implant. The presence of anechoic cysts or septations may be seen and are nonspecific.[11] Endometriosis nodules may be more prominent during the certain (catamenial) parts of the menstrual cycle.[19] Location is usually anterior and/or lateral relative to the rectum and rectosigmoid junction. The region of the rectovaginal septum has proven best visualized endosonographacially due to location and proximity to the EUS transducer.[18] Endometriotic nodules on the uterosacral ligament or in the ovaries (especially right ovary) are usually more distant than those occurring in the rectovaginal septum and consequently more difficult to visualize on EUS (sensitivity 42% and specificity 14% respectively in one study)[18] It may not be possible to follow the boundaries of the nodules fully beyond a diameter of 3-4 cm.[18] MRI may be better at detecting endometriotic nodules in the region of the uterosacral ligament and ovaries (including better than CT or transabominal CT[19] however MRI is less informative regarding the rectovaginal septum or infiltration of rectal wall.[16,18,20] Studies that have compared the two suggest that MRI is better at detecting nodules in the uterosacral ligaments and ovaries[4,16,18,20,27] although diagnostic accuracy not specified. Vaginal ultrasonography is limited because it cannot be applied above the vaginal cul de sac and does visualize posterior pelvic endometriosis or the rectal wall well.[12,18,19,21] Operator experience and proper use of improved ultrasound probes (reduced frequency of 5Mhz) may be more accurate than early experience has reported. Other endosonographic findings may be demonstrated in endometriosis including fluid in the uterine-rectum pouch of Douglas (present in up to two-thirds), ovarian cysts, or inflammatory lymph nodes.[18]

The role of EUS-guided FNA in the diagnosis of endometriosis has not been well studied.[7,22] Small retrospective series have suggested FNA to be a potentially accurate means to diagnose de novo endometriosis usually in the setting of an incidentally found subepithelial lesion during colonoscopy (Figure 35–6). In the majority of cases of endometrial infiltration of the intestinal wall, the mucosal and submucosal layers are not involved. Biopsy of overlying mucosa is often normal as typically. Cytopathologic evaluation of endometriotic implants may demonstrate the presence of glandular epithelial columnar cells and stroma (similar to the normal endometrium), connective/fibrous tissue fragments, blood, foamy macrophages with hemosiderin gran-

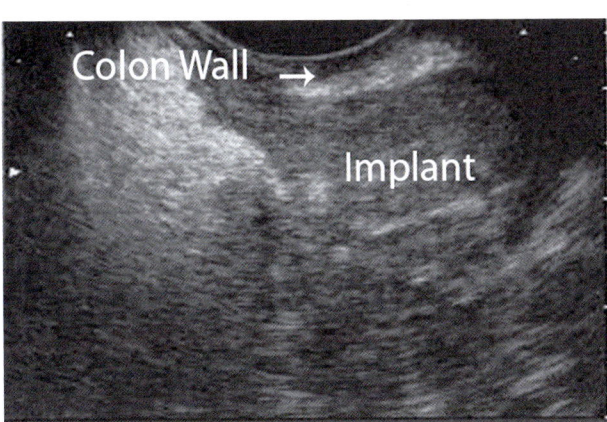

FIGURE 35–5. Linear array EUS from a woman with an extraluminal obstructing sigmoid colon lesion established as endometriosis by EUS FNA

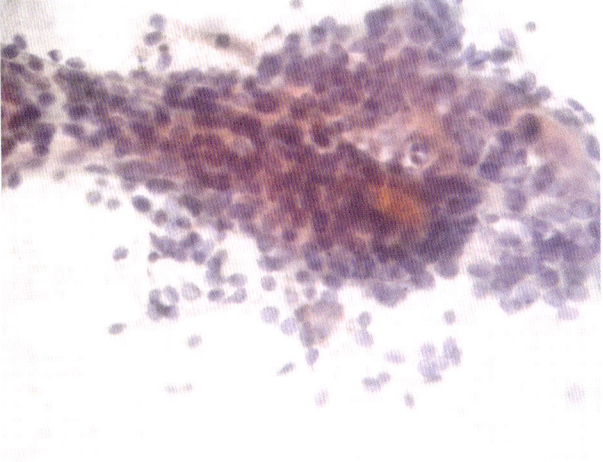

FIGURE 35–6. EUS FNA showing endometriosis from the EUS image shown in Figure 35–5

ules and cysts etc. Cytopathology may be indeterminant or nonspecific when suspicion is not high or number of cellular passes is suboptimal. In rare instances malignant transformation to adenocarcinoma or sarcomas may originate from endometriosis.

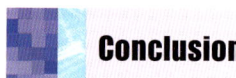
Conclusion

Potential limitations of rectal EUS include challenges related to locoregional anatomy. Only visualized lesions in the immediate perirectal region close to the probe are amenable to evaluation and sampling. Imaging at lower frequency may facilitate depth of visualization at expense of detail. Other challenges include the inability to reliably differentiate benign from malignant lesions especially in the presence of fibrotic or inflammatory tissue changes. This is particularly relevant in the evaluation of metastatic or restaging of recurrent disease after chemoradiation or postoperative residua. Morphology of recurrent or metastatic cancer may be indistinguishable from fibrotic (scar tissue) and inflammatory lesions for instance after chemoradiation or postoperatively.[1] This problem may be overcome by FNA. Increased awareness of the capacity and indications for EUS will enhance future utilization in the evaluation of pelvic/gynecological malignancies. Future studies will better define its role.

Video: Available at www.pmph-usa.com/bhutani
Video 35–1: Transrectal linear EUS of endometriosis involving the rectal wall. A hypoechoic mass is seen that is contiguous with the muscularis propria with similar EUS image as a rectal GI stromal tumor or myogenic tumor. Surgical resection proved this lesion to be endometriosis.

References

1. Hunerbein, M., Totkas, S., Balanou, P., Handke, T., et al.: EUS-guided fine needle biopsy: minimally invasive access to metastatic or recurrent cancer. Eur J Ultrasound 1999;10:151–157
2. Hoffman, B. J., Bhutani, M. S., Aabakken, L., Baron, P., et al.: Endoscopic ultrasound guided fine needle aspiration in the evaluation of extra-rectal pelvic masses. Gastrointestinal Endoscopy 1996;43.
3. St. Ville, E. W., Jafri, S. Z. H., Madrazo, B. L., Mezwa, D. G.., et al.: Endorectal Sonography in the evaluation of rectal and perirectal disease. AJR 1991;157:503–508.
4. Zwas, F. R., Lyon, F. R.: Endometriosis: an important condition in clinical gastroenterology. Dig Dis Sci 1991;36:353–364.
5. Roseau, G., Dumontier, I., Palazzo, L., Chapron, C., et al.: Rectosigmoid endometriosis: Endoscopic ultrasound features and clinical implications. Endoscopy 2000;32: 525–530.
6. Chapron, C., Dumontier, I., Dousset, B., Fritel, X., et al.: Results and role of rectal endoscopic ultrasonography for patients with deep pelvic endometriosis. Human Reproduction 1998;13:2260–2270.
7. Pishvaian, A. C., Ahlawat, S. K., Garvin, D., Haddad, N. G.: Role of EUS and EUS –guided FNA in the diagnosis of symptomatic rectosigmoid endometriosis. Gastrointestinal Endoscopy 2006;63:331–335.
8. Koga, K., Osuga, Y., Yano, T., Momoeda, M., et al.: Characteristic images of deeply infiltrating rectosigmoid endometriosis on transvaginal and transrectal ultrasonography. Hum Reprod 2003;18:1328–1833.
9. Schroder J., Lohnert, M., Doniec, J. M., et al.: Endoluminal ultrasound diagnosis and operative management of rectal endometriosis. Did Colon Rectum 1997;40:614–617.
10. Fedele, L., Bianchi, S., Portuee, A., et al.: Transrectal ultrasonography in the assessment of rectovaginal endometriosis. Obstet Gynecol 1998;91:444–448.
11. Doniec, J. M., Kahlke, V., Peetz, F., Schniewind, B., et al.: Rectal endometriosis: high sensitivity and specificity of endorectal ultrasound with an impact for the operative management. Dis Colon Rectum 2003;46:1667–173.
12. Bazot, M., Detchev, R., Cortez, A., et al.: Transvaginal sonography and rectal endoscopic sonography for the assessment of pelvic endometriosis: a preliminary comparison. Hum Reprod 2003;18:1686–1692.
13. Abrao, M. S., Neme, R. M., Averbach, M., Petta, C. A., et al.: Rectal endoscopic ultrasound with a radial probe in the assessment of rectovaginal endoemetriosis. J Am Assoc Gynecol Laparosc 2004;11:50–54.
14. Camagna, O., Dupuis, O., Soncini, E., et al.: Surgical treatment of rectovaginal septum endometriosis in infiltrating endometriosis: from a continuous series of 40 cases. Acta Endosc 2002;32:47–53.
15. Camagna, O., Dhainaut, C., Dupuis, O., et al.: Surgical management of rectovaginal septum endometriosis from a continuous series of 50 cases. Gynecol Obstet Fertil 2004;32:199–209.
16. Chapron, C., Viera, M., Chopin, N., et al.: Accuracy of rectal endoscopic ultrasonography and magnetic resonance imaging in the diagnosis of rectal involvement for patients presenting with deeply infiltrating endometriosis. Ultrasound Obstet Gynecol 2004;24:175–179.
17. Thomassin, I., Bazot, M., Detchev, R., Barranger, E., et al.: Symptoms before and after surgical removal of colorectal endometriosis that are assessed by magnetic resonance imaging and rectal endoscopic endosonography. Am J Obstet Gynecol 2004;190:1264–1271.
18. Delpy, R., Barthet, M., Gasmi, M., Berdah, S., et al.: Value of endorectal ultrasonography for diagnosing rectovaginal septal endometriosis infiltrating the rectum. Endoscopy 2005;37:357–361.
19. Bahr, A., de Parades, V., Gadonneix, P., Etienney, I., et al.: Endorectal ultrasonography in predicting rectal wall infiltration in patients with deep pelvic endometriosis: a modern tool for ancient disease. Dis Colon Rectum 2006;49:869–875.
20. Dumontier, I., Roseau, G., Vincent, B., et al.: Comparison of endoscopic ultrasound and magnetic resonance imaging in pelvic endometriosis. Gastroenterol Clin Biol 2000;24:1197–1204.
21. Dessole, S., Farina, M., Rubattu, G., Cosmi, E., et al.: Sonovaginography is a new technique for assessing rectovaginal endometriosis. Fertility and Sterility 2003;79:1023 1027.
22. Artifon, E. L., Franzini, T. A., Kumar, A., Matsura, P. F., et al.: EUS-guided FNA facilitates the diagnosis of retroperitoneal endometriosis. Gastrointestinal Endoscopy 2007;66:620–6222.

CHAPTER

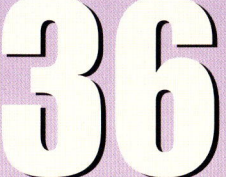

Subepithelial Colorectal Lesions/Colon Polyps/Adenomas

Dr. Irving Waxman
Dr. Jennifer Chennat
Dr. Alberto Herreros de Tejada

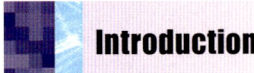

Introduction

With the evolution of endoscopic ultrasound (EUS) as a useful adjunctive tool for the acquisition of more detailed medical, radiologic, and pathologic information, more clinical applications have been found for lesions within the colorectal region. This chapter will focus on the endosonographic descriptions of various colorectal lesions, ranging from polyps to subepithelial lesions, and their differential diagnosis. Where pertinent, use of fine needle aspiration (FNA) will be reviewed, and correlating pathology will be described. Explanation of EUS techniques for imaging of these lesions will not be described.

Colonic Polyps and Adenomas

A colonic polyp is defined as a protuberant lesion rising into the lumen of the colon, although sometimes they may appear as a flat or depressed formation. They are usually asymptomatic, but may ulcerate and bleed; and when their size increases significantly, they may produce luminal obstruction. Polyps are classified based on their location, morphology, and histology. Morphology classification includes protruded, sessile, flat, and depressed polyps (Figure 36–1).[1,2]

From a histological point of view, we can differentiate the following types of polyps:

Endoscopic appearance	JRSC class		Description
Protruded lesions	Ip		Pedunculated polyps
	Ips		Subpedunculated polyps
	Is		Sessile polyps
Flat elevated lesions	IIa		Flat elevation of mucosa
	IIa / IIc		Flat elevation with central depression
Flat lesions	IIb		Flat mucosal change
	IIc		Mucosal depression
	IIc / IIa		Mucosal depression with raised edge

FIGURE 36–1. Classification of colorectal lesions based on morphology. Reprinted with permission from Ross et al. Am J Gastroenterol 2006;101:172–180.

Hyperplastic polyp: A nondysplastic, benign lesion, most of the time less than 5 mm in size with sessile morphology, which is usually encountered in the left colon and rectum. Microscopic evaluation shows a typical serrated pattern when seen sectioned along the crypt axis. Isolated hyperplastic polyps do not seem to be associated with a higher risk of colorectal cancer.[3]

Adenomatous polyp: By definition, a dysplastic polyp, with malignant potential to evolve into colorectal carcinoma, although only a small proportion eventually progresses to cancer (5%).[4] This type of polyp represents 70% of all colonic polyps, and it has been estimated that more than 30% of individuals 50 years or older have colonic adenomas.[5] About 30% of all adenomas are flat polyps, and 1% are depressed lesions; both types are associated with an increased risk of colorectal carcinoma.[6,7] Flat polyps are more difficult to identify during colonoscopy, and some special techniques, like chromoendoscopy or narrow banding imaging, are used to help in its diagnosis.[8] Histological features and size are the major determinants of their malignant potential. Histological classification is as follows:

Tubular adenoma (80%): Characterized by a network of branching adenomatous epithelium (Figure 36–2). To be classified as tubular, the adenoma should have a tubular component of at least 75%.

Villous adenoma (5–15%): Characterized by adjacent crypts or folia of dysplastic epithelium that, without branching, are elongated to at least twice the length of the normal crypt (Figure 36–3). The polyp should have a villous component of at least 75%.

Tubulovillous adenoma (5–15%): Defined by a percentage of villous component ranging between 26–75% of the entire histology (Figure 36–4).

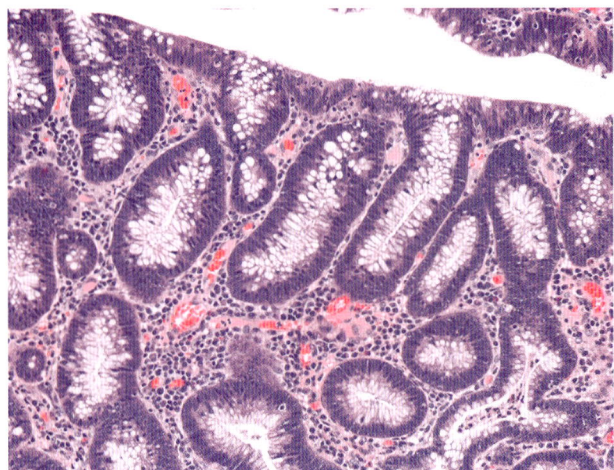

FIGURE 36–2. Microphotography (H/E) of a tubular adenoma. Courtesy of Dr. Noffsinger.

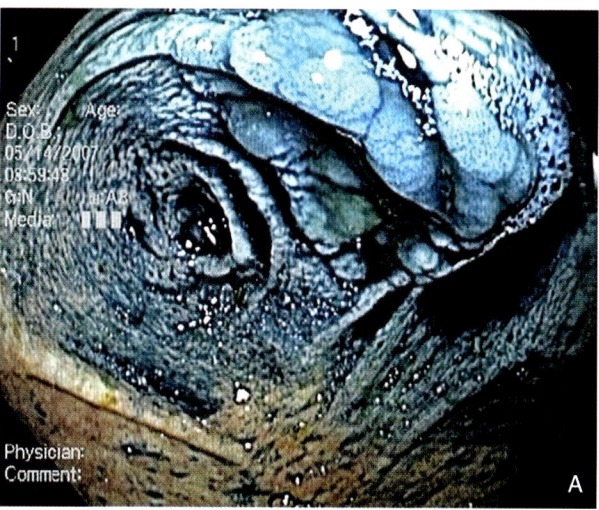
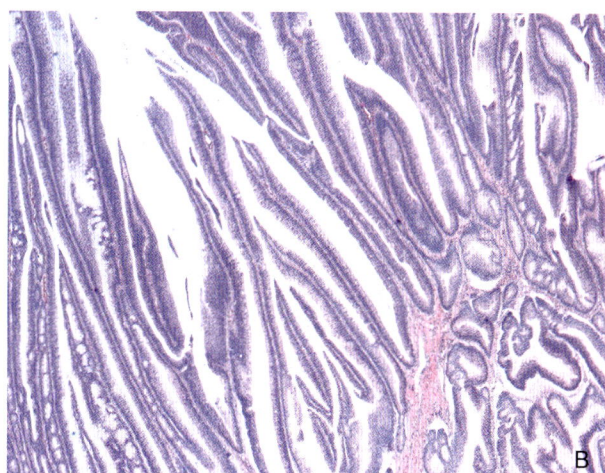

FIGURE 36–3. Flat polyp in the cecal region and correspondent histological microphotography (H/E) after endoscopic resection showing villous adenoma. Courtesy of Dr. Noffsinger.

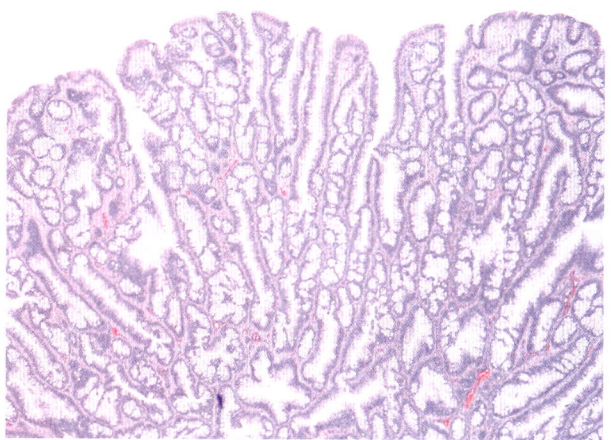

FIGURE 36–4. Microphotography (H/E) of a tubulovillous adenoma. Courtesy of Dr. Noffsinger

Hamartomatous polyp: Formed by an increased number of epithelial and muscular cells in a disorganized fashion, but without malignant behavior. There are different forms of hamartomatous polyps, and some particular syndromes associated with them.

Juvenile polyp: Histologically contain a congested lamina propria with significant dilatation of cystic mucosal glands. This type of polyp is more common in childhood, although it may appear in adults, and have a high risk of spontaneous bleeding. Familial juvenile polyposis is a rare hereditary disease associated with multiple juvenile polyps of the colon with increased risk of CRC.

Peutz-Jeghers polyp: Consists of increased glandular epithelium supported by smooth muscle cells, contiguous with the muscularis mucosa (Figure 36–5). It is associated with the Peutz-Jeghers syndrome, a familial hereditary disease associated with gastrointestinal and nongastrointestinal cancers.[9,10]

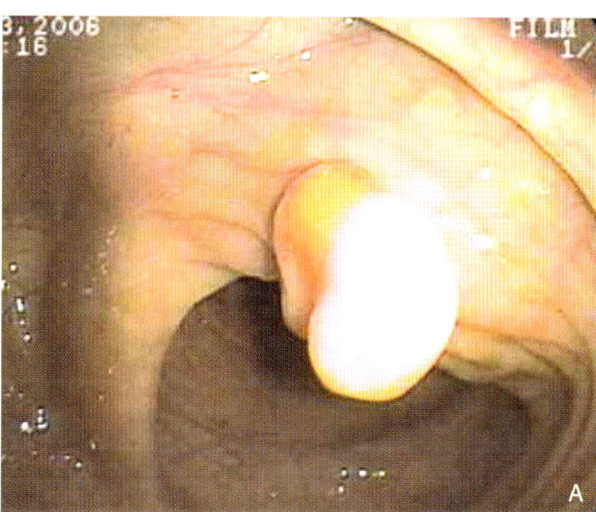
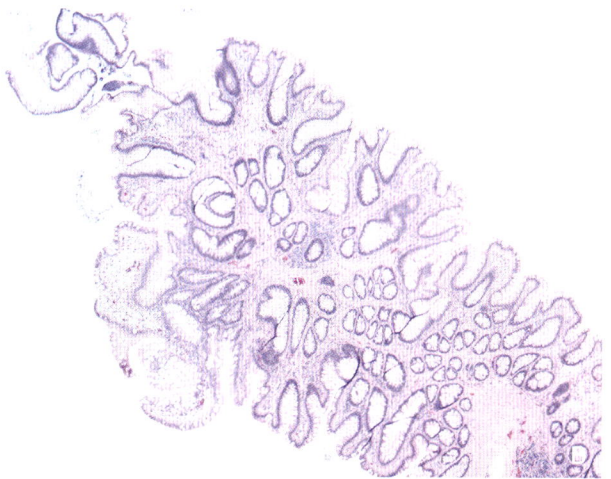

FIGURE 36–5. Peutz-Jeghers polyp in the transverse colon and correspondent histological microphotograph (H/E). Courtesy of Dr. Noffsinger

Cronkhite-Canada syndrome: Rare congenital disease associated with hamartomatous polyps, alopecia, cutaneous hyperpigmentation, onychodystrophy, and malabsorption.[11] Characteristically, the histological examination shows expansion of the lamina propria and increased eosinophils.

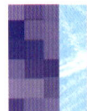

Endoscopic Ultrasound in Colonic and Rectal Adenomas

Colonic adenomas may have malignant histological degeneration, and endoscopic appearance alone may not be sufficiently accurate to identify this phenomenon. EUS has been used to evaluate depth of invasion and the presence of lymph node metastasis in colonic/rectal adenomas, which helps to stratify lesions suitable for endoscopic resection.[12] This is particularly important when nonsurgical treatment is clinically considered.[13]

Endoscopic ultrasound (EUS) examination can be performed either with a standard echoendoscope or a high-frequency ultrasound probe (HFUP). The standard EUS is more appropriate for large bulky lesions.[12,14] The HFUP probe can be used through a standard colonoscope, thus allowing scanning of proximal colonic lesions. The ideal targets for the HFUP are small, flat, or depressed tumors, where nearly 100% diagnostic accuracy can be reached.[15] HFUS imaging seems to be more accurate for T-staging than other endoscopic imaging techniques like magnification colonoscopy.[16,17]

Anatomy and Technique Tips

When considering the wall of the rectum under standard EUS, we can observe five alternating hyperechoic and hypoechoic layers.[12] The histological correlation is as follows (Figure 36–6):

1. First layer (hyperechoic)—interface between water or balloon and superficial mucosa
2. Second layer (hypoechoic)—deep mucosa and muscularis mucosa
3. Third layer (hyperechoic)—submucosa and its limits
4. Fourth layer (hypoechoic)—muscularis propria
5. Fifth layer (hyperechoic)—interface between serosa and perirectal fat

The image obtained with a HFUP has a depth of penetration limited to 2 to 3 cm from the surface, but its superior definition provides an ultrasound image of the wall structure resembling those seen on histology.[18] In the colon, the three layers of the muscularis propria may be visualized (Table 36–1). The detailed evaluation of the muscularis mucosa and muscularis propria is particularly useful in the evaluation of early cancers arising in adenomas prior to endoscopic resection.

Polyps are examined after the bowel had been filled with water and/or using the water-filled balloon juxtaposition technique.[19] Large pedunculated polyps are more difficult to visualize than flat or sessile lesions, mainly due to problems with visualization of the stalk.[20] The use of standard oblique-viewing EUS in sections of the colon proximal to the sigmoid is

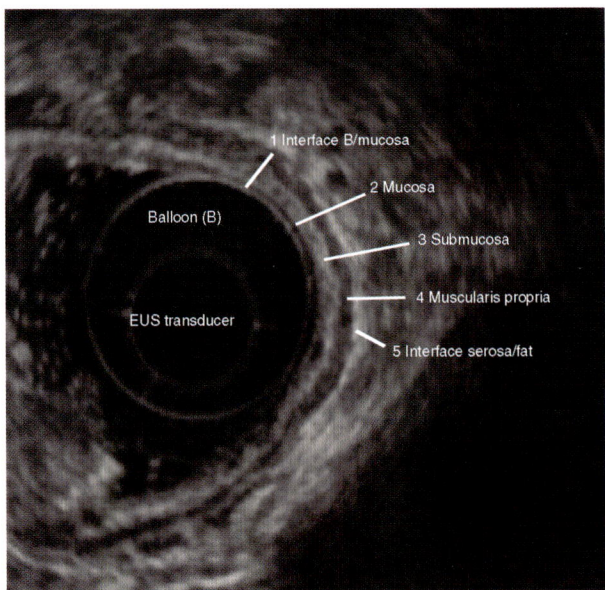

FIGURE 36–6. Ultrasonographic image of the rectal wall with the five echo-layers.

Table 36–1. Correlation Between HFUB Echogenic and Histological Layers of the Muscularis Propria

Location of the Layer in Relation with the HFUB	Echogenicity	Histological Correspondence
Inner	Hypoechoic	Circular muscle layer
Middle	Hyperechoic	Connective tissue
Outer	Hypoechoic	Longitudinal muscle layer

limited by its oblique optics and suboptimal maneuverability, thus making HFUB the better option.[21]

Applications of EUS

Colonic and rectal adenomas are polypoid lesions with potential to evolve into adenocarcinoma.[22] EUS is a useful tool to assess the presence of pathological echoic structures and evaluate their longitudinal and circumferential extent. When considering adenomas with submucosal invasion, assessment of the depth of invasion is key prior to treatment.[23-25] It has been proposed that a lesion invading less than 1000 μ of the submucosa layer (sm1) is feasible for endoscopic resection in the colon.[1] In rectal lesions, EUS can distinguish between noninvasive lesions and invasive early cancer of stage T0 or T1.[26]

In colonic adenomas, the presence of early cancer (T1 lesion) is observed with EUS as a hypoechoic mass limited to the mucosa or the submucosa (first three echo layers).[12] The echodensity of the suspected lesions should be compared with that of the third hyperechoic (submucosa) or fourth hypoechoic (muscularis propria) layers of the normal colorectal wall.[27]

Villous Adenomas

Villous adenomas are typically a protuberant soft and friable mass with a "shaggy" surface. As previously mentioned, villous adenomas are defined by the extent of the villous component.[27] A significant proportion of these adenomas have malignant transformation at the time of diagnosis, and their size is not a reliable predictor of presence of invasive carcinoma.[28] EUS is a useful tool in the preoperative workup of rectal villous adenomas, decreasing the need for additional surgery up to 24% of the cases.[29] (Figures 36–7A and 36–7B).

Location and size are significant factors in the accuracy of the EUS evaluation in villous lesions. In the study from Konishi et al, EUS was performed on 125 colorectal neoplastic lesions (35 villous and 90 nonvillous) and then compared with pathological results.[27] The overall accuracy of EUS-based evaluation of tumor invasion depth was 60% in villous lesions and 91% in nonvillous lesions. Overstaging in villous lesions reached 37%. Large (greater than 20 mm) or rectal villous lesions were more likely to be over/or understaged with regard to submucosal invasion. However, these differences seem to disappear when only colonic lesions are compared, in concordance with other studies.[30-32]

Other Clinical Applications of EUS of Colonic/Rectal Polyps

EUS has been used to assess the presence of vessels in rectal and colonic adenomatous polyps, prior to consideration for endoscopic polypectomy. Repeated results have shown imaging of a polyp and the corresponding deep vessels was not predictive of postpolypectomy bleeding risk.[19]

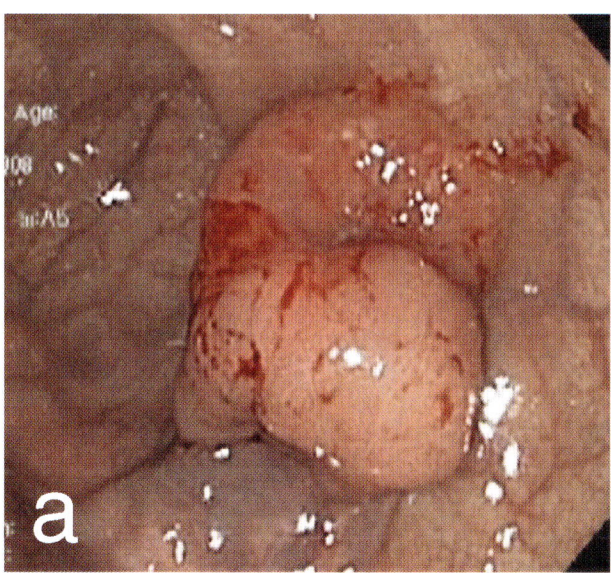
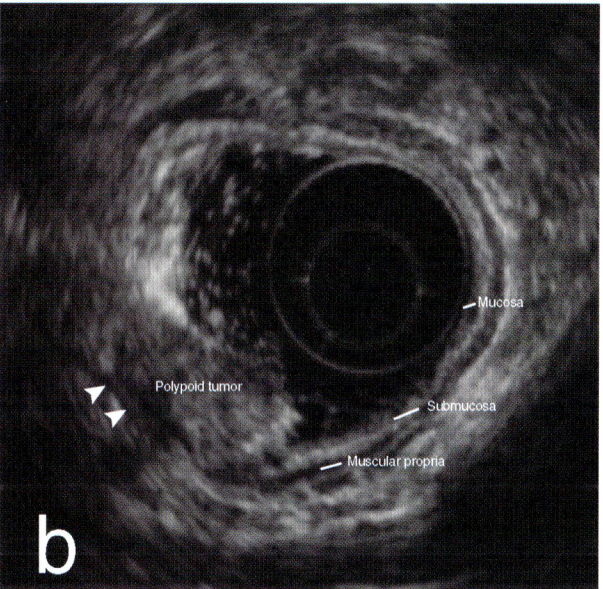

FIGURES 36–7 A and B Sessile polyp in the rectum: (A) endoscopic image; (B) EUS showing deep invasion of the muscular propria and serosa (stage T3). See also Video 36–1

Subepithelial Colorectal Lesions

Often found incidentally, subepithelial lesions of the colorectum can arise from any layer of the intestinal tract (intramural) or represent an extrinsic compression from outside the wall (extramural). Differentiating from which layer of the gastrointestinal tract the lesion originates is important for lesion characterization and management. Additionally, if the lesion is extramural in origin, then depending on the etiology, it may be therapeutically addressed using FNA.

The role of EUS in evaluation of similar upper gastrointestinal subepithelial lesions has been more clearly defined in the literature. Many of the same lesions do present in the large intestine and/or rectum. Flexible upper echoendoscopes have been utilized for evaluation of lesions not only in the rectum, but also in the sigmoid and left colon.[21] Through the scope HFUS probes can assist in evaluation of lesions throughout the colon as well.[33,34] Furthermore, high-frequency endosonographic miniprobes can help delineate which subepithelial lesions arise from the submucosa, and aid in the selection of these lesions for endoscopic resection.[35,36] Colorectal intramural lesions can be classified based on their wall layer origin (Table 36–2).

Table 36–2 Subepithelial Colorectal Lesions

Lesion	Wall Layer Involvement	Echo Features
Leiomyoma	Muscularis Propria, Muscularis Mucosae	Hypoechoic, well-defined margins
Leiomyosarcoma	Muscularis Propria	Hypoechoic, irregular margins, central hyperechoic necrosis
Lipoma	Submucosa	Hyperechoic, well-defined margins
Carcinoid	Muscularis Mucosae, Submucosa	Hypoechoic
Lymphangioma	Submucosa	Anechoic, cystic structure
Endometriosis	Muscularis Propria, Serosa	Hypoechoic

Gastrointestinal Stromal Tumors

Gastrointestinal stromal tumors (GISTs) are lesions of mesenchymal origin, derived from neural, muscular, or both types of cells. They are relatively rare lesions in the colon and rectum, comprising approximately 5% of total GIST incidence.[37] EUS characterization typically reveals a hypoechoic mass arising from most commonly the fourth (muscularis propria) and less commonly, the second (muscularis mucosae) layer of the normal gut wall with overlying smooth mucosa, that occasionally can be ulcerated. These lesions can grow endophytically (toward the intestinal lumen) or exophytically (growing outwardly). Occasionally, they can have bidirectional growth, yielding a dumbbell-shaped configuration.[38]

GISTs can be either benign or malignant, and their prognosis depends on size of the lesion, mitotic index, age of the patient, and location of the tumor. Endosonographic factors associated with malignant GIST lesions include EUS determined tumor size (diameter greater than 4 cm), irregular extraluminal border, heterogeneity, echogenic foci, and cystic spaces greater than 4 mm,[39] One study found that the combination of two out of three EUS features (irregular extraluminal margins, cystic spaces, and lymph nodes with a malignant pattern) had a positive predictive value of 100% for malignant or borderline GIST pathology. In the same study, tumors with diameter less than 30 mm, with regular margins, and a homogeneous echo pattern, were found to be usually benign.[40]

The overall accuracy for the diagnosis of malignant GIST was 78% by EUS imaging alone and 91% by histopathology obtained by EUS-FNA in one study. The addition of Ki-67 immunohistochemical staining to FNA specimens increased the accuracy to 100 percent.[41] If there is a strong clinical suspicion for GIST, then EUS-FNA with immunohistochemical staining should be performed for CD-117 (c-kit) (Figure 36–8). It has been demonstrated that C-kit positive tumors are more likely to have malignant features and should be resected and/or subjected to close clinical follow-up.[42]

Leiomyomas/Leiomyosarcomas

True smooth muscle neoplasms of mesenchymal origin such as leiomyomas and leiomyosarcomas should be included in the differential diagnosis of

Subepithelial Colorectal Lesions/Colon Polyps/Adenomas

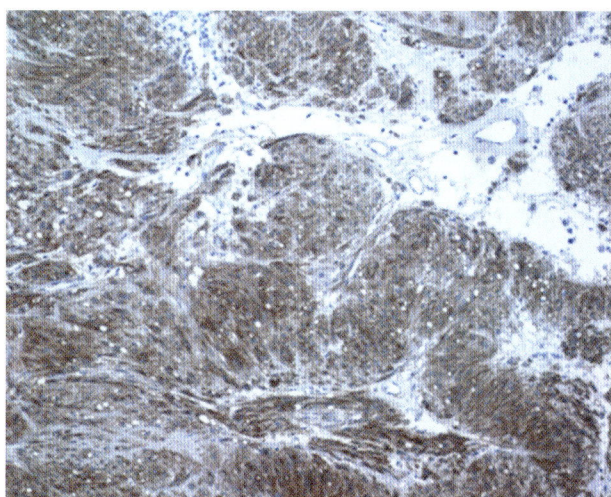

FIGURE 36–8. Rectal GIST: c-kit stain

GISTs. At endoscopy, these lesions are usually solitary and have overlying smooth mucosa. Leiomyomas and leiomyosarcomas usually arise from the fourth hypoechoic layer (muscularis propria) and occasionally from the muscularis mucosae (Figures 36–9A and 36–9B). Leiomyomas tend to have a well-demarcated, homogenous appearance with EUS imaging, sometimes having the same echogenicity as the muscularis propria. In contrast, the sarcoma variants tend to appear inhomogeneous, sometimes with hyperechoic necrotic central areas and lobulation.[43]

Schwannomas, Paragangliomas, and Fibrosarcomas

These are GISTs that are derived from neural cell origins. They should also be considered in the differential diagnosis of subepithelial lesions originating from the second or fourth layers of the intestinal wall and exhibiting a hypoechoic appearance on EUS.

Lipomas

Lipomas are subepithelial tumors comprised of adipose tissue that usually arise from the submucosal layer. The majority of them are found in the large intestine, namely the right colon. The lesions are usually solitary, with a yellowish hue to the overlying smooth mucosa on endoscopy. Sometimes they exhibit the classic "pillow sign," whereby the lesion forms an indentation with the application of gentle pressure using a closed cold endoscopic forceps. They may manifest clinically with bleeding and/or abdominal pain. EUS evaluation reveals a hyperechoic homogeneous lesion that originates most often from the third (submucosal) layer, with well-defined smooth margins.[38,43] (Figure 36–10).

Carcinoids

Gastrointestinal carcinoids are neoplasms that arise from a wide variety of specialized endocrine cells that populate the gastrointestinal mucosa and submucosa. Carcinoid tumors usually arise from enterochromaffin cells.[44] Modlin and colleagues reported that the incidence of carcinoids has increased over the past 30 years and that 41.8% of gastrointestinal carcinoids occurred in the small intestine, followed in decreasing order of frequency by the rectum (27.4%), appendix (24.1%), and stomach (8.7%).[45]

Carcinoid syndrome, characterized by cutaneous flushing, sweating, bronchospasm, abdominal pain,

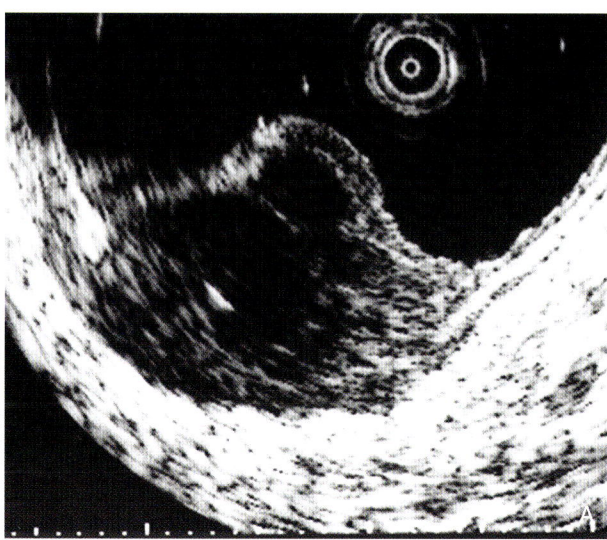
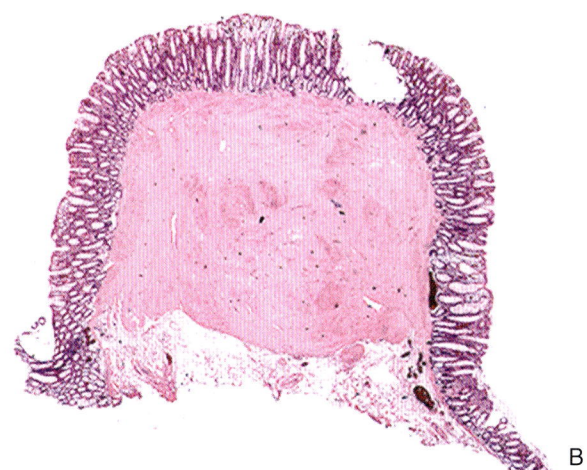

FIGURES 36–9 *A and B* (A) EUS visualized leiomyoma as a hypoechoic and homogeneous mass located in the fourth layer. (B) Photomicrography of the surgically resected tumor (H&E, original magnification ×3).

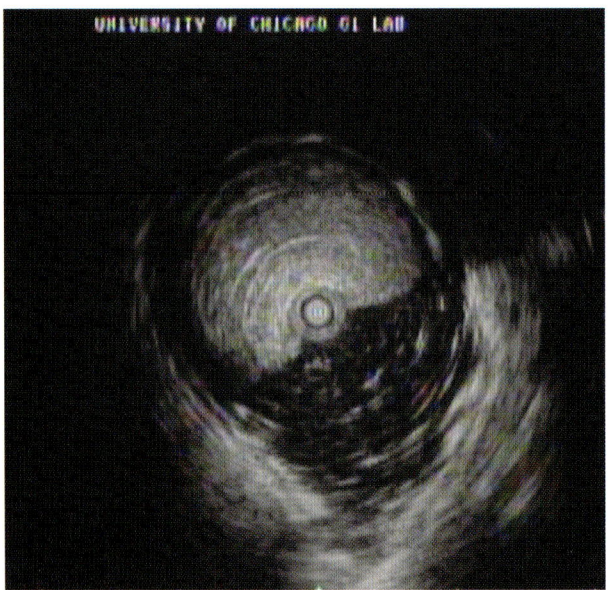

FIGURE 36–10. EUS image of lipoma visualized as a hyperechoic mass located in the third layer. See also Video 36–2

diarrhea, and right sided cardiac valvular fibrosis, occurs in less than 10% of patients with carcinoid tumors.[46] The syndrome develops because vasoactive substances produced by the carcinoid tumor enter into the systemic circulation without undergoing prior metabolic degradation. The syndrome most commonly occurs in patients with ileal carcinoids and/or hepatic/retroperitoneal metastases.[44]

The prognosis of carcinoid tumors relies on their size, with all metastatic presentations associated with tumors greater than 2 cm in size. Endoscopically, they are yellow to whitish in color. Endosongraphically, they appear hypoechoic, with well-defined borders, and generally arise from the second (muscularis mucosae) or third (submucosal) layers.

New treatment algorithms depend on the size of the lesion. Tumors that are less and 2 cm in size and not invading past the submucosal layer are potentially amenable to endoscopic resection. However, tumors greater than 2 cm, with invasion into the muscularis propria layer and/or deeper, or those demonstrating

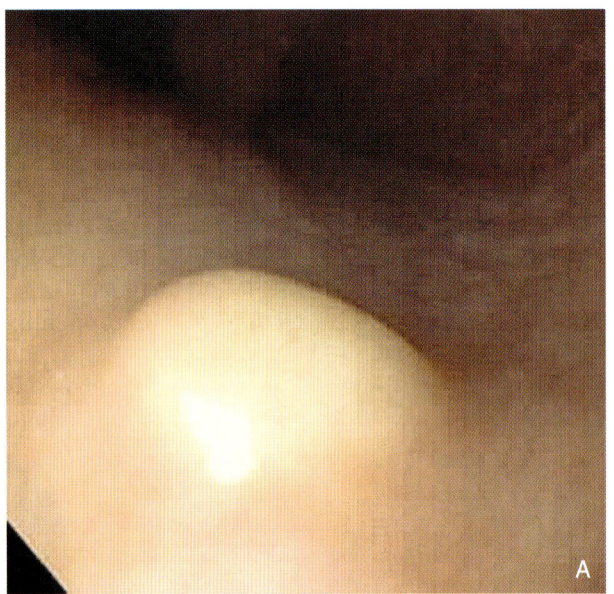

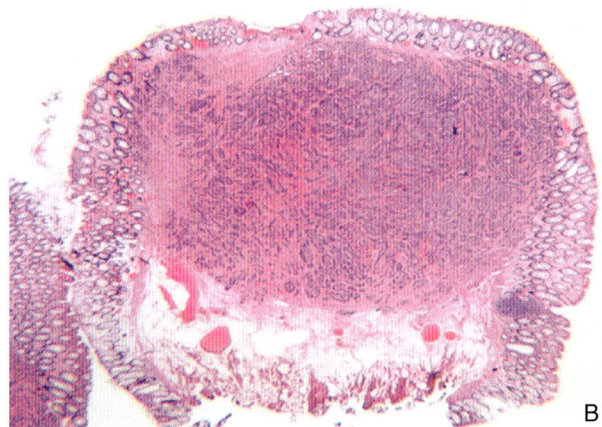

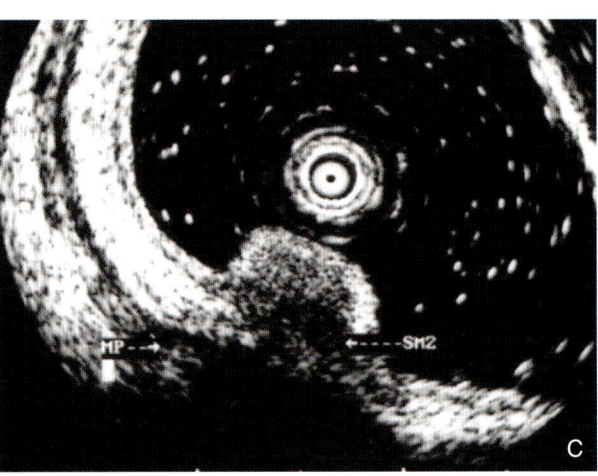

FIGURES 36–11 *A to C*. (A) Rectal carcinoid tumor, (B) endoscopic EUS, and (C) correspondent histologic image

lymph node involvement, should be surgically resected.[38]

Lymphangiomas

Colonic lymphangiomas are benign cystic lesions sometimes with septal structures that are located in the third (submucosal) layer. They are considered to be lymph vessel anomalies, and on endoscopy are usually solitary raised lesions with overlying normal appearing mucosa. On EUS, they appear as anechoic cystic structures with or without hypoechoic septations. Aspiration of these lesions yields clear yellow tinged fluid, similar in appearance to lymph.[47] Evaluation with a through the scope miniprobe can be useful in determining diagnosis and treatment management, which usually is conservative, if the patient is asymptomatic.[34]

Endometriosis

Up to 10–15% of all endometriosis cases have gastrointestinal involvement. Among female patients with intestinal endometriosis, the rectum and sigmoid colon are the most commonly involved areas (75–90%). The distal ileum (2–16%) and appendix (3–18%) are less commonly affected.[48] Although typically a disease of the young, gastrointestinal endometriosis can also affect postmenopausal women. The classic hallmark symptom is rectal bleeding during menstruation. However, intussusception, hemorrhage, perforation, small bowel or colonic obstruction have also been reported.[49]

On endoscopy, if these lesions are visible, they often have overlying normal appearing mucosa. The role of endoscopic ultrasound has expanded to applications in assessment of rectosigmoid endometriosis. EUS and confirmatory EUS-FNA of these lesions has been reported by Pishvaian and collegues. Endometriosis infiltrates either the fourth (muscularis propria) or fifth (serosal) layers. They have a hypoechoic appearance on EUS.[50]

Delpy and collegues reported on the value of endorectal ultrasonography for diagnosing rectovaginal septal endometriosis infiltrating the rectum. The sensitivity, specificity, and positive and negative predictive value of anorectal endoscopic ultrasonography as a means of diagnosing endometriosis of the rectovaginal septum and infiltration of the rectal wall were found to be 96%, 100%, 100%, and 83%, and 92%, 66%, 64% and 92%, respectively. The diagnostic accuracy was at 96% and 80%, respectively. Sensitivity of detection of endometriosis nodules farther from the rectal wall, such as in the uterosacral ligaments or ovaries was 42% and 14%, respectively, leading to diagnostic accuracy rates of 56% and 53%.[51]

Summary

Colonic polyps are lesions that are frequently found in the general population,. They are classified according to their shape, size, location, and histological features. One of the main concerns regarding colonic adenomas is their potential of malignant degeneration. Standard EUS and HFUS are diagnostic tools that image acquisition with accurate histological correlation. Their value in local staging of these lesions is paramount, helping in the decision making process for local resection. The role of endoscopic ultrasound in the assessment of colonic subepithelial lesions is advantageous in delineating the lesion's characterization. The use of EUS-guided FNA further solidifies diagnosis and management. Use of high-frequency miniprobes in the proximal colon has been clearly shown to aid in the diagnosis of lesions that otherwise might continue to be endoscopic and clinical conundrums. As endoscopic ultrasound technology continues to develop, expanding clinical applications will likely be found for both intrinsic and extrinsic colonic lesions.

Videos: Available at www.pmph-usa.com/bhutani

Video 36–1: Endoscopic video of a sessile polyp in the rectum, followed by radial and linear EUS examination of the lesion. Radial EUS shows the depth of the lesion, demonstrating the depth of invasion into the muscularis propria and serosal layers. Linear EUS is concordant with the radial exam findings.

Video 36–2: Endoscopic video of a lipoma in transverse colon, followed by High Frequency Ultrasound (HFUS) of the lesion. The large polyp with overlying smooth mucosa, is visualized under EUS as a hyperechoic mass located in the third layer (submucosa). There is a regular margin of the lesion, separating it from the muscular propria layer. Tunnel deep application of biopsy forceps reveals extrusion of pale pink lipoid tissue from within the submucosal space.

References

1. The Paris endoscopic classification of superficial neoplastic lesions: esophagus, stomach, and colon: November 30 to December 1, 2002. Gastrointest Endosc 2003;58(6 Suppl):S3-43.
2. Ross. A. S., Waxman, I.: Flat and depressed neoplasms of the colon in Western populations. *Am J Gastroenterol* 2006;101(1):172–180.

3. Rex, D. K., Smith, J. J., Ulbright, T. M., Lehman, G. A.: Distal colonic hyperplastic polyps do not predict proximal adenomas in asymptomatic average-risk subjects. Gastroenterology 1992;102(1):317–319.
4. O'Brien, M. J., Winawer, S. J., Zauber, A. G., Gottlieb, L. S., Sternberg, S. S., Diaz, B., et al.: The National Polyp Study. Patient and polyp characteristics associated with high-grade dysplasia in colorectal adenomas. Gastroenterology 1990;98(2):371–379.
5. Rex, D. K., Lehman, G. A., Ulbright, T. M., Smith, J. J., Pound, D. C., Hawes, R. H., et al.: Colonic neoplasia in asymptomatic persons with negative fecal occult blood tests: influence of age, gender, and family history. Am J Gastroenterol 1993;88(6):825–831.
6. Rembacken, B. J., Fujii, T., Cairns, A., Dixon, M. F., Yoshida, S., Chalmers, D. M., et al.: Flat and depressed colonic neoplasms: a prospective study of 1000 colonoscopies in the UK. Lancet 2000;355(9211):1211–1214.
7. Saitoh, Y., Waxman, I., West, A. B., Popnikolov, N. K., Gatalica, Z., Watari, J., et al.: Prevalence and distinctive biologic features of flat colorectal adenomas in a North American population. Gastroenterology 2001;120(7):1657–1665.
8. Su, M. Y., Hsu, C. M., Ho, Y. P., Chen, P. C., Lin, C. J., Chiu, C. T.: Comparative study of conventional colonoscopy, chromoendoscopy, and narrow-band imaging systems in differential diagnosis of neoplastic and nonneoplastic colonic polyps. Am J Gastroenterol 2006;101(12):2711–2716.
9. Giardiello, F. M., Welsh, S. B., Hamilton, S. R., Offerhaus, G. J., Gittelsohn, A. M., Booker, S. V., et al.: Increased risk of cancer in the Peutz-Jeghers syndrome. N Engl J Med 1987;316(24):1511–1514.
10. Gonzalez Munoz, J. L., Angoso Clavijo, M., Esteban Velasco, C., Rodriguez Perez, A., Munoz Bellvis, L., Gomez Alonso. L.: The diagnosis of Peutz-Jeghers syndrome. Rev Esp Enferm *Dig* 2007;99(3):167.
11. Cronkhite, L. W., Jr., Canada, W. J.: Generalized gastrointestinal polyposis; an unusual syndrome of polyposis, pigmentation, alopecia and onychotrophia. N Engl J Med 1955;252(24):1011–1015.
12. Ahmad, N. A., Kochman, M. L., Ginsberg, G. G.: Endoscopic ultrasound and endoscopic mucosal resection for rectal cancers and villous adenomas. Hematol Oncol Clin North Am 2002;16(4):897–906.
13. Hulsmans, F. H., Tio, T. L., Mathus-Vliegen, E. M., Bosma, A., Tytgat, G. N.: Colorectal villous adenoma: transrectal US in screening for invasive malignancy. Radiology 1992;185(1):193–196.
14. Saitoh, Y., Obara, T., Einami, K., Nomura, M., Taruishi, M., Ayabe, T., et al.: Efficacy of high-frequency ultrasound probes for the preoperative staging of invasion depth in flat and depressed colorectal tumors. Gastrointest Endosc 1996;44(1):34–39.
15. Hurlstone, D. P., Cross, S. S., Sanders, D. S.: 20-MHz high-frequency endoscopic ultrasound-assisted endoscopic mucosal resection for colorectal submucosal lesions: a prospective analysis. J Clin Gastroenterol 2005;39(7):596–599.
16. Matsumoto, T., Hizawa, K., Esaki, M., Kurahara, K., Mizuno, M., Hirakawa, K., et al.: Comparison of EUS and magnifying colonoscopy for assessment of small colorectal cancers. Gastrointest Endosc 2002;56(3):354–360.
17. Yoshida, M., Tsukamoto, Y., Niwa, Y., Goto, H., Hase, S., Hayakawa, T., et al.: Endoscopic assessment of invasion of colorectal tumors with a new high-frequency ultrasound probe. Gastrointest Endosc 1995;41(6):587–592.
18. Odegaard, S., Nesje, L. B., Ohm, I. M., Kimmey, M. B.: Endosonography in gastrointestinal diseases. Acta Radiol 1999;40(2):119–134.
19. Polkowski, M., Regula, J., Wronska, E., Pachlewski, J., Rupinski, M., Butruk, E.: Endoscopic ultrasonography for prediction of postpolypectomy bleeding in patients with large nonpedunculated rectosigmoid adenomas. Endoscopy 2003;35(4):343–347.
20. Polkowski, M., Regul,a J., Wronska, E.: Endosonography of large rectosigmoid adenomas is not useful for predicting postpolypectomy bleeding Gastrointest Endosc 1998; 47:AB152.
21. Bhutani, M. S., Nadella, P.: Utility of an upper echoendoscope for endoscopic ultrasonography of malignant and benign conditions of the sigmoid/left colon and the rectum. Am J Gastroenterol 2001;96(12):3318–3322.
22. Atkin, W. S., Morson, B. C., Cuzick, J.: Long-term risk of colorectal cancer after excision of rectosigmoid adenomas. N Engl J Med 1992;326(10):658–662.
23. Kudo, S., Kashida, H., Nakajima, T., Tamura, S., Nakajo, K.: Endoscopic diagnosis and treatment of early colorectal cancer. World J Surg 1997;21(7):694–701.
24. Conio, M., Repici, A., Demarquay, J. F., Blanchi, S., Dumas, R., Filiberti, R.: EMR of large sessile colorectal polyps. Gastrointest Endosc 2004;60(2):234-241.
25. Conio, M., Ponchon, T., Blanchi, S.: Filiberti R. Endoscopic mucosal resection. Am J Gastroenterol 2006;101(3):653–663.
26. Starck, M., Bohe, M., Simanaitis, M., Valentin, L.: Rectal endosonography can distinguish benign rectal lesions from invasive early rectal cancers. Colorectal Dis 2003;5(3):246–250.
27. Konishi, K., Akita, Y., Kaneko, K., Kurahashi, T., Yamamoto, T., Kusayanagi, S., et al.: Evaluation of endoscopic ultrasonography in colorectal villous lesions. Int J Colorectal Dis 2003;18(1):19–24.
28. Stulc, J. P., Petrelli, N. J., Herrera, L., Mittelman, A.: Colorectal villous and tubulovillous adenomas equal to or greater than four centimeters. Ann Surg 1988; 207(1):65–71.
29. Worrell, S., Horvath, K., Blakemore, T., Flum, D.: Endorectal ultrasound detection of focal carcinoma within rectal adenomas. Am J Surg 2004;187(5):625–629
30. Tio, T. L., Coene, P. P., van Delden, O. M., Tytgat, G. N.: Colorectal carcinoma: preoperative TNM classification with endosonography. Radiology 1991;179(1):165–170.
31. Pikarsky, A., Wexner, S., Lebensart, P., Efron, J., Weiss, E., Nogueras, J., et al.: The use of rectal ultrasound for the correct diagnosis and treatment of rectal villous tumors. Am J Surg 2000;179(4):261–265.
32. Adams, W. J., Wong, W. D.: Endorectal ultrasonic detection of malignancy within rectal villous lesions. Dis Colon Rectum 1995;38(10):1093–1096.
33. Fujimura, Y., Nishishita, C., Iida, M., Kajihara, Y.: Lymphangioma of the colon diagnosed with an endoscopic ultrasound probe and dynamic CT. Gastrointest Endosc 1995;41(3):252–254.
34. Irisawa, A., Bhutani, M. S.: Cystic lymphangioma of the colon: endosonographic diagnosis with through-the-scope catheter miniprobe and determination of further management. Report of a case. Dis Colon Rectum 2001;44(7):1040–1042.

35. Waxman, I., Saitoh, Y., Raju, G. S., Watari, J., Yokota, K., Reeves, A. L., et al.: High-frequency probe EUS-assisted endoscopic mucosal resection: a therapeutic strategy for submucosal tumors of the GI tract. Gastrointest Endosc 2002;55(1):44–49.
36. Waxman, I., Saitoh, Y.: Clinical outcome of endoscopic mucosal resection for superficial GI lesions and the role of high-frequency US probe sonography in an American population. Gastrointest Endosc 2000;52(3):322–327.
37. Feldman, Mea.: Sleisenger & Fordtran's Gastrointestinal and Liver Disease. 8 ed. Philadelphia: Saunders Elsevier, 2006.
38. Parmar Ka, I. W.: Endosonography in Submucosal Lesions: WB Saunders, 2000.
39. Chak, A., Canto, M. I., Rosch, T., Dittler, H. J., Hawes, R. H., Tio, T. L., et al.: Endosonographic differentiation of benign and malignant stromal cell tumors. Gastrointest Endosc 1997;45(6):468–473.
40. Palazzo, L., Landi, B., Cellier, C., Cuillerier, E., Roseau, G., Barbier, J. P.: Endosonographic features predictive of benign and malignant gastrointestinal stromal cell tumors. Gut 2000;46(1):88–92.
41. Ando, N., Goto, H., Niwa, Y., Hirooka, Y., Ohmiya, N., Nagasaka, T., et al.: The diagnosis of GI stromal tumors with EUS-guided fine needle aspiration with immunohistochemical analysis. Gastrointest Endosc 2002;55(1):37–43.
42. Hunt, G. C., Rader, A. E., Faigel, D. O.: A comparison of EUS features between CD-117 positive GI stromal tumors and CD-117 negative GI spindle cell tumors. Gastrointest Endosc 2003;57(4):469–474.
43. Kameyama, H., Niwa, Y., Arisawa, T., Goto, H., Hayakawa, T.: Endoscopic ultrasonography in the diagnosis of submucosal lesions of the large intestine. Gastrointest Endosc 1997;46(5):406–411.
44. Levy, A. D., Sobin, L. H.: From the archives of the AFIP: Gastrointestinal carcinoids: imaging features with clinicopathologic comparison. Radiographics 2007;27(1):237–257.
45. Modlin, I. M., Lye, K. D., Kidd, M.: A 5-decade analysis of 13,715 carcinoid tumors. *Cancer* 2003;97(4):934-59.
46. Sweeney JF, Rosemurgy AS. Carcinoid Tumors of the Gut. Cancer Control 1997;4(1):18–24.
47. Watanabe, T., Kato, K., Sugitani, M., Hasunuma, O., Sawada, T., Hoshino, N., et al.: A case of multiple lymphangiomas of the colon suggesting colonic lymphangiomatosis. Gastrointest Endosc 2000;52(6):781–784.
48. Miller, L. S.: Less frequent causes of lower gastrointestinal bleeding. Gastroenterology Clinics of North America, 1994:21–52.
49. Varras, M., Kostopanagiotou, E., Katis, K., Farantos, C., Angelidou-Manika, Z., Antoniou, S.: Endometriosis causing extensive intestinal obstruction simulating carcinoma of the sigmoid colon: a case report and review of the literature. Eur J Gynaecol Oncol 2002;23(4):353–357.
50. Pishvaian, A. C., Ahlawat, S. K., Garvin, D., Haddad, N. G.: Role of EUS and EUS-guided FNA in the diagnosis of symptomatic rectosigmoid endometriosis. Gastrointest Endosc 2006;63(2):331–235.
51. Delpy, R., Barthet, M., Gasmi, M., Berdah, S., Shojai, R., Desjeux, A., et al.: Value of endorectal ultrasonography for diagnosing rectovaginal septal endometriosis infiltrating the rectum. Endoscopy 2005;37(4):357–361.

CHAPTER 37

Prostate Lesions

Dr. Everson L. A. Artifon
Dr. Paulo Sakai
Dr. Manoop S. Bhutani

Urologic Echoendoscopy

There is limited published data on EUS of the prostate.[1] There may be potential for applying EUS for prostate imaging and intervention similar to application of EUS in the mediastinum and for lung pathologies. Urologic EUS aspects in relation to prostate are demonstrated in this chapter because this is an area of research and further development by the authors.

Echoendoscopy in Benign Prostate Pathologies

Most diseases affecting the prostate are benign. Benign neoplasias, inflammatory processes, cysts, and calculi are the most common. Benign prostate hyperplasia (BPH) represents the most common benign neoplastic disease. The other types of benign neoplasms being extremely rare (e.g. cystadenoma, smooth muscle myxoid tumors, and phyllode tumors).[7,8,13] However, the most important potential application of EUS is in the diagnosis and staging of prostate cancer.

Benign Prostate Hyperplasia (BPH)

The prevalence of this disease increases greatly with age at a rate of almost 90% in men older than 80.[3] In spite of the difference in the intensity and behavior in several racial groups, the symptoms are of an obstructive and irritating nature. The patients complain of weak or intermittent urinary flow, nocturia, urgency to urinate, difficulty in starting urination, incomplete emptying of the bladder, and consequently a higher frequency of urination episodes. These symptoms may lead to acute urinary retention, incontinence, and azotemia. An interesting observation in clinical practice is the lack of a linear relationship between the symptoms and the size of the gland.[3]

BPH histology is characterized by an alteration in prostate parenchyma architecture, which leads to global volumetric increase observed in the transition zone and to a lesser degree in the periurethral tissue. It is primarily an alteration of the internal gland. Histologic alterations occur due to androgenic stimulation. Hyperplasia corresponds to both components: glandular and stromal. Nodules of both elements and of varied proportions are formed. They may secrete corpora amylacea, a glycoproteic secretion that may become calcified. We may also find a diffusely increased aspect, due to fibromuscular nodules.[4,5]

Echoendoscopy for BPH evaluation may allow measurement of the gland dimensions to give the estimated volume by using mathematical formulas and computation.[12] The prostate has a relation of 1 cm^3 corresponding to 1 g. In fact, utilizing radial equipment we could measure the lateral-lateral and posterior-anterior diameter. Utilizing the sectorial equipment, we can measure the longitudinal diameter. Calculation of the volume is important because increase in gland dimensions is mainly in the anterior region, which cannot be evaluated by digital rectal exam.

Echoendoscopy basically gives us the image of an increased gland, with very well-defined contours that appears as a hyperechoic line corresponding to the anatomic capsule. The carcinoma frequently appears as a hypoechoic area in the peripheral zone (Figure 37–1).

The nodules are of varied sizes, and depending on the histological composition, may be hypo- or hyperechogenic or heterogeneous. Those with glandular predominance are hyperechogenic, while those with stromal predominance appear hypoechoic. However, the mixed type corresponds to the majority of nodules that appear heterogeneous.

In general, the contour tends to be symmetric. Asymmetry may be associated with suspected malignancy. Anterior growth in the middle line is due to hyperplasia of the periurethral stromal gland, a finding almost always associated with obstructive symptoms.

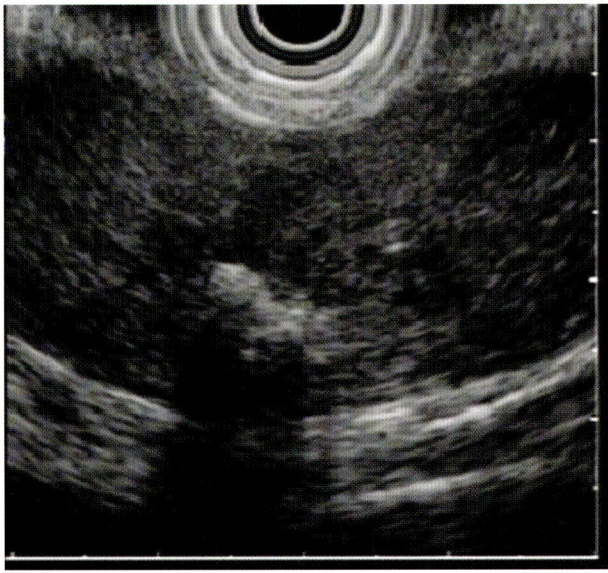

FIGURE 37–1. Radial EUS image demonstrating a heterogeneous area with calcifications in the midd-prostate corresponding to the BPH.

In BPH we observe an evident internal gland peripheral zone differentiation due to the difference in echogenicity subsequent to internal gland growth. The clear dividing line may be a hypoechogenic halo or a linear band with hyperechogenic areas, some with acoustic shadows corresponding to corpora amylacea deposits signifying a calcific focus.

Other BPH findings include acinar dilatations and infarcted areas with and without cystic degeneration. We may also find hyperplastic nodules in the peripheral zone, which corresponds to herniations of the internal gland into the peripheral zone. These are generally hypoechogenic images and cannot be distinguished from malignant lesions by ultrasonography. Studies with echo Doppler are not specific in BPH.[9,11]

Cysts

Degenerative cysts are the most commonly observed cystic structures in the prostate. Among the acquired cysts, the commonest are the ejaculatory duct cysts, due to an obstructive process.[2,5]

Congenital cysts are not rare and generally occur at a median site of the prostate.[5] Usually cysts are asymptomatic, and there may be obstructive symptoms or pain because of very large dimensions or secondary infection.

The prostatic utricle is a small sac, a normal remnant of Müller's tubercle, and it communicates with the posterior wall of the urethra at the level of the veromontanum, close to the ejaculatory ducts. When dilated, the utricle is present as a cystic structure of small dimensions at the median line. It may be associated with different congenital anomalies, the most frequent being hypospadias.[5]

Müller's duct cysts are usually voluminous and are observed at the median line or laterally to it. The fluid aspirated from these cysts does not contain spermatozoids and there is no association with congenital anomalies.[2]

Cyst dilatations of ejaculatory cysts are also usually observed at the median line and may be primary or secondary to obstructive processes. The aspirated fluid contains spermatozoids—in contrast to other cyst formations.[6] Cysts with voluminous dimensions make the analysis of the anatomical position difficult. In this case the diagnosis may be established by the analysis of the fluid aspirated from the cysts.[5,6] Most cysts appear on EUS as regular, anechoic, and mainly localized in the peripheral zone (Figure 37–2).

Other Lesions

Echoendoscopy has a high sensitivity but low specificity regarding focal lesions originating from the

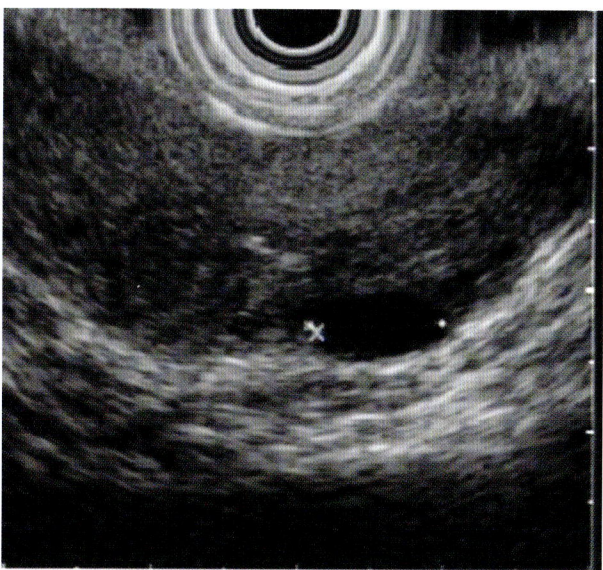

FIGURE 37–2. Radial EUS image demonstrating an anechoic area in the peripheral zone corresponding to a prostatic cyst.

peripheral zone. Thus not all peripheral hypochogenic areas correspond to carcinoma of the prostate. Anatomical structures, such as the urethra and periurethral fibromuscular tissues, ejaculatory duct complex, seminal vesicles. and vas deferens ampullae—structures of the interface between the prostate and surrounding fat—may present as hypochogenic areas. Other lesions that could be visualized in EUS include abscesses and ischemic areas.

Echoendoscopy in Loco-Regional Prostate Cancer Staging

Examination by digital exam is mandatory in the clinical evaluation of prostate cancer but the accuracy of this method to determine the extension of the lesion is limited. Rigid transrectal ultrasonography (TRUS) of the prostate is the most used supplementary examination for prostate cancer staging, besides directing the acquisition of biopsy specimens from gland regions with suspicion of cancer.[16,17] The usual equipment for performing TRUS is a transrectally introduced rigid probe of large diameter. Dimensions and rigidity of the equipment generate discomfort for the patients submitted to the examination and thus, in some situations the examinations are performed under deep sedation (Figure 37–3).

Linear and radial endoscopic ultrasonography is performed with flexible equipment of relatively reduced dimensions when compared to the TRUS

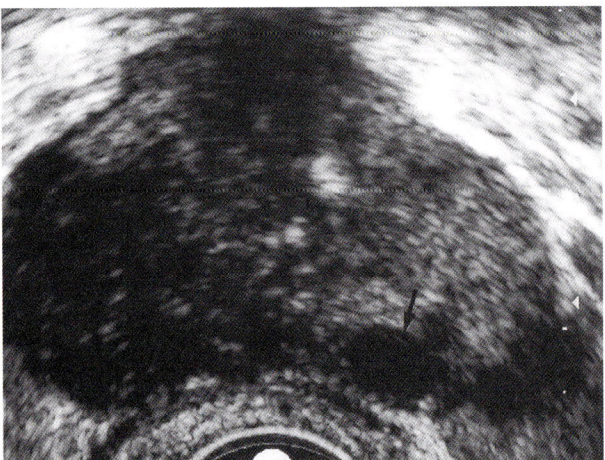

FIGURE 37–3. Sectorial TRUS image demonstrating a hypoechoic area corresponding to prostate cancer in the peripheric zone (black arrow).

equipment. The study of the prostate is an innovating application of echoendoscopy to be described in the following section based on our experience where some advantages of the use of the echoendoscopic modality as compared to TRUS in the assessment of prostate cancer were realized: An adequate assessment of the loco-regional extension of the disease with satisfactory accuracy, sensitivity, and specificity; the flexibility and reduced diameter of the equipment caused less discomfort and better acceptability by the patients submitted to the procedure.[1] (Figure 37–4)

Histopathologic Aspects of Prostate Cancer

Prostate adenocarcinoma is the most common neoplasm of the gland. During the examination one

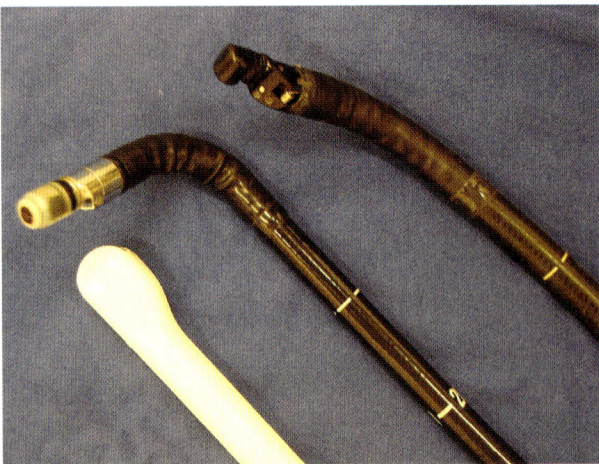

FIGURE 37–4. TRUS, radial, and linear equipment arranged sequentially from left to right.

may identify premalignant lesions and prostate cancer itself. The so-called intraepithelial neoplasms are lesions that are known to lead to prostate cancer development in an average period of 10 years after the diagnosis. They may be classified into ductal acinar dysplasia and atypical adenomatous hyperplasia. The former lesion type consists of epithelial proliferation of ducts and acini, mainly in the peripheral zone of the prostate determining the most incidence of the cancer in this area. The histologic images are usually small and maintain anarchitecture very similar to the normal prostate, being frequently confused with the normal prostatic tissue, and are not visible on ultrasound. They may occur as homogeneous and hypoechoic areas and thus are not different from carcinoma.[1] They may also coexist with carcinoma. Atypical adenomatous hyperplasia consists of proliferation of small glands of the central zone, covered by a single layer of epithelial cells, but no large nucleoli as typically observed in carcinoma.

Malignant tumors of the prostate have three types of echogenic findings: hyperechoic, isoechoic, and most frequently hypoechoic lesions.[20,21]

Echoendoscopic Examination Technique of the Prostate and Adnexa

The EUS examination should be performed by an experienced professional with adequate training in prostate and adnexa echoanatomy. Previous preparation of the patient regarding cleaning of the rectum, performed with 12% glycerine solution, with a maximum volume of 250 ml two hours before the procedure has a satisfactory effect (or two phosphosoda enemas may be given similar to preparation for flexible sigmoidoscopy). Examination is performed with the patient in left lateral decubitus and lower limbs in genupectoral position.[1] The structures that have to be visualized are shown in Figures 37–5 - 37–9. Some clinical conditions such as proctitis, acute bacterial prostatitis, rectum surgery, and acute anorectal diseases should be analyzed and may be relative or absolute contraindication for the examination. The echoendoscopic procedure is usually performed without sedation and with an average examination time of not more than 18 minutes.[1]

The equipment should be introduced in the rectum to approximately 8 to 10 cm from the anal margin. Initially the radial echoendoscopy equipment is used and then complemented with the linear equipment. After inflation of the transducer balloon, water is instilled in the rectum with the purpose of reducing the air window interposed between the probe and the rectum wall. We standardized a sequence of image acquisition and analysis: with the radial equipment we

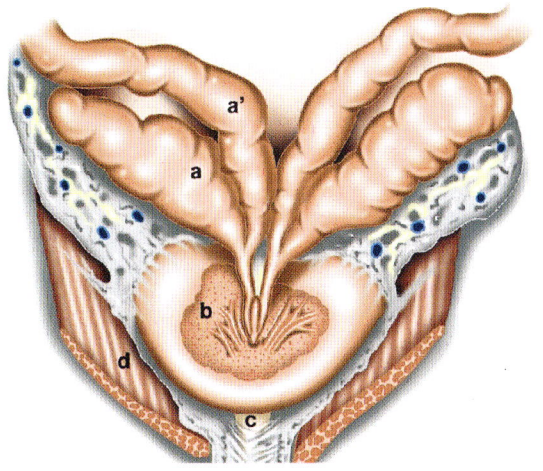

FIGURE 37–5. Diagram demonstrating the posterior-anterior structures around the prostate (a- seminal vesicle; a- deferens duct; b- prostate; c- urethra; d- elevator anus)

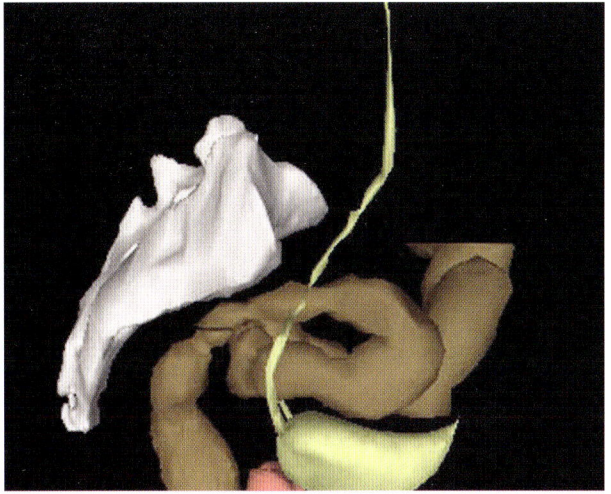

FIGURE 37–7. Visible Human Models of the prostate and rectum as seen from the right.

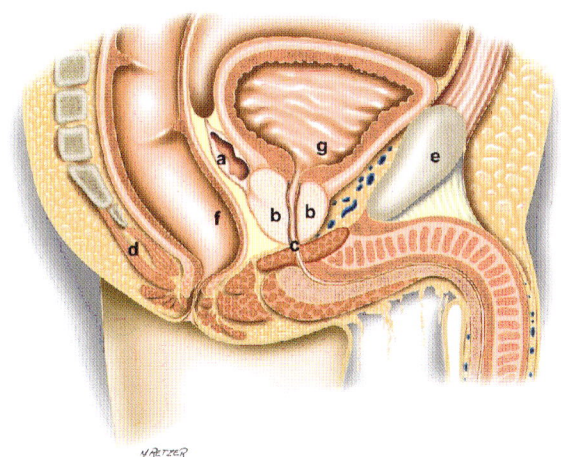

FIGURE 37–6. Diagram demonstrating the sagittal section of the structures around the prostate (a- seminal vesicle; b- prostate; c- urethra; d- elevator anus; e- pubis; f- rectum; g- bladder) (Reprinted from Gastrointestinal Endoscopy, Vol 65 /issue 3, Everson LA et al, EUS for locoregional staging of prostate cancer—a pilot study, Pages 440-477., March 2007, with permission from Elsevier)

obtain sequential images of the seminal vesicle, deferent duct, central and peripheral prostate zone, bladder base, anatomic capsule, and periprostatic lymph nodes. With the linear echoendoscope equipment images of the seminal vesicle and ejaculatory duct, central and peripheral prostate zone, anterior and posterior urethra, anatomic nodule are obtained, in addition to the longitudinal diameter and vascular study by using duplex scan.[1]

The examiner should obtain a panoramic window of the gland in order to observe its form and size, analyzing the presence of mass effect, imaging of peripheral zone, looking for areas of hypoechoic interruptions in the anatomic capsule, or dislocation of adjacent structures (Figures 37–10 and 37–11). Usually, the panoramic gland echostructure should be verified before the procedure. Distortion of gland contour by hyperplastic nodules and diffuse bilobar neoplasia are usually found. The limit between the internal margin of the gland and the peripheral zone (surgical capsule) may be altered by the presence of nodular hyperplasia or by bilobar infiltrating neoplasia. Hyperechoic and irregular alterations associated with the increase in heterogeneous areas and gland caliber may present as T1 stage neoplasias confirmed only by pathologic analysis after prostatectomy.[1]

Patients with T3 stage present with diffuse alterations in echogenicity, irregular contours, sometimes with invasion of the seminal vesicle, and increase in vascularization detectable by echo Doppler.

In our study, on echoendoscopy, lymph node metastases assessment showed rates of 62.5% sensitivity, 58.3% specificity, and 60% accuracy in N0 stages.[1] In cases classified as N1, sensitivity was 80.3%, specificity 52.5%, and accuracy 60%.[18]

On duplex scan, the finding of increase in gland vascularization is frequent in patients with adenocarcinoma.[9,11,15] (Figure 37–12) We observed that, of 20 patients, 17 presented with a diagnosis of cancer on echoendoscopy, confirmed by analysis of the surgical specimen, which confirmed hypervascularization. It was also verified that the finding of increase in vascularization on sectorial echoendoscopy did not occur in any of the patients with benign disease.[1]

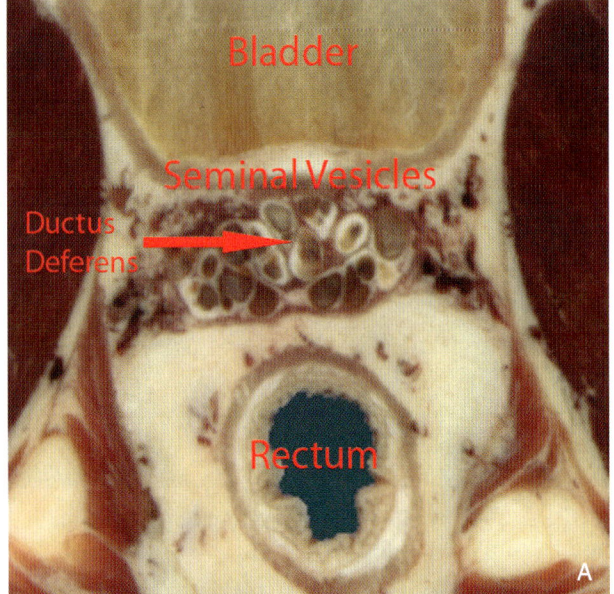
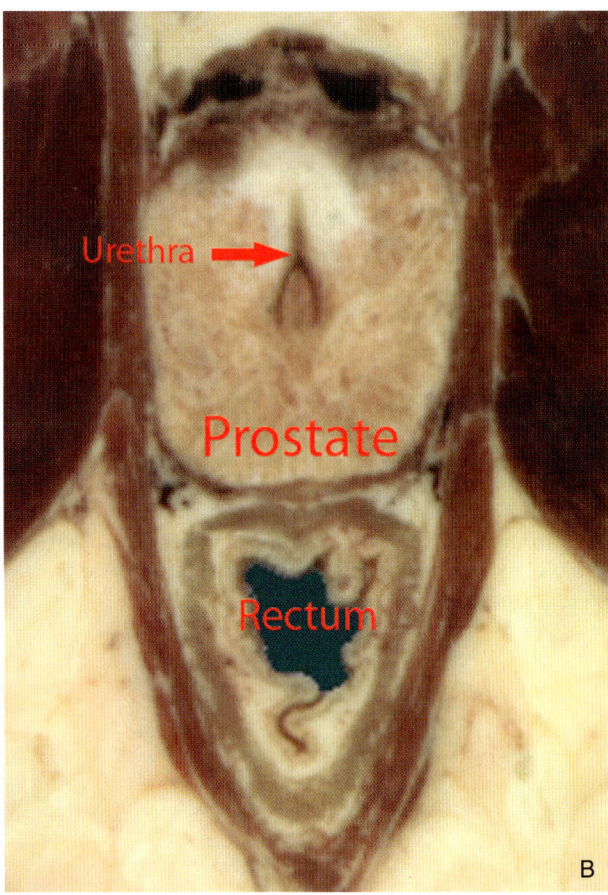
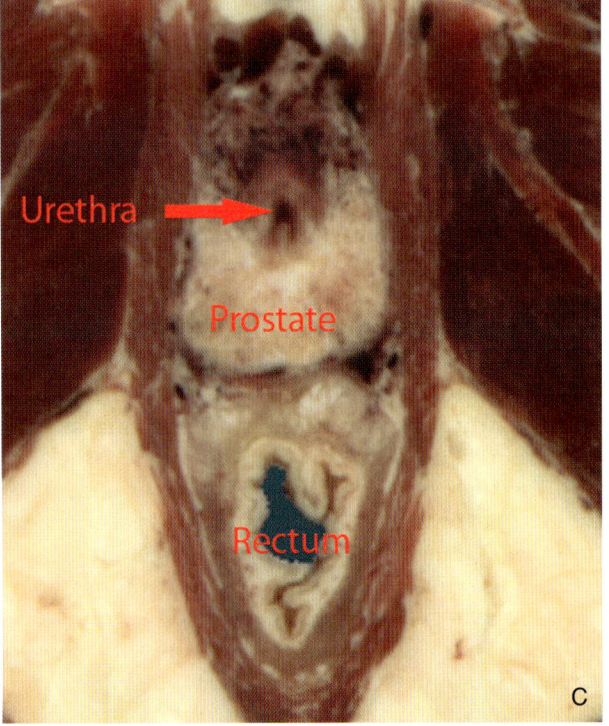

FIGURES 37–8. *A to C* Transaxial cross-sections of Visible Human Anatomy from the region of the prostate going from A (most proximal) to C (most distal). These views are similar to what is seen using radial array EUS.

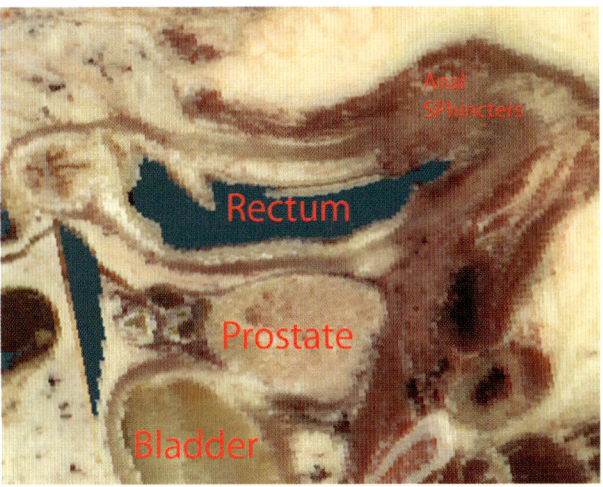

FIGURE 37–9. Visible Human sagittal view of rectum and prostate. This image is similar to what is seen using linear array EUS.

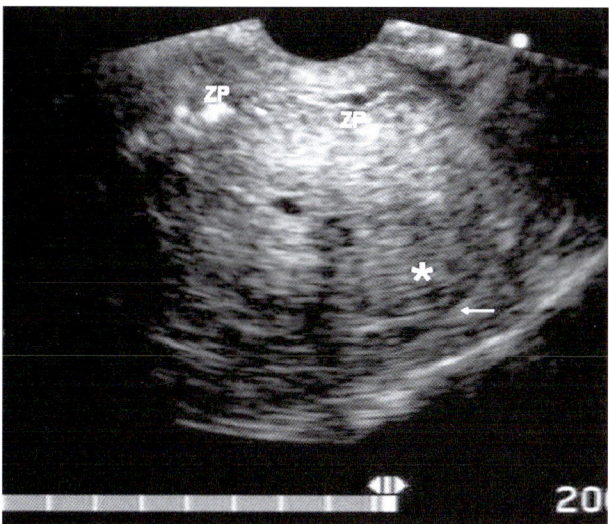

FIGURE 37–10. Linear image demonstrating hipoecoic lesion in the peripheral zone invading the anatomic capsule (STAGE IIB). Periferic zone (PZ), lesion and arrow showing the capsule invasion. (Reprinted from Gastrointestinal Endoscopy, Vol. 65 /issue 3, Everson LA et al, EUS for locoregional staging of prostate cancer—a pilot study, pp. 440-477, March 2007, with permission from Elsevier)

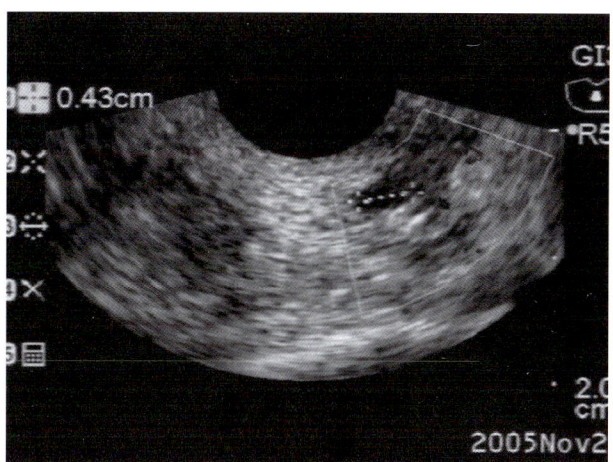

FIGURE 37–12. Linear image demonstrating a T2A adenocarcinoma and dupplex scan analysis in the lesion area (Reprinted from Gastrointestinal Endoscopy, Vol 65 /issue 3, Everson LA et al, EUS for locoregional staging of prostate cancer—a pilot study, pp, 440-477, March 2007, with permission from Elsevier)

Gross hyperechoic calcifications in the periurethral region and in the central parenchyma of the gland may be characterized in benign prostate hyperplasia. (Figure 37–13).

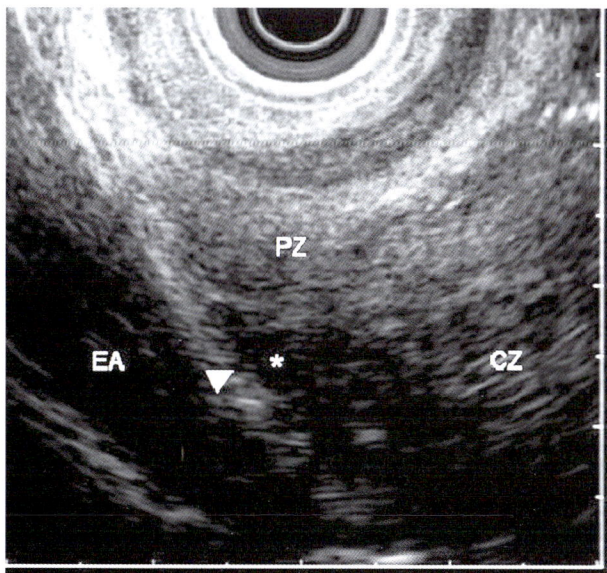

FIGURE 37–11. Radial image demonstrating an adenocarcinoma (T2B). Elevator anus (EA). Peripheral zone (PZ). Central zone (CZ) (Reprinted from Gastrointestinal Endoscopy, Vol 65 /issue 3, Everson LA et al, EUS for locoregional staging of prostate cancer—a pilot study, pp. 440 – 477, March 2007, with permission from Elsevier)

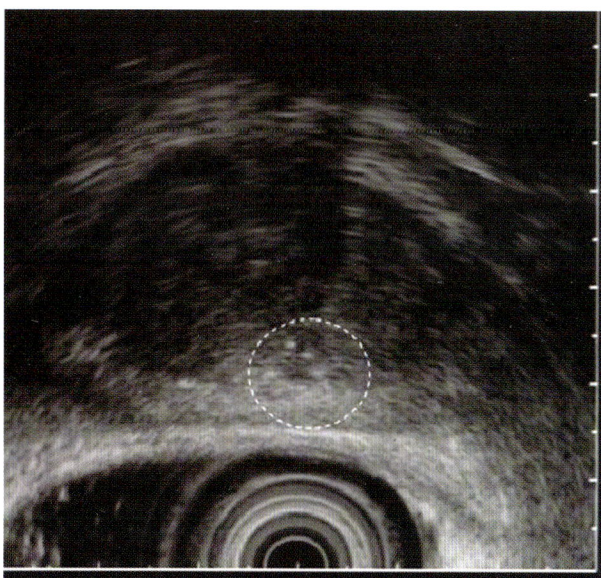

FIGURE 37–13. Radial image showing the Eiffel tower sign (Reprinted from Gastrointestinal Endoscopy, Vol 65 /issue 3, Everson LA et al, EUS for locoregional staging of prostate cancer—a pilot study, pp. 440-477, March 2007, with permission from Elsevier)

Discussion and Critical Analysis

Imaging methods such as magnetic resonance and positron emission tomography (PET SCAN) do not present adequate sensitivity for the detection of initial prostate cancer lesions.[13,18,19] We emphasize that T1 stage tumor is characterized, on echoendoscopy, as an irregular area that presents increase in vascularization in the central zone region close to the urethra, and usually difficulties occur in characterizing a defined area of the suspect prostatic lesion. Kelly at al[15] showed the importance of study by duplex scan in situations of findings of hypoechoic lesions and imprecise limits in the prostate peripheral zone; lesions with increased vascularization reinforce suspicion of malignant neoplasia. Prostate echoendoscopy was inadequate for findings of early prostate cancer processes, as in T1 stage tumors. But, in clinical practice, tumors classified as T1a and T1b are usually incidental findings and only proven at surgery.[14] In fact, this situation also occurred in our study.[1] The benefits of echoendoscopy applied to prostate cancer may include the flexibility of the equipment. This will allow for performing the procedure in the absence of sedation and will bring increased patient comfort. The possibility of acquisition of echoguided biopsy material may also be feasible.

In the T2a lesions, carcinoma appears very similar in both linear and radial array because the lesions are very close to the ecoendoscopic probe in the peripheral zone (Figures 37–14 and 37–15).

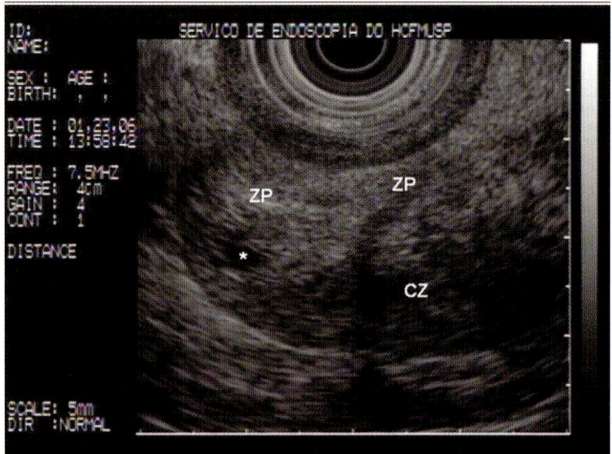

FIGURE 37–15. Radial image demonstrating a hypoechoic lesion in the ZP without anatomic capsule invasion (STAGE IIA). Central zone (CZ) and adenocarcinoma (Reprinted from Gastrointestinal Endoscopy, Vol 65 /issue 3, Everson LA et al, EUS for locoregional staging of prostate cancer—a pilot study, pp. 440-477, March 2007, with permission from Elsevier)

Our experience demonstrates that echoendoscopy applied to the study of prostate cancer presented a high diagnostic capacity in T2 and T3 stages and satisfactory accuracy in T1 stage, and in the analysis of loco-regional lymph nodes.[1] But, these data need to be compared to other imaging methods available for loco-regional assessment of prostate cancer.[19] In the future, other studies may directly compare EUS to TRUS regarding tolerability, accuracy in echo directed procedures, and cost effectiveness. Future comparative studies, and randomized and controlled trials should provide answers to the real value of application of echoendoscopy to prostate cancer.

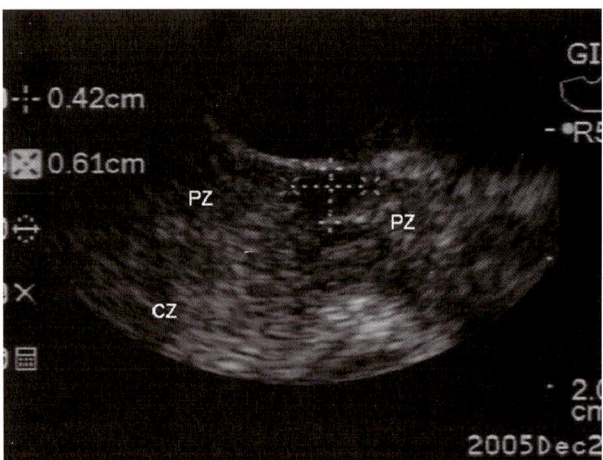

FIGURE 37–14. Linear image demonstrating a hypoechoic lesion in the peripheral zone (PZ) without anatomic capsule invasion (STAGE IIA). Central zone (CZ) (Reprinted from Gastrointestinal Endoscopy, Vol 65 /issue 3, Everson LA et al, EUS for locoregional staging of prostate cancer—a pilot study, pp. 440-477, March 2007, with permission from Elsevier)

References

1. Artifon, E. L. A., Sakai, P., Ishioka, S., Silva, A. F., Maluf, F., Chaves, D., Matuguma, S., Pompeo, A., Lucon, A. M., Srougi, M., Bhutani, M. S.: Endoscopic Ultrasonography for locoregional staging of prostate cancer – a pilot study. Gastrointest. Endosc. 2007 Mar; 65(3):440–447.
2. Ackerman, L. V.: Ackerman's Surgical Pathology 7th ed, St. Louis, Mosby, 1989.
3. Barry, M. J.: Epidemiology and natural history of benign prostatic hyperplasia. Urol. Clin. North Am. 1990;17(3): 495–507.
4. Campbell, M. F., Walsh, P. C., Resik, A. B.: Campbell's Urology. 6th ed. Philadelphia, WB Saunders, 1992.
5. Jakobsen, H., Torp-Pedersen, S., Juul, N.: Ultrasonic evaluation of age-related human prostatic growth and development of benign prostatic hyperplasia. Scand J Urol Nephrol. 1998;107(Suppl.):26–31.

6. Kirkali, Z., Yigitbasi, O., Diren, B., Hekimoglu, B., Ersoy, H.: Cysts of the prostatic, seminal vesicles and diverticulum of the ejaculatory ducts. Eur Urol. 1991;20:77–80.
7. Lim, D. J., Hayden, R. T., Murad, T., Nemcek, Jr., A. A., Dalton, D. P.: Multilocular prostatic cystadenoma presenting as a large complex pelvic cystic mass. J Urol. 1993;149:856–859.
8. Olson, E. M., Trambert, M. A., Mattrey, R. F.: Cystosarcoma phyllodes of the prostate: MRI findings. Abdom Imaging. 1994;19:180–181.
9. Rifkin, M. D., Alexander, A. A., Helinek, T. G., Merton, D. A.: Color Doppler as an adjunct to prostate ultrasound. Scand J Urol Nephrol. 1991;137(Suppl.):85–89.
10. Rifkin, M. D., Friedland, G. W., Shortliffe, L.: Prostatic evaluation by transrectal endosonography: detection of carcinoma. Radiology. 1986;158:85–90.
11. Rifkin, M.D., Sudakoff, G. S., Alexander, A. A.: Prostate: techniques, resultes and potential applications of color Doppler US scanning. Radiology. 1993;186:509–513.
12. Sehgal, C. M., Broderick, G. A., Whittington, R., Gorniak, R. J. T., Arger, P. H.: Three-dimensional US and volumetric assessment of the prostate. Radiology. 1994; 192:274–278.
13. Sudakoff, G. S.: Atypical myxoid smooth muscle tumor of the prostate: TRUS, CDI and MR findings. Abdom. Imaging. 1994;19:468–470.
14. Hasegawa, Y., Sakamoto, N.: Relationship of ultrasonographic findings to histology in prostate cancer. Eur Urol. 1994;26:10–17.
15. Kelly, I. M. G., Lees, W. R., Rickards, D.: Prostate cancer and the role of color Doppler US. Radiology. 1993; 189:153–156.
16. Lee, F., Torp-Pedersen, S. T., McLeary, R. D.: Diagnosis of prostate cancer by transrectal ultrasound. Urol Clin North Am. 1989;16(4):663–673.
17. Rifkin, M. D., McGlynn, E. T., Choi, H.: Echogenicity of prostate cancer correlated with histologic grade and stromal fibrosis: endorectal US studies. Radiology. 1989;170:549–552.
18. Leibovic, D., Kamat, A. M., Do, K. A., et al.: Transrectal ultrasound versus magnetic resonance imaging for detection of rectal wall invasion by prostate cancer. Prostate. 2005;62:101–104.
19. Hersh, M. R., Knapp, E. L., Choi, J.: Newer imaging modalities to assess tumor in the prostate. Cancer Control. 2004;11:353–357.
20. Egawa, S., Wheeler, T. M., Greene, D. R., et al.: Usual hyperechoic appearance of prostate on transrectal ultrasonography. Br J Urol. 1992;69:169–174.
21. Rifkin, M. D., Dahnert, W., Kurtz, A. B.: State of the art: endorectal sonography of the prostate gland. AJR. 1990;154:691–700.

… CHAPTER 38

Endoscopic Ultrasound (EUS) in Inflammatory Bowel Disease (IBD)

Dr. Brian R. Weston
Dr. Manoop S. Bhutani

Several studies have examined the role of rectal endoscopic ultrasound (EUS) in the evaluation of inflammatory bowel disease (IBD). The main established application for EUS at the present time is for evaluating perirectal and perianal complications of Crohn's disease.[1-4] Abscesses and fistulas occur commonly in IBD (up to 35–45% during the course of disease).[5]

Fistulae and Abscesses

The characteristic appearance of a fistula by EUS is that of a hypoechoic or anechoic duct-like 'serpignious' structure localized within the perianorectal region.[6] Air in the fistulous tract produces distinct sonographic images with reverberation echoes (from air bubbles) allowing visualization of the entire tract.[6] This is usually best seen with the linear versus radial probe, which may only show a limited cross-sectional view of the tract.[7] The characteristic appearance of an abscess by EUS is that of an anechoic or a hypoechoic cavity with irregular borders in the perianorectal region.[6] EUS has previously been demonstrated to be superior to imaging modalities such as fistulography and CT for evaluation of fistula.[3,8-10] EUS has also been shown to be essentially equivalent or better than CT for detection of perirectal abscess, likely depending on size.

In comparison with MRI, EUS was also shown to be either equivalent or better than MRI. One prospective study reported that EUS compared to MRI was 89% versus 48% sensitive and 66% versus 80% specific for fistulas, and 100% versus 55% sensitive and 77% versus 77% specific for abscesses respectively.[7] Another prospective triple-blind comparison study of pelvic MRI, EUS, and examination under anesthesia demonstrated similar high accuracy of performance for all three modalities (91%, 87%, and 91% respectively). Furthermore the authors noted that 100% accuracy could be attained if any two studies were used in combination.[11] Although high resolution CT and MRI imaging have improved in recent years, perineal complications may still be missed, and when clinical suspicion is high or otherwise indicated EUS imaging should be considered. The ability of EUS to define complex fistula and abscesses may facilitate surgical management.[12] Please refer to Chapter 32, Perirectal Abscesses, for details and images.

Luminal Inflammatory Bowel Disease

The role of EUS in evaluating luminal inflammatory bowel disease is less well defined. Numerous studies have demonstrated the ability of EUS to provide accurate transmural imaging of all layers of the intestinal wall. However the applicability or clinical utility of this information has not been reproducibly demonstrated. Much of the literature on this topic has been criticized on issues relating to measurement bias and interobserver or intraobserver variability.[4]

Several authors have examined bowel wall thickness and layer pattern to assess disease severity and possibly predict clinical course.[1,2,8,13-20] Tsuga et al developed a classification system based primarily on evaluation of intestinal wall layer interfaces (presence or absence of blurring) and correlation with an endoscopic grading system.[21] Yoshizawa et al[13] most recently examined the relationship between EUS appearance of the bowel wall, endoscopic appearance, and clinical severity in ulcerative colitis (Figures 38–1A - 38–1D and 3–2A - 38–2C). They demonstrated that concordance rates between the degree of vertical spread on histopathology and that of EUS in ulcerative colitis to be 95% for inflammation extending to the submucosa, 83% for

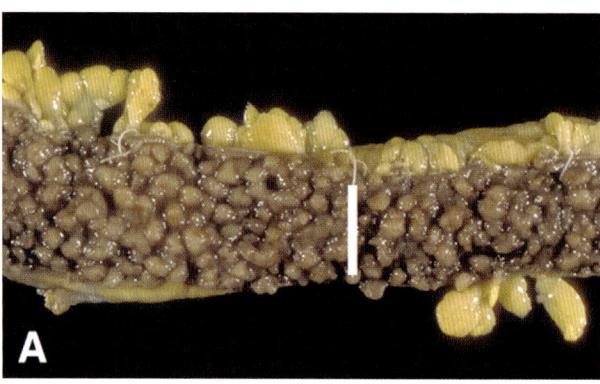
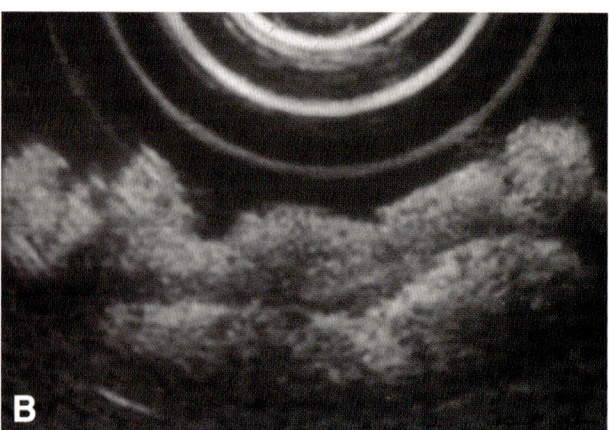

FIGURE 38–1 *A and B* Surgically resected specimen of UC scanned by EUS. (A) Macroscopic findings of the resected specimen revealed multiple deep ulcers in the descending colon; the intervening inflamed mucosa had pseudopolyposis. (B) EUS image of regions consisting primarily of deep ulcers demonstrated a thickened intestinal wall and a poorly demarcated structure from the first to fourth layers, suggesting that intestinal inflammation extended to the muscularis propria.

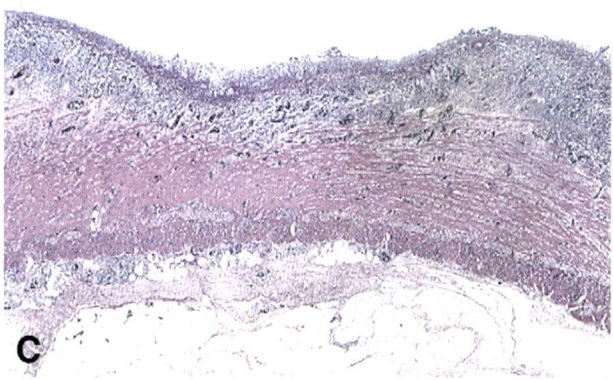
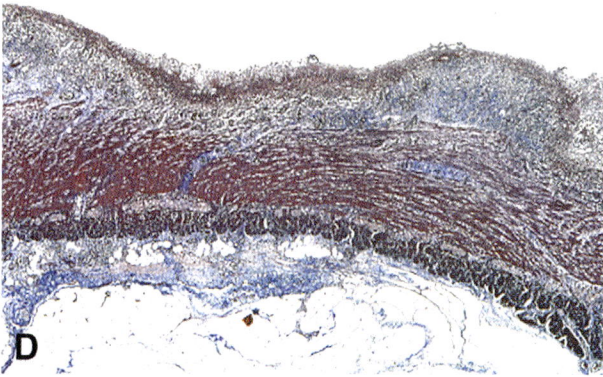

FIGURE 38–1 *C and D* (C and D) Histopathologic findings of the specimen scanned by EUS revealed extensive denuded areas of the mucosal surface, severe inflammatory cell infiltration extending to the muscularis propria, and partial loss and degeneration of the internal circular muscle layer. (C; H&E, orig. mag. X 40) (D; Masson's trichrome, orig. mag. X 40). *(Reprinted from Gastrointestinal Endoscopy, 2007;65:253-60, Yoshizawa et al, Clinical usefulness of EUS for active ulcerative colitis, with permission from Elsevier)*

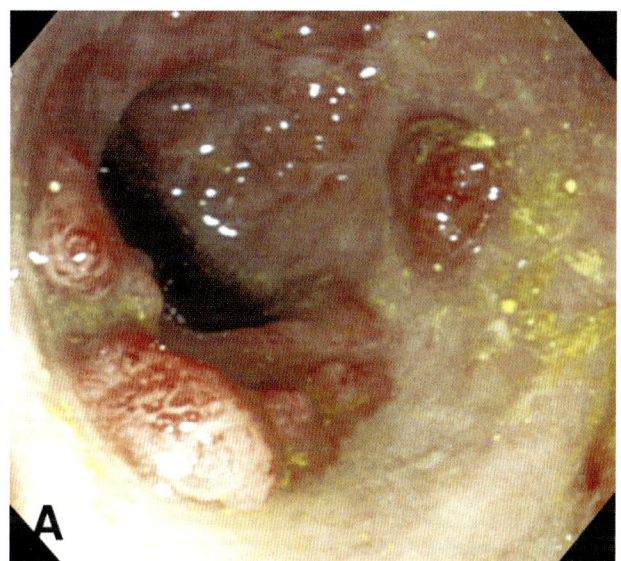
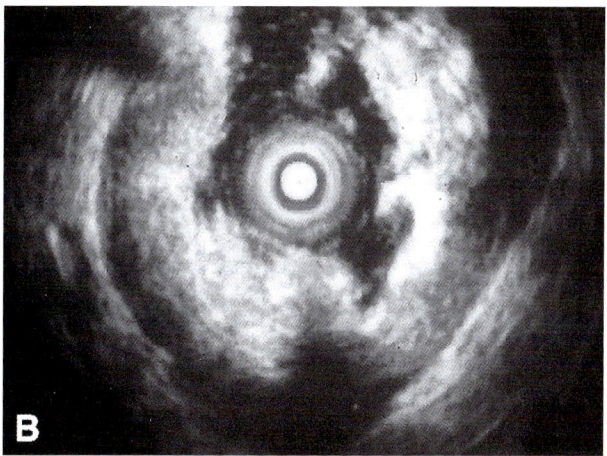
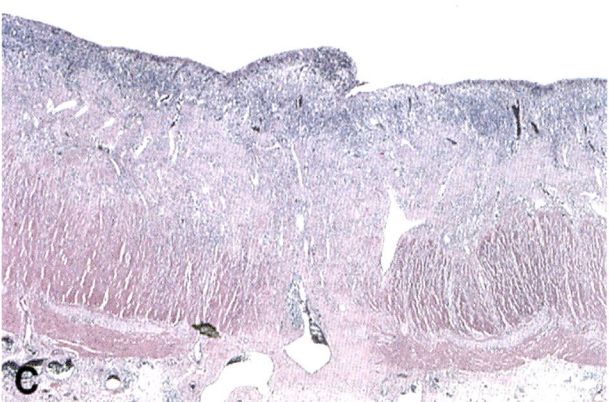

FIGURE 38–2 *A to C* A 56-year-old man with left-sided colitis. (A) Conventional colonoscopic view revealed deep ulcers in the descending colon; only island-shaped regions of mucosa remained. (B) EUS image demonstrated a markedly thickened bowel wall, with a poorly demarcated structure from the first to fourth layers, suggesting that intestinal inflammation extended to the muscularis propria. (C) Histopathologic evaluation of the surgically resected specimen revealed open ulcers extending to the muscularis propria, with inflammatory cell infiltration, consistent with EUS images (H&E, orig. mag. X40). *(Reprinted from Gastrointestinal Endoscopy, 2007;65:253-60, Yoshizawa et al, Clinical usefulness of EUS for active ulcerative colitis, with permission from Elsevier)*

that extending to the muscularis propria, and 100% for that extending to the subserosa. They suggest that inflammation extending to the muscularis propria or deeper had worse outcome with increased rates of surgical intervention. Unfortunately inconsistent results have been reported overall.

The ability to distinguish between Crohn's disease and ulcerative colitis based on the presence of transmural rectal wall involvement has also not been consistently demonstrated.[14-16,22,23] Indeterminate IBD occurs in approximately 10–20% of cases.[1] Inflammatory changes in ulcerative colitis are typically limited to the mucosa only, versus Crohn's, which is transmural. However, the extent of inflammation may not always be transmural in Crohn's disease; likewise severe ulcerative colitis may reach the muscularis propria or deeper with blurring of the wall layers and increased total mural thickness.[1,13,24] Different variations in the loss of the five-layer echopattern may occur in both types of inflammatory bowel disease making this factor a suboptimal diagnostic criterion. To date universally agreed EUS criteria have not been established that can be reliably used to differentiate indeterminate cases of colitis.

It remains to be seen whether the endosonographic measurement of intestinal inflammation by EUS will be of additional benefit or significantly impact management or outcome above and beyond current conventional management. The future of EUS in IBD will depend on local expertise at high-volume IBD centers.

References

1. Lew, R. J., Ginsberg, G. G.: The role of endoscopic ultrasound in inflammatory bowel disease. Gastrointest Endoscopy Clin N Am 2002;12:561–571.
2. Wijers, O. B., Tio, T. L., Tytgat, G. N.J.: Ultraonography and endosonography in the diagnosis and management of inflammatory bowel disease. Endoscopy 1992; 24:559–564.
3. Tio, T. L., Kallismanis, G. E.: Endoscopic ultrasonography of perirectal fistulas and abscesses. Endoscopy 1994;26:813–815.
4. Maple, J. T., Edmundowicz, S.: Using EUS to forecast the clinical course of ulcerative colitis: still a cloudy outlook. Gastrointestinal Endoscopy 2007;65:261–262.
5. Rankin, G. B., Watts, H. D., Melnyk, C. S., Kelley, M. L.: National Cooperative Crohn's Disease Study: extraintestinal manifestations and perianal complications. Gastroenterology 1979;77:914–920.
6. Bhutani, M. S., Hawes, R. H.: Endoluminal Ultrasound in Inflammatory Bowel Disease. In Inflammatory Bowel Disease, 3rd Edition. Eds: Allan, R. N., Keighley, M. R. B., Alexander-Williams, J., Rhodes, J. M., Hanauer, S. B., Fazio, V.: Edinburgh: Churchill Livingstone, 1997, pp. 285-290.
7. Orsoni, P., Barthet, M., Portier, F., Panuel, M., et al.: Prospective comparison of endosonography, magnetic resonance imaging and surgical findings in anorectal fistula and abscess complicating Crohn's disease. Br J Surgery 1999;86:360–364.
8. Van Outryv,e M.: Endoscopic ultrasonography in inflammatory bowel disease, para-colorectal inflammatory pathology and extramural abnormalities. Gastrointest Endosc Clin North Am 1995;5:861–867.
9. Schratter-Sehn, A. U., Lochs, H., Vogelsang, H., Schurawitzki, H., et al.: Endoscopic ultrasonography verses computed tomography in the differential diagnosis of perianorectal complication in Crohn's disease. Endoscopy 1993;25:582–586.
10. Tio, T. L., Mulder, C. J. J., Wijers, O. B., Sars, P. R. A., et al.: Endosonography of perianal and pericolorectal fistula and/or abscess in Crohn's disease. Gastrointest Endosc 1990;36:331–6.
11. Schwartz, D. A., Wiersema, M. J., Dudiak, K. M., Fletcher, J. G., et al.: A comparison of endoscopic ultrasound, magnetic resonance imaging, and exam under anesthesia for evaluation of Crohn's perinal fistulas. Gastroenterology 2001;121:1064–1072
12. Deen, K. I., Williams, J. G., Hutchinson, R., Keighley, M. R. B., Kumar, D.: Fistulas in Ano: endoanal ultrasonographic assessments assists decision making for surgery. Gut 1994; 35:391–394.
13. Yoshizawa, S., Kobayashi, K., Katsumata, T., Saigenji, K., et al.: Clinical usefulness of EUS for active ulcerative colitis. Gastrointestinal Endoscopy 2007;65:253–260.
14. Rasmussen, S. N., Riis, P.: Rectal wall thickness measured by ultrasound in chronic inflammatory disease of the colon. Scan J Gastroenterol 1985;20:109–114.
15. Dagli, U., Over, H., Tezel, A., et al.: Transrectal ultrasound in the diagnosis and management of inflammatory bowel disease. Endoscopy 1999;31:152–157.
16. Limberg, B.: Diagnosis of acute ulcerative colitis and colonic Crohn's disease by colonic sonography. J Clin Ultrasound. 1989;17:25–31.
17. Higaki, S., Nohara, H., Saitoh, Y., et al.: Increased rectal wall thickness may predict relapse in ulcerative colitis: a pilot follow-up study by ultrasonographic colonoscopy. Endoscopy 2002;34:212–319.
18. Shimuzu, S., Iso, A., Tada, M., Kawai, K.: Endoscopic ultrasonography in ulcerative colitis. Dig Endosc 1994;6:3–6.
19. Soweid, A. M., Chak, A., Katz, J. A., et al.: Catheter probe assisted endoluminal US in inflammatory bowel disease. Gastrointest Endosc 1999;50:41–46.
20. Hurlstone, D. P., Sanders, D. S., Lobo, A. L., et al.: Prospective evaluation of high frequency mini probe ultrasound colonoscopic imaging in ulcerative colitis; a valid tool for predicting clinical severity. Eur J Gastroenterol 2005;17:1325–1331.
21. Tsuga, K., Haruma, K., Fujimura, J., et al.: Evaluation of the colorectal wall in normal subjects and patients with ulcerative colitis using an ultrasonic catheter probe. Gastrointest Endosc 1998;48:477–484.
22. Kimmey, M. B., Wang, K. Y., Haggitt, R. C., Mack, L. A., et al.: Diagnosis of inflammatory bowel disease with ultrasound: an in vitro study. Invest Radiol 1990; 25:1085–1090.
23. Gast, P., Belaiche, J.: Rectal endosonography in inflammatory bowel disease: differential diagnosis and prediction of remission. Endoscopy 1999;31:158–166.
24. Buckell, N. A., Williams, G. T., Bartram, C.L., et al.: Depth of ulceration in acute colitis: correlation with outcome and clinical and radiologic features: Gastroenterology 1980;79:19–25.

SECTION IV

Miscellaneous

CHAPTER 39

EUS Elastography

Dr. Adrian Saftoiu
Dr. Peter Vilmann

Introduction

Palpation is defined as the act of feeling the surface of the body with the hands to determine the characteristics of the organs beneath the surface. It is an essential part of any clinical examination. Palpation has always been used to locate and characterize hard tissues, which are frequently determined by various disease processes, but especially malignant tumors. Although it is a subjective method, palpation is still considered useful for the screening and early diagnosis of breast cancer or prostate cancer.[1,2] Intraoperative palpation is also used by surgeons to locate and describe pancreatic tumors (adenocarcinomas and neuroendocrine tumors), and also to diagnose vascular invasion in pancreatic cancer.[3]

Developed recently, elasticity imaging is based on the hypothesis that the range of elastic moduli is different between normal and pathological human tissues. Various imaging methods have been consequently used to objectively depict differences in elasticity (strain) of the tissues. These include ultrasound elastography, optical coherence tomography elastography, and magnetic resonance elastography as noninvasive techniques that could show differences in tissue strain.[4,6] The major advantage of these methods consists in the extension of palpation to virtual any part of the body accessible to imaging, including the pancreas, lymph nodes, and liver.

Although ultrasound elastography was initially described more than 15 years ago, clinical applications developed only recently.[4] Initial applications were described for the diagnosis and differentiation of breast lesions[8-11] and prostate cancer.[12-14] Recent applications of elastography emerged in the cases where conventional ultrasound imaging is not useful, including the visualization of thermal lesions after radio frequency ablation (RFA) of liver lesions[15] or high intensity focused ultrasound (HIFU) of prostate lesions.[16] Based on the intrinsic deformation of tissues during cardiac movement and respiration, intravascular[17] and cardiac[18] applications of ultrasound elastography were also developed. Transient elastography was also used for the evaluation of fibrosis in chronic liver diseases by measurement of the liver stiffness,[19-23] although a recent meta-analysis of the studies showed mixed results.[24]

Real-Time Elastography

Real-time ultrasound elastography (sono-elastography) depicts the mechanical response of tissues by analyzing the backscattered ultrasound signals returned while tissue is slightly compressed and decompressed, thus offering complementary information to conventional ultrasonic imaging based on acoustic tissue scattering. Various improvements and adjustments of the method are currently under development, with a growing literature on clinical applications.[25]

Sono-elastography was initially developed to analyze breast tumors, showing similar accuracy with conventional ultrasound.[26] Because it provides additional information, real-time elastography might improve the specificity and decrease the rate of false positive results.[27-29] Real-time elastography in conjunction with B-mode ultrasonography significantly improved the detection rate of prostate cancer.[30-32] Several other potential clinical applications were also described, including real-time sono-elastography of the cervix[33] or thyroid.[34-36] Real-time ultrasound elastography was also successfully used for the evaluation of fibrosis in patients with chronic liver diseases.[37,38] This would have important consequences, especially for the noninvasive diagnosis of significant fibrosis in patients with a suspicion of liver cirrhosis. Most of the patients are correctly characterized by an imaging method, thus decreasing the proportion of unnecessary liver biopsies.

Method

The principle of real-time ultrasound elastography is based on initial tissue compression, which produces strain (deformation) within the tissue, while the strain is smaller in harder tissue as compared to softer tissue (Figure 39–1).[39,40] Consequently, by measuring the tissue strain induced by compression, it is possible to estimate the tissue mechanical properties, which may be useful in diagnosing and differentiating malignant tumors. Different computational models in conjunction with new data acquisition techniques are used to reconstruct images of tissue mechanical properties, an active area of research known as inverse problems.

Real-time ultrasound elastography (Hitachi Medical Systems Europe Holding AG, Zug, Switzerland) has two distinct phases: pressure application (tissue excitation) and information analysis for generating a specific image.[39-41] Information analysis is based on the premise that a stiff portion of tissue is less deformable as compared with an elastic portion of tissue. After pressure application, the distribution of induced deformation at the level of tissues is assessed by monitoring the movement. Practically, radio frequency waves are collected before and after the application of

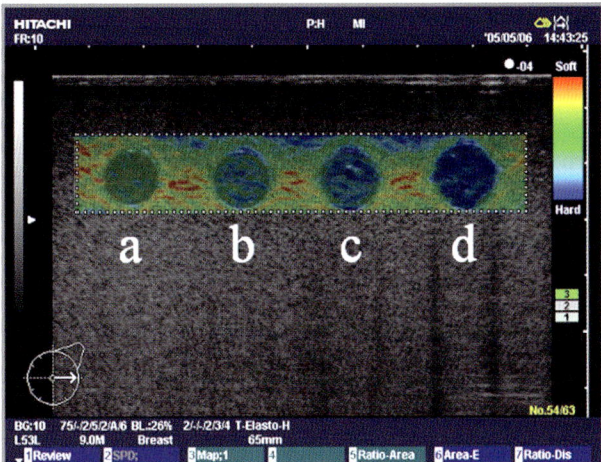

FIGURE 39–1. Principle of real-time ultrasound elastography, based on the visualization of the hardness of tissue due to different strains during compression. This is clearly evident on a quantitative elastography phantom with different elasticity gels (A–D) included in a low elasticity gel (© Hitachi Medical Systems Europe Holding AG, Zug, Switzerland. Reprinted by permission.).

the deformation stimulus and the longitudinal (axial) movement of tissues is assessed by following the movement of reflection, using auto-correlation methods.[41] The resulting deformation image is called an elastogram. The distribution of tissue elasticity is calculated in real-time and the result of the examination is displayed on the screen as a transparent overlay color-coded image, together with the conventional gray-scale image of the examined structure.[25] Normal linear transducers (including EUS linear transducers) are used for real-time ultrasound elastography, with the addition of special software that can specifically process ultrasound information in order to obtain the elastography image. The pressure applied with the transducer must be low, in order to keep the proportion between pressure and deformation. At high pressures, nonlinear manifestations of tissue elasticity appear, so that the application of a pressure exceeding a certain limit might provide false information.[4]

EUS elastography equipment includes a Hitachi 8500 ultrasound system with an embedded Sono-Elastography module (Hitachi Medical Systems Europe Holding AG, Zug, Switzerland), coupled with the EG-3830UT linear endoscope or the EG-3630UR radial endoscope (Pentax, Hamburg, Germany). Real-time EUS elastography can thus be performed with the conventional EUS probes, without any need for additional equipment that induces vibration or pressure. Due to its similarity with color Doppler examinations, EUS elastography is performed by using a two-panel image with the usual conventional gray-scale B-mode EUS image on the right side and the elastography image on the left side. A region of interest (ROI) for the elastography calculations is manually selected and should include the targeted lesion, as well as the soft surrounding tissues (Figure 39–2). The ROI needs to be set to include sufficient surrounding tissue because elasticity values are displayed relative to the average strain inside the ROI. The system also displays a compression threshold, which has to be set up between 3 and 4. To visualize tissue elasticity patterns, different elasticity values are marked with different colors (on a scale of 1 to 256) and the sonoelastography information is shown superimposed on the conventional gray-scale image. The system is set-up to use a hue color map (red-green-blue), where hard tissue areas are marked with dark blue, medium hard tissue areas with cyan, intermediate tissue areas with green, medium soft tissue areas with yellow, and soft tissue areas with red.

The same real-time ultrasound elastography technique is suited not only to improve the imaging diagnostic rate, but also to guide biopsies into stiffer areas of the tumor, in order to increase the accuracy of cytopathological diagnosis (Figure 39–3).[42-45] However, this hypothesis has not been yet validated in any prospective double-blinded study. The needle tract is sometime visible during the real-time guidance of biopsies (Figure 39–4), due to its hard signature relative to the surrounding soft tissues.[44]

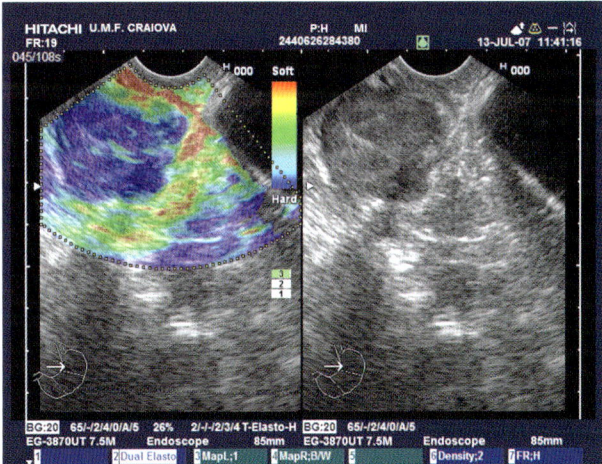

FIGURE 39–2. Typical settings of the real-time EUS elastography software, with the conventional EUS gray-scale image in the right pane, and the elastography information displayed in a transparent color overlay in the left pane. The elastography region of interest is set up to include the hard tumor mass (in this case a papillary tumor), as well as the soft surrounding tissues.

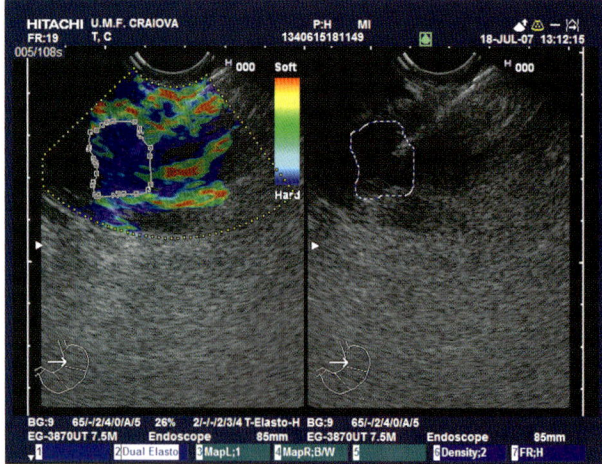

FIGURE 39-3. Real-time elastography guidance of EUS fine needle aspiration (FNA) into stiff (hard) areas of the pancreatic head, suspicious of malignancy.

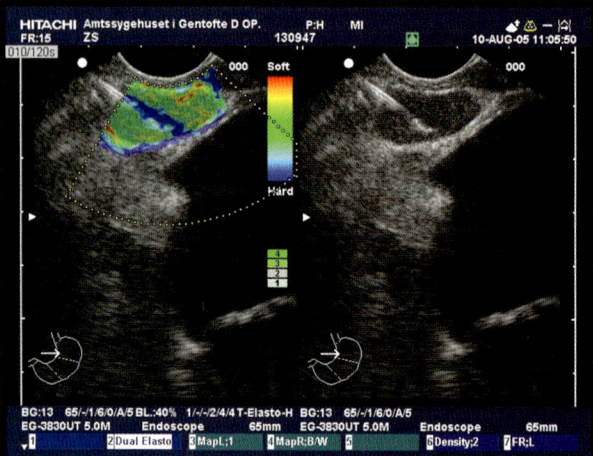

FIGURE 39-4. Visible needle tract during EUS-guided FNA, consistent with a hard signature inside the soft lymph node.

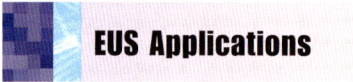

EUS Applications

The feasibility of real-time EUS elastography examinations was initially reported by Giovannini et al.[43] The study included 49 patients evaluated by EUS for pancreatic masses or lymph nodes. Although the sensitivity was 100% for both pancreatic masses and lymph nodes, the specificity was quite low—67% for pancreatic masses and 50% for lymph nodes, respectively. The study has been criticized strongly in an accompanying editorial, due to several methodological flaws.[45] These included bi-univocal relations between the color-coded elasticity information and histology (blue: malignant, green: fibrosis, yellow: normal, red: fat), definition of descriptive diagnostic patterns, lack of quantification of the elastography information, same group of patients used to develop the criteria and standards, as well as to subsequently test them, etc.

It is certainly difficult to postulate that a specific level of hardness is equivalent with the diagnosis of malignancy, because some of the benign lesions are very hard (focal chronic pancreatitis), while some of the tumors are very soft (mucinous or cystic adenocarcinomas, as well as tumors with extensive necrosis).[45] Nevertheless, a correlation between the elasticity imaging results and histology would be highly desirable, either to represent a "virtual" biopsy used for noninvasive characterization of lesions or for the real-time guidance of biopsies in stiffer areas of the lesions.[43] The potential of EUS elastography and the need for further studies including a larger number of patients lead to several other papers recently published.

Lymph Nodes

Another feasibility study described the potential of real-time elastography by using quantitative RGB histograms as compared to the qualitative pattern analysis previously used in most of the other studies.[44] RGB histogram analysis of the EUS elastography allowed an excellent discrimination between benign and malignant lymph nodes. Furthermore, an "elasticity ratio" was defined yielding a sensitivity, specificity and accuracy of 95.8%, 94.4%, and 95.2%, respectively. In this initial work we have acknowledged several limitations of this approach, including the use of static (still images) images, which are possibly associated with a significant selection bias induced by an arbitrary choice of the "best" frame from a dynamic sequence of EUS elastography frames. The presence of visual perception errors (caused by the mixture of green and blue in some lesions) and motion artifacts, as well as the impossibility to control tissue compression during EUS, are other confounding factors that might negatively impact the accuracy of EUS elastography.

The utility of computer-enhanced dynamic analysis of EUS elastography movies for the differential diagnosis of benign and malignant lymph nodes was further explored in a subsequent prospective study recently published by our research group.[46] We have initially obtained average images from EUS elastography movies of 78 lymph nodes, in order to eliminate possible operator-induced selection bias. Subsequent calculations were performed with a special plug-in written for a public domain JAVA-based image processing tool (ImageJ), developed at the National

Institutes of Health, Bethesda, Maryland. We have used hue histograms based on the rainbow color map used as a default setting in the EUS sono-elastography software, with the aim of better describing the elasticity of the lymph node as a monotone and bijective function. On the X axis of the histogram, the numeric values of the elasticity are displayed on a scale from 1 (softest) to 256 (hardest). On the Y axis, the height of the spikes displayed indicates the number of pixels of each elasticity level found in the region of interest (ROI). Consequently, the mean value of the histogram corresponds to the global hardness or elasticity of the lymph node while the standard deviation gives an indication on how homogenous is the strain inside the lymph node.

Based on this approach, we were able to differentiate benign (Figure 39–5) and malignant (Figure 39–6) lymph nodes with a high sensitivity, specificity and accuracy (85.4%, 91.9%, and 88.5%, respectively). Moreover, the area under the ROC curve of the mean hue values used for the discrimination of benign and malignant lymph nodes was 0.928 (p<0.0001). The complementary information provided by EUS elastography is not meant to replace tissue biopsy, but rather to help the targeting of the lymph nodes that are most probable malignant (based on the high positive predictive value), as well as to decrease the number of EUS-FNA procedures (based on the high negative predictive value).[46,47]

These results were recently confirmed in another prospective study, which included 50 consecutive patients with 66 mediastinal lymph nodes. Based on a pattern classification, the authors observed a variable accuracy for benign lymph nodes (81.8–87.9%) and malignant lymph nodes (84.6%–86.4%), with an excellent interobserver agreement (kappa = 0.84).[48]

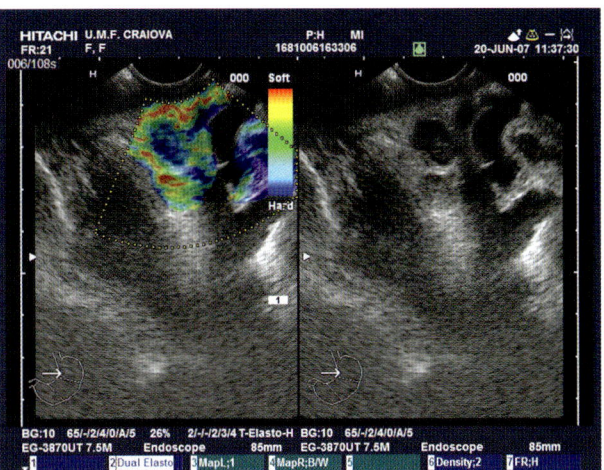

FIGURE 39–6. EUS elastography appearance of a malignant lymph node located near the celiac trunk, with a characteristic in-homogenous, hard pattern.

Although the reliability of EUS elastography has been clearly proved by this study, the results were considered inferior as compared to EUS-FNA. Consequently, the authors suggested that the method might be limited for targeting of the most suitable lymph node for biopsy.

Pancreatic Diseases

The feasibility of EUS elastography of the pancreas has also been demonstrated in a prospective study which included 73 patients (20 with normal pancreas, 20 with chronic pancreatitis, and 33 focal pancreatic lesions).[49] Although EUS elastography movies were deemed feasible and reproducible, the authors could not show any difference between chronic pancreatitis and hard tumors (pancreatic adenocarcinoma), probably because of their similar fibrous structure. Consequently, EUS elastography was considered limited in the ability to improve the diagnostic accuracy of tumors in patients with underlying chronic pancreatitis.[50]

Based on our experience with the method, we established that there is a clear difference between the patients with normal pancreas (Figure 39–7), chronic pseudotumoral pancreatitis (Figure 39–8), and pancreatic cancer (Figure 39–9). By using the same approach of post-processing analysis based on hue histograms of the EUS elastography average images, we have already shown that the sensitivity, specificity, and accuracy for the differentiation of malignant tumors is 91.4%, 87.9%, and 89.7%, respectively.[51] Furthermore, beside the differentiation of pancreatic tumors, the method might prove useful to target EUS-FNA biopsy into harder regions suspicious of

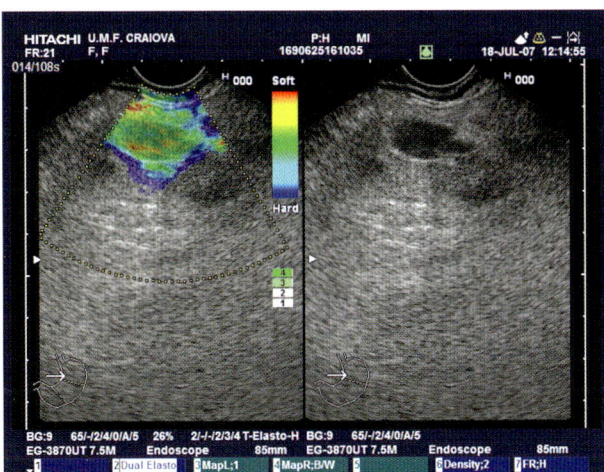

FIGURE 39–5. EUS elastography appearance of a mediastinal benign lymph node, with a characteristic in-homogenous, soft pattern (red-yellow-green).

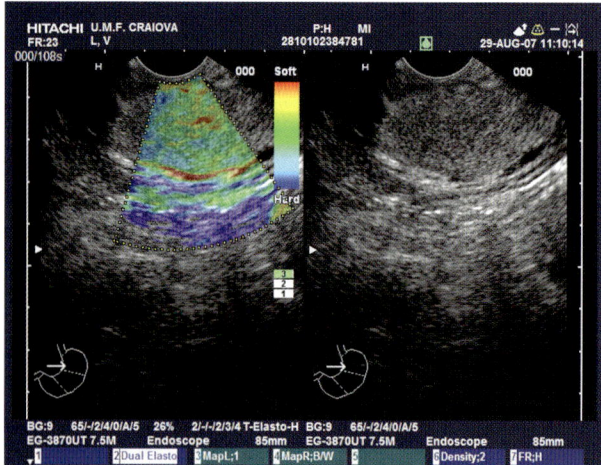

FIGURE 39–7. Normal pancreatic body imaged during EUS elastography as a soft structure (green-yelow). The normal pancreatic duct is frequently visible, as an extremely soft (red) structure in the middle of the pancreatic body.

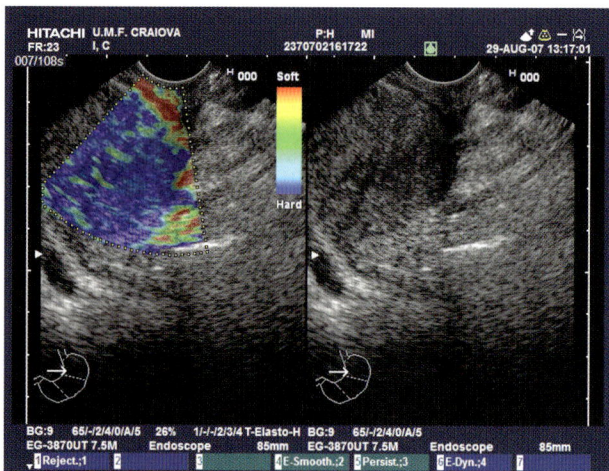

FIGURE 39–9. Pancreatic head adenocarcinoma confirmed by EUS-guided fine needle aspiration biopsy, depicted during EUS elastography as a homogenous hard mass (blue).

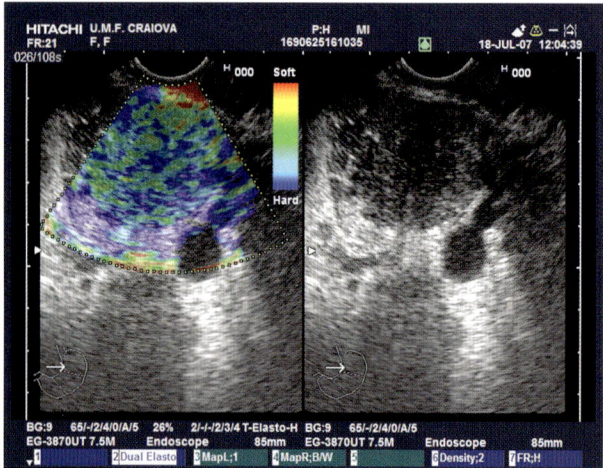

FIGURE 39–8. Chronic pseudotumoral pancreatitis in a young patient (38 years old), depicted by EUS elastography as an in-homogenous mass with mixed elasticity (blue-green).

malignancy (Figure 39–3). Further studies are needed before final conclusions can be made.

Focal Liver Lesions

The feasibility of EUS elastography for the visualization of liver lesions was reported in a case presentation, describing the appearance of granulomatous infiltration (liver sarcoidosis) or liver metastasis.[52] We have the same experience in examining the left liver lobe during staging of other GI tract tumors, with liver metastasis showing a consistent "hard" pattern surrounded by "soft" tissue (Figure 39–10). This pattern is also visible in small tumors, less than 5 mm in diameter (Figure 39–11).

Other Tumors

Different other solid tumors are visible and could be characterized by EUS elastography, including esophageal tumors, gastric tumors, GISTs (gastrointestinal stromal tumors), or adrenal masses.[53] Although these tumors usually have a characteristic "hard" EUS elastography pattern, the clinical utility of the findings remain to be established.

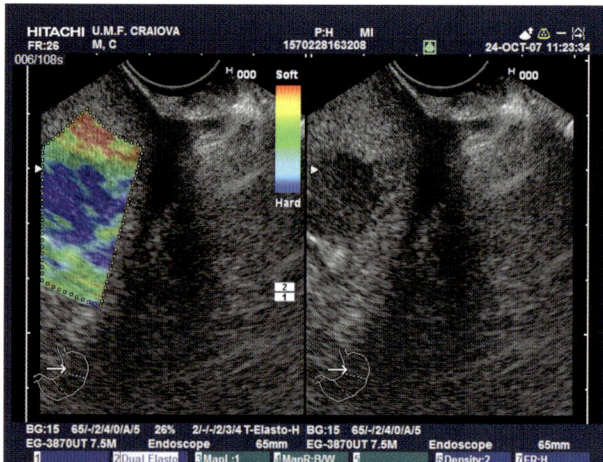

FIGURE 39–10. Liver metastasis in a patient with confirmed pancreatic head adenocarcinoma. The liver metastasis is depicted by EUS elastography as a homogenous hard (blue) mass as compared with the soft surrounding liver tissues.

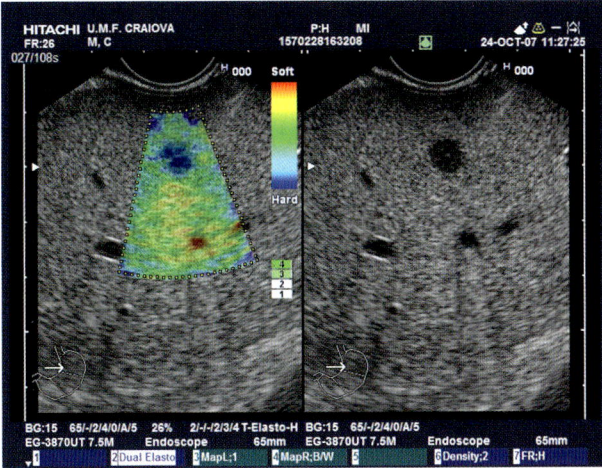

FIGURE 39–11. Small liver metastasis (~ 5 mm) depicted by EUS elastography as a homogenous hard (blue) mass as compared with the soft surrounding liver tissues.

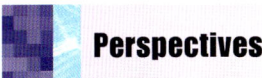

Perspectives

3-D Applications

Preliminary work has shown the feasibility of freehand 3-D ultrasound elastography, which is able to provide reliable and high quality images.[54] Three dimensional strain mapping was also performed after acquisition with a 3-D sectorial probe, by using cross-correlation of interpolated signals between adjacent radiofrequency lines.[55] Recently, near-real-time freehand ultrasound elastography system using a 3-D mechanical probe was also developed. The system generates a full 3-D axial strain volume, with estimates of lateral and elevational tissue movement in order to increase the accuracy of the axial strain measurement.[56]

Clinical applications of 3-D ultrasound elastography were also developed recently. The method might be useful for identifying and classifying the detected prostate lesions (invisible in sonograms) on the basis of their shape.[57] Likewise, the feasibility of a 3-D strain estimation algorithm was tested for the early diagnosis of pressure ulcers, which develop initially in the deep muscular tissues before they expand to the skin, being also harder than surrounding healthy tissues.[58]

Virtual Palpation

The development of "virtual elastography" might probably represent the final step toward tactile imaging, with the visualization and reconstruction of tissue elasticity distribution on haptically explorable surfaces or through force-feedback interaction devices.[59] The breakthrough of 3-D ultrasound elastography might confer the capability to characterize the entire region of high strain values. This could be translated into different virtual reality systems in order to haptically explore regions of the body normally inaccessible to direct palpation.[60–62] Consequently, the end-user would have the sensation of touch by applying forces or vibrations (force-feedback systems). Examples include the use of force-feedback gloves (Figure 39–12), which could be useful in the near future for the translation of virtual palpation into a meaningful clinical application using ultrasound elastography as the local receiver and a remote force-feedback glove as a haptic display. The feasibility of such an approach has been already confirmed more than 10 years ago in some preliminary work concerning tumor palpation simulation or training for the diagnosis of prostate cancer.[63–65]

Several clinical applications of these technologies could be easily foreseen, including training of palpatory diagnosis, as well as the development of remote surgery techniques. A clinician would be thus able to feel and palpate remotely, through the translation of ultrasound elastography information into haptic (touchable) information. Moreover, several organs/lesions that were previously inaccessible to direct palpation (for example the pancreas or intra-abdominal lymph nodes) would consequently be palpated through haptic force-feedback devices.

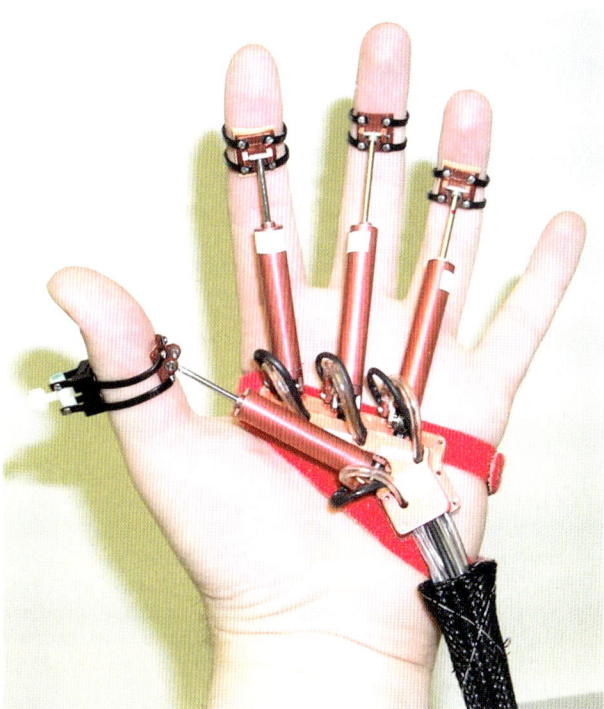

FIGURE 39–12. Example of a force-feedback glove used as a human-machine interface for haptic display in virtual palpation (Picture courtesy of Prof. Dr. G. Burdea, © Rutgers University CAIP Center. Reprinted by permission.).

References

1. McDonald, S., Saslow, D., Alciati, M. H.: Performance and reporting of clinical breast examination: a review of the literature. CA Cancer J Clin 2004; 54:345–361.
2. Partin, A. W., Stutzman, R. E.: Elevated prostate-specific antigen, abnormal prostate evaluation on digital rectal examination, and transrectal ultrasound and prostate biopsy. Urol Clin North Am 1998; 25:581–589, viii.
3. Aslanian, H., Salem, R., Lee, J., Andersen, D., Robert, M., Topazian, M.: EUS diagnosis of vascular invasion in pancreatic cancer: surgical and histologic correlates. Am J Gastroenterol. 2005; 100: 1381–1385.
4. Ophir, J., Céspedes, I., Ponnekanti, H., Yazdi, Y., Li, X.: Elastography: a quantitative method for imaging the elasticity of biological tissues. Ultrason Imaging 1991;13:111–134.
5. Khalil, A. S., Chan, R. C., Chau, A. H., Bouma, B. E., Mofrad, M. R.: Tissue elasticity estimation with optical coherence elastography: toward mechanical characterization of in vivo soft tissue. Ann Biomed Eng 2005; 33:1631–1639.
6. Bishop, J., Samani, A., Sciarretta, J., Plewes, D. B.: Two-dimensional MR elastography with linear inversion reconstruction: methodology and noise analysis. Phys Med Biol. 2000; 45:2081–2091.
7. Konofagou, E. E.: Quo vadis elasticity imaging? Ultrasonics 2004;42: 331–336.
8. Céspedes, I., Ophir, J., Ponnekanti, H., Maklad, N.: Elastography: elasticity imaging using ultrasound with application to muscle and breast in vivo. Ultrason Imaging 1993; 15:73–88.
9. Garra, B. S., Céspedes, E. I., Ophir, J., et al.: Elastography of breast lesions: initial clinical results. Radiology 1997;202: 79–86.
10. Hiltawsky, K. M., Kruger, M., Starke, C., et al.: Freehand ultrasound elastography of breast lesions: clinical results. Ultrasound Med Biol 2001;27:1461–1467.
11. Bercoff, J., Chaffai, S., Tanter, M., et al.: In vivo breast tumor detection using transient elastography. Ultrasound Med Biol 2003; 29:1387–1396.
12. Cochlin, D. L., Ganatra, R. H., Griffiths, D. F. R.: Elastography in the detection of prostatic cancer. Clinical Radiology 2002; 57:1014–1020.
13. Sommerfeld, H. J., Garcia-Schurmann, J. M., Schewe, J., et al.: Prostate cancer diagnosis using ultrasound elastography. Introduction of a novel technique and first clinical results. Urologe A 2003; 42:941–945.
14. König, K., Scheipers, U., Pesavento, A., Lorenz, A., Ermert, H., Senge, T.: Initial experiences with real-time elastography guided biopsies of the prostate. J Urol 2005;174:115–117.
15. Varghese, T., Techavipoo, U., Liu, W., Zagzebski, J. A., Chen, Q., Frank, G., Lee, F. T., Jr.: Elastographic measurement of the area and volume of thermal lesions resulting from radiofrequency ablation: pathologic correlation. AJR Am J Roentgenol 2003; 181:701–707.
16. Souchon, R., Rouvière, O., Gelet, A., et al.: Visualization of HIFU lesions using elastography of the human prostate in vivo: preliminary results. J Ultrasound Med Biol 2003;29: 1007–1015.
17. Schaar, J. A., de Korte, C. L., Mastik, F., Strijder, C., Pasterkamp, G., Boersma, E., Serruys, P. W., van der Steen, A. F. W.: Characterizing vulnerable plaque features with intravascular elastography. Circulation 2003;108:2636–2641.
18. Varghese, T., Zagzebski, J. A., Rahko, P., Breburda, C. S.: Ultrasonic imaging of myocardial strain using cardiac elastography. Ultrason Imaging 2003;25:1–16.
19. Sandrin, L., Fourqet, B., Hasquenoph, J. M., et al.: Transient elastography: a new noninvasive method for assessment of hepatic fibrosis. Ultrasound Med Biol 2003;29:1705–1713.
20. Ziol, M., Handra-Luca, A., Kettaneh, A., et al.: Noninvasive assessment of liver fibrosis by measurement of stiffness in patients with chronic hepatitis C. Hepatology 2005;41:48–54.
21. Castera, L., Vergniol, J., Foucher, J., et al.: Prospective comparison of transient elastography, Fibrotest, APRI, and liver biopsy for the assessment of fibrosis in chronic hepatitis C. Gastroenterology 2005;128:343–350.
22. Colletta, C., Smirne, C., Fabris, C., et al.: Value of two noninvasive methods to detect progression of fibrosis among HCV carriers with normal aminotransferases. Hepatology 2005;42:838–845.
23. Foucher, J., Chanteloup, E., Vergniol, J., et al.: Diagnosis of cirrhosis by transient elastography (Fibroscan (R): a prospective study. Gut 2006;55:403–408.
24. Shaheen, A. A., Wan, A. F., Myers, R. P.: FibroTest and FibroScan for the prediction of hepatitis C-related fibrosis: a systematic review of diagnostic test accuracy. Am J Gastroenterol 2007;102:2589–2600.
25. Săftoiu, A., Vilman, P.: Endoscopic ultrasound elastography—a new imaging technique for the visualization of tissue elasticity distribution. J Gastrointestin Liver Dis 2006;15:161–5.
26. Itoh, A., Ueno, E., Tohno, E., Kamma, H., Takahashi, H., Shiina, T., Yamakawa, M., Matsumura, T.: Breast disease: clinical application of US elastography for diagnosis. Radiology. 2006; 239:341–350.
27. Thomas, A., Fischer, T., Frey, H., Ohlinger, R., Grunwald, S., Blohmer, J. U., Winzer, K. J., Weber, S., Kristiansen, G., Ebert, B., Kümmel, S.: Real-time elastography—an advanced method of ultrasound: First results in 108 patients with breast lesions. Ultrasound Obstet Gynecol. 2006;28:335–340.
28. Zhi, H., Ou, B., Luo, B. M., Feng, X., Wen, Y. L., Yang, H. Y.: Comparison of ultrasound elastography, mammography, and sonography in the diagnosis of solid breast lesions. J Ultrasound Med. 2007;26: 807–815.
29. Tardivon, A., El Khoury, C., Thibault, F., Wyler, A., Barreau, B., Neuenschwander, S.: Elastography of the breast: a prospective study of 122 lesions. J Radiol 2007; 88: 657–62.
30. Miyanaga, N., Akaza, H., Yamakawa, M., Oikawa, T., Sekido, N., Hinotsu, S., Kawai, K., Shimazui, T., Shiina, T.: Tissue elasticity imaging for diagnosis of prostate cancer: a preliminary report. Int J Urol 2006;13: 1514–1518.
31. Tsutsumi, M., Miyagawa T, Matsumura T, Kawazoe N, Ishikawa S, Shimokama T, Shiina T, Miyanaga N, Akaza, H.: The impact of real-time tissue elasticity imaging (elastography) on the detection of prostate cancer: clinicopathological analysis. Int J Clin Oncol. 2007; 12(4):250–255.
32. Sumura, M., Shigeno, K., Hyuga, T., Yoneda, T., Shiina, H., Igawa, M.: Initial evaluation of prostate cancer with real-time elastography based on step-section pathological analysis after radical prostatectomy: a preliminary study. Int J Urol. 2007 Sep;14(9):811–816.
33. Thomas, A., Kümmel, S., Gemeinhardt, O., Fischer, T.: Real-time sonoelastography of the cervix: tissue

elasticity of the normal and abnormal cervix. Acad Radiol 2007; 14:193–200.
34. Lyshchik, A., Higashi, T., Asato, R., Tanaka, S., Ito, J., Mai, J. J., Pellot-Barakat, C., Insana, M. F., Brill, A. B., Saga, T., Hiraoka, M., Togashi, K.: Thyroid gland tumor diagnosis at US elastography. Radiology 2005;237: 202–211.
35. Bae, U., Dighe, M., Dubinsky, T., Minoshima, S., Shamdasani, V., Kim, Y.: Ultrasound thyroid elastography using carotid artery pulsation: preliminary study. J Ultrasound Med 2007; 26:797–805.
36. Rago, T., Santini, F., Scutari, M., Pinchera, A., Vitti, P.: Elastography: new developments in ultrasound for predicting malignancy in thyroid nodules. J Ultrasound Med. 2007;26:807–815.
37. Friedrich-Rust, M., Ong, M. F., Herrmann, E., Dries, V., Samaras, P., Zeuzem, S., Sarrazin, C.: Real-time elastography for noninvasive assessment of liver fibrosis in chronic viral hepatitis. AJR Am J Roentgenol 2007; 188:758–764.
38. Săftoiu, A., Gheonea, D. I., Ciurea, T.: Hue histogram analysis of real-time elastography images for noninvasive assessment of liver fibrosis. AJR Am J Roentgenol. 2007;189:W232–233.
39. Frey, H.: Real-time elastography. A new ultrasound procedure for the reconstruction of tissue elasticity. Der Radiologe 2003;43:850–855.
40. Yamakawa, M., Nitta, N., Shiina, T., Matsumura, S., Tamano, S., Mitake, T., Ueno, E.: High-speed Freehand Tissue Elasticity Imaging for Breast Diagnosis. Jpn J Appl Phys 2003; 42:3265–3270.
41. Shiina, T., Nitta, N., Ueno, E. I., Bamber, J. C.: Real-time tissue elasticity imaging using the combined autocorrelation method. J Med Ultrason 2002; 29:119–128.
42. König, K., Scheipers, U., Pesavento, A., Lorenz, A., Ermert, H., Senge, T.: Initial experiences with real-time elastography guided biopsies of the prostate. J Urol 2005; 174:115–117.
43. Giovannini, M., Hookey, L. C., Bories, E., Pesenti, C., Monges, G., Delpero, J. R.: Endoscopic ultrasound elastography: the first step towards virtual biopsy? Preliminary results in 49 patients. Endoscopy 2006;38: 344–348.
44. Săftoiu, A., Vilmann, P., Hassan, H., Gorunescu, F.: Analysis of endoscopic ultrasound elastography used for characterization and differentiation of benign and malignant lymph nodes. Ultraschall Med 2006; 27:535–342.
45. Fritscher-Ravens, A.: Blue clouds and green clouds: virtual biopsy via EUS elastography? Endoscopy. 2006; 38:416–417.
46. Săftoiu, A., Vilmann, P., Ciurea, T., Popescu, G. L., Iordache, A., Hassan, H., Gorunescu, F., Iordache, S.: Dynamic analysis of EUS used for the differentiation of benign and malignant lymph nodes. Gastrointest Endosc. 2007; 66:291–300.
47. Jacobson, B. C.: Pressed for an answer: has elastography finally come to EUS? Gastrointest Endosc. 2007;66: 301–303.
48. Janssen, J., Dietrich, C. F., Will, U., Greiner, L.: Endosonographic elastography in the diagnosis of mediastinal lymph nodes. Endoscopy 2007;39:952–957.
49. Janssen, J., Schlörer, E., Greiner, L.: EUS elastography of the pancreas: feasibility and pattern description of the normal pancreas, chronic pancreatitis, and focal pancreatic lesions. Gastrointest Endosc. 2007;65: 971–978.
50. Micames, C. G., Gress, F. G.: EUS elastography: a step ahead? Gastrointest Endosc. 2007;65:979–981.
51. Săftoiu, A., Vilmann, P., Gorunescu, F., Gheonea, D.I., Gorunescu, M., Ciurea, T., Popescu, G. L., Iordache, A., Hassan, H., Iordache, S.: Neural network analysis of dynamic sequences of EUS elastography used for the differential diagnosis of chronic pancreatitis and pancreatic cancer. Gastrointest Endosc. 2008;68: 1086–94.
52. Nadan, R., Irena, H., Milorad, O., Rajko, O., Jasminka, J. R., Marino, K., Roland, P., Boris, V.: EUS elastography in the diagnosis of focal liver lesions. Gastrointest Endosc 2007;66(4):823–824.
53. Gheorghe, L., Gheorghe, C., Cotruta, B., Carabela, A.: CT aspects of gastrointestinal stromal tumors: adding EUS and EUS elastography to the diagnostic tools. J Gastrointestin Liver Dis. 2007;16(3):346–347.
54. Lindop, J. E., Treece, G. M., Gee, A. H., Prager RW. 3D elastography using freehand ultrasound. Ultrasound Med Biol 2006; 32:529–545.
55. Said, G., Basset, O., Mari, J. M., Cachard, C., Brusseau, E., Vray, D.: Experimental three dimensional strain estimation from ultrasonic sectorial data. Ultrasonics 2006;44 Suppl 1: 189–193.
56. Treece, G. M., Lindop, J. E., Gee, A. H., Prager, R. W.: Freehand ultrasound elastography with a 3-D probe. Ultrasound Med Biol. 2008;34:463–74.
57. Patil, A. V., Garson, C. D., Hossack, J. A.: 3D prostate elastography: algorithm, simulations and experiments. Phys Med Biol. 2007;52:3643–663.
58. Deprez, J. F., Cloutier, G., Schmitt, C., Gehin, C., Dittmar, A., Basset, O., Brusseau, E.: 3D Ultrasound Elastography for Early Detection of Lesions. Evaluation on a Pressure Ulcer Mimicking Phantom. Conf Proc IEEE Eng Med Biol Soc. 2007;1:79–82
59. Gilja, O. H., Hatlebakk, J. G., Odegaard, S., Berstad, A., Viola, I., Giertsen, C., Hausken, T., Gregersen, H.: Advanced imaging and visualization in gastrointestinal disorders. World J Gastroenterol 2007;13:1408–1421.
60. Khaled, W., Reichling, S., Bruhns, O. T., Boese, H., Baumann, M., Monkman, G., Egersdoerfer, S., Klein, D., Tunayar, A., Freimuth, H., Lorenz, A., Pessavento, A., Ermert, H.: Palpation imaging using a haptic system for virtual reality applications in medicine. Stud Health Technol Inform. 2004; 98:147–153.
61. Monkman, G. J., Boese, H., Ermert, H., Klein, D., Freimuth, H., Baumann, M., Egersdoerfer, S., Bruhns, O. T., Meier, A., Raja, K.: Technologies for haptic systems in telemedicine. Stud Health Technol Inform 2003;97:83–93.
62. Khaled, W., Ermert, H., Bruhns, O., Boese, H., Baumann, M., Monkman, G. J., Egersdoerfer, S., Meier, A., Klein, D., Freimuth, H.: A haptic sensor-actor-system based on ultrasound elastography and electrorheological fluids for virtual reality applications in medicine. Stud Health Technol Inform. 2003; 94:144–150.
63. Burdea, G., Patounakis, G., Popescu, V., Weiss, R. E.: Virtual reality-based training for the diagnosis of prostate cancer. IEEE transactions on biomedical engineering 1999;46:1253–1260.
64. Langrana, N., Burdea, G., Ladeji, J., Dinsmore, M.: Human performance using virtual reality tumor palpation simulation. Comput & Graphics 1997;21:451–458.
65. Bouzit, M., Burdea, G., Popescu, G., Boian, R.: The Rutgers Master II – New Design Force-Feedback Glove. IEEE/ASME Transactions on Mechatronics 2002;7: 256–263.

CHAPTER 40

EUS Contrast Agents

Dr. Nischita K. Reddy
Dr. Adrian Săftoiu
Dr. Manoop S. Bhutani

The use of intravenous contrast agents in ultrasonography first came about in echocardiography where they were used to improve imaging of the cardiac chambers and great vessels.[1] Since then, their use has been described in transabdominal ultrasonography and now in endoscopic ultrasonography (EUS). Use of contrast agents in EUS has shown to improve characterization of vasculature inside the organ of interest, better delineate benign from malignant pathology,[2–8] aid in staging and directing therapeutic procedures and thereby alter prognosis.

Contrast Agents

Contrast agents are made of gas-filled microbubbles encapsulated by a phospholipid or albumin shell. They are categorized into first, second, and third generation based on their capability of transpulmonary passage and half-life in the human body. Commonly used first generation agents include Albunex, Levovist, Echovist. Second generation agents include SonoVue, Sonazoid, and Optison among others.[9,10] The only third generation agent currently available is Echogen, capable of phase-shift from liquid to gas form once it attains body temperature.[11] Contrast agents in use today are relatively safe and have demonstrated no severe, long-lasting adverse effects in humans.[12,13]

Mechanisms of Action

Contrast agents were specifically developed to image vascularity and vessel patterns, especially for small volume and slow velocity blood flow. This is highly important in tumors, where angiogenesis alters completely the vascular structure. The principle of ultrasound contrast agents is that they create multiple small interfaces with high echogenicity, a process best achieved by gaseous microbubbles, surrounded by a shell used to increase stability.[14] Microbubbles are very good at backscattering ultrasound, effectively reflecting the ultrasound waves. However, the microbubbles respond and oscillate to the sound pressure in a nonlinear fashion, with an asymetrical diameter cause by ultrasound pressure. The diameter is variable between 2–10 μm, about the size of red blood cells. Consequently, they do not leave the vascular system (blood pool contrast agents). The ultrasound contrast agents are administered through intravenous bolus injection, in a large arm vein. Second-generation contrast agents pass through the lungs, allowing the contrast enhancement of the entire vascular system.

Contrast agents were used initially as Doppler signal enhancers, including in contrast-enhanced EUS examinations (CE-EUS). Both color Doppler and power Doppler can be used, especially for regions with very low flow volumes, where the unenhanced signal is too weak or the signal-noise ratio is too poor. Although the contrast agent selectively enhances the useful signal in the detriment of the noise, the main disadvantage of these techniques is the presence of artifacts. Both tissue motion (flash) artifacts and blooming artifacts appear and impede the examinations. Flash artifacts are specific to the Doppler mode, appearing as color signals caused by tissue motion, being most commonly seen in hypoechoic areas, induced by cardiac or respiratory motion.[15] Blooming artifacts appear as a consequence of the high amplification of the backscattered signal, which saturates the receiver and causes smearing of the color signal. They appear immediately after the wash-in phase and disappear when the concentration of contrast is lower.[16]

Contrast specific imaging techniques were developed to gain advantage of the nonlinear behavior of the contrast agents (microbubbles). Different technical approaches were used to separate contrast echoes from tissue and artifacts echoes, one of the most used being contrast harmonic imaging (pulse inversion, phase inversion or wide band harmonic imaging). All examinations use a high mechanical index (with destruction of the microbubbles) or a low mechanical index (with constant oscillation of the microbubbles). Newer contrast agents (Sonovue, Definity, etc.) have flexible outer shells, which allow the use of a mechanical index below 0.1, with continuous transmission and visualization of parenchymal blood flow (real-time perfusion imaging). Contrast harmonic imaging examinations with a low-mechanical index are recently available for use with EUS technology.[17,18] The main advantage is the absence of sensitivity to motion artifacts (cardiac or respiratory) movements.

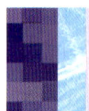

Clinical Uses of Contrast Enhanced Endoscopic Ultrasonography (CE-EUS)

Differentiating Benign from Malignant Mediastinal Lymphadenopathy

EUS-guided fine-needle aspiration (FNA) represents the current "gold-standard" for the diagnosis of malignant mediastinal lymphadenopathy,[19,20] further improved by on-site cytopathologic assessment of the specimens.[21] Although, studies have not been consistent in their findings,[6,22] there are suggestions that CE-EUS may offer a noninvasive method to increase the specificity of diagnosing benign lymph nodes, and aid in targeting aspiration of only high-yield lymph nodes.

However, differentiating benign from malignant lymph nodes using appearance and type (arterial, venous) of vascularity may not be reliable since nonlymphomatous cancer cells invade lymph nodes heterogeneneously.[23] Currently, CE-EUS can not replace EUS-guided FNA in confirming malignant mediastinal lymph nodes. The combination of CE-EUS and EUS-FNA will possibly improve diagnostic accuracy.

Esophageal and Gastric Cancer

EUS can provide cross-sectional imaging of the wall of the gastro-intestinal tract, and determine the depth of invasion of cancers. The normal esophageal and gastric walls consist of five layers on EUS images with enhancement of the third and fifth layers (submucosa and adventitia or serosa, respectively). Esophageal cancers do not enhance with CE-EUS due to relative avascularity.[8] In gastric cancer, assessment of depth of invasion can be improved with CE-EUS, especially for depressed, endophytic cancers. Use of CE-EUS improves the overall accuracy for assessment of depth of invasion of gastric carcinoma from 70% to 90%. Active ulcers and scars in both malignant and nonmalignant lesions do not enhance post-contrast. This has been attributed to the nature of vascularity (linear convergence) and foci of fibrosis. Gastric myogenic tumors appear as hypoechoic masses linked to the fourth layer on EUS.[8] Hirooka et al demonstrated that poorly differentiated gastric carcinomas enhanced by infusion of Albunex whereas well differentiated ones did not. However, prediction of histologic type of gastric carcinoma by nature of enhancement has been inconsistent.[24]

Gallbladder Diseases

CE-EUS has the potential to differentiate gallbladder lesions and assess the depth of tumor infiltration in gallbladder carcinomas.[5] It can differentiate chronic cholecystitis and cholesterol polyps from infiltrating and exophytic gallbladder cancer, respectively, since the three-layer structure remains intact in the benign conditions. Majority of gallbladder adenocarcinomas enhance with EUS on administration of Albunex,[5] unlike other gallbladder diseases including adenosquamous carcinoma cholesterol polyps, chronic cholecystitis.[5,24] CE-EUS is also able to clearly differentiate the depth of invasion in the gallbladder wall from T1b from T1a, improving accuracy over standard EUS.[5]

Pancreatic Diseases: First Generation

CE-EUS has been used in pancreatic cancer to demarcate vascular landmarks, detect vascular obliteration by thrombus or tumor, and examine microvascular blood flow to organs and lesions.

Albunex was the earliest contrast agent used to enhance EUS images. Hirooka et al (1997) demonstrated that peripheral injection of Albunex can enhance B-mode images of pancreatic pathology during high-frequency EUS.[24] Enhancement was marked in cases of pancreatic islet cell tumor. Pancreatic ductal cell carcinomas remained unenhanced compared to surrounding normal parenchyma and fibrosis thereby making boundaries clearer.[24]

A study by the same authors in 1998 demonstrated similar findings with 100% image enhancement (at 12 Hz) using Albunex in islet cell carcinomas and serous cystadenomas, 80% enhancement in mucin-producing tumors, and 75% in chronic pancreatitis. Also, no enhancement was noted with ductal cell carcinomas and pancreatic pseudocysts, consistent with hypovascularity. Differences in vascularity as demonstrated on angiography paralleled the enhancement patterns during CE-EUS, except in 20% and 25% of cases with mucin-producing tumors and chronic pancreatitis, respectively. In addition, they demonstrated that areas of normal parenchyma and fibrosis around a lesion can enhance, demarcating boundaries. This could lead to accurate pre-operative staging and planning of surgical resection lines, in the case of mucinous tumors involving the main pancreatic duct.[4]

The authors propose that enhancement after Albunex maybe related atleast in part to the nature of microcirculation and vascular permeability of the lesion, which determine the concentration of constrast agent within the lesion. This could account for the less predictive pattern of angiography with sonographic enhancement.[4]

Pancreatic Diseases: Second Generation

Using an experimental second generation microbubble contrast agent, Wong et al demonstrated hypoechogenicity in normal pancreatic tissue after a bolus but not with continuous infusion. This could be related to greater intravascular density of contrast material with bolus injection compared to a continuous infusion. Decreased echo signal from the pancreatic parenchyma after contrast injection maybe due to increased signal from the pancreatic interface with adjacent structures.[25] Whether this will have a clinical useful application remains to be determined. Certainly, lesions that enhance with contrast will be easier to distinguish from the surrounding normal pancreas.

CE-EUS reveals the characteristic vascularity and can diagnose and follow-up Intraductal Papillary Mucinous Neoplasms of the Pancreas (IPMN). Enlargement or enhancement of a mural nodule accurately indicated the presence of atypical malignant epithelium and determined need for surgical resection.[26] Mural nodules were classified into four types based on morphology during EUS, before and after contrast: Type 1 (low papillary type), Type 2 (polypoid type), Type 3 (villous type) and Type 4 (invasive type with blurred hypoechoic area between lesion and parenchyma). IPMNs with Type 3/4 features more accurately identified as having higher grade dysplastic or malignant features histologically.[27]

Color Doppler:

Combining B-mode EUS with CE- Doppler ultrasound improves the visualization of vascularity of a pancreatic lesion with malignant ductal adenocarcinoma demonstrating low flow and relatively avascular pattern. Bhutani et al[28] described enhancement of color-Doppler signals from the celiac artery, superior mesenteric artery, and portal vein during EUS in a swine model on administration of Levovist. This effect was easily appreciated without the need for complex quantitative measurements. No visually obvious enhancement was evident in vessels like the aorta that already had pronounced unenhanced color Doppler signal. Using Optison (FS069), Becker et al[29] demonstrated that sensitivity and specificity of echo-enhanced color-Doppler EUS are comparable with cytopathology results. Ueno et al differentiated islet cell tumors and ductal cell cancer with color-Doppler EUS. Islet cell tumors had marked hypervascularization whereas patients with adenocarcinoma had vascularity only around the tumor.[30] These results have been confirmed by several other investigators. Hypovascularity as a sign of malignancy in CE-EUS can obtain a 92% sensitivity and 100% specificity (89%–100%).[2] Using CE-Doppler EUS hypovascularized malignant ductal adenocarcinoma and hypervascularized benign tumor entities, mostly neuroendocrine tumors, and serous microcystic adenomas of the pancreas can be easily differentiated. This is of pivotal importance since serous microcystic adenomas can be observed due to low growth potential, neuroendocrine tumors may be enucleated or otherwise less radically resected compared to ductal adenocarcinoma.

Power Doppler:

Unenhanced power Doppler ultrasonography is unable to provide tumor differentiation, as a previous study showed a very low specificity (77%) of unenhanced power Doppler EUS.[31] Although other factors like the presence of peripancreatic collaterals, might improve the specificity, this wasn't confirmed in larger studies. It is possible to misdiagnose necrotic pancreatitis as ductal adenocarcinoma and also to find inflammation surrounding ductal adenocarcinomas? Indeed, the presence of power Doppler inside the inflammatory masses is variable as a function of inflammation and necrosis, thus complicating the differential diagnosis.[31]

The sensitivity of power Doppler sonography to depict tumor neovascularization can be increased by contrast agents. In an animal model of pancreatic vascular disruption using 50% ethanol plus purified carbon particle solution, standard EUS demonstrated hypoechogenecity in the ethanol treated area. With injection of Definity, power Doppler EUS revealed marked contrast enhancement of normal pancreatic parenchyma from the ethanol-treated area.[32] Several studies using CE-EUS with power Doppler scanning also demonstrated an improvement in discrimination of pancreatic cancer from chronic pancreatitis [28,33–37] and may also help in localizing small benign tumors like insulinomas.[7]

Hocke et al[35], using pulsed Doppler analysis with CE-Doppler EUS demonstrated an improvement in the differentiation between chronic pancreatitis and malignancy. They used specific criteria to define malignancy: lack of vascularisation before injection of SonoVue, irregular appearance of arterial vessels over a short distance post-injection and absence of detection of venous vessels in the lesion.[35] In contrast to the technique described by Becker et al, Hocke et al combined the analysis of the detected vessels with pulsed wave Doppler analysis. They concluded that the use of second-generation contrast agents with low mechanical index techniques will possibly allow real-time imaging with or without three dimensional reconstructions in EUS imaging.

With contrast-enhanced power Doppler sonography, the signal intensity from flowing blood is lower compared to that of moving solid tissue structures. Harmonic imaging was specifically developed to overcome these obstacles, since tissue particles have fewer harmonic waves than intravascular microbubbles, thus avoiding flash and blooming artifacts.[17,18]

Harmonic Imaging:

Contrast enhanced harmonic imaging techniques are currently available for EUS, due to the improvement in transducer technology. The use of adequate broadband transducers that can detect harmonic signals was recently reported.[17,18] A pilot study previously described an experimental technique with low mechanical index, which allowed the differentiation between chronic pancreatitis and pancreatic cancer, based on tissue microperfusion characteristics.[17] Another feasibility study demonstrated both parenchymal perfusion and microvasculature in the pancreas.[18] Both intermittent homogenous parenchymal perfusion images and real-time continuous images of finely branching vessels of the pancreas were obtained with a mechanical index of 0.4. Although the initial study included a small number of patients with pancreatic lesions, it seemed that tumor characterization was possible based on vascular or perfusion pattern. Thus, pancreatic carcinomas had absent or heterogenous perfusion images in the intermittent mode, while the vessels were visualized like irregular "network like" structures in real-time mode. Both neuroendocrine tumors and chronic pseudotumoral pancreatitis were homogenous and iso- or hypervascular.

Several other research groups are testing the feasibility of CE-EUS.[36,37]

CE-EUS with low mechanical index (0.4) was tested in 25 patients, after peripheral injection of Sonovue. The method seemed feasible to differentiate adenocarcinoma from other focal mass lesions, being proposed as the method of choice to establish the management of the patients when EUS-FNA is noncontributive.[36] Harmonic imaging has been also used with CE-EUS after peripheral injection of Sonazoid in two settings, WPI (wide-band pulse inversion harmonic) and EXPHD (extended pure harmonic detection). The change in echo-intensity was evaluated. Ductal carcinomas, IPMNs, chronic pancreatitis and endocrine tumors demonstrate varied echo-intensities after infusion of contrast agent.[37]

Esophageal Varices and Portal Hypertension

B-mode EUS can detect grade II varices or larger. After administration of Levovist, flow signals can become evident beneath the third echogenic layer of the esophageal wall and help visualize perforating veins and periesophageal vessels.[38] EUS-guided portal vein (PV) angiography by using CO_2 as a contrast agent, has been evaluated in a porcine model. This is less viscous making it easier to inject through small-caliber needles, minimizing damage to the vascular wall compared to iodinated contrast.[39] Figures 40–1A - 40–1C through 40–3A - 40–3C provide examples of contrast enhanced EUS in gastric cancer and pancreas.

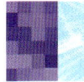

Future Perspectives

Tumor blood flow was previously linked in several studies with both metastasis potential and poor prognosis. A clear correlation was also proven between microvessel density, different angiogenic factors (for example vascular endothelial growth factor, etc.) and the tumors with definite vascular signals demonstrated by contrast-enhanced ultrasound.[40] Quantification of tumor perfusion has been proven feasible for the early assessment and monitoring of the efficacy of antiangiogenic agents in quantitative terms

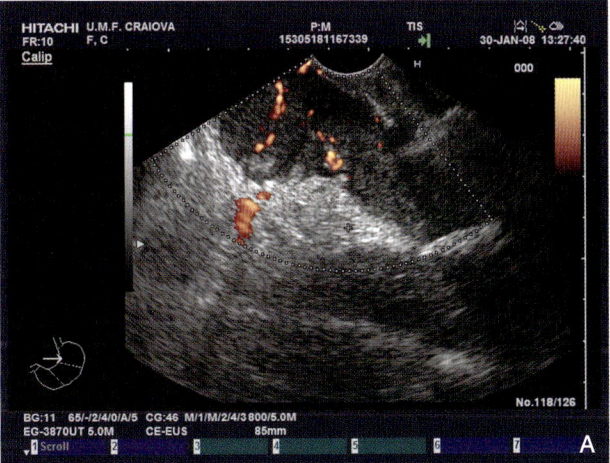 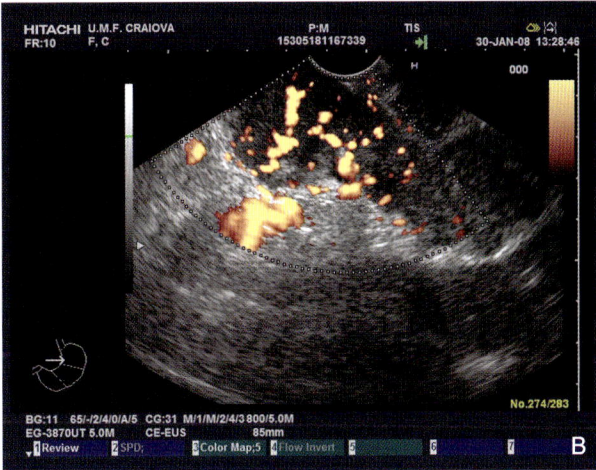

FIGURE 40–1. *A and B* (A) Unenhanced power Doppler endoscopic ultrasound (EUS) of a gastric adenocarcinoma. (B) Contrast-enhanced power Doppler EUS of the same gastric tumor showing a better visualization of tumor vasculature.

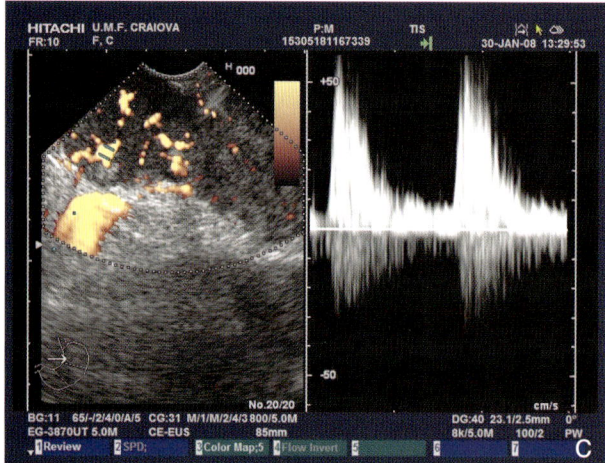

FIGURE 40–1C. Pulsed Doppler analysis of the intratumoral vessels showing arterial signals with a high pulsatility index.

based on changes in vascularity, before morphological changes become apparent.[41]

The feasibility of new technologies using contrast-enhanced ultrasound with microbubbles targeted to vascular endothelial growth factor receptor type 2 (VEGFR2) are currently being tested.[42-44] Several applications of molecular imaging and targeted ultrasound therapy can be also envisioned in the near future, while the detailed physical processes behind sonoporation (increased uptake of drugs inside the cell through transient porosities in the cell membrane in the presence of contrast agents.[45]

In this context, the development of contrast-enhanced endoscopic ultrasound will be clearly beneficial for targeted ultrasound imaging and ultrasound-assisted drug-delivery applications in gastrointestinal tract tumors, as well as other tumors accessible by EUS (pancreatic, lung tumors, etc.).

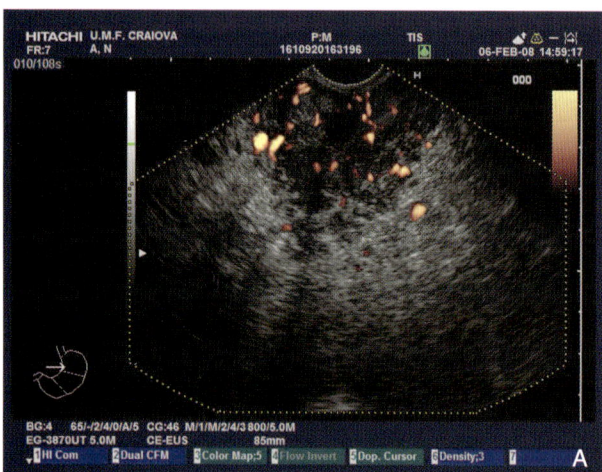

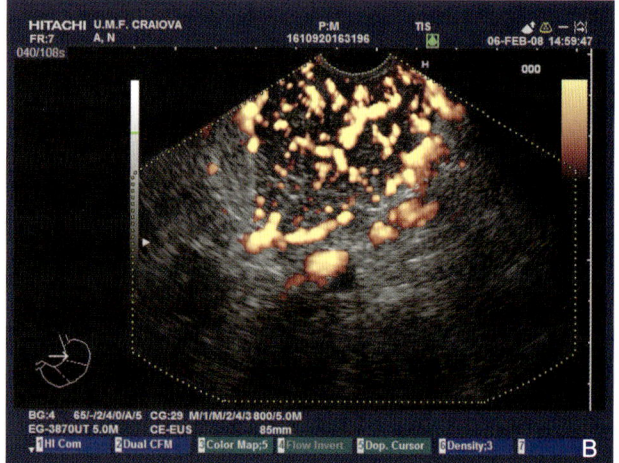

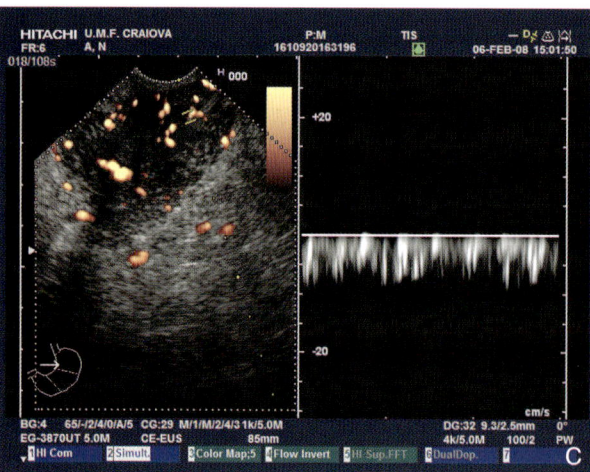

FIGURE 40–2. *A to C* (A) Unenhanced power Doppler endoscopic ultrasound (EUS) of a pseudotumoral chronic pancreatitis mass. (B) Contrast-enhanced power Doppler EUS of the same gastric tumor showing a better visualization of tumor vasculature, with a high vascularity index. (C) Pulsed Doppler analysis analysis of the intratumoral vessels showing venous signals.

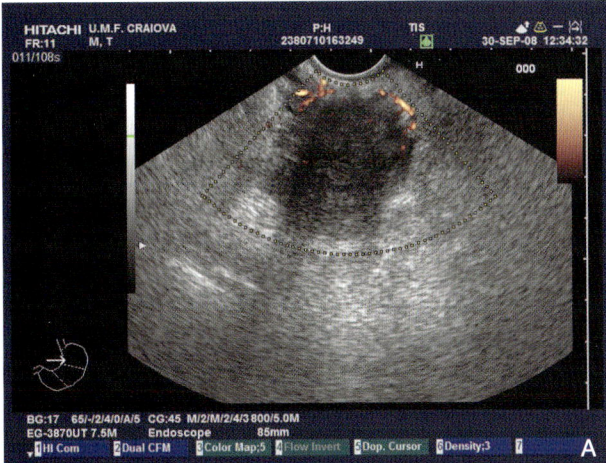
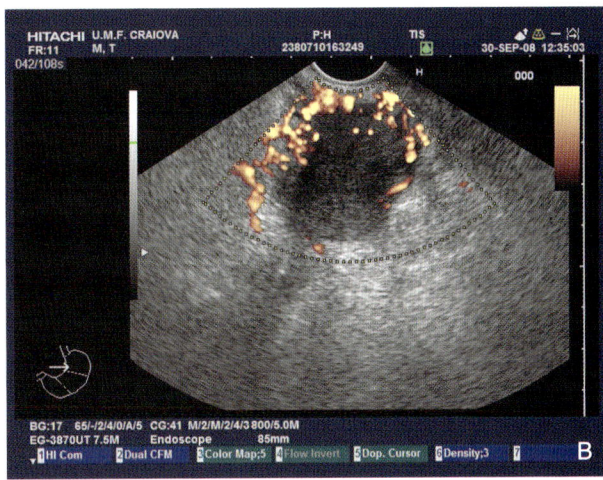
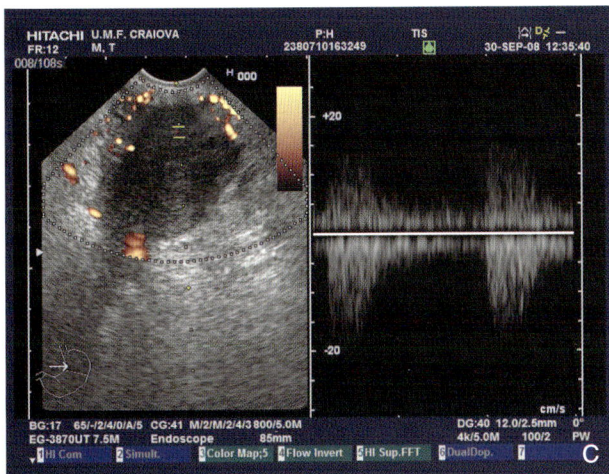

FIGURE 40–3 A to C. (A) Unenhanced power Doppler endoscopic ultrasound (EUS) of a pancreatic adenocarcinoma mass. (B) Contrast-enhanced power Doppler EUS of the same pancreatic adenocarcinoma mass showing a better visualization of tumor vasculature, with a very low vascularity index and enhancement of the peritumoral collaterals. (C) Pulsed Doppler analysis analysis of the intratumoral vessels showing arterial signals with a high pulsatility index.

References

1. Keller, M. W., Feinstein, S. B., Watson, D. D.: Successful left ventricular opacification following peripheral venous injection of sonicated contrast agent: an experimental evaluation. American Heart Journal 1987;114(3):570–575.
2. Dietrich, C. F., Ignee, A., Braden, B., Barreiros, A. P., Ott, M., Hocke, M.: Improved differentiation of pancreatic tumors using contrast-enhanced endoscopic ultrasound. Clin Gastroenterol Hepatol 2008;6(5):590–597.
3. Goldberg, B. B., Hilpert, P. L., Burns, P. N., et al.: Hepatic tumors: signal enhancement at Doppler US after intravenous injection of a contrast agent. Radiology 1990;177(3):713–717.
4. Hirooka, Y., Goto, H., Ito, A., et al.: Contrast-enhanced endoscopic ultrasonography in pancreatic diseases: a preliminary study. American Journal of Gastroenterology 1998;93(4):632–635.
5. Hirooka, Y., Naitoh, Y., Goto, H., et al.: Contrast-enhanced endoscopic ultrasonography in gallbladder diseases. Gastrointest Endosc 1998;48(4):406–410.
6. Hocke, M., Menges, M., Topalidis, T., Dietrich, C. F., Stallmach, A.: Contrast-enhanced endoscopic ultrasound in discrimination between benign and malignant mediastinal and abdominal lymph nodes. Journal of Cancer Research and Clinical Oncology 2008;134(4):473–480.
7. Kasono, K., Hyodo, T., Suminaga, Y., et al.: Contrast-enhanced endoscopic ultrasonography improves the preoperative localization of insulinomas. Endocrine Journal 2002;49(4):517–522.
8. Nomura, N., Goto, H., Niwa, Y., Arisawa, T., Hirooka, Y., Hayakawa, T.: Usefulness of contrast-enhanced EUS in the diagnosis of upper GI tract diseases. Gastrointest Endosc 1999;50(4):555–560.
9. Straub, J. A., Chickering, D. E., Church, C. C., Shah, B., Hanlon, T., Bernstein, H.: Porous PLGA microparticles: AI-700, an intravenously administered ultrasound contrast agent for use in echocardiography. J Control Release 2005;108(1):21–32.
10. Klibanov, A. L.: Ultrasound molecular imaging with targeted microbubble contrast agents. J Nucl Cardiol 2007;14(6):876–884.
11. Geiser, E. A., Buss, D. D., Wible, J. H., Jr., et al.: Evidence for a relation between inspired gas mixture and the left ventricular contrast achieved with Albunex in a canine model. Clinical Cardiology 1996;19(4):289–295.
12. Wolf K-J, Fobbe F.: Color Duplex Sonography Principles and Clinical Applications: New York: Thieme Publishing Group; 1995.

13. Quaia, E.: Microbubble ultrasound contrast agents: an update. European radiology 2007;17(8):1995–2008.
14. Greis, C., Dietrich, C. F.: Ultrasound contrast agents and contrast-enhanced ultrasonography. In Endoscopic Ultrasound—An Introductory Manual and Atlas, Dietrich C Ed., Thieme 2006; 44–59.
15. Campbell, S. C., Cullinan, J. A., Rubens, D. J.: Slow flow or no flow? Color and Power Doppler US pitfalls in the abdomen and pelvis. Radiographics 2004;24: 497–506.
16. Forsberg, F., Liu, J. B., Burns, P. N., Merton, D. A., Goldberg, B. B.: Artifacts in ultrasonic contrast agent studies. J Ultrasound Med 1994;13:357–365.
17. Dietrich, C. F., Ignee, A., Frey, H.L Contrast-enhanced endoscopic ultrasound with low mechanical index: a new technique. Z Gastroenterol 2005; 43:121–1223.
18. Kitano, M., Sakamoto, H., Matsui, U., et al.: A novel perfusion imaging technique of the pancreas: contrast-enhanced harmonic EUS (with video). Gastrointest Endosc 2008;67(1):141–150.
19. Micames, C. G., McCrory, D. C., Pavey, D. A., Jowell, P. S., Gress, F. G.: Endoscopic ultrasound-guided fine-needle aspiration for non-small cell lung cancer staging: A systematic review and metaanalysis. Chest 2007;131(2):539–548.
20. Yasuda, I., Tsurumi, H., Omar, S., et al.: Endoscopic ultrasound-guided fine-needle aspiration biopsy for lymphadenopathy of unknown origin. Endoscopy 2006;38(9):919–924.
21. Tournoy, K. G., Praet, M. M., Van Maele, G., Van Meerbeeck, J. P.: Esophageal endoscopic ultrasound with fine-needle aspiration with an on-site cytopathologist: high accuracy for the diagnosis of mediastinal lymphadenopathy. Chest 2005;128(4):3004–3009.
22. Kanamori, A., Hirooka, Y., Itoh, A., et al.: Usefulness of contrast-enhanced endoscopic ultrasonography in the differentiation between malignant and benign lymphadenopathy. The American journal of gastroenterology 2006;101(1):45–51.
23. Nakase, K., Yamamoto, K., Hiasa, A., Tawara, I., Yamaguchi, M., Shiku, H.: Contrast-enhanced ultrasound examination of lymph nodes in different types of lymphoma. Cancer detection and prevention 2006; 30(2):188–191.
24. Hirooka, Y., Naitoh, Y., Goto, H., Ito, A., Taki, T., Hayakawa, T.: Usefulness of contrast-enhanced endoscopic ultrasonography with intravenous injection of sonicated serum albumin. Gastrointest Endosc 1997; 46(2):166–169.
25. Wong, R., Tarcin, O., Reddy, N. K., et al.: Contrast-Enhanced EUS (CE-EUS) Using a New Microbubble Contrast Agent (MRX-815)—A Feasibility Study in a Porcine Model Gastroenterology Endoscopy 2006; 63(5):AB274.
26. Ohno, E., Hirooka, Y., Itoh, A., et al.: Usefulness of Contrast-Enhanced Endoscopic Ultrasonography for the Initial Diagnosis and Long-Term Follow-Up of Intraductal Papillary Mucinous Neoplasms of the Pancreas. Gastrointestinal Endoscopy 2007;65(5): T1577.
27. Ohno, E., Hirooka, Y. A. I. et al.: Usefulness of Contrast-Enhanced Endoscopic Ultrasonography (CE-EUS) in the Diagnosis of Mural Nodule of Intraductal Papillary Mucinous Neoplasms of the Pancreas. The Comparison of the CE-EUS Findings with the Pathological Findings. Gastrointestinal Endoscopy 2008;67(5):AB209.
28. Bhutani, M. S., Hoffman, B. J., van Velse, A., Hawes, R. H.: Contrast-enhanced endoscopic ultrasonography with galactose microparticles: SHU508 A (Levovist). Endoscopy 1997;29(7):635–639.
29. Becker, D., Strobel, D., Bernatik, T., Hahn, E. G.: Echo-enhanced color- and power-Doppler EUS for the discrimination between focal pancreatitis and pancreatic carcinoma. Gastrointest Endosc 2001;53(7): 784–789.
30. Ueno, N., Tomiyama, T., Tano, S., Wada, S., Aizawa, T., Kimura, K.: Utility of endoscopic ultrasonography with color Doppler function for the diagnosis of islet cell tumor. American Journal of Gastroenterology 1996; 91(4):772–776.
31. Săftoiu, A., Popescu, C., Cazacu, S., et al.: Power Doppler Endoscopic Ultrasonography for the Differential Diagnosis Between Pancreatic Cancer and Pseudotumoral Chronic Pancreatitis. J Ultrasound Med 2006; 25:363–372.
32. Giday, S. A., Canto, M. I., Magno, P., et al.: Contrast-Enhanced Endoscopic Ultrasonography (CE-EUS) Improves Visualization of Pancreatic Vasculature. Gastrointestinal Endoscopy 2006;63(5):AB266.
33. Rosch, T., Lorenz, R., Braig, C., Feuerbach, S., Siewert, J. R., Classen, M.: Endosonographic diagnosis of pancreatic tumors. Deutsche Medizinische Wochenschrift (1946) 1990;115(36):1339–1347.
34. Okamoto, Y., Kawamoto, H., Takaki, A., et al.: Contrast-enhanced ultrasonography depicts small tumor vessels for the evaluation of pancreatic tumors. European Journal of Radiology 2007;61(1):163–169.
35. Hocke, M., Schulze, E., Gottschalk, P., Topalidis, T., Dietrich, C. F.: Contrast-enhanced endoscopic ultrasound in discrimination between focal pancreatitis and pancreatic cancer. World J Gastroenterol 2006;12(2): 246–250.
36. Napoleon, B., Gincoul, R., Lefort, C., et al.: Contrast-enhanced endoscopic ultrasonography (CE-EUS) in solid tumors of the pancreas: results of a pilot study. Gastrointest Endosc 2008;67:AB202.
37. Hirooka, Y., Itoh, A., Kawashima, H., et al.: Utility of Contrast-Enhanced Endoscopic Ultrasonography (CE-EUS) in the Diagnosis of Pancreatic Diseases Using Perflubutane Microbubbles. Gastrointestinal Endoscopy 2008;67(5):AB214.
38. Ernst, H., Nusko, G., Hahn, E. G., Heyder, N.: Color Doppler endosonography of esophageal varices: signal enhancement after intravenous injection of the ultrasound contrast agent Levovist. Endoscopy 1997;29(7): S42–S43.
39. Giday, S. A., Ko, C. W., Clarke, J. O., et al.: EUS-guided portal vein carbon dioxide angiography: a pilot study in a porcine model. Gastrointestinal Endoscopy 2007; 66(4):814–819.
40. Ohshima, T., Yamaguchi, T., Takeshi, I., et al.: Evaluation of bloody flow in pancreatic ducal carcinoma using contrast-enhanced, wide-band Doppler ultrasonography. Correlation with tumor characteristics and vascular endothelial growth factor. Pancreas 2004; 28: 335–343
41. Lassau, N., Brule, A., Chami, L., Benatsou, B., Péronneau, P., Roche, A.: Evaluation of early response to antiangiogenic treatment with dynamic contrast enhanced ultrasound. J Radiol 2008; 89: 549–555.
42. Lyshchik, A., Fleischer, A. C., Huamani, J., Hallahan, D. E., Brissova, M., Gore, J. C.: Molecular imaging of vascular endothelial growth factor receptor 2 expression

using targeted contrast-enhanced high-frequency ultrasonography. J Ultrasound Med 2007;26(11):1575–1586.
43. Palmowski, M., Huppert, J., Ladewig, G., et al.: Molecular profiling of angiogenesis with targeted ultrasound imaging: early assessment of antiangiogenic therapy effects. Mol Cancer Ther 2008;7(1):101–109.
44. Willmann, J. K., Lutz, A. M., Paulmurugan, R., Patel, M. R., Chu, P., Rosenberg, J., Gambhir, S. S.: Dual-targeted contrast agent for US assessment of tumor angiogenesis in vivo. Radiology 2008;248(3):936–944.
45. Postema, M., Gilja, O. H.: Ultrasound-directed drug delivery. Curr Pharm Biotechnol 2007;8(6):355–361.

Index

Figures are denoted by *f*; tables by *t*.

A

Abdominoperineal resection, 337, 340
Abscess
  anorectal (perirectal), 345–353
    horseshoe, 352*f*
    inflammatory bowel disease-related, 398
    intersphincteric, 346, 350*f*, 351*f*
    ischorectal, 346, 350*f*, 352*f*
    perianal, 346, 350*f*, 352*f*
    submucosal, 350*f*
    supralevatoric, 346, 350*f*, 352*f*
    surgical drainage of, 346
  pelvic, 372
  prostatic, 389
  splenic, 303–304, 304*f*
Adenocarcinoma
  ampullary, 280*f*
    differentiated from pancreatic head cancer, 278, 278*f*
  cholangiocarcinoma as, 293
  colonic/colorectal, 379
    metastatic to the liver, 294, 295*f*
  esophageal, 20, 22*f*
    pleural effusions associated with, 327*f*
  of the gallbladder, 264–265, 269–271*f*
    contrast-enhanced EUS of, 415
  gastric
    contrast-enhanced EUS of, 417*f*
    as large gastric folds cause, 58*t*, 59*t*
    with lymph node metastases, 51*f*
    surgical resection of, 50
  of the gastroesophageal junction, 50
  metastatic, 143*f*
    to the liver, 157*f*, 294, 294*f*, 295*f*, 296*f*
    to the spleen, 309*f*
  pancreatic, 156
    contrast-enhanced EUS of, 416, 418*f*
    with liver metastases, 157*f*
  as mortality cause, 150
  staging of, 158*f*
  prostatic, 391, 393*f*
  pulmonary
    cytological features of, 134
    metastatic, 143*f*
Adenoma
  adrenal metastatic, 315
  ampullary, 277–278, 277*f*, 279*f*
    endoscopic removal of, 283
  of the bile ducts, 288
  colonic, 378–379
    malignant degeneration of, 376, 378, 379, 383
    tubular, 376, 376*f*
    tubulovillous, 376, 377*f*
    villous, 376, 377*f*, 379*f*
  of the gallbladder, 264, 267–268*f*, 269*f*
  liver cell, 288, 290*f*, 291*f*
  pancreatic
    as chronic pancreatitis cause, 151, 152*f*
    differential diagnosis of, 151, 153
    real-time elastography of, 407, 408*f*
  rectal, 379
  superficial villous rectal, 337
Adenomyomatosis, 259–260, 262*f*, 263–264*f*
  coexistent with anomalous pancreaticobiliary junction, 232–233
Ad.IL-12, 161
Adrenal glands
  identification of, 314–315, 314*f*
  lesions of, 313–317
    adenoma, 315
    EUS-guided fine-needle aspiration biopsy of, 316, 317*f*
    metastatic disease of, 316, 316*f*
    real-time elastography of, 408
    Trucut biopsy of, 316–317
  morphology of, 315, 316*f*
  Visible Human Data Set Models of, 218*f*, 314*f*, 315*f*
Adventitia, in esophageal cancer, 27*f*
Albunex, 414, 415
Ampulla of Vater, 273–286
  benign lesions, 275–277
  common bile duct lesions adjacent to, 250, 251*f*
  definition of, 274
  edema of, 277*f*
  EUS evaluation of, 251*f*, 274–275
  fibrosis and stenosing papillitis of, 275–276
  inflammatory lesions of, 275–277
  interventional EUS of, 283–285, 284*f*
  malignant lesions of, 277–282, 277–282*f*
    adencarcinoma, 278, 278*f*, 280*f*
    endoscopic management of, 282–283
    EUS-guided fine-needle aspiration biopsy of, 281
    intraductal ultrasonography of, 279
    tumors, 277–278
  mucus secretion from, 192*f*, 194
  normal, 276*f*
  surgical removal of, 283
  Visible Human Data Set Model of, 275*f*
Ampullectomy, 283
  with methylene blue pancreatic stenting, 283–285, 284*f*
Amyloidosis, as large gastric folds cause, 58*t*
Anal canal
  distal, 350*f*
  layers of, 350*f*, 356*f*
  normal ultrasound anatomy of, 362*f*, 364*f*
  Visible Human Data Set Models of, 336*f*, 349*f*
Anal sphincters
  defects of, 361–368
    magnetic resonance imaging of, 367

Anal sphincters *(continued)*
  external, Visible Human Data Set Models of, 346*f*, 347*f*, 349*f*
  internal, Visible Human Data Set Models of, 346*f*, 348*f*, 349*f*
  normal ultrasound anatomy of, 363*f*
  preservation in abdominoperineal resection, 337, 340
Anastomotic sites, gastric cancer of, 54*f*
Aneurysm
  aortic, 111, 112*f*
  of the celiac artery, 113, 114*f*
  of the splenic artery, 113, 114*f*, 115, 115*f*
Angiogenic factors, 417–418
Angioma, littoral cell, 306, 306*f*
Angiosarcoma, hepatic, 294
Anisakiasis, as large gastric folds cause, 58*t*, 59*t*, 60, 72
Anorectum. *See also* Anal canal; Anal sphincters; Anus; Rectum
  anatomy of
    in females, 336, 337*f*
    in males, 336, 336*f*
Ansa pancreatica, 229*f*
Antibiotic prophylaxis, for fine-needle aspiration biopsy, 81, 301, 330
Antibiotic therapy, for MALT lymphoma, 64, 65
Anus. *See also* Abscess, anorectal (perirectal); Anal canal; Anal sphincters; Fistulae, anorectal
  elevator, 391*f*
Aorta
  accessory, 108
  ascending, Visible Human Data Set Model of, 108*f*
  calcification of, 112*f*
  in esophageal cancer, 27*f*
  in lung cancer, 134
  primary lung cancer adjacent to, 133*f*
  Visible Human Data Set Models of, 2, 3, 108*f*, 139*f*, 151*f*, 167*f*
Aortic arches, 108*f*
  anomalies of, 108–111, 109*f*, 110*f*
  right-sided, 108, 109, 110, 110*f*
  normal, 111*f*
  Visible Human Data Set Model of, 111*f*
Arterial tree, 108*f*
Ascites
  malignant, 326
    gastric cancer-related, 50, 54*f*
    pancreatic adenocarcinoma-related, 329*f*
    prognostic and therapeutic implications of, 330
    tumors markers for, 329

portal vein thrombosis-related, 320, 321*f*
  transduodenal, 326, 329*f*
Aspergillosis, as large gastric folds cause, 58*t*
Atherosclerotic plaques, 111, 112*f*
Azygous vein, Visible Human Data Set Models of, 100*f*, 328*f*

B
Barrett's esophagus
  definition of, 20
  dysplasia associated with, 15–16, 20–22, 21*f*
  EUS-assisted staging of
    high-frequency probes for, 11
    overstaging in, 15
  intramucosal carcinoma associated with, 22*f*
Benign prostate hyperplasia (BPH), 388–389, 388*f*
Bile ducts. *See also* Common bile duct
  adenomas of, 288
  ampullary tumors of, 281*f*, 283
  benign lesions of, 243–248
  cholangiocarcinoma of, 249–256
  cystic, 238, 239*f*
  gallstones (choledocholithiasis) of, 245–248, 277
  hamartomas of, 288
  malignant lesions of, 249–256
  strictures of
    autoimmune pancreatitis-related, 215, 216, 216*f*, 220
    cholangiocarcinoma-related, 249–256
    misdiagnosed as cholangiocarcinoma, 216*f*
  Visible Human Data Set Models of, 245*f*, 258*f*, 259*f*
Biliary system, embryological development of, 226
Biliary tree
  magnetic resonance cholangiopancreatography of, 244–245, 244*f*
  relationship to the liver, 259*f*
  Visible Human Data Set Models of, 166*f*, 234–235*f*, 244–245, 244*f*, 250*f*, 258*f*
Biopsy. *See also* Fine-needle aspiration biopsy, EUS-guided
  EUS-guided core needle
    of gastrointestinal stromal tumors (GIST), 86–87, 88*f*
    of gastrointestinal subepithelial lesions, 81
  stacked forceps, of gastrointestinal subepithelial lesions, 82
  Trucut
    of adrenal lesions, 316–317

of autoimmune pancreatitis, 215, 217, 218*f*, 219, 221–222
    of chronic pancreatitis, 208
    of mediastinal cysts, 121
    of mediastinal masses and lesions, 119, 126
    of pancreatic cancer, 178, 179–181, 180*f*
Blastomycosis, 121
Brachiocephalic artery, Visible Human Data Set Models of, 108*f*, 130*f*
Brachiocephalic vein, left, Visible Human Data Set Model of, 130*f*
Breast cancer
  metastatic, 90
    as large gastric folds cause, 66
    to the liver, 294
    to the mediastinum, 124
    to the pancreas, 151, 153*f*, 174, 174*t*
    to the pleura, 326
  palpation of, 404
Bronchial tree, Visible Human Data Set Model of, 139*f*
"Bubble test," 236, 237, 238*f*
Budd-Chiari syndrome, 84

C
Calcification
  aortic, 112*f*
  cavernous hemangioma-related, 288, 290*f*
  of the celiac artery, 111, 113*f*, 114*f*
  prostatic, 393, 393*f*
  of the superior mesenteric artery, 111, 113*f*, 114*f*
Carcinoembryonic antigen (CEA), as malignant effusion tumor marker, 329, 330
Carcinoid syndrome, 381–382
Carcinoid tumors
  colorectal, 381–383, 382*f*
  duodenal, 171, 172*f*
  gastric, 171, 171*f*
    presenting as subepithelial lesions, 87–88, 89*f*
  metastatic to the liver, 297*f*
Carotid artery
  left, Visible Human Data Set Models of, 108*f*, 130*f*
  right, Visible Human Data Set Model of, 108*f*
Celiac artery
  aneurysm of, 113, 114*f*
  bifurcation of, Visible Human Data Set Model of, 151*f*
  calcification and obstruction of, 111, 113*f*, 114*f*
  pancreatic cancer adjacent to, 178*f*
  pancreatic cancer invasion of, 153

relationship to the esophagus, 26f
Visible Human Data Set Models of, 108f, 151f
Center for Human Simulation, 2, 3
Cervix, Visible Human Data Set Models of, 337f, 370f
Chemotherapy, contrast-enhanced EUS-assisted, 418
Childbirth, as anal sphincter injury cause, 363, 365f, 386f
Children
  colonic polyps in, 377
  portal vein thrombosis in, 320
Cholangiocarcinoma, 249–256
  bile duct strictures misdiagnosed as, 216f
  biliary, 232
  coexistent with
    anomalous pancreaticobiliary junction, 232–233
    hepatocellular carcinoma, 293
  curvilinear endoscopic evaluation of, 250, 252
  endoscopic cholangiopancreatography of, 251, 253, 253f, 255f
  EUS-guided fine-needle aspiration biopsy of, 252, 252f, 253f, 254–256
  immunohistochemistry of, 252f
  intraductal ultrasound of, 251–252, 253–254
  intrahepatic, 292–293, 293f
  magnetic resonance cholangiopancreatography of, 253, 255–256f
  radial endoscopic evaluation of, 250–251, 251f, 252
Cholangitis, 277f
  acute, 245
  recurrent, 292–293
  sclerosing, 276
Cholecystectomy, papillary stenosis after, 276
Cholecystitis, 260, 264, 265f, 266f
  chronic, 260, 264, 265f
  pericholecystic fluid associated with, 326
  xanthogranulomatous, 264, 266f
Choledochocele, 233, 235–236, 237, 238, 253f
  type I, 253f
Choledocholithiasis, 245–248, 276f, 277
  computed tomography of, 246
  endoscopic retrograde cholangiopancreatography of, 244–246, 247f, 248
  intraductal ultrasound of, 248
  magnetic resonance cholangiopancreatography of, 247–248
  treatment of, 245–246
Choledochopancreatic junction, 274

Cholesterolosis, 259, 260f, 261f
  as ampullary papillitis cause, 276
Ciprofloxacin, 330
Cirrhosis
  as gastric varices cause, 71
  as portal vein thrombosis cause, 320
Clonorchis sinensis, 292–293
Coccidiomycosis, 119
Coccyx, Visible Human Data Set Models of, 336f, 346f, 347f, 348f
Colitis, ulcerative, 398t, 399
  anorectal fistulae associated with, 359
  differentiated from Crohn's disease, 400
  muscularis propria involvement in, 398–399f, 400
Colon cancer. *See also* Colorectal cancer
  management of, 337
  metastatic
    to the liver, 294, 295f
    to the mediastinum, 124
    to the pancreas, 151
    to the spleen, 306, 309f, 310
Colorectal cancer. *See also* Rectal cancer
  colonic adenoma-related, 376, 378, 379
  metastatic
    to the ovary, 371f, 372f
    to the pancreas, 174
  subepithelial, 380–383, 380t
    carcinoid tumors, 381–383
    fibrosarcomas, 381
    gastrointestinal stromal tumors (GISTs), 380
    leiomyomas/leiomyosarcomas, 380–381, 381f
    lipomas, 381, 382f
    lymphangiomas, 383
    paragangliomas, 381
    schwannomas, 381
Colorectal lesions, 375–385
  colonic adenomas, 376–379
  colonic polyps, 376–379
    classification of, 376, 376f, 377
Common bile duct
  in autoimmune pancreatitis, 161f
  cholangiocarcinoma of, 249–256
  cholestasis-related microstones in, 278
  computed tomography of, 246
  debris/sludge in, 246
  differentiated from the gallbladder, 253f
  dilation of, 151, 244, 253f
  EUS examination of, 243–248, 276–277
  gallstones in, 276f

magnetic resonance cholangiopancreatography of, 247–248
metastatic cancer of, 151
microlithiasis of, 246, 247f
obstruction of, 244
  ampullary inflammation-related, 276f, 277, 277f
  ampullary neoplasia-related, 278
  posterior-to-anterior view of, 244–245
short, 238, 239f
small lesions of, 250
stenting of, 246f
stones in, 244
strictures of
  benign differentiated from malignant, 254–256
  malignant. *See* Cholangiocarcinoma
Visible Human Data Set Models of, 151f, 175f, 250–251f, 275f
Computed tomography (CT)
  of advanced pancreatic cancer, 26
  of aortic arch anomalies, 110
  of choledolithiasis, 246
  of the common bile duct, 246
  of esophageal cancer, 8, 17
  of gastric cancer, 51, 52f, 60
  of lung cancer, 130f, 138, 143
  of mediastinal lymph nodes and masses, 138, 143
  of pancreatic cancer, 150, 151–156, 152f, 153f, 154f, 155f, 158–160, 161, 174, 175, 176f, 177f
Contrast agents, use in EUS, 413–421
  action mechanism of, 414
  current applications of, 414–417
  future applications of, 417–418
Crohn's disease
  anorectal abscesses associated with, 346, 352f
  anorectal fistulae associated with, 359, 359f
  differentiated from ulcerative colitis, 400
  as large gastric folds cause, 58t
  perirectal and perianal complications of, 398
Cronkhite-Canada syndrome, 378
"Crossed duct/stack sign," 226, 230f
Cryptococcosis, as large gastric folds cause, 58t
Cystadenoma, serous, 184t, 185, 193
Cysts/cystic lesions
  biliary (choledochal), 233–236, 233–236f
    classification of, 233
    coexistent with anomalous pancreaticobiliary junction, 231, 232–233

Cysts/cystic lesions *(continued)*
　embryological origin of, 226
　Visible Human Data Set Models of, 234–235*f*
　duplication
　　duodenal, 236–237, 238*f*
　　esophageal, 121, 122*f*
　　presenting as subepithelial lesions, 82*t*, 85, 86*f*
　EUS-guided fine-needle aspiration biopsy of, 81
　gastritis cystica profunda-related, 72, 73*f*
　hepatic, 291, 291*f*
　mediastinal, 121–122, 122*f*, 127*t*
　neuroendocrine tumor-related, 169, 169*f*
　neuroenteric, 121
　pancreatic, 183–189
　　chronic pancreatitis-associated, 210*f*, 212
　　cystic endocrine tumors, 184*t*, 187–188m 187*f*
　　demographics and characteristics of, 184*t*
　　differential diagnosis of, 193–194, 195*t*
　　EUS-guided fine-needle aspiration biopsy of, 184, 210*f*
　　intraductal papillary mucinous tumors, 184*t*, 185, 187*f*, 188, 191–204
　　lymphoepithelial cysts, 188*f*
　　mucinous cystic tumors, 184*t*, 185–186, 186*f*, 188, 193
　　pseudocysts, 185, 185*t*, 193
　　serous cystadenomas, 184*t*, 185*t*, 193
　　solid pseudopapillary neoplasm, 184*t*, 185–186
　　presenting as subepithelial lesions, 85, 86*f*
　prostatic, 389, 389*f*
Cytomegalovirus infections
　as large gastric folds cause, 58*t*, 69, 70, 72
　as Menetrier's disease cause, 69, 70

D

Diaphragm, in gastric cancer, 54*f*
Dieulafoy lesions, 115–116, 115*f*
Digital Human Anatomy and Endoscopic Ultrasonography (Spitzer and Reinig), 2
Diverticula, duodenal, 227
Doppler ultrasound, contrast-enhanced, of pancreatic lesions, 416, 417*f*, 418*f*, 419*f*
Dorsal duct syndrome, 226
Drug delivery, ultrasound-assisted, 418

Duct of Santorini
　embryological development of, 226
　Visible Human Data Set Model of, 227*f*
Duct of Wirsung
　embryological development of, 226
　Visible Human Data Set Model of, 227*f*
Duodenal bulb, ascites adjacent to, 327, 328*f*, 329*f*
Duodenum
　ampullary tumor invasion of, 278, 282*f*
　diverticula of, 227
　duplication cyst-related obstruction of, 236
　gastrinomas of, 70
　metastatic cancer of, 151
　neuroendocrine tumors adjacent to, 170–171, 171*f*
　Visible Human Data Set Models of, 151*f*, 166*f*, 167*f*, 175*f*, 227*f*, 228*f*, 244–245, 244*f*
"Dypsphagia lusoria," 108
Dysplasia, esophageal, 15–16, 20–22, 21*f*

E

Echoendoscopes, types of, 244
　endobronchial ultrasound (EBUS), 141*f*
　endoscopic ultrasound (EUS), 141*f*
Echogen, 414
Echovist, 414
Ejaculatory duct complex, 389, 391
Elastography, EUS, 403–411
　real-time, 404–409
　　applications of, 404, 406–409, 407*f*, 408*f*, 409*f*
　　method of, 404–407, 405*f*, 406*f*
　3-D applications of, 409
　"virtual," 409, 409*f*
Endocrine tumors, cystic pancreatic, 184*t*, 187–188, 187*f*
Endometriosis, 372–374, 372*t*, 373*f*, 383
　EUS-guided fine-needle aspiration biopsy of, 373–374, 373*f*
Endoscopic mucosal dissection (EDR), of gastrointestinal subepithelial lesions, 82
Endoscopic mucosal resection (EMR)
　of esophageal adenocarcinoma, 20
　of esophageal dysplasia, 20
　of gastrointestinal subepithelial lesions, 82
　of pancreatic rests, 85, 85*f*
　of rectal villous adenomas, 337

Endoscopic retrograde cholangiopancreatography (ERCP). *See also* Magnetic resonance cholangiopancreatography (MRCP)
　of anomalous pancreaticobiliary junction, 232, 232*f*
　of autoimmune pancreatitis, 215, 215*f*, 221, 221*t*
　of bile ducts, 244–245
　　biliary cysts, 233
　　cholangiocarcinoma, 251, 253, 253*f*
　　choledocholithiasis, 245–246, 247*f*
　of duodenal duplication cysts, 237
　of extrahepatic biliary anomalies, 238, 239*f*
　failure of, 283, 284
　of intraductal papillary mucinous tumors, 194, 196*f*
　of pancreas divisum, 226
　of pancreatic agenesis, 233
　of pancreatic cancer, 158
Endoscopic therapy, for early gastric cancer, 45
Endoscopic ultrasonography (EUS)
　complications of, 161
　introduction of, 50
　overview of, 1–3
Enteritis granulomatosis. *See* Crohn's disease
Enterochromaffin-like (ECL) cells, 70
Epitheloid cell granuloma, 301*f*
Esophageal cancer
　definition of, 8*t*
　metastatic
　　to the liver, 294
　　to the mediastinum, 124
　as mortality cause, 8
　mucosal, differentiated from submucosal, 22
　real-time elastography of, 408
　relative avascularity of, 415
　submucosal, differentiated from mucosal, 22
　survival rate in, 8, 8*t*
Esophageal cancer, advanced, 25–32
　EUS-assisted staging of, 26–32
　　of adventitial metastases, 27*f*
　　after neoadjuvant radiochemotherapy, 29–30
　　of aortic metastases, 27*f*
　　comparison with computed tomography, 26
　　comparison with positron emission tomography, 26
　　of lymph node metastases, 28–29, 28*f*
　　M-staging, 29
　　muscularis propria in, 27*f*
　　N-staging, 28–29
　　of pleural metastases, 27*f*

radial *versus* linear scanners in, 26–27, 27*f*, 28*f*
in squamous cell carcinoma, 28*f*
in stricturing tumors, 29
T-staging, 27, 27*f*, 28*f*, 30
incidence of, 26
as mortality cause, 26
prevalence of, 8
Visible Human Data Set Models of, 26–27, 26*f*
Esophageal cancer, early, 7–18
EUS-assisted staging of, 8–15
accuracy of, 13, 16*t*, 17
comparison with computed tomography, 8, 17
dedicated endoscope use in, 11, 11*t*
equipment for, 10–11, 10*t*
factors affecting, 9–11
high-frequency probe use in, 10–11, 11*t*, 13, 15*f*, 16, 16*t*, 17
of mucosal cancer, 12, 14*f*, 16–17
nomenclature of, 12, 12*t*
operator expertise in, 9
over- or understaging in, 15, 16, 29
"Salami Effect" in, 9
of submucosal cancer, 12, 13*f*, 14*f*, 15*f*, 16, 17
technique, 9–10
photodynamic therapy (PAT) for, 8
subclassification of, 12, 12*f*, 13*f*
submucosal dissection of (ESD), 8
treatment of, 9
Esophageal-gastric junction, venous system of, 102, 102*f*
Esophageal varices
contrast-enhanced EUS of, 417
portal-systemic collateral venous system of, 96–103, 99–103*f*
Doppler endoscopic ultrasound of, 96
portal vein thrombosis-related, 320
Esophageal wall
layers of, 415
metastases to, 90, 91*f*
normal, 20*f*
Esophagectomy, 15, 20
Esophagus. *See also* Barrett's esophagus
aspiration of lung tumors from, 131
duplication cysts of, 121, 122*f*
granular cell tumors of, 90, 90*f*
leiomyoma of, 83, 86
pleural fibrosis-related displacement of, 111, 112*f*
primary lung cancer adjacent to, 130, 130*f*, 131*f*
relationship to
celiac artery, 26*f*
lymph nodes, 26*f*
pleura, 326, 327*f*
Visible Human Data Set Models of, 130*f*, 139*f*, 149*f*
EUS. *See* Endoscopic ultrasonography (EUS)

F

Fecal incontinence, 363, 364*f*, 365–368
Fibroma, presenting as intramural subepithelial lesion, 82*t*
Fibrosarcoma, colorectal, 381
Fine-needle aspiration biopsy, EUS-guided
accuracy of, effect of chronic pancreatitis on, 160–161
of adrenal lesions, 316, 317*f*
of advanced esophageal cancer, 29, 30
of autoimmune pancreatitis, 217, 219, 221
of cholangiocarcinoma, 252, 252*f*, 253*f*, 254–256
complications of, 81
of cysts, 81
of early gastric cancer, 44
of gastrointestinal stromal tumors (GIST), 81, 86–87, 87*f*, 380
of gastrointestinal subepithelial lesions, 81
of glomus tumors, 89
as infection cause, 330
of large gastric folds, 59, 59*f*
of linitis plastica, 68
of lung cancer, 129–134, 130*f*, 131–133*f*, 135
false-negative results in, 133
non-small-cell lung cancer, 139, 143
of lymphoma, 88
mediastinal, 118, 118*f*, 414–415
of lymphoma, 124, 126
of malignant lesions, 122, 123*t*
of mediastinal cysts, 121, 122
as mediastinitis cause, 121, 122
in tuberculosis, 121
of neuroendocrine tumors, 166, 166*f*
of pancreatic cancer, 158, 160–161
of pancreatic cysts, 210*f*
of pancreatic intraductal papillary mucinous tumors, 192, 199–200, 199*f*, 200*f*
of pancreatic metastases, 174–175, 174–175*t*, 176, 176*f*, 177*f*, 178, 179–180
of pleural effusions, 326, 327*f*, 329–330
real-time elastography-guided, 406*f*
of rectal cancer, 339
risks of, 126
of splenic lesions, 300–310
Fine-needle aspiration injection (FNI), as pancreatic cancer treatment, 161–162
Fistulae
anorectal, 355–360
definition of, 356
extrasphincteric, 356, 356*f*, 357*f*
intersphincteric, 356, 356*f*, 357*f*, 358*f*
magnetic resonance imaging of, 356
peroxide-enhanced EUS of, 356, 358*f*
superficial, 359*f*
suprasphincteric, 356, 356*f*
3-D EUS of, 356
transperianal ultrasound (TPUS) of, 359
transsphincteric, 356, 356*f*, 357*f*, 358*f*
Crohn's disease-associated, 359, 359*f*
pelvic, 372
Fungal infections. *See also specific fungal infections*
as large gastric folds cause, 58*t*

G

Gallbladder, 257–272
adenomyomatosis of, 232–233, 259–260, 262*f*, 263–264*f*
cholecystitis of, 260, 264, 265*f*, 266*f*
cholesterolosis/cholesterol polyps of, 259, 260*f*, 261*f*
differentiated from common bile ducts, 253*f*
enlarged, as subepithelial lesion cause, 80*f*
EUS examination of, 276–277
inflammatory polyps of, 264, 267–268*f*
"strawberry," 260*f*
Visible Human Data Set Models of, 250–251*f*, 258*f*
Gallbladder cancer
adenocarcinoma, 264–265, 269–271*f*
adenoma, 264, 267–268*f*, 269*f*
coexistent with anomalous pancreaticobiliary junction, 232–233
contrast-enhanced EUS of, 415
Gallbladder wall, normal, 258
Gallstones
as ampullary papillitis cause, 276, 276*f*
of the bile ducts (choledocholithiasis), 245–248
chronic cholecystitis-related, 260
coexistent with anomalous pancreaticobiliary junction, 232–233
Gastrectomy, Bilroth II, 160

Gastric artery, left, Visible Human Data Set Model of, 108f
Gastric cancer
  adenocarcinoma
    contrast-enhanced EUS of, 417f
    as large gastric folds cause, 58t, 59t
    with lymph node metastases, 51f
    surgical resection of, 50
  ascites associated with, 328f
  computed tomography of, 51, 52f, 60
  contrast-enhanced EUS of, 415, 418f
  diagnostic criteria for, 37, 41f
  differentiated from large gastric folds, 60
  incidence of, 34, 50
  as large gastric folds cause, 58t, 59
  lymphoma
    B-cell, 88
    diagnosis and staging of, 65
    differentiated from Menetrier's disease, 69
    EUS-guided fine-needle aspiration biopsy of, 88
    gastric carcinoma associated with, 62, 63f
    immunohistochemistry of, 64f
    large B-cell, 62
    as large gastric folds cause, 58t, 59t, 60, 62–66
    mantle cell, 62, 63f
    non-Hodgkin's, 62
    presenting as subepithelial lesions, 88
    staging of, 60–61
    staging systems for, 61, 61t, 62t
    T-cell, 62
  magnetic resonance imaging of, 51
  metastatic
    to the pancreas, 151
    to the spleen, 309f
  as mortality cause, 50
  mucosal lesions of, 36
  overstaging of, 60
  positron emission tomography of, 51, 53f
  real-time elastography of, 408
  submucosal lesions of, 36
  survival rates in, 34
  TNM staging of, 60, 61t
    M-staging, 50
    N-staging, 50
    T-staging, 50
Gastric cancer, advanced, 38f, 49–56
  ascites associated with, 54f
  diaphragmatic involvement in, 54f
  differentiated from early gastric cancer, 51, 60
  endoscopic views of, 40f
  with lymph node metastases, 51, 51f, 52f
  muscularis propria in, 36, 37
  N1 stage of, 50
  N2 stage of, 50
  N3 stage of, 50
  overstaging of, 40–41, 41f, 43f, 44f, 45f
  prognosis for, 50
  recurrent, 54f
  surgical anastomotic sites in, 54f
  surgical treatment for, 50
  survival rate in, 50
  Visible Human Data Set Models of, 53f
Gastric cancer, early, 33–48
  definition of, 33
  diagnostic criteria for, 37, 42f
  differentiated from advanced gastric cancer, 51, 60
  endoscopic therapy for, 45
  EUS-based detection and staging of
    EUS-guided fine-needle aspiration biopsy of, 44
    instruments for, 34–35
    literature summary of, 42t
    miniprobe use in, 34–35, 35t
    N-staging, 37
    radial *versus* linear scanner use in, 34
    radial videoscope examination of, 43–44
    staging errors in, 45t
    technique, 35, 36f
    3-D EUS, 47
    T1 stage, 37–38
    T-staging, 37–38
    understaging, 41–42f
  lymph node metastases of, 42–44
  mucosal, 34, 37–38, 38f, 39f
  muscularis mucosa in, 45, 47
  submucosal, 34, 37–38, 39f, 40f, 46t
Gastric folds, large, 57–77
  amyloidosis-related, 58t
  anisakiasis-related, 58t, 59t, 60
  aspergillosis-related, 58t
  barium upper GI (UGI) series of, 58f
  blastomycosis-related, 121
  coccidiomycosis-related, 119
  cryptococcosis-related, 58t
  cytomegalovirus infections-related, 58t, 69, 70, 72
  diagnostic criteria for, 58t
  differential diagnosis of, 58–60
  differentiated from gastric cancer, 60
  etiology of, 58–59, 58t
  gastric adenocarcinoma-related, 58t, 59t
  Helicobacter pylori infection-related, 58, 59t, 60, 69, 70, 72, 73f
  linitis plastica, 60, 66, 68, 69f
  linitis plastica-related, 58f, 59t, 60, 66, 68, 69f
  Zollinger-Ellison syndrome-related, 70, 71f
Gastric varices
  biopsy-related hemorrhage of, 71, 72f
  cirrhosis-associated, 71
  classification of, 71, 72t
  as contraindication to endoscopic biopsy, 59
  esophageal varices associated with, 71
  hemodynamics of, 99f
  as large gastric folds cause, 58t, 59t, 71
  portal hypertension associated with, 71
    venous collaterals in, 103–105, 104–105f
  portal vein thrombosis-related, 320, 322f
  presenting as subepithelial lesions, 82, 84f
Gastric veins
  left, 98, 99f, 105
  post, 98, 105
  short, 98, 98f, 99f, 105
  Visible Human Data Set Model of, 97–98f
Gastric wall
  ascites adjacent to, 328f
  layers of, 244, 415
  linitis plastica of, 66, 68, 68f, 69f
  metastases to, 90
  normal, 35–36, 37f, 58f
Gastrinoma
  duodenal, 171, 172f
  location of, 166
  as Zollinger-Ellison syndrome cause, 70
Gastrinoma triangle, 166, 166f
Gastritis
  Helicobacter pylori infection-related, 72, 73f
  hyperrugosity, as large gastric folds cause, 58t, 59t
  as large gastric folds cause, 58t, 59t, 60, 72, 73f
  lymphocytic, differentiated from Menetrier's disease, 60
Gastritis cystica profunda, as large gastric folds cause, 58t, 59t, 72, 73f
Gastroduodenal artery, pancreatic cancer adjacent to, 157f
Gastroesophageal junction
  adenocarcinoma of, 50
  anatomy of, 20, 20f
Gastrointestinal stromal tumors (GIST), 82t, 86–87, 87f
  accessory spleen misdiagnosed as, 311
  of ampulla of Vater, 277

benign, 380
colorectal, 380
differentiated from glomus tumors, 89
EUS-guided core biopsy of, 86–87, 88f
EUS-guided fine-needle aspiration biopsy of, 81, 86–87, 87f, 380
immunohistochemical staining of, 81, 90t, 380, 381f
malignant, 380
malignant potential of, 86
metastatic to the liver, 294, 296f
misclassification as leiomyoma or leiomyosarcoma, 83, 86
real-time elastography of, 408
Gastrointestinal wall, layers of, 81, 81t
Gastro-renal shunt, 105
Genitourinary tract cancers. *See also* Gynecological lesions; Ovarian cancer
metastatic to the liver, 294
Giant cell carcinoma, 132f
Glomus tumors
EUS-guided fine-needle aspiration biopsy of, 89
immunohistochemical staining of, 81, 89
metastatic, 88–89
differentiated from gastrointestinal stromal tumors, 89
presenting as subepithelial lesions, 82t, 88–89
Glucogonoma, 167–168, 168f
Granular cell tumors, 90, 90f
Granuloma
epithelioid cell, 301f
of mediastinal lymph nodes, 119–120, 121, 121f
Gynecological lesions, 369–400
endometriosis, 372–374, 372t, 373f
ovarian cancer
metastatic, 90
of metastatic origin, 371f, 372f
pelvic inflammatory disorders, 372–374
pelvic tumors, 371–372, 371f

H

Hamartoma, of the bile ducts, 288
Harmonic imaging, contrast-enhanced, 416–417
Helicobacter pylori infections, 58, 59t, 60
eradication of, 64, 70
as gastritis cause, 72, 73f
as large gastric folds cause, 58, 59t, 60, 69, 70, 72, 73f
as Menetrier's disease cause, 69, 70
Hemangioendothelioma, epithelioid, 294
Hemangioma

cavernous, 288, 290f
splenic, 304, 305f, 306, 306f
Hemiazygous vein, Visible Human Data Set Model of, 100f
Hemorrhoidal veins, 336
Hemorrhoidectomy, as anal sphincter injury cause, 363, 365f
Hepatic arteries
common, Visible Human Data Set Model of, 108f
in pancreatic cancer, 153
Hepatic duct
aberrant right, 238, 240f
Visible Human Data Set Model of, 250–251f
Hepatocellular carcinoma, 292f
coexistent with cholangiocarcinoma, 293
definition of, 291
differentiated from liver cell adenoma, 288
fibrolamellar, 292
metastatic, to the spleen, 179
morphologic variations of, 291–292
as portal vein thrombosis cause, 320
Herpes simplex virus infections, as large gastric folds cause, 58t
Histoplasmosis
as large gastric folds cause, 58t
mediastinal, 119, 121, 121f
Hydrogen peroxide injection, 356, 358f
Hyperplasia
benign prostate (BPH), 388–389, 388f
hepatic focal nodular, 288, 290f
Hypertension, portal, 320, 417
esophageal and gastric varices-related, 71, 84, 95–104
large gastric folds associated with, 58t

I

Immunohistochemistry
of cholangiocarcinoma, 252f
of gastric lymphoma, 64f
of gastrointestinal stromal tumors, 86, 87f, 90t, 380, 381f
of glomus tumors, 89, 90t
of granular cell tumors, 90
of hypoechoic intramural masses, 81
of leiomyoma, 83
of pancreatic metastases, 178–179, 178f, 179f
of primary lung cancer, 134
of schwannomas, 90t
of smooth muscle tumors, 90t
Infarction, splenic, 304, 305f
Infection
fine-needle aspiration biopsy-related, 330
as large gastric folds cause, 58t
as portal vein thrombosis cause, 320

Inferior mesenteric vein, Visible Human Data Set Model of, 196f
Inferior vena cava, Visible Human Data Set Models of, 151f, 196f, 275f, 314f, 315f
Inflammatory bowel disease, 397–400
Insulinoma, 167, 167f, 168, 168f
Interleukin-12 adenoviral vector (ad.IL.12), 161
Intersphincteric space, 350f
Intraductal papillary mucinous tumors (IPMTs), of the pancreas, 191–204
branch duct type of, 192, 192f, 196f, 197f, 198, 198t, 199f, 202
clinical manifestations of, 192–193
contrast-enhanced EUS of, 416
definition of, 192
EUS-guided fine-needle aspiration biopsy of, 192, 199–200, 199f, 200f
intraductal EUS imaging of, 200–202, 201f
main duct type of, 192, 192f, 194, 195f, 196f, 197f, 202
malignant transformation of, 198, 198f, 199, 199f, 202
resembling a serous cystadenoma, 195f
survival rate in, 202
therapy for, 202
3-dimensional EUS imaging of, 202
Intraductal ultrasound (IDUS)
of ampullary lesions, 279
of cholangiocarcinoma, 251–252, 253–254, 254
of choledocholithiasis, 248
of intraductal papillary mucinous tumors, 200–202, 201f
Ischemia
gastrointestinal, 112f, 114
prostatic, 389
Islet cell tumors
contrast-enhanced EUS of, 416
as pancreatic cancer mimic, 151, 153

J

Japan Pancreas Society, autoimmune pancreatitis diagnostic criteria of, 214, 214t, 221
Jaundice, autoimmune pancreatitis-related, 214

K

Kidney, Visible Human Data Set Models of, 175f, 218f
Kidney cancer, metastatic, 90
to the mediastinum, 124
to the pancreas, 174

L

Lactate dehydrogenase, as pleural fluid tumor marker, 330
Laryngeal cancer, metastatic, 124

Leiomyoma
  colorectal, 380–381, 381f
  immunohistochemical staining of, 81
  presenting as subepithelial lesions, 82t, 83
Leiomyosarcoma, colorectal, 380–381
Levator ani, 336
  Visible Human Data Set Models of, 347f, 348f, 349f
Levovist, 414, 417
Linitis plastica, as large gastric folds cause, 58t, 59t, 60, 66, 68, 68f, 69f
Lipoma
  of ampulla of Vater, 277
  colorectal, 381, 382f
  presenting as subepithelial lesions, 82t, 83, 84f
Littoral cell angioma, 306, 306f
Liver
  anatomic relationships of, 288, 289f
  radiofrequency ablation of, 404
Liver cancer
  angiosarcoma, 294
  coexistent with hepatocellular and cholangiocarcinoma, 293
  epitheloid hemangioendothelioma, 294
  hepatocellular carcinoma, 29, 179, 291–292, 292t, 320
  intrahepatic cholangiocarcinoma, 292–293, 293f
  lymphoma, 293–294, 293f
  metastatic, 409f
    cholangiocarcinoma-related, 255f
    to the mediastinum, 124, 294–297
    neuroendocrine tumor-related, 169–170, 171f
    pancreatic cancer-related, 153, 156, 157f, 408f
Liver lesions
  benign tumors and tumor-like lesions, 288, 290–291
    bile duct adenomas, 288
    bile duct hamartomas (von Meyerburg complexes), 288
    cavernous hemangiomas, 288, 290f
    cystic lesions, 291, 291f
    focal nodular hyperplasia, 288, 290f
    liver cell adenoma, 288, 290f, 291f
    sarcoidosis-related, 408
  focal, real-time elastography of, 408, 408f, 409f
  malignant. See Liver cancer
Lung cancer, 129–135
  bronchoscopy of, 130
  cell block sections of, 131f, 132f, 134
  computed tomography of, 130f
  cytopathology of, 133–134
  differentiated from mediastinal lymph nodes, 130, 132f
  EUS-guided fine-needle aspiration biopsy of, 129–134, 130f, 131–133f, 135
  incidence of, 130
  large-cell, cytological features of, 134
  metastatic, 90
    to the adrenal glands, 315
    to the liver, 294, 295f
    to the mediastinum, 134–135
    to the pancreas, 151, 174–175t, 179
    of pancreatic cancer origin, 153, 154, 155f
    to the pleura, 326
  non-small-cell
    EUS-guided fine-needle aspiration biopsy of, 130–131, 143
    EUS-guided treatment of, 143
    mediastinal, 118, 122, 123–124f, 124, 125f
    mediastinal lymph node staging in, 137–146
    metastatic to the liver, 294, 295f
    rapid onsite cytopathology (ROSE) of, 142, 143f
    surgical resection of, 138
    survival rate in, 138
    treatment of, 138
  small-cell, 130, 170, 170f
    cytological features of, 134
    metastatic to the liver, 294, 297f
    metastatic to the spleen, 306, 309f
  World Health Organization (WHO) classification of, 134
Lymphangioma
  colonic, 383
  presenting as subepithelial lesions, 82t
Lymph nodes
  celiac, in esophageal cancer, 28–29, 28f
  real-time elastography of, 406–407, 407f
Lymphoma
  Burkitt, 293
  gastric
    B-cell, 88
    diagnosis and staging of, 65
    differentiated from Menetrier's disease, 69
    EUS-guided fine-needle aspiration biopsy of, 88
    gastric carcinoma associated with, 62, 63f
    immunohistochemistry of, 64f
    large B-cell, 62
    as large gastric folds cause, 58t, 59t, 60, 62–66
    mantle cell, 62, 63f
    non-Hodgkin's, 62
    presenting as subepithelial lesions, 88
    staging of, 60–61
    staging systems for, 61, 61t, 62t
    T3 stage, 69f
  hepatic, 293–294, 293f
  Hodgkin's, splenic, 306, 307f, 308f
  intrapulmonary, 131
  large B-cell, 293f
    splenic, 307f
  mediastinal, 118, 124, 125–126f, 126
  metastatic
    to the liver, 294
    to the pancreas, 152f
  mucosa-associated lymphoid tissue (MALT), 88, 293
    high-grade, 66, 66f, 67f, 68f
    as large gastric folds cause, 60, 62
    low-grade, 64, 64f, 65f, 66f
    perigastric lymph nodes in, 61f
    T1m stage, 65, 65f
    treatment of, 64, 65
    T2 stage, 66, 67f
    T3 stage, 66, 67f
    T4 stage, 66, 68f
  non-Hodgkin's, as large gastric folds cause, 62–63f, 62–66, 64f
  pancreatic, 156
  presenting as subepithelial lesions, 82t
  splenic, 306, 307f, 308f
  T-cell, 293

M

Magnetic resonance cholangiopancreatography (MRCP), 156
  of annular pancreas, 227
  of biliary cysts, 233
  of the biliary tree, 244–245, 244f
  of cholangiocarcinoma, 253
  of extrahepatic biliary anomalies, 238
  of gastric cancer, 51
  of intraductal papillary mucinous tumors, 194, 197t
Magnetic resonance imaging (MRI), of aortic arch anomalies, 110
Mayo Clinic HISORt diagnostic criteria, for autoimmune pancreatitis, 214, 221, 221t
Mediastinal lymph nodes and masses, 117–128
  benign differentiated from malignant, 414–415
  differential diagnosis of
    coccidiomycosis, 119

histoplasmosis, 119, 121, 121f
mediastinal cysts, 121–122, 122f
sarcoidosis, 119, 120–121, 120f
tuberculosis, 119
differentiated from primary lung cancer, 130, 132f
EUS-guided fine-needle aspiration biopsy of, 118, 118f, 414–415
of cysts, 121, 122
of lymphoma, 121, 122, 123t, 124, 126, 414–415
of malignant lesions, 122, 123t
as mediastinitis cause, 121, 122
in tuberculosis, 121
granulomatous lymph nodes, 119–121, 120f, 121f
in lung cancer, 122, 123
malignant posterior mediastinal lesions, 122–126
in non-small-cell lung cancer, 137–146
blind transbronchial needle aspiration biopsy (TBNA) of, 138–139, 143
computed tomography-guided transthoracic needle aspiration (TTNA) of, 138
computed tomography of, 138, 143
EUS-guided fine-needle aspiration biopsy of, 139, 143
EUS-guided transbronchial needle aspiration biopsy (EUS-TBNA) of, 140–143, 141–143f
18-fluoro-deoxyglucose positron emission tomography of, 138, 143
invasive staging modalities for, 138–140
mediastinoscopy of, 138, 139
noninvasive staging modalities for, 138
paratracheal nodes
hilar, 142f, 143f
interlobar, 142f
left lower, 141f
right lower, 142f
right upper, 141f
posterior lymph nodes
lymphoma, 124, 125–126f, 126
normal benign reactive, 119–122, 119f
Visible Human Data Set Models of, 139–140f
Mediastinitis, EUS-guided fine-needle aspiration biopsy-related, 121, 122, 126, 127
Mediastinoscopy, 138, 139
Mediastinum
lung cancer invasion of, 134–135
strictures of, 112f

Melanoma, metastatic, 90
to the adrenal glands, 315
to the liver, 294, 296f, 297f
to the pancreas, 174, 175t, 178t, 179
Menetrier's disease
differentiated from
gastric lymphoma, 69
lymphocytic gastritis, 60
as large gastric folds cause, 58t, 59, 59t, 60, 69–70, 70f
Mesorectum, in rectal cancer, 342f
Metastases. *See also* metastatic *under specific types of cancer*
as large gastric folds cause, 58t
of neuroendocrine tumors, 169–170, 170f
perirectal or pelvic, 371–372
presenting as intramural subepithelial lesions, 82t
Microlithiasis, 246, 247f
Multiple endocrine neoplasia (MEN)
metastatic, 315
type 1, 70
Muscularis mucosa
correlation between echogenic and histological layers of, 378, 378t
definition of, 45
in early gastric cancer, 45, 47
in gastrointestinal stromal tumors, 86
in leiomyoma, 83
Peutz-Jeghers polyps of, 377
Muscularis propria
in ampullary tumors, 278, 280f
colonic polyps of, 379f
in esophageal cancer, 15f, 16f, 17, 27f
in gastric carcinoma, 37
in gastrointestinal stromal tumors, 86
in leiomyoma, 83
in linitis plastica, 66, 68
of normal gastric wall, 36
in rectal cancer, 338
subepithelial lesions of, 81
in ulcerative colitis, 398–399f, 400
Mycobacterium tuberculosis, 121. *See also* Tuberculosis

N

Needles
for endobronchial ultrasound (EBUS), 141f
for endoscopic ultrasound (EUS), 141f
Trucut, 81, 119. *See also* Biopsy, Trucut
Neuroendocrine tumors
of ampulla of Vater, 277
metastatic to the liver, 294
pancreatic, 165–172

definition of, 166
EUS-guided fine-needle aspiration biopsy of, 166, 166f
localized functional, 167–168, 167f, 168f
localized nonfunctional, 168–169, 169f
luminal, 170–173, 171f, 172f
metastatic, 169–170, 170f
Neurofibroma, presenting as subepithelial lesions, 82t

O

Omentum, in gastric cancer, 50, 54f
OncoGel, 162
Opisthorchis viverrini, 292–293
Optison, 414, 416
Osteochondroma, presenting as subepithelial lesions, 82t
Ovarian cancer
metastatic, 90
of metastatic origin, 371f, 372f

P

Palpation. *See also* Elastography, EUS
definition of, 404
"virtual," 409, 409f
Pancreas
agenesis of, 226, 233
annular
embryological origin of, 226
Visible Human Data Set Model of, 227, 231f.
autoimmune pancreatitis-related enlargement of, 214, 215, 217f, 220
benign lesions of, real-time elastography of, 406
cystic lesions of, 183–189
demographics and characteristics of, 184t
differential diagnosis of, 193–194, 195t
intraductal papillary mucinous tumors, 191–204
mucinous cystic tumors, 193, 195t
pseudocysts, 193, 195t
serous cyst adenomas, 193, 195t
embryological development of, 226
Pancreas divisum, 226–227, 228f, 230f
acquired (pseudodivisum), 226
coexistent with pancreatic agenesis, 233
embryological origin of, 226
santorinicele associated with, 231f
Pancreatic buds, 226
Pancreatic cancer, 149–163, 158–162, 158t, 159f, 160f, 161f
adenocarcinoma, 156
contrast-enhanced EUS of, 416, 418f

Pancreatic cancer *(continued)*
  with liver metastases, 157f
  as mortality cause, 150
  staging of, 158f
 adenoma
  as chronic pancreatitis cause, 151, 152f
  differential diagnosis of, 151, 153
  real-time elastography of, 407, 408f
 annular pancreas associated with, 227
 anomalous pancreatobiliary junction associated with, 232
 bile duct strictures misdiagnosed as, 216f
 computed tomography of, 150, 151–156, 152f, 153f, 154f, 155f, 158–160, 161
 contrast-enhanced EUS of, 415–416
 differentiated from benign lesions, 158, 159f, 160f
 ductal
  autoimmune pancreatitis as mimic of, 214, 217, 218f
  contrast-enhanced EUS of, 416
 eccrine, 150
 EUS-guided fine-needle aspiration biopsy of, 158, 160–161
 EUS-guided fine-needle injection (FNI) treatment of, 161–162
 exocrine, 150
 gastrinoma, 70
 imaging equipment and techniques for, 150
 immunohistocytology of, 178, 179, 179f
 intraductal papillary mucinous tumors (IPMTs), 191–204
  branch duct type of, 192, 192f, 196f, 197f, 198, 198t, 199f, 202
  clinical manifestations of, 192–193
  contrast-enhanced EUS of, 416
  definition of, 192
  differential diagnosis of, 193–194
  EUS-guided fine-needle aspiration biopsy of, 192, 199–200, 199f, 200f
  main duct type of, 192, 192f, 194, 195f, 196f, 197f, 202
  malignant transformation of, 198, 198f, 199, 199f, 202
  pathology of, 193, 193f
  resembling a serous cystadenoma, 195f
  survival rate in, 202
  therapy for, 202
  3-dimensional EUS imaging of, 202
 magnetic resonance imaging of, 150, 156–157, 156f, 157f, 158, 160, 161
 metastatic, 173–181, 174t
  to the adrenal glands, 315
  of ampullary cancer, 279f
  computed tomography of, 174, 175, 176f, 177f
  EUS-guided fine-needle aspiration biopsy of, 174–175, 174–175t, 176, 176f, 177f, 178, 179–180
  to the liver, 294, 295f, 408f
  to the mediastinum, 124
 pancreatic duct dilation and, 251
 pseudopapillary tumors, 159f
 real-time elastography of, 406, 407–408, 408f
 secondary effects of, 151, 152f
 short, 229f
 Visible Human Data Set Models of, 2, 3, 151f, 166f, 167f, 175f, 209f, 210, 218f
Pancreatic diseases, real-time elastography of, 407–408, 408f
Pancreatic duct
 ampullary tumor infiltration of, 281f, 283
 dilation of, 206, 207t, 209f, 210f, 251
  autoimmune pancreatitis-related, 214
  cancer-related, 151, 152f
  EUS evaluation of, 251
  pancreas divisum anomaly of, 226–227, 228f
  Visible Human Data Set Models of, 175f, 227f, 228f, 231f, 275f
Pancreatic duct stones, 211, 212f
Pancreatic head cancer, 151, 152f, 153f, 155f
 adenocarcinoma
  ascites associated with, 329f
  real-time elastography of, 408, 408f, 409f
 differentiated from ampullary adenocarcinoma, 278, 278f
 glucogonoma, 167–168, 168f
 neuroendocrine tumors, 170, 171f, 172f
 nonfunctional neuroendocrine tumors of, 168–169, 169f
 Visible Human Data Set images of, 175f
Pancreatic neck cancer, 152f
Pancreaticobiliary anomalies, 225–241
 annular pancreas, 226, 227, 231f
 biliary cysts, 233–236, 233–236f
 duodenal duplication cysts, 236–237, 238f
 miscellaneous extrahepatic biliary anomalies, 238–240
 pancreas divisum, 226–227, 228f, 230f
 pancreatic agenesis, 26, 233
 santorinicele, 231, 231f

Pancreaticobiliary channel, common, 239, 240f
Pancreaticobiliary junction
 anomalous, 231–233, 232f, 238, 239f
  embryological origin of, 226
 normal, 232f
 Visible Human Data Set Model of, 232f
Pancreaticoduodenectomy, 282
Pancreatic rests
 endoscopic mucosal resection (EMR) of, 85, 85f
 presenting as subepithelial lesions, 84–85, 85f
Pancreatic tail
 cancer of, 156f
  glucogonoma, 167–168, 168f
  insulinoma, 167, 168f
  neuroendocrine tumors, 166
  nonfunctional neuroendocrine tumors, 169, 169f
 Visible Human Data Set Model of, 167f
Pancreatic tissue, heterotopic. *See* Pancreatic rests
Pancreatitis
 acute. as ampullary papillitis cause, 276
 alcoholic. differentiated from autoimmune pancreatitis, 215
 annular pancreas associated with, 227
 anomalous pancreatobiliary junction associated with, 232
 autoimmune, 161, 161f, 213–224
  clinical features of, 214
  definition of, 214
  diagnostic criteria for, 214, 214t, 216–217, 219, 221–222, 222t
  EUS-guided fine-needle aspiration biopsy of, 217, 219
  extra-pancreatic organ involvement in, 214, 220
  serology of, 219–220
  steroid therapy for, 214, 220
  Trucut biopsy of, 217, 218f, 219
  "tumefactive," 221
 choledocholithiasis-related, 245
 chronic, 205–212
  computed tomography of, 215–216, 215f
  contrast-enhanced EUS of, 415, 416
  definition of, 206
  ductal features of, 206, 207t, 208t, 209f, 210f, 211, 212f
  effect on EUS imaging, 160–161
  endoscopic retrograde cholangiopancreatography of, 215, 215f
  EUS-based diagnostic features of, 206, 207–208t

histological findings in, 214–215
magnetic resonance imaging of, 215–216, 215f
minimal change, 206
pancreatic cancer-related, 151, 152f, 156
parenchymal features of, 207t, 208t, 210f, 211, 211f, 212f
real-time elastography of, 406, 407
"Rosemont criteria," for diagnosis of, 212
secretin test for, 206
severity index for, 206
splenic vein thrombosis associated with, 321
duodenal duplication cysts associated with, 236
gastric varices associated with, 84
intraductal papillary mucinous tumors-related, 192–193
lymphoplasmacytic sclerosing, 214–215
pseudotumoral, real-time elastography of, 407, 408f
recurrent, 192–193
Pancreatography, EUS-guided methylene blue, 283–284
Papilla of Vater. See Ampulla of Vater
Papillectomy, endoscopic, 283
Para-esophageal collateral veins, 102, 103f
Paraganglioma, 381
metastatic, 315
Paris staging system, for primary gastrointestinal lymphoma, 61, 62t
Pelvic bones, Visible Human Data Set Model of, 336f
Pelvic disorders, in females, 369–374
Pelvic inflammatory disorders, 372–374
Pelvic tumors, 371–372, 371f
Pelvis
female, Visible Human Data Set Model of, 370f
male, Visible Human Data Set Model of, 336f
metastatic invasion of, 153, 371–372
Peptic ulcer disease, as ampullary papillitis cause, 276
Perforating veins, 102, 104f
Perfusion studies, with contrast-enhanced EUS, 417–418
Pericardial effusions, 326
Visible Human Data Set Model of, 328f
Pericholecystic fluid, 326
Peri-esophageal collateral veins, 102, 103f
Perirectal fluid retention, 372
Peritoneal cancer, of metastastic origin, 153, 155–156, 155f
Peritoneal fluid, 326

Peutz-Jeghers syndrome, 377, 377f
Pheochromocytoma, metastatic, 315
"Pillow sign," 80, 83, 381
Pleura
in esophageal cancer, 27f
relationship to the esophagus, 326, 327f
Pleural effusions
benign, 326, 330
EUS-guided detection of, 326
EUS-guided fine-needle aspiration biopsy of, 326, 327, 327f, 329–330
malignant, 326
gastric cancer-related, 50
tumor markers for, 329–330
Polypectomy, bleeding risk associated with, 379
Polypectomy site, Dieulafoy lesions of, 115–116, 115f
Polypectomy snares, 283
Polyposis, familial adenomatous, 278
Polyps
cholesterol, 259, 260f, 261f
colonic
adenomatous, 376–377
classification of, 376f, 383
definition of, 376
EUS examination of, 378–379, 379f
hamartomatous, 377f
hyperplastic, 376
juvenile, 377f
Peutz-Jeghers, 377, 377f
fibrovascular, 82t
gastric inflammatory, 264, 267–268f
fibroid, 85, 86f
as large gastric folds cause, 72, 74f
Portal vein
cholangiocarcinoma invasion of, 253f
EUS-guided angiography of, 417
extrahepatic, Visible Human Data Set Model of, 96f
thrombosis of, 319–323, 320f, 321–322f
in children, 320
gastric varices associated with, 84
as portal hypertension cause, 320
venous angiography of, 320
Visible Human Data Set Model of, 320f
Visible Human Data Set Models of, 100f, 151f, 196f, 314f, 315f
Portal venous system, Visible Human Data Set Model of, 96–98f
Positron emission tomography (PET)
of gastric cancer, 51, 53f
of lung cancer, 138, 143
of mediastinal lymph nodes and masses, 138, 143
of pancreatic cancer, 26

Proctodeal gland
infections of, 346
inflammation of, 356
Prostate cancer
digital examination of, 389
EUS imaging of, 390–394, 393f, 394f
high-intensity focused ultrasound (HIFU) of, 404
metastatic, 391
N0 stage, 391
N1 stage, 391
palpation of, 404
T1a stage, 394
T1b stage, 394
transrectal ultrasonography (TRUS) of, 389–390, 390f, 394
T1 stage, 391, 394
T2 stage, 393f, 394
T3 stage, 391, 394
Prostate gland
cystic lesions of, 389, 389f
EUS imaging of, 390–394, 391f, 392f, 393f, 394f
Visible Human Data Set Models of, 391f, 392f
Prostate lesions
benign, 388–389, 388f, 389f
benign prostatic hyperplasia (BHP), 388–389, 388f
cysts, 389, 389f
malignant. See Prostate cancer
Pseudocysts, pancreatic, 185, 185t
Pseudopapillary tumors, pancreatic, 159f
Pubis, male, 391f
Pulmonary artery, lung cancer invasion of, 132f

R

Rectal cancer, 335–344
abdominoperineal resection of, 337, 340
EUS detection and staging of, 337t
accuracy of, 339–340
comparison with computed tomography, 340
comparison with magnetic resonance imaging, 340
equipment and techniques for, 337–338, 337f
fine-needle aspiration biopsy of, 339
in local recurring cancer, 340–341, 340f
lymph node staging, 339, 339f
restaging after neoadjuvant therapy, 340
3-D EUS, 341–342, 342f
T3/N1 stage, 339f
T1 stage, 338f
T2 stage, 339f, 340

Rectal cancer *(continued)*
  T3 stage, 338–339, 339*f*, 340
  T4 stage, 339, 339*f*
  neoadjuvant therapy of, 337, 340
  prognosis for, 336–337
  rigid probe use in, 337*f*
Rectal wall
  echo-layers of, 378*f*
  normal, 338*f*
  rectal cancer invasion of, 338–339
Rectosigmoid cancer, 371*f*
Rectum, 391*f*. *See also* Abscess, anorectal (perirectal); Fistulae, anorectal
  anatomy of, 336, 336*f*
  3-D EUS imaging of, 342*f*
  in endometriosis, 383
  Visible Human Data Set Models of, 336*f*, 337*f*, 346*f*, 347*f*, 391*f*, 392*f*
Reinig, Karl, 2
Renal cell carcinoma, metastatic
  to the adrenal glands, 315
  to the pancreas, 174–175*t*, 176, 177*f*, 179
Renal vein, left, Visible Human Data Set Models of, 100*f*, 196*f*
Rokitansky-Aschoff sinuses, 259–260, 262*f*, 263*f*, 264*f*

S

"Salami Effect," 9
Santorinicele, 231, 231*f*
Sarcoidosis
  as large gastric folds cause, 58*t*
  of the liver, 408
  mediastinal lymph nodes in, 119, 120–121, 120*f*
  of the spleen, 303–304, 303*f*
Sarcoma
  Ewing, metastatic to the pancreas, 153*f*
  metastatic to the pancreas, 151, 153*f*
Schwannoma
  colorectal, 381
  immunohistochemical staining of, 81, 90*t*
Seminal vesicles, 336, 389, 390–391, 391, 391*f*
Sigmoidoscopy, for recurrent rectal cancer detection, 340
Sinuses, Rokitansky-Aschoff, 259–260, 262*f*, 263*f*, 264*f*
Sjogren's-like syndrome, 220
Smokers
  esophageal cancer overstaging in, 29
  lung cancer in, 130*f*
Smooth muscle tumors, immunohistochemical staining of, 90*t*
Sonazoid, 414
Sonoporation, 418
Sonovue, 414

Sphincter of Oddi
  dysfunction of, 232, 277
  intraductal ultrasonography of, 279
Spitzer, Vic, 2
Spleen, 299–311
  abscess of, 303–304, 304*f*
  accessory, 311, 311*f*
  anatomic relationships of, 300, 300*f*
  benign lesions of, 303–306, 304*f*, 305*f*, 306*f*
  EUS-guided fine-needle aspiration biopsy of, 300–311
  hemangioma of, 304, 305*f*, 306, 306*f*
  infarction of, 304, 305*f*
  littoral cell angioma, 306, 306*f*
  malignant diseases of, 306–310, 307–310*f*
  sarcoidosis of, 303–304, 303*f*
  in tuberculosis, 301*f*, 302*f*, 303–304
  Visible Human Data Set Models of, 2, 3, 167*f*, 300*f*
Splenic artery
  aneurysm of, 113, 114*f*, 115, 115*f*
  insulinoma adjacent to, 167, 167*f*
  pseudoaneurysm of, 115, 115*f*
  Visible Human Data Set Models of, 2, 3, 108*f*, 151*f*, 218*f*, 300*f*
Splenic hilum, Visible Human Data Set Model of, 167*f*
Splenic vein
  in portal vein thrombosis, 321*f*
  thrombosis of, 321, 321*f*
  Visible Human Data Set Models of, 97*f*, 100*f*, 151*f*, 196*f*, 218*f*, 300*f*
Squamous cell carcinoma
  esophageal, 28*f*
  pulmonary, 134
"Stack sign," 226, 230*f*
Stenting
  aortic, 112*f*
  in common bile duct, 246*f*
  pancreatic, after ampullectomy, 283–285, 284*f*
Steroid therapy, for autoimmune pancreatitis, 220
Stomach
  ascites adjacent to, 327
  large gastric folds of. *See* Gastric folds, large
  Visible Human Data Set Model of, 300*f*
  Visible Human Data Set Models of, 314*f*, 315*f*
Subcarinal space
  anatomy of, 118–119*f*
  caudal to tracheal carina, 142*f*
  Visible Human Data Set Models of, 139*f*
Subclavian artery

  left, Visible Human Data Set Models of, 108*f*, 130*f*
  right
    anomalies of, 108, 109*f*, 110*f*
    Visible Human Data Set Model of, 108*f*
Subepithelial lesions, 380–383, 380*t*
  carcinoid tumors, 381–383
  fibrosarcomas, 381
  gastrointestinal stromal tumors (GISTs), 380
  leiomyomas/leiomyosarcomas, 380–381, 381*f*
  lipomas, 381, 382*f*
  lymphangiomas, 383
  paragangliomas, 381
  schwannomas, 381
  upper gastrointestinal, 79–93
    differential diagnosis of, 82–83*t*, 82–91
    endoscopic assessment of, 80
    endoscopic mucosal dissection (EDR) of, 82
    endoscopic mucosal resection (EMR) of, 82
    EUS-guided core needle biopsy of, 81
    gastrointestinal stromal tumors (GISTs), 86–87, 87*f*
    intramucosal differentiated from extramucosal, 80
    "pillow sign" of, 80
    as "submucosal" lesions, 80
Superior mesenteric artery
  calcification and obstruction of, 111, 113*f*, 114*f*
  in pancreatic cancer, 153, 153*f*, 154*f*
  pancreatic cancer adjacent to, 176*f*
  Visible Human Data Set Models of, 96*f*, 108*f*, 151*f*, 167*f*, 175*f*, 196*f*, 275*f*, 314*f*, 315*f*
Superior mesenteric vein
  in pancreatic cancer, 153*f*, 154*f*, 157*f*
  Visible Human Data Set Models of, 100*f*, 151*f*, 175*f*, 196*f*, 275*f*
Superior vena cava, Visible Human Data Set Model of, 100*f*
Syphilis, as large gastric folds cause, 58*t*, 72

T

Teratoma, mediastinal, 127*t*
Testicular cancer, with mediastinal metastases, 124
Thoracentesis, EUS-guided, 330
Thorotrast, as intraheptic cholangiocarcinoma cause, 292–293
Tissue perfusion studies, with contrast-enhanced EUS, 417–418

TNFerade, 161–162
Trachea, Visible Human Data Set Models of, 130*f*, 139*f*, 140*f*
Transbronchial needle aspiration biopsy (EUS-TBNA), EUS-guided, 140–143, 141–143*f*
Transbronchial needle aspiration biopsy (TBNA), 138–139, 143
Transbronchial ultrasound, 137–146
Transperianal ultrasound (TPUS), of anorectal fistulae, 359
Transrectal ultrasound (TRUS), of prostate cancer, 389–390, 390*f*, 394
Transthoracic needle aspiration (TTNA) biopsy, computed tomography-guided, 138
Tuberculosis
  as large gastric folds cause, 58*t*, 72
  mediastinal lymph nodes in, 119, 121
  splenic lesions associated with, 301*f*, 302*f*

U
Ulcers, esophageal, 15
Umbilical cord sepsis, as portal vein thrombosis cause, 320
University of Colorado
  Center for Human Simulation, 2, 3
  Visible Human Data Set, 2–3
Upper gastrointestinal tract, subepithelial lesions of, 79–93
  differential diagnosis of, 82–83*t*, 82–91
  endoscopic assessment of, 80
  endoscopic mucosal dissection (EDR) of, 82
  endoscopic mucosal resection (EMR) of, 82
  EUS-guided core needle biopsy of, 81
  gastrointestinal stromal tumors (GISTs), 86–87, 87*f*
  intramucosal differentiated from extramucosal, 80
  "pillow sign" of, 80
  as "submucosal" lesions, 80
Urethra, 336, 389, 391, 391*f*
Urinary bladder, 336
Uterus, 336

V
Vagina, 336
Varices. *See also* Esophageal varices; Gastric varices
  Visible Human Data Set Models of, 96–98*f*
Vascular anomalies, 107–116
  acquired, 111–115
    aortic aneurysms, 111, 112*f*
    atherosclerotic plaques, 111, 112*f*
    gastrointestinal ischemia-related, 112*f*, 114
  Dieulafoy lesions, 115–116, 115*f*
  right subclavian artery anomalies, 108, 109*f*, 110*f*
Vascular diseases, as large gastric folds cause, 58*t*
Vascular endothelial growth factor receptor type 2 (VEGFR2), 418
Vas deferens ampullae, 389
Vas deferens duct, 391*f*
VIPoma, location of, 166
Visible Human Data Set, 2–3
von Meyerburg complexes, 288

W
Water-immersion technique, for miniprobe use, 35, 35*t*, 36*f*

Z
Zollinger-Ellison syndrome, 58*t*, 70, 71*f*